Instant Medicine for NEET SS

(DM/DNB Entrance Exam)

Authentic Answers with Explanations

Extensively Cross-referenced with
Harrison Principles of Internal Medicine, 21st Edition

SECOND EDITION

EXPERT TEAM

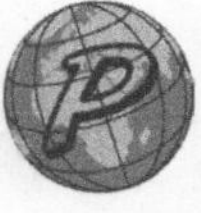

Peepee Publishers and Distributors (P) Ltd.®

Instant Medicine for NEET SS Exam

Editor: Dr. Teja Kantamani

Published by
Pawaninder P. Vij and Anupam Vij

Peepee Publishers and Distributors (P) Ltd.
Head Office: 160, Shakti Vihar, Pitam Pura, Delhi-110 034 (India)

Correspondence Address:
7/31, First Floor, Ansari Road, Daryaganj
New Delhi-110 002 (India)
Ph: 41512412, 23246245, 9811156083
e-mail: peepee160@yahoo.co.in
e-mail: peepee160@gmail.com
www.peepeepub.com
join us on facebook.com/pp.publishers

First Edition: 2022
Second Edition: 2023

ISBN: 978-81-9523-447-9

Dedicated to

My beloved parents and family,
P. Lakshmi Aishwarya – Wife, K. V. Raghavulu – Father, K. Panitha Lakshmi – Mother,
K. Bhanu Teja and K. Rama Lakshmi and K.Tapaswini

Chief Author and Editor: Dr. Kantamani Bala Teja, Oncologist

Expert Team Members:

Dr. Lakshmi Aishwarya, DM Nephrology, Tirupati

Dr. Krishna Sai, MD General Medicine, Bhubaneswar

Dr. Rakesh Chintala, DM Endocrinology, Vijayawada

Dr. Kishore, DM Gastroenterology, SGPGI

Dr. Praveen Meduri, DM, Neurology, Guntur

Dr. Ramprakash, Gastroenterologist, Vijayawada

Dr. Satish, MD General Medicine, Vijayawada

Dr. Deepthi Alla, MD General Medicine, Guntur

Dr. Mahesh, MD, Guntur

Dr. Ashok, MBBS, MD

Other Contributors:

Dr. Rajesh Vepuri, MS

Dr. Venkateswarulu, MS

Dr. Pavan, MS

PREFACE

On viewing the pattern of many NEET SS Exam patterns, we felt that there is no book available in the market for the best preparation to crack the exam. Many of the exams had repeats all the time. This book is started with sole purpose of clearing various aspects of General Medicine and guide aspirants for their preparation. These questions had been solved by experts of India from reputed institutes. For controversial questions, every attempt has been made to trace the source and solve the questions.

This 2nd edition has been updated based on Harrison 21st edition – As per need and advises by students who purchased 1st edition.

- We have included Tables, Magical Points, Illustrations and Flowcharts for the better understanding.
- We have highlighted all repeat questions so that aspirants will concentrate on them.
- We would like to congratulate all the contributors for their commitment and hard work.

NOTE: This book is only preparation purposes. We recommend Harrison 21st edition Textbook to be used at the time of using this book for quick reference and understanding concepts for long run time. Our motto is to reduce your preparation time (TIME–VERY VALUABLE FOR PREPARATION)–Not to replace textbook reading policy.

"Team work always wins"

The only option for success in our exam is to "READ REVISE REPEAT".

Have faith in you, your parents and Almighty God.

All the best!

EXPERT TEAM

ACKNOWLEDGEMENTS

I thank Mr. Pawaninder Paul Vij, Director of Peepee Publishers and Distributors (P) Ltd., who has always been with me and supported me. I would also like to thank entire publishing team for their efforts in bringing this excellent book to this stage.

Note: This book abides to the rules of NEET SS Non Disclosure Agreement (NDA). If MCQs simulate the NEET SS pattern, they are just mere resemblance and are handpicked questions from standard textbooks by the author.

CONTENTS

"He who makes us understand is not the teacher, but who moulds us to the best is the one." These words played a crucial role in my life and I expect the same in yours too.

MODEL QUESTION

Q. Identify the image shown below:

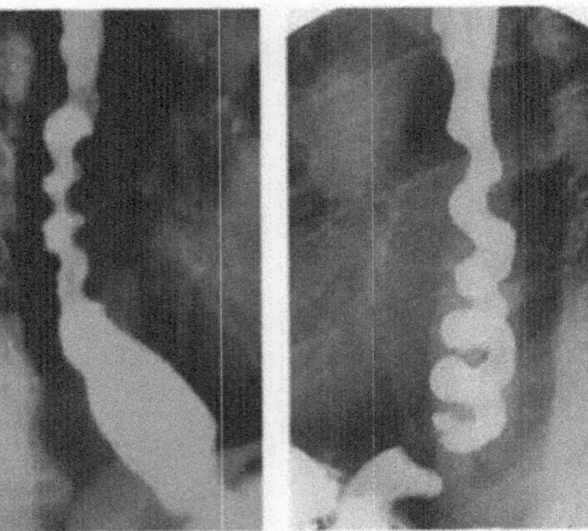

A. Schatzki ring

B. Achalasia

C. Diffuse esophageal spasm

D. Carcinoma esophagus

Explanation:

- In the image cork screw appearence of esophagus is seen due to spastic contraction of circular muscle in esophageal wall.
- In achalasia there will be dilation of esophagus with tappering of gastroesophageal junction with air fluid level in esophagus.

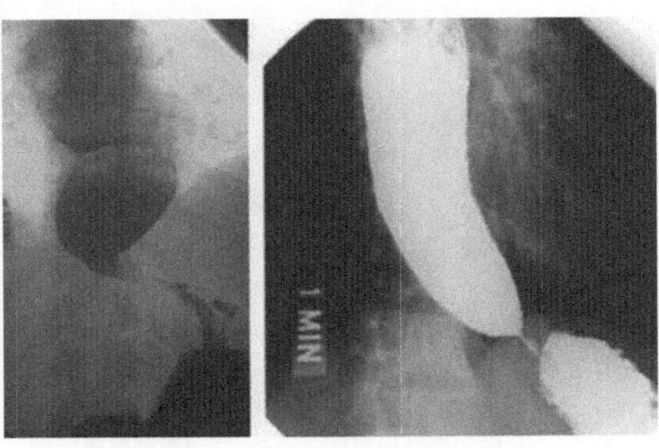

- In some individuals there is circular indentation of esophagus leading to dysphagia.

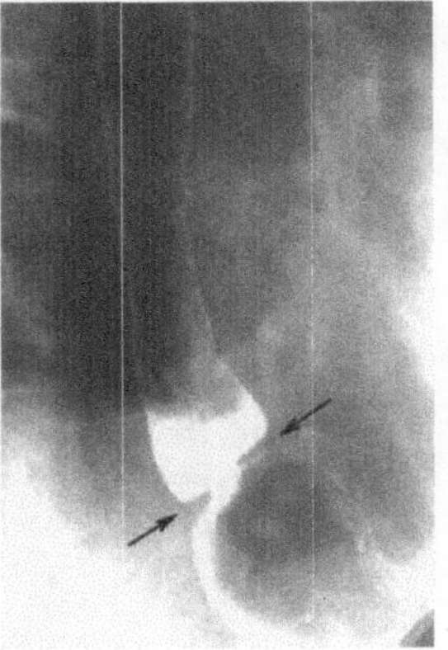

Ans. C Ref. Harrison 21st Edition Chapter Gastroenterology

CHAPTER 1

GENERAL
(Infectious Diseases, Autoimmunity, Transplant, Fever & Others)

1. A 50 year old with past history of diabetes for past 20 years and right lower limb necrotizing fasciitis, with fever for past 3 days, BP- 70/50 mm Hg, HR- 120mt, RR- 20/mt with altered mentation. Early treatment of sepsis and septic shock management includes:

A. Patient should receive first dose of antibiotic as soon as possible after which blood culture should be collected

B. Patient must receive an IV fluid bolus of within 6 hours of presentation

C. Lactate elevations are the stand alone biomarker for sepsis

D. SOFA score > 5 indicates 10% risk of in hospital death

Explanation:

Early treatment of sepsis and septic shock is best summarized by two "bundles" of care:

1. Within 3 h of presentation (ideally within the first hour), the pt should be given appropriate broad-spectrum antibiotics, with collection of blood for culture before antibiotic administration and measurement of serum lactate levels.
   - For every 1-h delay in the initiation of antibiotic administration to pts with sepsis, there is a 3–7% increase in the odds of in-hospital death.
2. Within 6 h of presentation, the pt should receive an IV fluid bolus and treatment with vasopressors for persistent hypotension or shock, and serum lactate levels should be re-measured.
   - More than 30% of pts with severe sepsis require source control, mainly for abdominal, urinary, and soft-tissue infections.

Ans. B

2. A 67 yr old man presents to emergency department with shortness of breath. He is found to have elevated serum BNP. All the following cause this elevation except (NEET SS Pattern):

A. Advanced age

B. Female sex

C. Obesity

D. Pulmonary embolism with right heart strain

Explanation:

- Levels of BNP are falsely low in Obesity
- High BNP levels are seen in Heart failure, Advanced age, Renal impairment, Females and Right heart failure.

Ans. C

3. Which option best explains 'flipping effect'?

A. LDH 1 > LDH 2

B. LDH 2 > LDH 1

C. LDH 2 > LDH 3

D. LDH 3 > LDH 2

An LDH-1 level higher than the LDH-2 level (a "flipped** pattern") suggests myocardial infarction (damage to heart tissues releases heart **LDH, which is rich in LDH-1, into the bloodstream).
Flipping can also occur in Renal infarcts, Hemolysis, Hypothyroidism & CA Stomach

Normal ratios: LDH-1 less than LDH-2 & LDH-5 less than LDH-4

LDH-1 is greater than your LDH-2 is referred to as "flipped LDH" →Indicates myocardial damage
LDH-5 is greater than your LDH-4 →Indicates cirrhosis and hepatitis.

- LDH-1—In heart and in RBC (red blood cells), as well as the brain
- LDH-2—In reticuloendothelial system
- LDH-3—In lungs
- LDH-4—In the kidneys, placenta and pancreas
- LDH-5—In the liver and striated muscle

Uses:

- LDH levels are more in RBC
- Helpful in assessment of Hemolysis/Tissue breakdown

Ans. A

4. **Low Brain natriuretic peptide is associated with:**

A. Renal failure
B. Advanced age
C. Use of Acute receptor neprilysin inhibitor (ARNI)
D. Obesity

Explanation:

- BNP levels are high in Advanced age, Women, Patients taking ANRI. Falsely low in Obese patients

Ans. D

5. **A 64-year-old woman presents to the emergency room with confusion and difficulty walking. Her examination shows nystagmus, limited ocular movements on lateral gaze, and ataxia. Given her daughter's report of chronic alcoholism, intoxication is suspected. Labs return showing a blood alcohol content of zero and slight hyponatremia. What is the next best step?**

A. Give intravenous (IV) thiamine 500 mg tid × 3–5 days followed by maintenance thiamine thereafter
B. Continue metabolic workup as the patient is admitted
C. Rule out infectious causes of her altered mental status
D. Obtain an electroencephalogram

Explanation:

- Most likely diagnosis in this woman with chronic alcoholism who presents with encephalopathy, nystagmus, ophthalmoparesis, and ataxia is Wernicke encephalopathy secondary to thiamine deficiency.
- Chronically, Wernicke encephalopathy can develop into Korsakoff syndrome, manifested by anterograde amnesia.
- Magnetic resonance imaging most often shows petechial hemorrhages in mammillary bodies, hypothalamus, medial thalami, and periaqueductal gray matter. Before any glucose is given to this patient, IV thiamine should be supplemented first and foremost, as glucose metabolism further depletes thiamine.
- Given that this patient is symptomatic from thiamine deficiency, treatment doses should be administered preferably with the IV formulation.
- Obtaining GQ1b antibodies (often helpful in Miller-Fisher syndrome) should be considered in cases of ataxia and ophthalmoparesis, but is not the best answer in this case because there is no mention of peripheral neuropathy.
- Other choices mentioned are also reasonable in anyone with altered mentation, but it is important to recognize syndrome and treat with thiamine early and first.

Ans. A

6. Most common type of leprosy in India is:

A. Tuberculoid
B. Borderline tuberculoid
C. Mid borderline
D. Borderline lepromatous

Explanation:

- Most common type is Tuberculoid leprosy in India

Ans. A

7. Which statements correctly describes role of PCR in diagnosis of HIV infection?

A. Should be used if western blot is indeterminate
B. Useful screening test
C. Should be used if 2 consecutive serologic tests are +ve
D. Should be used if initial serologic test is +ve but 2nd is -ve

Explanation:

- PCR Should be used if western blot is indeterminate

Ans. A

8. Which is not true regarding Primary chancre in syphilis?

A. Painless papule
B. Usually multiple
C. Erosions & Indurations are common
D. Cartilaginous consistency on palpation

Explanation:

- Usually chancre is single painless papule that rapidly erodes & usually becomes indurated
- Cartilaginous consistency on palpation
- Heterosexual men: Usually seen on penis

Ans. B

9. Hecht pneumonia is caused by:

A. Measles virus
B. CMV
C. VZV
D. HIV

Explanation:

Measles

- Characteristic rash of measles is a consequence of the cellular immune response, it may not develop in persons with impaired cellular immunity (e.g., those with AIDS).
- These persons have a high case-fatality rate and frequently develop Giant-cell pneumonitis (Hecht pneumonia) caused by measles virus.
- T lymphocyte defects (e.g., cancer chemotherapy) also are associated with increased severity of measles.

Ans. A

10. Drug that causes bone marrow depression in patients with HIV infection include all except:

A. Zidovudine
B. Didanosine
C. Dapsone
D. Ganciclovir

Explanation:

Table: Causes of bone marrow suppression in patients with HIV infection	
HIV Mycobacterial infections Fungal infections B_{19} parvovirus infection Lymphoma	**Medications** • Zidovudine • Dapsone • Trimethoprim/sulfamethoxazole • Pyrimethamine • 5-Flucytosine • Ganciclovir • Interferon α • Trimetrexate • Foscarnet

Ans. B

11. Which of the following is not a characteristic of Immune Reconstitution inflammatory syndrome?

A. Paradoxical worsening of existing clinical condition or abrupt appearance of new clinical finding following ART therapy

B. Occurs within days following initiation of ART

C. Most common in patients starting therapy with CD4 T cell count <50u/L who experience a precipituous drop in viral load

D. Can be fatal

Explanation:

Table: Characteristics of immune reconstitution inflammatory syndrome (IRIS)
• Paradoxical worsening of an existing clinical condition or abrupt appearance or a new clinical finding (unmasking) is seen following the initiation of antiretroviral therapy
• Occurs weeks to months following the initiation of antiretroviral therapy
• Is most common in patients starting therapy with a CD4+ T cell count < 50/μl who experience a precipitous drop in viral load
• Is frequently seen in the setting of tuberculosis; particularly when cART is starting soon after initiation of anti-TB therapy
• Can be fatal

Ans. B

12. According to American college of Obstetrics & Gynecology safest part of pregnancy in which to travel

A. 10-16 wks
B. 16-20 wks
C. 18-24 wks
D. 24-28 wks

Explanation:

- According to the American College of Obstetrics and Gynecology, safest part of pregnancy in which to travel is between 18 and 24 weeks, when there is least danger of spontaneous abortion or premature labor.
- Some obstetricians prefer that women stay within a few hundred miles of home after 28th wk of pregnancy in case problems arise.

Ans. C

13. Which of the following is not a tick borne organism cause for Relative Bradycardia?

A. Coxiella
B. Orientia
C. Rickettsia
D. Babesia

Explanation:

Table: Causes of relative bradycardia	
Infectious Causes	
Intracellular organisms • Gram-negative bacteria	*Salmonella typhi* *Francisella tularensis* *Brucella spp.* *Coxiella burnetii* (Q fever) *Leptospira interrogans* *Legionella pneumophila* *Mycoplasma pneumoniae*
• Tick-borne organisms	*Rickettsia* spp. *Orientia tsutsugamushi* (scrub typhus) *Babesia* spp.
• Other	*Corynebacterium diphtheriae* *Plasmodium* spp. (malaria)
Viruses/Viral infections	Yellow fever virus Dengue virus Viral hemorrhagic fevers[a] Viral myocarditis
Noninfectious Causes	
	Drug fever Beta blocker use Central nervous system lesions Malignant lymphoma Factitious fever

Ans. A

14. A 33-year-old male recently started a migraine preventive medication. Two weeks later he presents to the emergency department with severe abdominal pain, nausea, and vomiting. His complete blood count has normal white blood cells and hemoglobin, and a mildly low level of platelets. A complete metabolic panel is normal, including liver enzymes. Amylase and lipase are both elevated. Which of the following is the most likely cause of his condition?

A. Valproic acid
B. Topiramate
C. Propranolol
D. Amitriptyline

Explanation:

- Valproic acid has been shown to have a slight, but significant, risk of pancreatitis, among many other side effects, including hepatoxicity, thrombocytopenia, teratogenicity, and milder effects like tremor and weight gain.
- Topiramate has an increased risk of teratogenicity, metabolic acidosis, nephrolithiasis, anhydria, and cognitive slowing.

- Propranolol has an increased risk of worsening depression, cardiac arrhythmias, and worsening asthma.
- Amitriptyline has an increased risk of depression, QT prolongation, and other cardiac arrhythmias. Verapamil has an increased risk of cardiac arrhythmias, hepatotoxicity, and paralytic ileus.

Ans. A

15. Interleukin not produced by TH2 is:

A. IL 4

B. IL 5

C. IL 13

D. IL 17

Explanation:

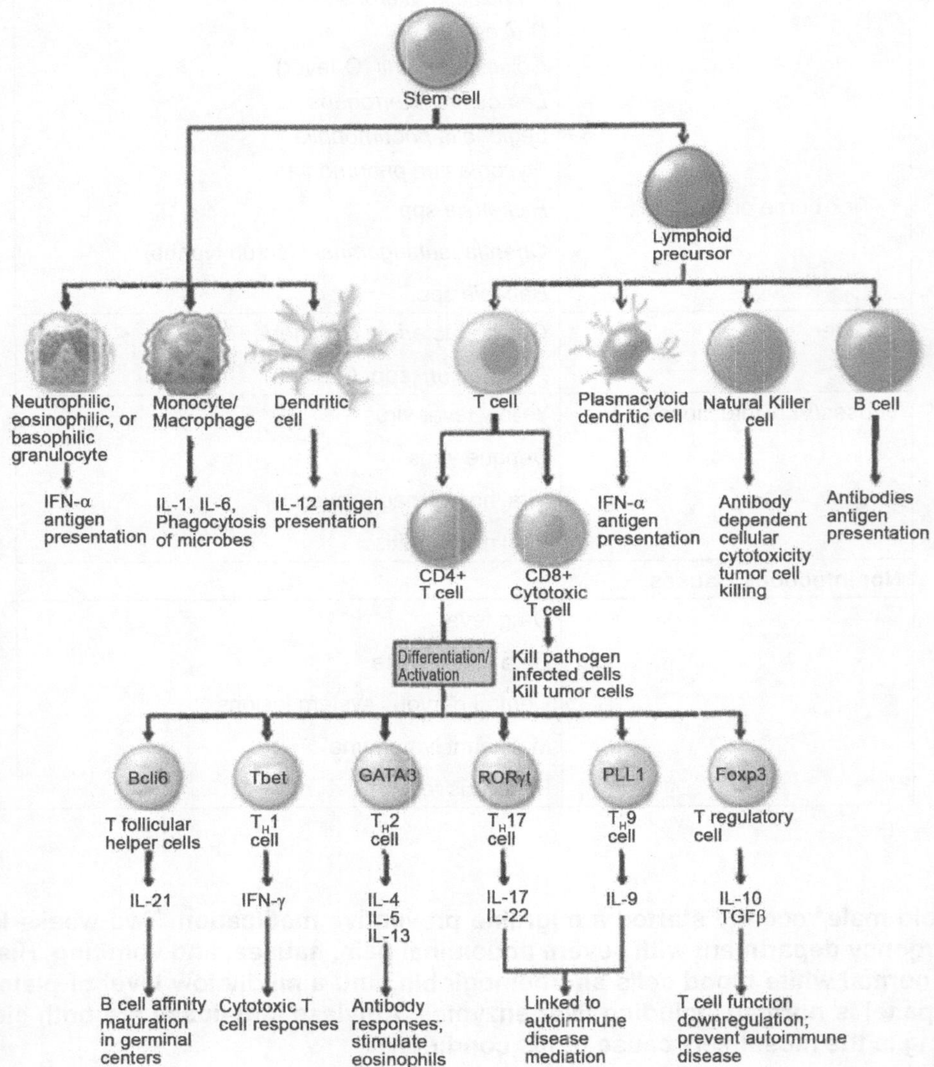

Ans. D

16. A 45-year-old man presents to the emergency room with 1 day of headache and several hours of left arm heaviness. He notes that he fell off a ladder and hurt his neck the day before. In completing a full neurological examination, the emergency room physician additionally notes the abnormality shown here. Which of the following is the most likely test to demonstrate the etiology of the patient's symptoms?

A. Magnetic resonance imaging (MRI) of the brain
B. Magnetic resonance angiogram of the neck
C. Electroencephalogram
D. Edrophonium test

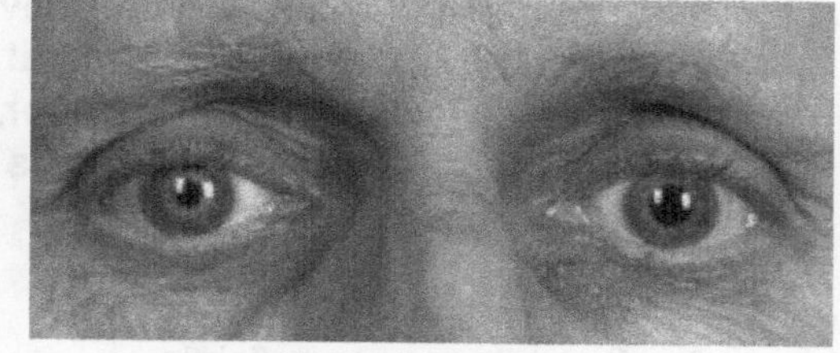

Explanation:

- Given the history of recent trauma, the most likely cause of this patient's left arm weakness and right Horner syndrome is right carotid artery dissection.
- Sympathetic chain runs inside the carotid sheath in neck and, in the case of cervical carotid dissection, may cause an ipsilateral Horner syndrome with contralateral symptoms of anterior ischemia.
- MRI of the brain may demonstrate evidence of ischemia related to the carotid dissection, but would not be the most direct means of diagnosing the problem.
- Chest X-ray would be a reasonable test to look for a Pancoast tumor, which may cause ipsilateral Horner syndrome. However, in event that the brachial plexus were also affected by a Pancoast tumor, the weakness would also be ipsilateral.
- Further, the recent trauma in this patient reduces the likelihood of a tumor.
- Electroencephalogram would not be a useful test in this patient, because seizure would be quite unlikely to cause Horner syndrome.
- Edrophonium test would be useful to diagnose myasthenia gravis, although that would present with ptosis without miosis

Ans. B

17. Babes nodules are seen in:

A. Mumps
B. Rabies
C. HIV
D. HTLV

Explanation:

- Pathologic studies show mild inflammatory changes in CNS in rabies, with mononuclear inflammatory infiltration in leptomeninges, perivascular regions, and parenchyma, including microglial nodules called *Babes nodules.*
- Degenerative neuronal changes usually are not prominent, and there is little evidence of neuronal death; neuronophagia is observed occasionally.
- Pathologic changes are surprisingly mild in light of the clinical severity and fatal outcome of the disease.
- Most characteristic pathologic finding in rabies is the *Negri body.*
- Negri bodies are eosinophilic cytoplasmic inclusions in brain neurons that are composed of rabies virus proteins and viral RNA.
- These inclusions occur in a minority of infected neurons, are commonly observed in Purkinje cells of the cerebellum and in pyramidal neurons of the hippocampus, and are less frequently seen in cortical and brainstem neurons.
- **Negri bodies are not observed in all cases of rabies.**
- Lack of prominent degenerative neuronal changes has led to the concept that neuronal dysfunction—rather than neuronal death—is responsible for clinical disease in rabies.
- Basis for behavioral changes, including the aggressive behavior of rabid animals, is not well understood but may be related to infection of serotonergic neurons in the brainstem.

Ans. B

18. A 42-year-old diabetic woman develops maxillary pain and rhinorrhea. Four days later, she notes epistaxis, diplopia, and retroorbital pain. On presentation to the emergency room, she is noted to have a dark mass in each nostril. Further, she has bilateral ptosis, numbness in V1 and V2 distributions, and bilateral ophthalmoplegia. There is no proptosis. Which of the following is the most likely etiology for her symptoms?

A. Tolosa-Hunt syndrome
B. Idiopathic intracranial hypertension
C. Carotid-cavernous fistula
D. Mucormycosis infection

Explanation:

- Mucormycosis classically affects diabetic patients, involving invasion of the cavernous sinuses. Tolosa Hunt syndrome is an idiopathic, recurrent, steroid responsive granulomatous disease that usually affects the cavernous sinuses.
- Idiopathic intracranial hypertension may cause abducens palsy due to tension on the nerve, but is not associated with cavernous sinus syndrome. Pituitary adenomas may invade cavernous sinuses and cause compressive cranial neuropathies. However, the rapidity of symptom onset, epistaxis, and nasal mass noted in the question stem make this less likely. Rather than cavernous sinus symptoms, carotid-cavernous fistulae more commonly present with pain, pulsatile proptosis, ocular injection, progressive vision loss, and an ocular bruit on careful auscultation.

Ans. D

19. Not a part of qSOFA Score is:

A. PaO2/FiO2 ration
B. Respiratory rate
C. Bilirubin
D. Serum creatinine

Explanation:

Table: Calculation of SOFA score[a]

System	0	1	2	3	4
Respiration PaO_2/FiO_2, mm Hg (kPa)	≥ 400 (53.3)	< 400 (53.3)	< 300 (40)	< 200 (26.7) with respiratory support	< 100 (13.3) with respiratory support
Coagulation Platelets, × 10^3/µl	> 150	< 150	< 100	< 50	< 20
Liver Bilirubin mg/dl (µmol/l)	< 1.2 (20)	1.2-1.9 (20-32)	2.0-5.9 (33-101)	6.0-11.9 (102-204)	> 12.0 (204)
Cardiovascular	MAP > 70 mm Hg	MAP < 70 mm Hg	Dopamine < 5 or dobutamine (any dose)[a]	Dopamine 5.1-15 or epinephrine < 0.1 or norepinephrine < 0.1[a]	Dopamine > 15 or epinephrine > 0.1 or norepinephrine > 0.1[b]
Central Nervous System Glasgow Coma Scale[4]	15	13-14	10-12	6-9	< 6
Renal Creatinine, mg/dl (µmol/l)	<1.2 (110)	1.2-1.9 (110-170)	2.0-3.4 (171-299)	3.5-4.9 (300-440)	> 5.0 (440)
Urine output, ml/dl				<500	< 200

Ans. B

20. Overcorrection of acidosis by bicarbonate infusion can cause:

A. Hyperkalemia
B. Hypercalcemia
C. Volume overload
D. All of the above

Explanation:

- Metabolic acidosis is generally not treated unless severe (pH <7.20 and serum bicarbonate <15 mmol/L).
- Acidosis can be treated with oral or intravenous sodium bicarbonate but overcorrection should be avoided because of possibility of metabolic alkalosis, hypocalcemia, hypokalemia, and volume overload.

Ans. C

21. Cell that will not secrete TNF alpha is:

A. Fibroblasts
B. Eosinophils
C. Erythrocyte
D. Macrophages

Explanation:

Cytokine	Receptor	Cell Source	Cell Target	Biologic Activity
TNF-α	TNFrI, TNFrII	Monocytes-macrophages, mast cells, basophils, eosinophils, NK cells, B cells, T cells, keratinocytes, fibroblasts, thymic epithelial cells	All cells except erythrocytes	Fever, anorexia, shock, capillary leak syndrome, enhanced leukocyte cytotoxicity, enhanced NK cell function, acute phase protein synthesis, proinflammatory cytokine induction
TNF-β	TNFrI, TNFrII	T cells, B cells	All cells except erythrocytes	Cell cytotoxicity, lymph node and spleen development

Ans. C

22. Marker for Osteoclasts is:

A. CD5
B. CD1a
C. CD103
D. CD68

Explanation:

- Osteoclasts are multinucleated giant cells that can be identified by their expression of CD68, tartrate-resistant acid phosphatase, cathepsin K, and the calcitonin receptor.
- They appear at the pannus-bone interface where they eventually form resorption lacunae

Ans. D

23. A 43-year-old man recently returned from military deployment overseas. While there, he was involved in an improvised explosive device explosion resulting in injury to his right lower extremity, which ultimately required amputation. Since his surgery, he has had increased pain in his lower extremity, despite amputation. Which of the following is not a possible treatment for his condition?

A. N-methyl-D-aspartate (NMDA) receptor antagonists
B. Tricyclic antidepressants
C. Gabapentin
D. Valproic acid

Explanation:

- Patient has phantom limb pain, a condition that commonly follows amputation The onset of pain is often early, but may be delayed for months or years.

- It is most common in patients who suffered pain before their amputation. Pain is described as sharp, stabbing, shooting, or squeezing, and patients may also have vivid feelings of the previously amputated limb (phantom limb sensation).
- Exact pathophysiology is unknown, but many factors may contribute to phantom limb pain, such as vascular etiology for amputation, lower limb amputation, prior use of prosthesis, and prior history of stump pain.
- Treatment can include opiates, tricyclic antidepressants, antiepileptics such as carbamazepine (not calcium channel blockers), lidocaine, and NMDA receptor antagonists such as memantine or ketamine, as well as beta-blockers. Nonmedicinal treatments can also be of benefit, such as acupuncture, biofeedback, and massage. Finally, surgical treatments may provide benefit in refractory cases, including surgical dorsal root entry zone lesions, rhizotomies, or sympathectomies.

Ans. D

24. All are hereditary cause of Angioedema except:

A. Hereditary angioedema
B. C3b Inhibitor deficiency
C. Schnitzler syndrome
D. Muckle Wells syndrome

Explanation:

Table: Classification of urticaria and/or angioedema	
Acute	**Chronic**
• Drug Reactions – NSAIDS, IV contrast angiotensin-converting enzyme (ACE) inhibitors, etc. • Foods • Inhalation or contact with environmental allergens • Transfusion reactions • Insects • Infections–viral, bacterial, parasitic	• Idiopathic–a subset with autoimmune component • Collagen vascular disease–urticarial vasculitis • Physical stimuli – Dermatographism – Cholinergic urticaria – Vibration, cold, pressure, water (aquagenic) – Sun (Solar) • Mastocytosis/Urticaria pigmentosa • Hereditary – Hereditary angioedema (HAE) – Familial cold urticaria – C3b inhibitor deficiency – Muckle-Wells syndrome • Schnitzler syndrome • Hypereosinophilic syndrome • Gleich syndrome

Ans. C

25. An 8-year-old boy has a history of developmental delay with an intelligence quotient (IQ) of 45. His pediatrician also notes that he has an elongated face with protuberant ears and enlarged testicles. His family has a long history of mental retardation. Which of the following is true regarding his condition?

A. He has mild mental retardation
B. He has moderate mental retardation
C. He has severe mental retardation
D. He has the least common inherited cause of mental retardation

Explanation:

- The patient has moderate mental retardation (MR) based on his IQ of 45. Normal IQ is >70, mild MR has an IQ range of 55–70, moderate MR has a range of 40–55, and severe MR has a range of 25–40.

- Based on included description of his habitus along with a strong family history of MR, fragile X syndrome is most likely.
- This is the most commonly inherited form of MR and is due to a CGG expansion in FMR1 on the X chromosome.
- Common physical signs include elongated face, high forehead, protuberant ears, and enlarged testicles. There is often a strong family history of MR, and men are most often affected (due to the dysfunction of a single X chromosome).
- Females may also be affected by fragile X syndrome due to X inactivation (lyonization) of the normal X copy. Their phenotype is generally less severe, though it often includes premature ovarian failure.
- Other causes of MR include chromosomal abnormalities such as Down syndrome (trisomy 21), Rett syndrome, Prader-Willi syndrome, Angelman syndrome, toxic disturbances, metabolic disturbances, and pre/perinatal birth injuries or infections.

Ans. B

26. Endocrine and metabolic disorder abnormality common in HIV. Which of the following statements is not correct?

A. Predominant abnormality is Subclinical hypothyroidism

B. Lipoatrophy changes are particularly severe un patients receiving thymidine analogues stavudine

C. HIV infection seems to have significant effect on menstrual cycle

D. Immune reconstruction graves disease may occur as late (9-48 months) complication of cART

Explanation:

Table: Nucleoside or nucleotide reverse transcriptase inhibitors

Drug	Status	Indication	Dose in Combination	Supporting Data	Toxicity
Zidovudine (AZT, azidothymidine, *Retrovir, 3' azido-3'-deoxythymidine)	Licensed	Treatment of HIV infection in combination with other antiretroviral agents	200 mg q8h or 300 mg bid	19 vs 1 death in original placebo-controlled trial in 281 patients with AIDS or ARC	Anemia, granulocytopenia, myopathy, lactic acidosis, hepatomegaly with steatosis, headache, nausea, nail pigmentation, lipid abnormalities, lipoatrophy, hyperglycemia
		Prevention of maternal-fetal HIV transmission		In pregnant women with CD4+ T cell count ≥ 200/μl, AZT PO beginning at weeks 14-34 of gestation plus IV drug during labor and delivery plus PO AZT to infant for 6 weeks decreased transmission of HIV by 67.5% (from 25.5% to 8.3%); n=363	

- *Thyroid function* may be altered in 10–15% of patients with HIV infection. Both hypo- and hyperthyroidism may be seen.
- Predominant abnormality is subclinical hypothyroidism.

- In the setting of cART, up to 10% of patients have been noted to have elevated thyroid stimulating hormone levels, suggesting that this may be a manifestation of immune reconstitution.
- Immune-reconstitution Graves' disease may occur as a late (9–48 months) complication of cART.
- In advanced HIV disease, infection of the thyroid gland may occur with opportunistic pathogens, including *P. jirovecii*, CMV, mycobacteria, *Toxoplasma gondii*, and *Cryptococcus neoformans*.
- These infections are generally associated with a nontender, diffuse enlargement of the thyroid gland.
- Thyroid function is usually normal. Diagnosis is made by fine-needle aspirate or open biopsy

Ans. C

27. In Orthostatic hypotension with intractable symptoms are commonly treated by which of the following?

A. Pyridostigmine
B. Midodrine
C. Atomoxetine
D. Erythropoietin

Explanation:

- If these nonpharmacologic measures fail, pharmacologic intervention with fludrocortisone acetate and vasoconstricting agents such as midodrine, l-dihydroxyphenylserine, and pseudoephedrine should be introduced.
- Some patients with intractable symptoms require additional therapy with supplementary agents that include pyridostigmine, atomoxetine, yohimbine, desmopressin acetate (DDAVP) and erythropoietin.

Ans. B

28. COX 1 is expressed in all except:

A. Stomach
B. Kidney
C. Platelets
D. Brain

Explanation:

- COX-1 is expressed in a host of tissues, including the stomach, platelets, kidneys, and endothelial cells.
- This isoform is expressed in a constitutive manner and plays an important role in maintaining the integrity of renal function, platelet aggregation, and gastrointestinal (GI) mucosal integrity.
- In contrast, the expression of COX-2 is inducible by inflammatory stimuli, and it is expressed in macrophages, leukocytes, fibroblasts, and synovial cells.
- Beneficial effects of nonsteroidal anti-inflammatory drugs (NSAIDs) on tissue inflammation are due to inhibition of COX-2; the toxicity of these drugs (e.g., GI mucosal ulceration and renal dysfunction) is related to inhibition of the COX-1 isoform.
- Highly COX-2–selective NSAIDs have potential to provide the beneficial effect of decreasing tissue inflammation while minimizing toxicity in the GI tract.
- Selective COX-2 inhibitors have had adverse effects on the cardiovascular (CV) system, leading to increased risk of myocardial infarction.

Ans. D

29. After a bat bite, a rural farmer suffers from flu-like symptoms. Over the following days he develops diffuse weakness and confusion and is dead within 1 month. The following image was taken from autopsy. What is the name of the pathognomonic findings indicated by the arrows?

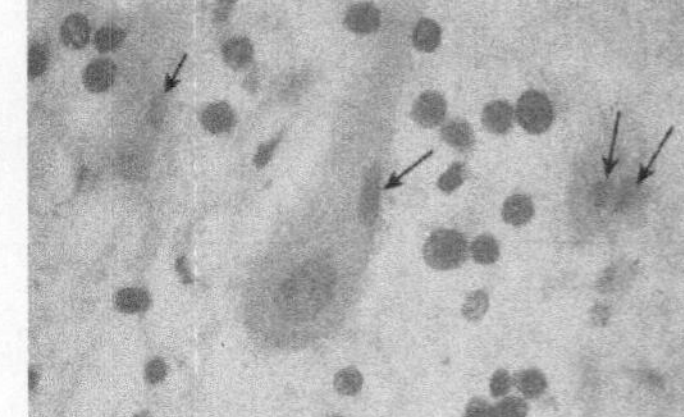

A. Negri bodies
B. Cowdry type A
C. Cowdry type B
D Howell-Jolly bodies

Explanation:

- Negri bodies (eosinophilic intracytoplasmic inclusions) are found in the pyramidal cells and in Purkinje cells of the cerebellum and are associated with rabies virus infection. Cowdry type A inclusions are eosinophilic nuclear inclusions seen in cells infected with herpes simplex virus.
- Cowdry type B inclusions are also eosinophilic nuclear inclusions associated with margination of chromatin on the nuclear membrane and are associated with adenovirus or poliovirus infection. Howell-Jolly bodies are small, round, basophilic nuclear inclusions found in erythrocytes associated with splenic dysfunction.
- Rosenthal fibers are extracellular, eosinophilic bundles that often appear like a corkscrew and may be seen with long-standing gliosis, some low-grade tumors, or some metabolic disorders.

Ans. A

30. All the following acts on G protein coupled seven transmembrane receptor (GPCR) except:

A. FSH
B. TSH
C. LH
D. Glucagon

Explanation:

Table: Examples of membrane receptor families and signaling pathways		
Receptors	**Effectors**	**Signaling Pathways**
G Protein-Coupled	**Seven-Transmembrane**	**Receptor (GPCR)**
β-Adrenergic, LH, FSH, TSH	$G_s\alpha$, adenylate cyclase	Stimulation of cyclic AMP production, protein kinase A
Glucagon, PTH, PTHrP, ACTH, MSH, GHRH, CRH	Ca^{2+} channels	Calmodulin, Ca^{2+}-dependent kinases
α-Adrenergic, somatostatin	$G_i\alpha$	Inhibition of cyclic AMP production Activation of K^+, Ca^{2+} channels
TRH, GnRH	G_q, G_{11}	Phospholipase C, diacyl-glycerol, IP_3, protein kinase C, voltage-dependent Ca^{2+} channels
Receptor Tyrosine Kinase		
Insulin, IGF-I	Tyrosine kinases, IRS	MAP kinases, PI 3-kinase; AKT
EGF, NGF	Tyrosine kinases, ras	Raf, MAP kinases, RSK
Cytokine Receptor–Linked Kinase		
GH, PRL	JAK, tyrosine kinases	STAT, MAP kinase, PI 3-kinase, IRS-1
Serine Kinase		
Activin, TGF-β, MIS	Serine kinase	Smads

Ans. D

31. Not true about tangier disease is:

A. Rare autosomal dominant disorder
B. Presents as slowly progressive symmetric polyneuropathy predominantly in legs.
C. Pseudo syringomyelia pattern with dissociated sensory loss
D. Caused by mutation in ATP Binding cassette transporter 1 (ABC1) Gene

Explanation:

- Tangier disease is a rare autosomal recessive disorder that can present as (1) asymmetric multiple mononeuropathies, (2) a slowly progressive symmetric polyneuropathy predominantly in the legs, or (3) a pseudo-syringomyelia pattern with dissociated sensory loss (i.e., abnormal pain/temperature perception but preserved position/ vibration in the arms

- Tonsils may appear swollen and yellowish-orange in color, and there may also be splenomegaly and lymphadenopathy.
- Tangier disease is caused by mutations in the ATP-binding cassette transporter 1 (ABC1) gene, which leads to markedly reduced levels of high-density lipoprotein (HDL) cholesterol levels, whereas triacylglycerol levels are increased. Nerve biopsies reveal axonal degeneration with demyelination and remyelination. Electron microscopy demonstrates abnormal accumulation of lipid in Schwann cells, particularly those encompassing unmyelinated and small myelinated nerves. There is no specific treatment.

Ans. A

32. Which of the following statements regarding S aureus is true?

A. Infections due to S aureus among colonized individuals are almost always due to a strain distinct from their colonizing strain

B. S aureus is always a pathogen when detected in any human culture

C. Anterior nares and oropharynx are the most common sites of colonization with S aureus

D. Colonization rate in the population is independent of patient factors

Explanation:

- S aureus is both a commensal and an opportunistic pathogen. Approximately 30% of healthy persons are episodically colonized with S aureus, with a smaller percentage (~10%) persistently colonized.
- Rate of colonization is elevated among insulin-dependent diabetics, HIV-infected patients, patients undergoing hemodialysis, injection drug users, and individuals with skin damage.
- Anterior nares and oropharynx are frequent sites of human colonization, although the skin (especially when damaged), vagina, axilla, and perineum may also be colonized.
- These colonization sites serve as a reservoir for future infections.
- Transmission of S aureus most frequently results from direct personal contact.
- Colonization of different body sites allows transfer from one person to another during contact. Spread of staphylococci in aerosols of respiratory or nasal secretions from heavily colonized individuals has also been reported.
- Most individuals who develop S aureus infections become infected with a strain that is already a part of their own commensal flora.
- Breaches of the skin or mucosal membrane allow S aureus to initiate infection.
- Some diseases increase the risk of S aureus infection; diabetes, for example, combines an increased rate of colonization and the use of injectable insulin with the possibility of impaired leukocyte function.
- Individuals with congenital or acquired qualitative or quantitative defects of polymorph nuclear leukocytes (PMNs) are at increased risk of S aureus infections; this group includes neutropenic patients (e.g., those receiving chemotherapeutic agents), those with chronic granulomatous disease, and those with Job or Chédiak-Higashi syndrome.
- Other groups at risk include individuals with end-stage renal disease, HIV infection, skin abnormalities, or prosthetic devices

Ans. C

33. Which of the following disorders is responsible for orthostatic hypotension:

A. Parkinson's disease

B. Shy drager syndrome

C. Hereditary amyloidosis

D. All of the above

Explanation:

- Primary autonomic failure due to idiopathic central and peripheral neurodegenerative diseases--the synucleinopathies Lewy body diseases Parkinson's disease Lewy body dementia Pure autonomic failure Multiple system atrophy (Shy-Drager syndrome)
- Secondary autonomic failure due to autonomic peripheral neuropathies Diabetes Hereditary amyloidosis familial amyloid polyneuropathy Primary amyloidosis (AL amyloidosis: immunoglobulin light chain associated) Hereditary sensory and autonomic neuropathies (HSAN) (especially type III-familial dysautonomia) Idiopathic immunemediated autonomic neuropathy Autoimmune autonomic ganglionopathy Sjögren's syndrome Paraneoplastic autonomic neuropathy HIV neuropathy Postprandial hypotension iatrogenic (drug-induced) Volume depletion.

Ans. D

34. Jung, 18-year-old previously healthy woman who presents with fever and hypotension. On the morning of admission, she felt quite ill with fevers, rigors, nausea, vomiting, and diarrhea. As the day progressed, she developed redness of her skin all over and became lethargic and ultimately quite difficult to arouse. She has no notable past medical history and takes no medications. She does not use alcohol or illicit drugs and is not sexually active. Her parents brought her to the emergency department in the late afternoon where her BP was noted to be 70/50 mmHg, with a HR of 140 bpm, temperature of 39.5°C, and RR of 24 breaths/min. Oxygen saturation is 94% on room air. She is minimally responsive. Skin examination reveals generalized erythroderma but no signs of skin tears or infection. Genitourinary examination reveals a retained tampon that is immediately removed. Blood Gram stain and culture are negative at 12 hours. You suspect staphylococcal toxic shock syndrome (TSS). Which of the following statements regarding staphylococcal TSS is true?

A. Skin site infection is clinically apparent in most cases
B. Blood cultures will likely return positive by 24–36 hours given her grave clinical presentation
C. Desquamation of the skin will occur within 1–2 days
D. Caused by a toxin that binds to the invariant region of the major histocompatibility complex and directly stimulates T-cell replication

Explanation:

- S aureus produces three types of toxin: cytotoxins, pyrogenic toxin superantigens, and exfoliative toxins.
- Toxic shock syndrome (TSS) results from the ability of enterotoxins and TSS toxin-1 to function as T-cell mitogens. In the normal process of antigen presentation, antigen is first processed within the cell, and peptides are then presented in the major histocompatibility complex (MHC) class II groove, initiating a measured T-cell response.
- In contrast, enterotoxins bind directly to the invariant region of MHC—outside MHC class II groove. The enterotoxins can then bind T-cell receptors via the vβ chain; this binding results in a dramatic overexpansion of T-cell clones (up to 20% of the total T-cell population).
- Consequence of this T-cell expansion is a "cytokine storm," with the release of inflammatory mediators that include interferon-γ, IL-1, IL-6, TNF-α, and TNF-β. Resulting multisystem disease produces a constellation of findings that mimic those in endotoxin shock; however, the pathogenic mechanisms differ.
- For TSS, investigators recommend a combination of clindamycin and a semisynthetic penicillin or vancomycin (if the isolate is resistant to methicillin). Clindamycin is advocated because, as a protein synthesis inhibitor, it reduces toxin synthesis in vitro.
- Linezolid also appears to be effective. In most cases of staphylococcal TSS (including nonmenstrual cases), a skin site of infection is not clinically apparent. Because this disease is mediated by toxin formation, blood cultures are almost always negative.
- Desquamation of the skin often occurs 1–2 weeks after the onset of the illness. Staphylococcal scalded skin syndrome, which affects primarily newborns and children, exhibits skin desquamation very early in disease.

Ans. D

35. A 50 year old male who is a hypertensive presents to the OPD with dry hacking cough. Which among the following drugs is responsible for this symptom?

A. Nifedipine
B. Lisinopril
C. Furosemide
D. Propanolol

Explanation:

- A dry hacking cough is seen in patients treated with ACE inhibitors. The cough usually begins 1 to 2 weeks after starting treatment, but it can be delayed upto 6 months. Women are more frequently affected than males. Pathophysiology of the ACE inhibitor induced cough is due to increased concentration of bradykinin, substance P and prostaglandins. Stopping the ACE inhibitor leads to the resolution of cough.

Ans. B

36. An anxiety disorder patient comes to the OPD with hyper ventilation. Which of the following is not seen in this disease?

A. Tetany
B. Respiratory alkalosis
C. Low serum bicarbonate
D. Metabolic alkalosis

Explanation:

- Hyperventilation is caused by ventilation in excess of requirements based on CO_2 production, leading to a reduced $PaCO_2$. Although anxiety can contribute to the initiation and progression of hyperventilation, hyperventilation is not always related to anxiety. Hyperventilation can precede systemic illnesses such as diabetic ketoacidosis. Symptoms of chronic hyperventilation can include dyspnea, paresthesias, headache, tetany, visual disturbances, and atypical chest pain. Laboratory findings of chronic hyperventilation include a reduced $PaCO_2$, but low serum bicarbonate level and near normal pH on arterial blood gas analysis. Treatment of chronic hyperventilation is problematic. Identification of initiating factors and excluding alternative diagnoses can be helpful.

Ans. D

37. Isolated angioedema is seen in which drug patients:

A. ACE inhibitor
B. Calcium channel inhibitors
C. Vasopressin analogues
D. Thiazide diuretics

Explanation:

- Use of ACE inhibitors results in impaired bradykinin degradation and explains the angioedema that occurs idiosyncratically in ACE inhibitor exposed patients with a normal C1INH.
- Bradykinin mediated angioedema, whether caused by ACE inhibitors or by C1INH deficiency, is noteworthy for conspicuous absence of concomitant urticaria or pruritus, frequent involvement of the gastrointestinal tract, and duration of symptoms >24h.

Ans. A

38. Following picture shows vesicular eruptions and shedding of finger nails. Which organism is responsible for this condition?

A. Measles virus
B. Varicella zoster virus
C. Coxsackievirus
D. Herpes simplex 1

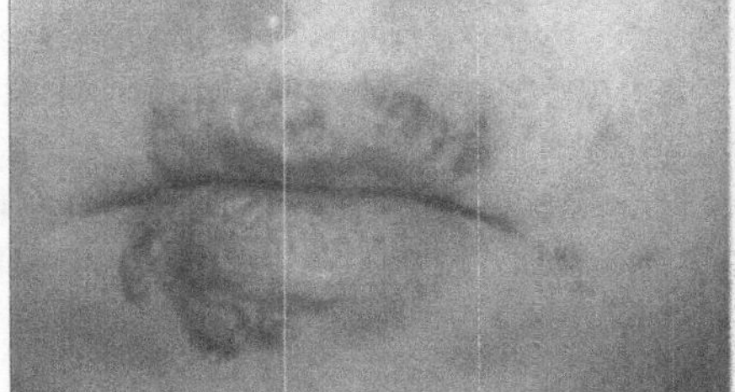

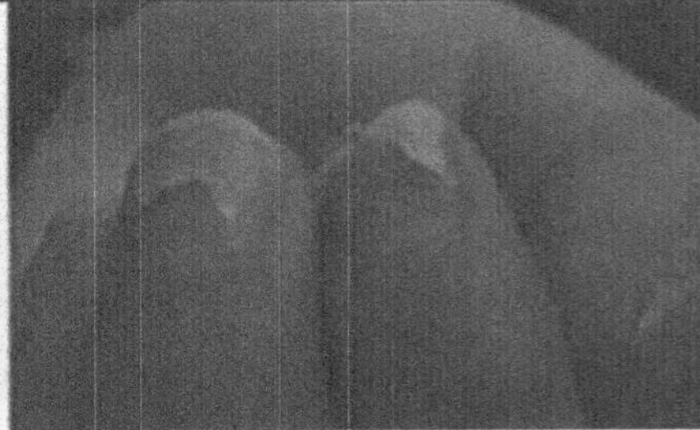

Explanation:

- Vesicular eruptions of the hand (A), knee (B), and mouth (C) of a 6-year old boy with Coxsackievirus A6 infection.
- Several of his fingernails were shed 2 months later (D).
- **HAND-FOOT-AND-MOUTH DISEASE** - After an incubation period of 4–6 days, patients with hand-foot-and-mouth disease present with fever anorexia, and malaise; these manifestations are followed by development of sore throat and vesicles on buccal mucosa and often on the tongue and then by appearance of tender vesicular lesions on the dorsum of hands, sometimes with involvement of the palms.
- Vesicles may form bullae and quickly ulcerate.
- About one-third of patients also have lesions on the palate, uvula, or tonsillar pillars, and one-third have a rash on the feet (including soles) or on the buttocks.
- Generalized rashes also have been reported.
- Disease is highly infectious, with attack rates of close to 100% among young children. The lesions usually resolve in 1 week. Most cases are due to Coxsackievirus A16 or enterovirus 71.

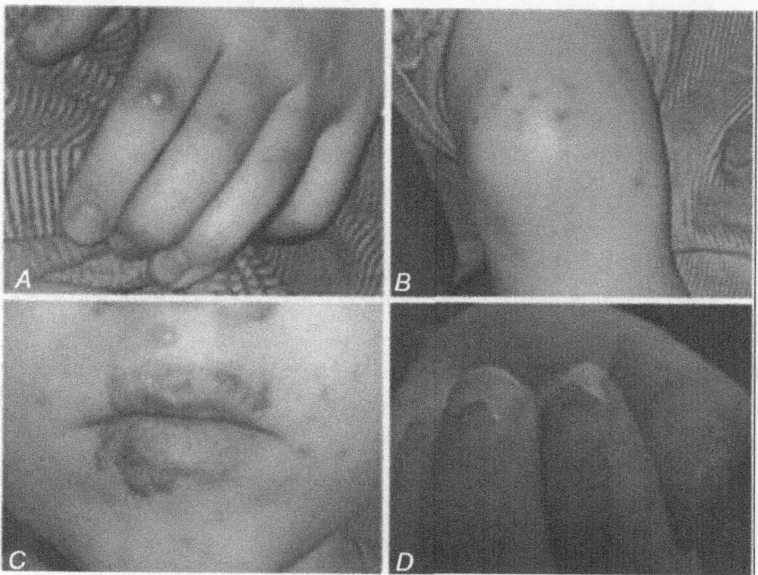

Ans. C

39. Which of the following analgesic medication act by inhibiting cyclooxygenase?

A. Aspirin
B. Acetaminophen
C. NSAIDS
D. All of the above

Explanation:

- All these drugs act by inhibiting the enzyme cyclooxygenase and they also have anti inflammatory action except for acetaminophen.

Ans. D

40. A 52 year old male presents to the OPD with sudden onset rhinorrhoea, sore throat, conjunctivitis and cough. RTPCR of the respiratory samples revealed influenza viral infection. Which among the following statements is true regarding this disease?

A. It is a segmented double stranded DNA virus
B. Influenza A viruses are sub typed by H and N antigen

C. A typical outbreak usually occurs in the summer season

D. Oseltamivir is given once a day for 3 days

Explanation:

- Influenza A, B, and C viruses are segmented, single-stranded, negative-sense RNA viruses that have on their outer surface prominent spikes formed by two surface glycoproteins, hemagglutinin (H) and neuraminidase (N). Influenza A and B viruses are major human pathogens, but influenza C virus causes only intermittent mild disease. Influenza A viruses are subtyped by the H and N antigens. Influenza outbreaks occur during cooler months. A typical outbreak begins in early winter and lasts 4–5 weeks in a given community, although its impact on the entire country lasts considerably longer.
- Oseltamivir and intranasal zanamivir are given twice a day for 5 days.

Ans. B

41. Most common clinical manifestation of Clostridium difficile infection?

A. Diarrhea

B. Fever

C. Abdominal pain

D. Leukocytosis

Explanation:

- Diarrhea is the most common manifestation caused by C. difficile. Stools are almost never grossly bloody and range from soft and unformed to watery or mucoid in consistency, with a characteristic odor.
- Clinical and laboratory findings include fever in 28% of cases, abdominal pain in 22%, and leukocytosis in 50%.
- When adynamic ileus (which is seen on X-ray in ~20% of cases) results in cessation of stool passage, the diagnosis of CDI is frequently overlooked.
- A clue to the presence of unsuspected CDI in these patients is unexplained leukocytosis, with ≥15,000 white blood cells (WBCs)/μL. Such patients are at high risk for complications of C. difficile infection, particularly toxic megacolon and sepsis.

Ans. A

42. Most common cause of Septic arthritis in adult:

A. Staph.aureus

B. Strep.pyogenes

C. Strep.pneumoniae

D. Staph. epidermidis

Explanation:

- Staphylococcus aureus is the most common cause of septic arthritis (native joints) in adults.
- This infection is rapidly progressive and may be associated with extensive joint destruction if left untreated.
- It presents with intense pain on motion of the affected joint, swelling, and fever.
- Aspiration of the synovial fluid reveals turbid fluid, with >50,000 PMNs/μL and gram positive cocci in clusters on Gram's stain.
- In adults, septic arthritis may result from trauma, surgical intervention of joints, or hematogenous dissemination.
- **Most commonly involved joints include the knee.**
- Infection frequently develops in joints previously damaged by osteoarthritis or rheumatoid arthritis.
- Staphylococcus aureus is the most common cause of septic arthritis (native joints) in children.

Ans. A

43. Ligand for TLR (Toll Like Receptor)-4 is:

A. dsRNA
B. Flagellin
C. LPS
D. CpG DNA

Explanation:

- TLRs (Toll Like Receptors) are part of innate immune system. As it recognizes foreign material, TLRs are called as Pattern Recognition Receptors (PRRs).
- In humans, 10 TLRs are present (TLR-1 to TLR-10)
- **TLR4 plays a major role in Septic shock.**
- **TLR 9 plays a major role in SLE.**

Important TLRs and their ligands as follows:

- TLR-3 - dsRNA
- TLR-4 - LPS
- TLR-5 - Flagellin
- TLR-9 - CpG DNA

PRR Family	PRRS	Ligand	DC or Macrophage Cytokine Response	Adaptive Immune Response
TLRs	TLR2 (heterodimer with TLR1 or 6)	Lipopeptides Pam-3-cys (TLR 2/1)	Low IL-12p70 High IL-10 IL-6	T_H1 T_H2 T regulatory
	TLR3	dsRNA	IL-12p70 IFN-α IL-6	T_H1
	TLR4	*Escherichia coli* LPS	High IL-12p70 Intermediate IL-10 IL-6	T_H1
	TLR5	Flagellin	High IL-12p70 Low IL-12p70	T_H1 T_H2
	TLR 7/8	ssRNA Imidazoquinolines	High IL-12p70 IFN- α IL-6	T_H1
	TLR9	CpG DNA	High IL-12p70 Low IL-10 IFN- α	T_H1
	TLR10	?	?	?
	TLR11	Profilin-like molecule uropathogenic bacteria	?	?

Ans. C

44. MRI of a 35-year-old woman with progressive myoclonus and apathy showing cortical ribboning. Most likely diagnosis is:

A. Herpes simplex encephalitis
B. Subacute sclerosing panenchepalitis
C. Alziehmers disease
D. Creutzfeldt-jakob disease

Explanation:

- Image shows cortical ribboning with clinical features of myoclonus and apathy favours Creutzfeldt-jakob disease

- Herpes simplex involves temporal lobe
- Subacute sclerosing panencephalitis seen in children and associated with mumps virus infection
- Alziehmers seen in old age people associated with corrical degeneration

Ans. D

45. A 70 year old male was given iloprost to reduce his pulmonary arterial pressure. He developed flushing as a side effect post treatment with iloprost. What is the mode of administration of iloprost?

A. Subcutaneous
B. Inhalation
C. IM
D. IV

Explanation:

- Prostaglandins (iloprost by inhalation, epoprostenol by continuous IV infusion, and treprostinil by IV, SC, or inhalation routes) improve symptoms, exercise tolerance, and, in the case of epoprostenol, survival. The most common side effect is flushing.

Ans. B

46. Following pesion seen in 26-year-old female patient with,yellowish discolouration of skin,tremors, psychiatric problems presented to medicine OPD and ophthalmological examination shown is likely to be:

A. Kayser Fleischer ring
B. Arcus senilis
C. Pterygium
D. Cataract

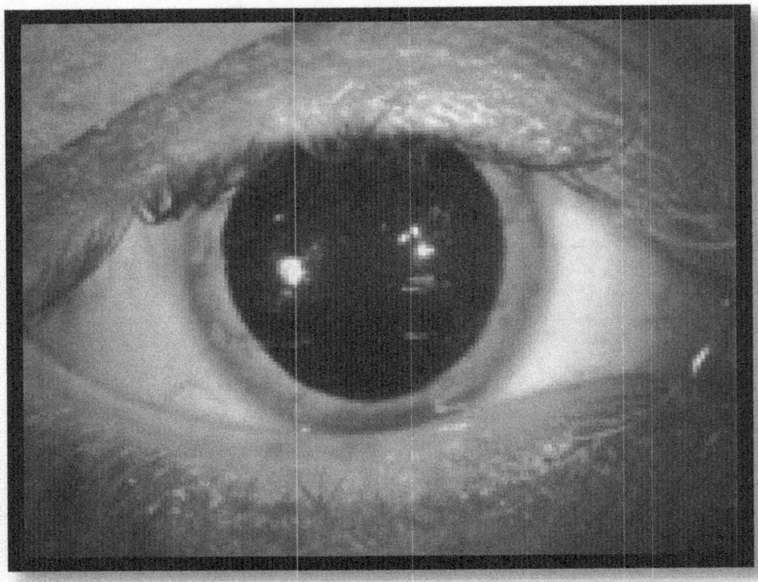

Explanation:

- Young female with jaundice,tremors,nuero psychiatric symptoms with golden yellow ring on ophthalmological examination is Kayser-Fleischer ring.
- Arcus senilis is whitish fat deposition which is senile seen in old age.
- Pterygium is degenerative condition of conjuctiva which is bilateral usually.
- Cataract is opacification of lens which is commonly seen in old age.

Ans. A

47. A 42-year-old surveyor from Western state presents with a 2 day history of the rash seen in Figure. Which of the following signs or symptoms is also likely to develop in this patient?

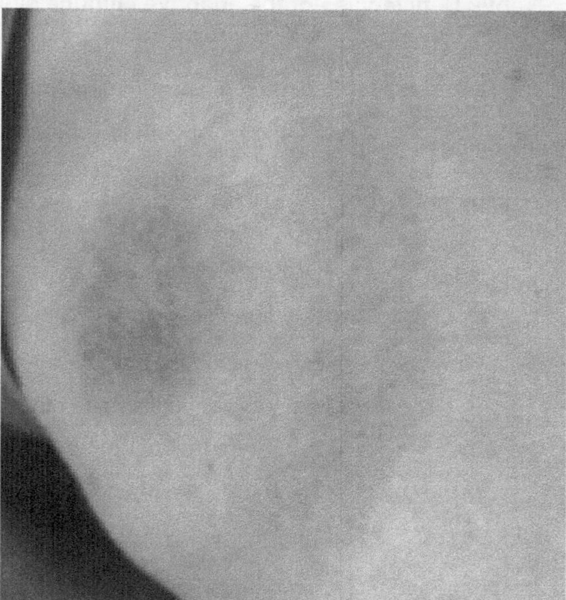

A. Holosystolic murmur loudest at the cardiac apex and radiating to the axilla

B. Fissured lip, strawberry tongue, and coronary aneurysms

C. Bradycardia with an electrocardiogram finding of complete atrioventricular dissociation

D. Diffuse exanthematous rash with eventual desquamation of the hands and feet

Explanation:

- Patient exhibits classic findings of the drug reaction with eosinophilia and systemic symptoms syndrome (DRESS). Some individuals are genetically unable to detoxify arene oxides present in some anticonvulsants (e.g., phenobarbital) and are susceptible to this dire syndrome.
- Confluence of this desquamative rash, eosinophilia, hepatic involvement, facial edema, and hypotension are all typical of this disease.
- Sweet syndrome, or acute febrile neutrophilic dermatosis, is characterized by erythematous indurated plaque with a pseudovesicular border. In 20% of cases, it is associated with malignancy (usually hematologic) but can also be associated with infections, inflammatory bowel disease, or pregnancy.
- Erythema multiforme is characterized by target lesions (central erythema surrounded by area of clearing and another rim of erythema) up to 2 cm, which are symmetric on knees, elbows, palms, and soles and spread centripetally. It is often confused with Stevens-Johnson syndrome, although erythema multiforme lacks the m arked skin sloughing seen in Stevens-Johnson syndrome.
- Staphylococcus toxic shock syndrome is a consideration here, as the hypotension and skin rash are typical. However, the lack of a cutaneous lesion or other risk factors and the concomitant eosinophilia and hepatitis make DRESS the more likely diagnosis.

Ans. A

48. Disorder related to T lymphocytes is:

A. Hyper IgE syndrome

B. X linked & Autosomal recessive agammaglobulinemia

C. Hyper IgM syndrome

D. IgA deficiency

Explanation:

Table: Deficiencies of the adaptive immune system	
• T lymphocytes: – Impaired development – Impaired survival, migration, function	Severe combined immune deficiencies (SCIDs) DiGeorge's syndrome Combined immunodeficiencies Hyper-IgE syndrome (autosomal dominant) DOCK8 deficiency CD40 ligand deficiency Wiskott-Aldrich syndrome Ataxia-telangiectasia and other DNA repair deficiencies
• B lymphocytes: – Impaired development – Impaired function	XL and AR agammaglobulinemia Hyper-IgM syndrome Common variable immunodeficiency (CVID) IgA deficiency

Ans. A

49. Patient has headache, fever, lethargy but no meningismus symptoms. What is the causative organism?

A. Cryptococcus neoformans
B. Cryptococcus gatti
C. Histoplasma capsulatum
D. N.meningiditis

Explanation:

- Clinical manifestations of cryptococcosis reflect the site of fungal infection.
- Spectrum of disease caused by Cryptococcus species consists of meningoencephalitis and pneumonia predominantly, but skin and soft tissue infections also occur; in fact, cryptococcosis can affect any tissue or organ.
- CNS involvement usually presents as signs and symptoms of chronic meningitis, such as headache, fever, lethargy, sensory deficits, memory deficits, cranial nerve paresis, vision deficits, and meningismus.
- Cryptococcal meningitis differs from bacterial meningitis in that many Cryptococcus-infected patients present with symptoms of several weeks duration. In addition, classic characteristics of meningeal irritation, such as meningismus, may be absent in cryptococcal meningitis.
- Indolent cases can present as subacute dementia.
- Meningeal cryptococcosis can lead to sudden catastrophic vision loss.
- Patients infected with C. gattii can present with granulomatous pulmonary masses known as cryptococcomas.

Ans. A

50. Synovial fluid culture of a patient with Fever, chills and knee pain have a negative for any organism. What is the causative organism?

A. N.meningiditis
B. N.gonorrhea
C. H.influenzae
D. S.aureus

Explanation:

- Most common manifestation of Disseminated Gonococcal Infection is a syndrome of fever, chills, rash, and articular symptoms.
- Small numbers of papules that progress to hemorrhagic pustules develop on the trunk and the extensor surfaces of the distal extremities.
- Migratory arthritis and tenosynovitis of the knees, hands, wrists, feet, and ankles are prominent.
- Cutaneous lesions and articular findings are believed to be the consequence of an immune reaction to circulating gonococci and immunecomplex deposition in tissues.
- Thus, cultures of synovial fluid are consistently negative, and blood cultures are positive in fewer than 45% of patients.
- Synovial fluid may be difficult to obtain from inflamed joints and usually contains only 10,000–20,000 leukocytes/μL.

Ans. B

51. Which Opportunistic infection is common in peritransplant and late transplant?

A. Herpes
B. Aspergillus
C. CMV
D. Nocardia

Explanation:

Table: The most common opportunistic infections in renal transplant recipients	
Peritransplant (<1 month)	**Late (> 6 months)**
• Wound infections	• *Aspergillus*
• Herpesvirus	• *Nocardia*
• Oral candidiasis	• BK virus (polyoma)
• Urinary tract infection	• Herpes zoster
Early (1-6 months)	• Hepatitis B
• *Pheumocystis carinii*	• Hepatitis C
• Cytomegalovirus	
• *Legionella*	
• *Listeria*	
• Hepatitis B	
• Hepatitis C	

Ans. A

52. Which of the following Category C pregnancy drug?

A. Rituximab
B. Azathioprine
C. Cyclophosphamide
D. Methotrexate

Explanation:

- Glucocorticoids are listed by the FDA as pregnancy category A (no evidence of teratogenicity in human studies); cyclosporine, tacrolimus, and rituximab are listed as category C (may be teratogenic in animals but no good evidence in humans); azathioprine, hydroxychloroquine, mycophenolate mofetil, and cyclophosphamide are category D (there is evidence of teratogenicity in humans, but benefits might outweigh risks in certain situations); and methotrexate is category X (risks outweigh benefits).

Ans. A

53. Amyloid precursor protein related to CNS disease include all *except:*

A. Cystatin C
B. Prion protein
C. Gelsolin
D. Amyloid Beta protein

Explanation:

Table: Amyloid precursor proteins and their clinical syndromes

Designation	Precursor	Clinical Syndrome	Clinical Involvement
Systemic Amyloidoses			
AL	Immunoglobulin light chain	Primary or myeloma-associated[a]	Any
AH	Immunoglobulin heavy chain	Rare variant of primary or myeloma-associated	Any
AA	Serum amyloid A protein	Secondary; reactive[b]	Renal, heart, other
$A\beta_2M$	β_2-Microglobulin	Hemodialysis-associated	Synovial tissue, bone
ATTR	Transthyretin	Familial (mutant) Age-related (wild type)	Cardiac, peripheral and autonomic nerves
AApoAI	Apolipoprotein AI	Familial	Hepatic, renal
AApoAII	Apolipoprotein AII	Familial	Renal
AGel	Gelsolin	Familial	Cornea, cranial nerves, skin, renal
AFib	Fibrinogen $A\alpha$	Familial	Renal
ALys	Lysozyme	Familial	Renal, hepatic
ALECT2	Leukocyte chemotactic factor2	Undefined	Renal
Localized Amyloidoses			
$A\beta$	Amyloid β protein	Alzheimer's disease; Down's syndrome	Central nervous system
ACys	Cystatin C	Cerebral amyloid angiopathy	Central nervous system, vascular
APrP	Prion protein	Spongiform encephalopathies	Central nervous system
AIAPP	Islet amyloid polypeptide (amylin)	Diabetes-associated	Pancreas
ACal	Calcitonin	Medullary carcinoma of the thyroid	Thyroid
AANF	Atrial natriuretic factor	Atrial fibrillation	Cardiac atria
APro	Prolactin	Endocrinopathy	Pituitary
ASgI	Semenogelin I	Age-related; incidental autopsy or biopsy finding	Seminal vesicles

Ans. C

54. Parrot's pseudoparalysis is associated with:

A. Lyme arthritis
B. Syphilitic arthritis
C. Fungal arthritis
D. Gonococcal arthritis

Explanation:

- Articular manifestations occur in different stages of syphilis.

- In early congenital syphilis, periarticular swelling and immobilization of the involved limbs *(Parrot's pseudoparalysis)* complicate osteochondritis of long bones.
- *Clutton's joint,* a late manifestation of congenital syphilis that typically develops between ages 8 and 15 years, is caused by chronic painless synovitis with effusions of large joints, particularly knees and elbows.
- Secondary syphilis may be associated with arthralgias, with symmetric arthritis of the knees and ankles and occasionally of the shoulders and wrists, and with sacroiliitis.
- Arthritis follows subacute to chronic course with a mixed mononuclear and neutrophilic synovial-fluid pleocytosis (typical cell counts, 5000–15,000/μL).
- Immunologic mechanisms may contribute to the arthritis, and symptoms usually improve rapidly with penicillin therapy. In tertiary syphilis, Charcot joint results from sensory loss due to tabes dorsalis. Penicillin is not helpful in this setting.

Ans. B

55. A 30 year old male presents with complaints of acute onset breathing difficulty , fever , myalgia, loss of taste and smell sensation. His CT chest reveals bilateral peripheral ground glass opacities with 50% lung involvement. Which among the following CO-RADS score is typical of COVID 19 infection?

A. CO-RADS 1
B. CO-RADS 2
C. CO-RADS 4
D. CO-RADS 5

Explanation:

- Based on the CT findings, the level of suspicion of COVID-19 infection is graded from very low or CO-RADS 1 up to very high or CO-RADS 5 and the severity and stage of the disease is determined with remarks on comorbidity and a differential diagnosis.

Co-RADS* Level of suspicion COVID-19 infection		
		CT findings
CO-RADS 1	No	Normal or non-infectious abnormalities
CO-RADS 2	Low	Abnormalities consistent with infections other than COVID-19
CO-RADS 3	Indeterminate	Unclear whether COVID-19 is present
CO-RADS 4	High	Abnormalities suspicious for COVID-19
CO-RADS 5	Very high	Typical COVID-19
CO-RADS 6	PCR +	

- CO-RADS 6 is CT picture typical of COVID 19 infection with RT=PCR test positive for COVID 19 infection.

Ans. D

56. A 60 year old obese female visits the fever clinic with complaints of 3 days history of fever, cough, breathing difficulty, loose stools and myalgia. Which among the following tests is not useful in diagnosing COVID 19 infection in this patient?

A. RT-PCR
B. CT CHEST
C. ABG
D. Antibody testing with IgM and IgG

Explanation:

- The possibility of coronavirus disease 2019 (COVID-19) should be considered in patients with the above mentioned complaints, those who reside in or have travelled to areas with community transmission or who have had recent close contact with a confirmed or suspected case of COVID-19. Clinicians should also be aware of the possibility of COVID-19 in patients with severe respiratory illness when no other etiology can be identified.

- Nucleic acid amplification testing (NAAT), most commonly with a reverse-transcription polymerase chain reaction (RT-PCR) assay, to detect SARS-CoV-2 RNA from the upper respiratory tract is the preferred initial diagnostic test for COVID-19.
- Serologic tests detect antibodies to SARS-CoV-2 in the blood and can help identify patients who previously had COVID-19.
- Patients can be treated as Covid 19 infection if the clinical symptoms and CT chest are consistent with Covid 19 infection.

Ans. C

57. Identify the condition:

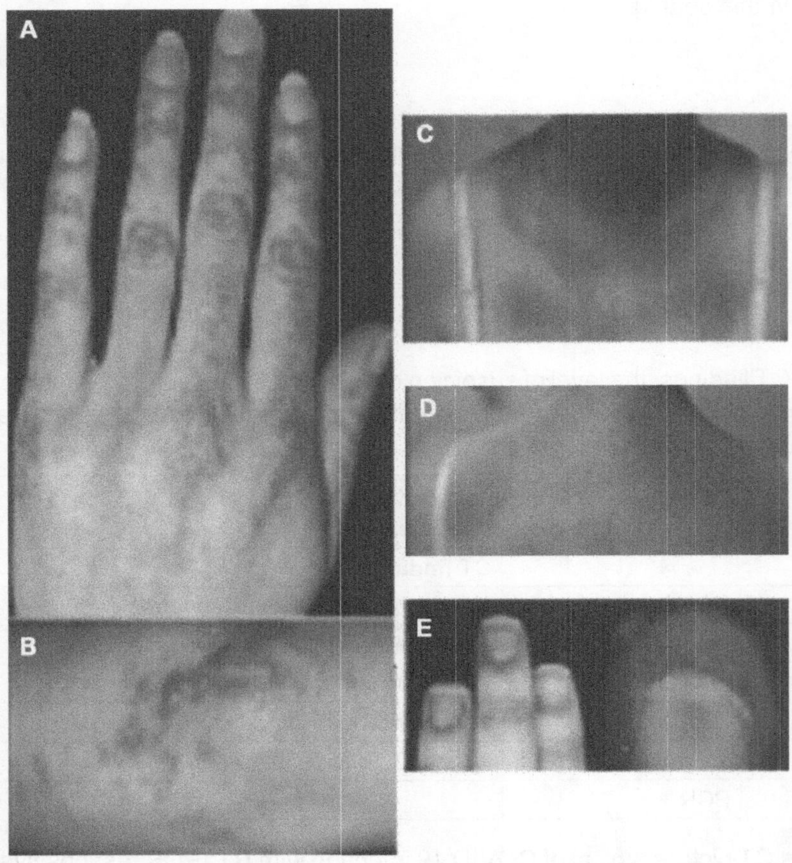

A. Lichen planus
B. Psoriasis
C. Dermatomyositis
D. Sarcoidosis

Explanation:

- Macular erythematous plaques (gottron sign) erythematous papules (gottrons papules) on extensor surface of fingers and elbow.
- Macular erythematous plaques over anterior chest and neck (V sign) and posterior neck and shoulder (Shawl sign).
- Dilated capillaries over nail bed are seen in favour of dermatomyositis.
- In psoriasis slivery, mica crusting is seen.
- Lichen planus: flat topped, purple, polygonal, pruritic, papules and plaques mucous membrane also involved usually.

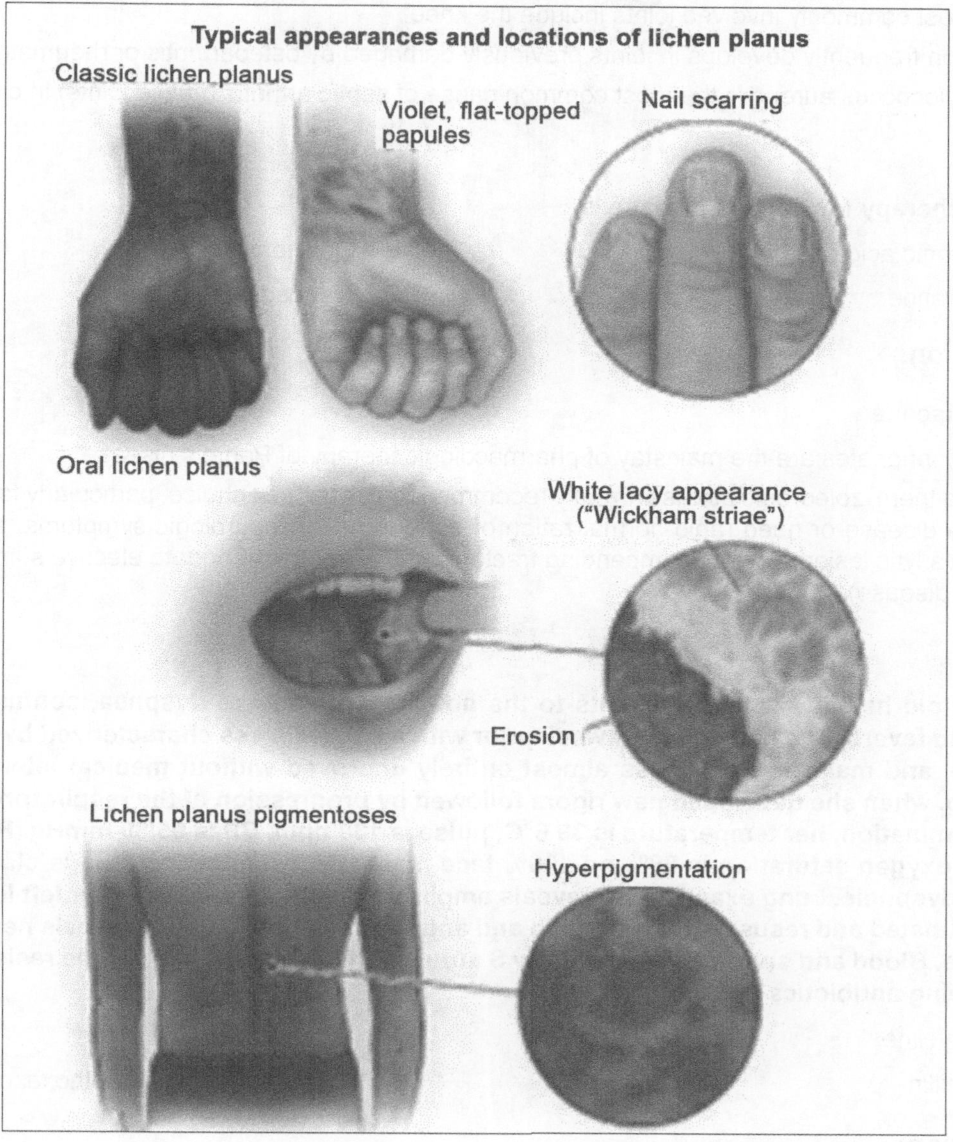

Ans. C

58. Most common cause of Septic arthritis in adult:

A. Staph. aureus
B. Strep. pyogenes
C. Strep. pneumoniae
D. Staph. epidermidis

Explanation:

- Staphylococcus aureus is the most common cause of septic arthritis (native joints) in adults.
- This infection is rapidly progressive and may be associated with extensive joint destruction if left untreated.
- It presents with intense pain on motion of the affected joint, swelling, and fever.
- Aspiration of the synovial fluid reveals turbid fluid, with >50,000 PMNs/μL and gram positive cocci in clusters on Gram's stain.
- In adults, septic arthritis may result from trauma, surgical intervention of joints, or hematogenous dissemination.

- The most commonly involved joints include the knee.
- Infection frequently develops in joints previously damaged by osteoarthritis or rheumatoid arthritis.
- Staphylococcus aureus is the most common cause of septic arthritis (native joints) in children.

Ans. A

59. First line therapy for Paget's disease is:

A. Zoledronic acid
B. Calcitonin
C. Teriparatide
D. Denosumab

Explanation:

Paget's Disease

- Bisphosphonates are the mainstay of pharmacologic therapy of Paget's disease.
- Among them, zoledronic acid is currently recommended as the first choice, particularly for those who have severe disease or need rapid normalization of bone turnover (neurologic symptoms, severe bone pain due to a lytic lesion, risk of an impending fracture, or pre-treatment prior to elective surgery in an area of active disease).

Ans. A

60. A 30-year-old healthy woman presents to the hospital with severe dyspnea, confusion, productive cough, and fevers. She had been ill 1 week prior with a flulike illness characterized by fever, myalgias, headache, and malaise. Her illness almost entirely improved without medical intervention until 36 hours ago, when she developed new rigors followed by progression of the respiratory symptoms. On initial examination, her temperature is 39.6°C, pulse is 130 bpm, BP is 95/60 mmHg, RR is 40 breaths/min, and oxygen saturation is 88% on 100% face mask. On examination, she is clammy, confused, and very dyspneic. Lung examination reveals amphoric breath sounds over her left lower lung fields. She is intubated and resuscitated with fluid and antibiotics. Chest CT scan reveals necrosis of her left lower lobe. Blood and sputum cultures grow S aureus. This isolate is likely to be resistant to which of the following antibiotics?

A. Doxycycline
B. Linezolid
C. Methicillin
D. Trimethoprim-sulfamethoxazole

Explanation:

- In the past 10 years, numerous outbreaks of community-based infection caused by MRSA in individuals with no prior medical exposure have been reported.
- These outbreaks have taken place in both rural and urban settings in widely separated regions throughout the world. The reports document a dramatic change in the epidemiology of MRSA infections.
- Outbreaks have occurred among such diverse groups as children, prisoners, athletes, Native Americans, and drug users. Risk factors common to these outbreaks include poor hygienic conditions, close contact, contaminated material and damaged skin.
- Community-associated infections have been caused by a limited number of MRSA strains. In the United States, strain USA300 (defined by pulsed-field gel electrophoresis) has been the predominant clone.
- While the majority of infections caused by this community-based clone of MRSA have involved the skin and soft tissue, 5%–10% have been invasive, including severe necrotizing lung infections, necrotizing fasciitis, infectious pyomyositis, endocarditis, and osteomylitis.
- Most feared complication is a necrotizing pneumonia that often follows influenza upper respiratory infection and can affect previously healthy people.
- This pathogen produces the Panton-Valentine leukocidin protein that forms holes in the membranes of neutrophils as they arrive at the site of infection and serves as a marker for this pathogen.

- An easy way to identify this strain of MRSA is its sensitivity profile. Unlike MRSA isolates of the past, which were sensitive only to vancomycin, daptomycin, quinupristin/dalfopristin, and linezolid, community-acquired MRSA is almost uniformly susceptible to trimethoprim-sulfamethoxazole and doxycycline.
- Organism is also usually sensitive to clindamycin. The term community-acquired has probably outlived its usefulness because this isolate has become the most common S aureus isolate causing infection in many hospitals around the world.

Ans. C

61. A 50 year old male who is a known case of PTB defaulter before 5 years is now diagnosed with XDR TB (Extensive drug resistant TB). He was treated with bedaquiline and other second line ATT drugs. Which among the following is the mechanism of action of bedaquiline?

A. Inhibits ATP synthase
B. Inhibits mitochondrial cell wall synthesis
C. Inhibits DNA gyrase
D. Inhibits DNA dependent RNA polymerase

Explanation:

- Bedaquiline and delamanid are the newer drugs approved for the management of drug resistant tuberculosis.
- Bedaquiline inhibits ATP synthase, an enzyme necessary for the generation of energy in mycobacterium tuberculosis. Dose- 400mg once daily for the first 2weeks followed by 200mg three times per week from week 3-week 24.
- Delamanid: The mechanism of action of delaminid is by inhibiting the synthesis of mycobacterial cell well components.
- Fluoroquinolones inhibit DNA gyrase.
- Rifampicin acts by inhibiting the DNA dependant RNA polymerase.

Ans. A

62. A 42-year-old man with poorly controlled diabetes (hemoglobin A1C = 13.3%) presents with thigh pain and fever over several weeks. Physical examination reveals erythema and warmth over the thigh with notable woody nonpitting edema. There are no cutaneous ulcers. CT of the thigh reveals several abscesses located between the muscle fibers of the thigh. Orthopedics is consulted to drain and culture the abscesses. Which of the following is the most likely pathogen?

A. Clostridium perfringens
B. Group A Streptococcus
C. Polymicrobial flora
D. S aureus

Explanation:

- This patient has infectious pyomyositis, a disease of the tropics and of immunocompromised hosts such as patients with poorly controlled diabetes mellitus or AIDS.
- Pathogen is usually S aureus.
- Management includes aggressive debridement, antibiotics, and attempts to reverse the patient's immunocompromised status.
- Clostridium perfringens may cause gas gangrene, particularly in devitalized tissues.
- Streptococcal infections may cause cellulitis or an aggressive fasciitis, but the presence of abscesses in a patient with poorly controlled diabetes makes staphylococcal infection more likely.
- Polymicrobial infections are common in diabetic ulcers, but in this case, the imaging and physical examination show intramuscular abscesses.

Ans. D

63. All are entry inhibitors except:

A. Rilpivirine

B. Maraviroc

C. Enfuviritide

D. Ibalizumab

Explanation:

Table: Entry inhibitors

Drug	Status	Indication	Dose in Combination	Supporting Data	Toxicity
Enfuvirtide (Fuzeon)	Licensed	In combination with other agents in treatment–experienced patients with evidence of HIV-1 replication despite ongoing anti-retroviral therapy	90 mg SC bid	In treatment of experienced patients, superior to placebo when added to new optimized background (37% vs 16% with < 400 HIV RNA copies/ml at 24 weeks; + 71 vs + 35 CD4 + T cells at 24 weeks)	Local injection reactions, hypersensitivity reactions, increased rate of bacterial pneumonia
Maraviroc (Selzentry)	Licensed	In combination with other antiretroviral agents in adults infected with only CCR5-tropic HIV-1	150-600 mg bid depending on concomitant medications (see text)	At 24 weeks, among 635 patients with CCR5-tropic virus and HIV-1 RNA > 5000 copies/ml despite at least 6 months of prior therapy with at least 1 agent from 3 of the 4 antiretroviral drug classes, 61% of patients randomized to maraviroc achieved HIV RNA levels < 400 copies/ml compared with 28% of patients randomized to plaebo	Hepatotoxicity, nasopharyngitis, fever, cough, rash, abdominal pain, dizziness, musculoskeletal symptoms
Ibalizumab (Trogarzo)	Licensed	In combination with other antiretroviral agents in patients with multidrug-resistant HIV-1	Single loading dose of 2000 mg followed by a maintenance dose of 800 mg every 2 weeks	At 25 weeks, 50% of patients with multi-drug resistant HIV-1 with HIV-1 RNA > 1000 copies/ml treated with an optimized background of 1 active drug and ibalizumab achieved HIV RNA levels < 200 copies/ml	Rash, diarrhea, nausea

Ans. A

64. Most useful laboratory indicator of systemic inflammation is:

A. Increased serum CRP

B. Increased serum albumin

C. Increased ESR

D. Increased serum creatinine

Explanation:

- Presence or absence of systemic inflammation distinguishes SM from CDM/cachexia.
- Most useful laboratory indicators of systemic inflammation are a reduced serum albumin concentration and an increased serum C-reactive protein concentration.

- Systemic inflammation increases the permeability of capillary walls to large molecules; the resulting osmotic shift increases the ECF volume.
- Intravascular albumin pool redistributes into this large volume, decreasing the serum albumin concentration. Increased albumin catabolism likely also contributes.
- Muscle atrophy and dietary protein deficiency perpetuate inflammation-induced hypoalbuminemia, because muscle protein and the diet provide the amino acids required for hepatic albumin synthesis

Ans. A

65. 5-HT1F receptor agonist:

A. Rimegepant
B. Ubrogepant
C. Lasmiditan
D. Sumatriptan

Explanation:

- Mainstay of pharmacologic therapy is the judicious use of one or more of the many medicines that are effective in migraine. Selection of the optimal regimen for a given patient depends on a number of factors, the most important of which is the severity of the attack. Mild migraine attacks can usually be managed by oral agents; the average efficacy rate is 50–70%.
- Severe migraine attacks may require parenteral therapy. Most drugs effective in the treatment of migraine are members of one of three major pharmacologic classes: nonsteroidal anti-inflammatory drugs.
- 5-HT1B/1D receptor agonists, and dopamine receptor antagonists.
- **Two new classes of therapeutic agents, CGRP receptor antagonists, such as rimegepant and ubrogepant, and 5-HT1F receptor agonists, such as lasmiditan, should soon be available.**

Ans. C

66. Adenosine is a potent vasoconstrictor of:

A. Afferent arteriole
B. Vasa recta
C. Efferent arteriole
D. Renal vein

Explanation:

- TGF changes the rate of filtration and tubular flow by reflex vasoconstriction or dilatation of the afferent arteriole.
- TGF is mediated by specialized cells in the thick ascending limb of loop of Henle called *macula densa* that act as sensors of solute concentration and tubular fluid flow rate. With high tubular flow rates, a proxy for an inappropriately high filtration rate, there is increased solute delivery to the macula densa that evokes vasoconstriction of the afferent arteriole causing GFR to return toward normal.
- One component of the soluble signal from the macula densa is adenosine triphosphate (ATP) released by the cells during increased NaCl reabsorption. ATP is metabolized in extracellular space to generate **adenosine, a potent vasoconstrictor of the afferent arteriole.**
- During conditions associated with a fall in filtration rate, reduced solute delivery to the macula densa attenuates TGF, allowing afferent arteriolar dilatation and restoring GFR to normal levels.
- Angiotensin II and reactive oxygen species enhance, while nitric oxide (NO) blunts TGF

Ans. A

67. A 65 year old male presents to the ER with fever and confusion. His respiratory rate is 40 breaths/minute and blood pressure is 80/50mmHg. Chest radiograph is suggestive of community acquired pneumonia. Which among the following bio markers helps to identify between bacterial or other citology?

A. NT-PRO BNP
B. Pro calcitonin
C. CRP
D. ESR

Explanation:

- Serial measurements of C-reactive protein (CRP) levels in serum may help identify worsening disease or treatment failure. Measurement of serum procalcitonin (PCT) levels can help distinguish bacterial from viral infection, determine the need for antibacterial therapy, or determine when to discontinue treatment.
- NT-PRO BNP is raised in heart failure.

Ans: B

68. All Mediate phagocytosis and ADCC (antibody-dependent cell-mediated cytotoxicity) except:

A. CD16a

B. CD32a

C. CD64

D. CD86

Explanation:

Table: Human leukocyte surface antigens–The CD classification of leukocyte differentiation antigens

Surface Antigen (Other Names)	Family	Molecular Mass, kDa	Distribution	Ligand(s)	Function
CD1a (T6, HTA-1)	Ig	49	CD, cortical thymocytes, Langerhans type of DCs	TCRγδ T cells	CD1 molecules present lipid antigens of intracellular bacteria such as Mycobacterium leprae and M. tuberculosis to TCR γδ T cells
CD1b	Ig	45	CD, cortical thymocytes, Langerhans type of DCs	TCRγδ T cells	
CD1c	Ig	43	DC, cortical thymocytes, subset of B cells, Langerhans type of DCs	TCRγδ T cells	
CD1d	Ig	37	Cortical thymocytes, intestinal epithelium, Langerhans type of DCs	TCRγδ T cells	
CD2 (T12, LFA-2)	Ig	50	T, NK	CD58, CD48, CD59, CD15	Alternative T cell activation, T cell anergy, T cell cytokine production, T- or NK-mediated cytolysis, T cell apoptosis, cell adhesion
CD3 (T3, Leu-4)	Ig	γ:25-28, δ:21-28, τ:20-25, η:21-22, ς:16	T	Associates with the TCR	T cell activation and function; ς is the signal transduction component of the CD3 complex

Contd.

Contd.

CD4 (T4, Leu-3)	Ig	55	T, myeloid	MHC-I, HIV, gp120, IL-16, SABP	T cell selection, T cell activation, signal transduction with p56lck, primary receptor for HIV
CD7 (3A1, Leu-9)	Ig	40	T, NK	K-12 (CD7L)	T and NK cell signal transduction and regulation of IFN-γ, TNF-α production
CD8 (T8, Leu-2)	Ig	34	T	MHC-I	T cell selection, T cell activation, signal transduction with P56lck
CD14 (LPS-receptor)	LRG	53−55	M, G (weak), not by myeloid progenitors	Endotoxin (lipopolysaccharide), lipoteichoic acid, PI	TLR4 mediates with LPS and other PAMP activation of innate immunity
CD16a (FcγRIIIa)	Ig	50−80	NK, Macrophages, neutrophils	Fc portion of IgG	Mediates phagocytosis and ADCC
CD19 B4	Ig	95	B (except plasma cells), FDC	Not known	Associates with CD21 and CD81 to form a complex involved in signal transduction in B cell development, activation, and differentiation
CD20 (B1)	Unassigned	33-37	B (except plasma cells)	Not known	Cell signalling, may be important for B cell activation and proliferation
CD21 (B2, CR2, EBV-R, C3dR)	RCA	145	Mature B, FDC, subset of thymocytes	C3d, C3dg, iC3b, CD23, EBV	Associates with CD19 and CD81 to form a complex involved in signal transduction in B cell development, activation and differentiation; Epstein-Barr virus receptor
CD22 (BL-CAM)	Ig	130-140	Mature B	CDw 75	Cell adhesion, signalling through association with p72sky, p53/56lyn P13 kinase, SHP1, fLCγ

Contd.

Contd.

CD23 (FcεRII, B6, Leu-20, BLAST-2)	C-type lectin	45	B,M, FDC	IgE, CD21, CD11b CD11c	Regulates IgE synthesis, cytokine release by monocytes
CD28	Ig	44	T, plasma cells	CD80, CD86	Co-stimulatory for T cell activation; involved in the decision between T cell activation and anergy
CD32a (FcγRIIa)	Ig	40	NK, macrophages, neutrophils	Fc portion of IgG	Mediates phagocytosis and ADCC
CD40	TNFR	48–50	B, DC, EC, thymic epithelium, MP, cancers	CD154	B cell activation, proliferation and differentiation; formation of GCs; isotype switching; rescue from apoptosis
CD45 (LCA, T200, B220)	PTP	180, 200, 210, 220	All leukocytes	Galectin-1, CD2, CD3, CD4	T and B activation thymocyte development, signal transduction, apoptosis
CD45RA	PTP	210, 220	Subset T, medullary thymocytes, "naïve" T	Galectin-1, CD2, CD3, CD4	Isoforms of CD45 containing exon4 (A), restricted to a subset of T cells
CD45RB	PTP	200, 210, 220	All leukocytes	Galectin-1, CD2, CD3, CD4	Isoforms of CD45 containing exon 5 (B)
CD45RC	PTP	210, 220	Subset T, medullary thymocytes, "naïve" T	Galectin-1, CD2, CD3, CD4	Isoforms of CD45 containing exon 6 (C), restricted to a subset of T cells
CD45RO	PTP	180	Subset T, cortical thymocytes, "memory" T	Galectin-1, CD2, CD3, CD4	Isoforms of CD45 containing no differentially spliced exons, restricted to a subset of T cells
CD64 (FcγRI)	Ig	45–55	Macrophages and monocytes	Fc portion of IgG	Mediates phagocytosis and ADCC
CD80 (B7-1 B81)	Ig	60	Activated B and T, MP, DC	CD28, CD152	Co-regulator of T cells activation; signaling through CD28 stimulates and through CD152 inhibits T cell activation

Contd.

Contd.

CD86 (B7-2, B70)	Ig	80	Subset B, DC, EC, activated T, thymic epithelium	CD28, CD152	Co-regulator of T cell activation; signaling through CD28 stimulates and through CD152 inhibits T cell activation
CD89 (FCαR)	Ig	55-100	Neutrophils, esoinophils, monocytes and MP	Fc portion of IgG	Mediates phagocytosis and ADCC of IgA-coated pathogens
CD95 (APO-1, Fas)	TNFR	43	Activated T and B	Fas ligand	Mediates apoptosis
CD152 (CTLA-4)	Ig	30-33	Activated T	CD80, CD86	Inhibits T cell proliferation
CD154 (CD40L)	TNF	33	Activated CD4+ T, subset CD8+ T, NK, M, basophil	CD40	Co-stimulatory for T cell activation, B cell proliferation and differentiation
CD279 (PD-1)	Ig	50−55	B, T, TfH	PD-L1, PD-L2	Inhibits T cell proliferation

Ans. D

69. IL-1 cytokine is structurally similar to all except:

A. IL-18
B. ECGF
C. PDGF
D. FGF

Explanation:

Table: Cytokine families grouped by structural similarity	
Hematopoietines	IL-2, IL-3, IL-4, IL-5, IL-6, IL-7, IL-9, IL-11, IL-12, IL-15, IL-16, IL-17, IL-21, IL-23, EPO, LIF, GM-CSF, G-CSF, OSM, CNTF, GH and TPO TNF-α, LT-α, LT-β, CD40L, CD30L, CD27L, 4-1BBL, OX40, OPG and FasL
IL-1	IL-1α, IL-1β, IL-1ra, IL-18, bFGF, aFGF and ECGF
PDGF	PDGF A, PDGF B and M-CSF
TGF-β	TGF-β and BMPs (1, 2, 4 etc.)
C-X-C chemokines	IL-8, Gro-α/β/γ, NAP-2, ENA 78, GCP-2, PF4, CTAP-3, MIG and IP-10
C-C chemokines	MCP-1, MCP-2, MCP-3, MIP-1α, MIP-1β, RANTES

Ans. C

70. Golden rice is enriched with:

A. Vitamin D
B. Vitamin A
C. Vitamin C
D. Vitamin E

Explanation:

- Selective plant-breeding techniques that lead to a higher provitamin A carotenoid content in staple foods may decrease vitamin A malnutrition in low-income countries. Moreover, a recently developed genetically modified food (Golden Rice) has an improved β-carotene–to–vitamin A conversion ratio of ~3:1.

Ans. B

71. Carbohydrate in parenteral nutrition is:

A. Glucose
B. Lactose
C. Dextrose
D. Fructose

Explanation:

- PN delivers a complete nutritional regimen directly into the bloodstream in the form of crystalline amino acids, dextrose, triglyceride emulsions, minerals (calcium, phosphate, magnesium, and zinc), electrolytes, and micronutrients.
- Because of its high osmolarity (>1200 mOsm/L) and often large volume, PN is infused into a central vein in adults. Ready-to-use PN admixtures typically containing 4–7% hydrous amino acids and 20–25% dextrose (with or without electrolytes) are available in 2-chamber (amino acids and dextrose) or 3-chamber (amino acids, dextrose, and lipid) bags that are intermixed and vitamins, trace minerals and additional electrolytes added just prior to infusion. Although convenient and cost-effective, these products have fixed nutrient composition and thus are dosed according to the volume required to meet calorie requirements.
- In some situations—especially ADM—a costlier approach is justified that uses a computer-controlled sterile compounder to generate combinations of amino acid and dextrose that meet the precise protein and energy requirements of individual patients.

Ans. C

72. A 40 year old male who is a known diabetic and an alcoholic comes to the OPD with chest radiograph showing homogenous right upper lobar consolidation. Bulging fissure sign is positive. He is diagnosed to have Klebsiella pneumonia in sputum culture. Which among the following statements is false?

A. It is a gram-negative bacilli
B. Most frequently occurs as a nosocomial infection.
C. Lung abscess is common.
D. Carbapenemase resistance has not been noted

Explanation:

- *Klebsiella pneumoniae*, a gram-negative bacillus, most frequently causes infection in hospitalized patients and in those with impaired host defenses, including patients with diabetes mellitus, alcoholism, malignancy, hepatobiliary disease, chronic obstructive pulmonary disease, renal failure, and glucocorticoid therapy.
- *K. pneumoniae* is a relatively common cause of nosocomial bacteremia.
- Diagnosis of *K. pneumoniae* is generally made by isolation of the organism from culture of the relevant specimen. On Gram stain, *Klebsiella* species typically appear as short, plump, gram-negative bacilli, which are usually surrounded by a capsule that appears as a clear space.
- The antibiotic regimen for infections with *K. pneumoniae* is usually determined by the results of susceptibility testing. Outbreaks of strains that produce an extended-spectrum beta-lactamase or a carbapenemase have been reported worldwide.

Ans. D

73. Gene products implicated in enhancing or maintaining self renewal capacity of cells except:

A. Bmi-1
B. Gfi-1
C. Bax-1
D. HoxB4

Explanation:

- HoxB4 is capable of inducing extensive self renewal of stem cells through its DNA-binding motif.
- Other members of hox family of genes have been noted to affect normal stem cells, but they are also associated with leukemia.

- External signals that may influence the relative self-renewal versus differentiation outcomes of stem cell cycling include specific Wnt ligands.
- Intracellular signal transducing intermediates are also implicated in regulating self-renewal. They include PTEN, an inhibitor of the AKT pathway and STAT5, both of which are downstream of activated growth factor receptors and necessary for normal stem cell functions including self-renewal, at least in mouse models.

Ans. C

74. All are causes of absolute erythrocytosis except:

A. Carbon monoxide intoxication
B. High altitude
C. Tobacco abuse
D. Meningioma

Explanation:

Table: Relative erythrocytosis	
Hemoconcentration secondary to dehydration, diuretics, ethanol abuse, androgens, or tobacco abuse	
Absolute Erthrocytosis	
Hypoxia	**Tumors**
Carbon monoxide intoxication	Hypernephroma
High-oxygen-affinity hemoglobins	Hepatoma
High altitude	Cerebellar hemangioblastoma
Pulmonary disease	Uterine myoma
Right-to-left cardiac or vascular shunts	Adrenal tumors
Sleep apnea syndrome	Meningioma
Hepatopulmonary syndrome	Pheochromocytoma
Renal Disease	**Drugs**
Renal artery stenosis	Androgens
Focal sclerosing or membranous glomerulonephritis	Recombinant erythropoietin
Postrenal transplantation	**Familial (with normal hemoglobin function)**
Renal cysts	Erythropoietin receptor mutations
Bartter's syndrome	VHL mutations (Chuvash polycythemia)
	2,3-BPG mutation
	PHD2 and HIF2α mutations
	Polycythemia vera

Ans. C

75. Postoperative low cardiac output syndrome is seen after:

A. Drainage of massive pleural effusion
B. Drainage of massive ascites
C. Drainage of pericardial effusion
D. Drainage of spinal fluid

Explanation:

- "Postoperative low cardiac output syndrome" occurs in up to 10% of patients undergoing surgical drainage and carries poor short-term survival.

Ans. C

76. All are correct combinations except:

A. Often exertional pain, felt as pressure on chest with raised JVP is PAH

B. Tearing or ripping pain often between blades of shoulder is aortic dissection

C. Heaviness of chest with dyspnea and tachycardia is small pulmonary embolism

D. Pleuritic sharp pain relieved by sitting and bending forward is acute pericarditis

Explanation:

System	Condition	Onset/Duration	Quality	Location	Associated Features
Cardiopulmonary					
Cardiac	Myocardial ischemia	*Stable angina:* Precipitated by exertion, cold or stress: 2-10 min *Unstable angina:* Increasing pattern or at rest *Myocardial infarction:* Usually > 30 min	Pressure, tightness, squeezing, heaviness, burning	Retrosternal; often radiation to neck, jaw, shoulders, or arms; sometimes epigastric	S_4 gallop or mitral regurgitation murmur (rare) during pain: S_1 or rales if severe ischemia or complication of myocardial infarction
	Pericarditis	Variable; hours to days; may be episodic	Pleuritic, sharp	Retrosternal or toward cardiac apex; may radiate to left shoulder	May be relieved by sitting up and leaning forward; pericardial friction rub
Vascular	Acute aortic syndrome	Sudden onset of unrelenting pain	Tearing or ripping knifelike	Anterior chest, often radiating to back, between shoulder blades	Associated with hypertension and/ or underlying connective tissue disorder; murmur of aortic insufficiency; loss of peripheral pulses
	Pulmonary embolism	Sudden onset	Pleuritic; may manifest as heaviness with massive pulmonary embolism	Often lateral, on the side of the embolism	Dyspnea, tachypnea, tachycardia and hypotension
	Pulmonary hypertension	Variable; often exertional	Pressure	Substernal	Dyspnea, signs of increased venous pressure
Pulmonary	Pneumonia or pleuritics	Variable	Pleuritic	Unilateral, often localized	Dyspnea, cough, fever, rales, occasional rub
	Spontaneous pneumothorax	Sudden onset	Pleuritic	Lateral to side of pneumothorax	Dyspnea, decreased breath sound on side of pneumothorax

Contd.

Contd.

Non-cardiopulmonary					
Gastrointestinal	Esophageal reflux	10-60 min	Burning	Substernal, epigastric	Worsened by postprandial recumbency; relieved by antacids
	Esophageal spasm	2-30 min	Pressure, tightness, burning	Retrosternal	Can closely mimic angina
	Peptic ulcer	Prolonged; 60-90 min after meals	Burning	Epigastric, substernal	Relieved with food or antacids
	Gallbladder disease	Prolonged	Aching or colicky	Epigastric, right upper quadrant; sometimes to the back	May follow meal
Neuromuscular	Costochondritis	Variable	Aching	Sternal	Sometimes swollen, tender, warm over joint; may be reproduced by localised pressure on examination
	Cervical disk disease	Variable; may be sudden	Aching; may include numbness	Arms and shoulders	May be exacerbated by movement of neck
	Trauma or strain	Usually constant	Aching	Localized to area of strain	Reproduced by movement of palpation
	Herpes zoster	Usually prolonged	Sharp or burning	Dermatomal distribution	Vesicular rash in area of discomfort
Psychological	Emotional and psychiatric conditions	Variable: may be fleeting or prolonged	Variable: often manifests as tightness and dyspnea with feeling of panic or doom	Variable; may be retrosternal	Situational factors may precipitate symptoms; history of panic attacks, depression

Ans. C

77. In mechanically ventilated patient, Hypotension resulting from elevated intrathoracic pressures with decreased venous return is almost always responsive to:

A. Vasopressors
B. Intravascular volume repletion
C. Decreasing PEEP
D. Ketamine

Explanation:

- Hypotension resulting from elevated intrathoracic pressures with decreased venous return is almost always responsive to intravascular volume repletion.
- In patients who are judged to have respiratory ailure on the basis of alveolar edema but in whom the cardiac or pulmonary origin of the edema is unclear, hemodynamic monitoring with a pulmonary arterial catheter may be of value in helping to clarify cause of the edema.
- Gastrointestinal effects of positive-pressure ventilation include stress ulceration and mild to moderate cholestasis.

Ans. B

78. Under normal conditions, lactate is produced from all except:

A. Skeletal muscle
B. Brain
C. Skin
D. Heart

Explanation:

- Lactate measurement has a role in the diagnosis, risk stratification, and, potentially, the treatment of shock.
- Increased lactate (hyperlactemia) and lactic acidosis (hyperlactemia and pH <7.35) are common in shock.
- Lactate is a product of anaerobic glucose metabolism. In glycolysis, enzyme phosphofructokinase metabolizes glucose to pyruvate.
- Under aerobic conditions, the pyruvate is then converted (in the mitochondria) to acetyl CoA and enters the Krebs cycle with resulting ATP generation through oxidative phosphorylation.
- In the setting of cellular hypoxia, the Krebs (tricarboxylic acid) cycle cannot oxidize pyruvate, and thus, pyruvate is converted to lactate by enzyme lactate dehydrogenase.
- Under normal conditions, lactate is produced from skeletal muscle, brain, skin, and intestine.
- In the setting of reduced oxygen delivery and cellular hypoxia, the amount of lactate produced from these tissues increases (and other tissue can begin to produce lactate).
- While most of the studies have been performed in patients with septic shock, there is evidence that elevated lactate correlates with a worse outcome.
- A recent systematic literature review evaluating the role of lactate measurement in a variety of critically ill populations supported the value of serial lactate measurements in the evaluation of critically ill patients and their response to therapy.

Ans. D

79. Infection transmitted by tick bite is:

A. Rickettsial pox
B. Rocky Mountain spotted fever
C. Q fever
D. Scrub typhus

Explanation:

Table: Features of selected rickettsial infections

Disease	Organism	Transmission	Geographic Range	Incubation Period, Days	Duration, Days	RASH %	ESCHAR %	Lymphadenopathy[a]
Rocky mountain spotted fever	*Rickettsia rickettsii*	Tick bite: *Dermacentor andersoni*, *D. variabilis*	United States	2-14	10-20	90	<1	+
		Amblyomma cajennense sensu lato, *A. aureolatum*	Central/South America					
		Rhipicephalus sanguineus	Mexico, Brazil, United States					
Mediterranean spotted fever	*R. conoril*	Tick bite: *R. sanguineus*, *R. pumilio*	Southern Europe, Africa, Middle East, Central Asia	5-7	7-14	97	50	+

Contd.

Contd.

African tick-bite fever	*R. africae*	Tick bite: *A, hebraeum, A. variegatum*	Sub-Saharan Africa, West Indies	4-10	4-19	50	90	+++
Maculatum disease	*R. parkeri*	Tick bite: *A. maculatum, A. triste, A. tigrinum*	United States, South America	2-10	6-16	88	94	++
Pacific Coast tick fever	*Rickettsia 364D*	Tick bite: *D. occidentalis*	United States	3-9	5-14	14	100	+++
Rickettsialpox	*R. akari*	Mite bite: *Liponyssoides sanguineus*	United States, Ukraine, Turkey, Mexico, Croatia	10-17	3-11	100	90	+++
Tick-borne lymphadeno-pathy	*R. slovaca*	Tick bite: *D. marginatus, D. reticularis*	Europe	7-9	17-180	5	100	++++
Flea-borne spotted fever	*R. felis*	Flea (mechanism undeter-mined): *Ctenocephalides felis*	Worldwide	8-16	8-16	80	15	–
Epidemic typhus	*R. prowazekii*	Louse *feces: Pediculus humanus corporis,* fleas and lice of flying squirrels, or recrudescence	Worldwide	7-14	10-18	80	None	–
Murine typhus	*R.typhi*	Flea feces: *Xenopsylla cheopis, C. felis, others*	Worldwide	8-16	9-18	80	None	–
Human mono-cytotropic ehrlichiosis	*Ehrlichia chaffeensis*	Tick bie: *A americanum, D. variabilis*	United States	1-21	3-21	26	None	++
Ewingii ehrlichiosis	*E.ewingii*	Tick bite: *A. americanum*	United States	1-21	4-21	0	None	None
Unnamed ehrlichiosis	*E. muris eauclairensis*	Tick bite: *Ixodes scapularis*	United States	Unknown	3-14	12	None	
Human granulocytotropic anaplasmosis	*Anaplasma phagocytophilum*	Tick bite: *I. scapularis, I. ricinus, I. pacificus, I. persulcatus*	United States, Europe, Asia	4-8	3-14	Rare	None	–
Unnamed disease	*A. capra*	I. persulcatus	Northeastern China	Unknown	11-21	17	9	+

Contd.

Contd.

Neoehrlichiosis	*"Candidatus Neoehrlichia mikurensis"*	Tick bite: *I. ricinus, I. persulcatus, Haemaphysalis concinna*	Europe, China	≥8	11-75	10	None	
Scrub typhus	*Orientia tsutsugamushi*	Mite bite: *Leptotrombidium delicense,* others	Asia, Australia, Pacific and Indian Ocean islands	9-18	6-21	50	35	+++
Q fever	*Coxiella burnetii*	Inhalation of aerosols of infected parturition material (goats, sheep, cattle, cats, others), ingestion of infected milk or milk products	Worldwide except New Zealand, Antarctica	3-30	5-57	<1	None	–

Ans. B

80. All are possible mechanism of resistance to aminoglycosides except:

A. Drug-modifying enzymes

B. Methylation at ribosome binding site

C. Decreased permeation to target due to active efflux

D. Ribosomal protection proteins

Explanation:

Antibacterial Agent(s)	Major Target	Machanism(s) of Action	Mechanism(s) of Resistance
β-Lactams (penicillins, cephalosporins, monobactams, carbapenems	Cell wall sythesis	Bind cell wall cross-linking enzymes (PBPs, transpeptidases)	1. Drug inactivation by β-lactamases 2. Altered PBP targets 3. Reduced diffusion through porin channels
Glycopeptides and lipoglycopeptides (vancomycin, teicoplanin, telavancin, dalbavancin, oritavancin)	Cell wall synthesis	Block cell wall glycosyltransferases by binding D-Ala-D-Ala stem-peptide terminus Teicoplanin, telavancin, dalbavancin, and oritavancin: affect membrane function	1. Altered D-Ala-D-Ala target (D-Ala-D-Lac) 2. Increased D-Ala-D-Ala target binding at sites distant from cell wall synthesis enzymes
Bacitracin	Cell wall synthesis	Blocks lipid carrier of cell wall precursors	Active drug efflux
Fosfomycin	Cell wall synthesis	Blocks linkage of stem peptide to NAG by enoyltransferase	1. Target enzyme overexpression 2. Drug-modifying enzymes

Contd.

Contd.

Aminoglycosides (gentamicin, tobramycin, amikacin)	Protein synthesis	Bind 30S ribosomal subunit Block translocation of peptide chain Cause misreading of mRNA	1. Drug-modifying enzymes 2. Methylation at ribosome binding site 3. Decreased permeation to target due to active efflux
Tetracyclines (tetracycline, doxycycline, minocycline)	Protein synthesis	Bind 30S ribosomal subunit Inhibit peptide elongation	1. Active drug efflux 2. Ribosomal protection proteins
Tigecycline	Protein synthesis	Same as tetracyclines	Active drug efflux (pumps different from those affecting tetracyclines)
Macrolides (erythromycin clarithromycin, azithromycin) and the ketolide telithromycin	Protein synthesis	Bind 50S ribosomal subunit Block peptide chain exit	1. Methylation at ribosome binding site 2. Active drug efflux
Lincosamides (clindamycin)	Protein synthesis	B50S ribosomal subunit Block peptide bond formation	Methylation at ribosome binding site
Streptogramins (quinupristin, dalfopristin)	Protein synthesis	Same as macrolides	1. Same as macrolides 2. Drug-modifying enzymes
Chloramphenicol	Protein synthesis	Binds 50S ribosomal subunit Blocks aminoacyl tRNA positioning	Drug-modifying enzymes
Oxazolidinones (linezolid, tedizolid)	Protein synthesis	Bind 50S ribosomal subunit Inhibit initiation of peptide synthesis	1. Altered rRNA binding site 2. Methylation of ribosome binding site
Mupirocin	Protein synthesis	Blocks isoleucyl tRNA synthetase	1. Acquired resistant tRNA synthetase (drug bypass) 2. Altered native tRNA synthetase target
Sulfonamides (sulfadiazine, sulfisoxazole and sulfamethoxazole)	Folate synthesis	Inhibit dihydropteroate synthetase	Acquired resistant dihydropteroate synthetase (drug bypass)
Trimethoprim	Folate synthesis	Inhibits dihydrofolate reducatase	Acquired resistant dihydrofolate reductase (drug bypass)
Quinolones (norfloxacin, ciprofloxacin, ofloxacin, levofloxacin, moxifloxacin, gemifloxacin, delafloxacin)	DNA synthesis	Inhibit DNA gyrase and DNA topoisomerase IV Enzyme-DNA-drug complex: blocks DNA replication apparatus	1. Altered target(s) 2. Active efflux 3. Protection of target from drug 4. Drug-modifying enzyme (ciprofloxacin)
Rifamycins (rifampin, rifabutin, rifapentine)	RNA synthesis	Inhibit RNA polymerase	Altered target

Contd.

Contd.

Nitrofurantoin	Nucleic acid synthesis	Reduces reactive drug derivatives that damage DNA	Altered drug-activating enzymes
Metronidazole	Nucleic acid synthesis	Reduces reactive drug derivatives that damage DNA	1. Altered drug-activating enzyme 2. Acquired detoxifying enzymes 3. Active efflux
Polymyxins (polymyxin B and polymyxin E [colistin])	Cell membrane	Bind LPS and disrupt both outer and cytoplasmic membranes	Altered cell-membrane charge with reduced drug binding
Daptomycin	Cell membrane	Produces membrane channel and membrane leakage	Altered cell-membrane charge with reduced drug binding

Ans. D

81. A 50 year old male after a cosmetic surgery develops painful erythematous draining subcutaneous nodules. Th aetiology was found to be due to rapidly growing non tubercular mycobacterium. Which among the following is a slow growing mycobacterium?

A. M. abscesses B. M. fortuitum

C. Chelonae D. M. avium complex

Explanation:

- Mycobacteria other than those of the M. tuberculosis complex and M. leprae are referred to as nontuberculous or atypical mycobacteria and are ubiquitous in soil and water.
- NTM are broadly differentiated into rapidly and slowly growing forms(<7 days and ≥7 days, respectively). M. abscessus, M. fortuitum, and M. chelonae are examples of rapid growers; species such as M. avium and M. intracellulare (the M. avium complex, or MAC), M. kansasii, M. ulcerans, and M. marinum are slow growers.
- Rapidly growing NTM are associated with outbreaks of infection acquired via skin contamination from surgical instruments (especially in cosmetic surgery), injections, and other procedures. These infections are typically accompanied by painful, erythematous, draining SC nodules, usually without associated fever or systemic symptoms.

Ans. D

82. There is less safety information about all below drugs when used in pregnancy for asthma except:

A. LABA B. Theophylline

C. Antileukotrienes D. Anti IgE

Explanation:

- Approximately one-third of asthmatic patients who are pregnant improve during the course of a pregnancy, one third deteriorate, and one-third are unchanged. It is important to maintain good control of asthma as poor control may have adverse effects on fetal development.
- Adherence may be a problem as there is often concern about the effects of antiasthma medications on fetal development.

- Drugs that have been used for many years in asthma therapy have now been shown to be safe and without teratogenic potential.
- These drugs include **SABA, ICS, and theophylline**; there is less safety information about newer classes of drugs such as LABA, antileukotrienes, and anti-IgE. If an OCS is needed, it is better to use prednisone rather than prednisolone as it cannot be converted to the active prednisolone by fetal liver, thus protecting fetus from systemic effects of corticosteroid.
- There is no contraindication to breast-feeding when patients are using these drugs.

Ans. B

83. Mixed opioid/adrenergic action is seen with:

A. Meperidine
B. Tramadol
C. Morphine
D. Codeine

Explanation:

Table: Narcotic Analgesics: Usual doses and intervals			
Generic Name	**Parenteral Dose, mg**	**PO Dose, mg**	**Comments**
Codeine	30–60 q4h	30–60 q4h	Nausea common
Oxycodone	–	5–10 q4–6h	Usually available with acetaminophen or aspirin
Morphine	5 q4h	30 q4h	
Morphine sustained release	–	15-60 bid to tid	Oral slow-release preparation
Hydromorphone	1–2 q4h	2–4 q4h	Shorter acting than morphine sulfate
Levorphanol	2 q6–8h	4 q6–8h	Longer acting than morphine sulfate; absorbed well PO
Methadone	5–10 q6–8h	5–20 q6–8h	Due to long half-life, respiratory depression and sedation may persist after analgesic effect subsides; therapy should not be initiated with >40 mg/d, and dose escalation should be made no more frequently than every 3 days
Meperidine	50–100 q3–4h	300 q4h	Poorly absorbed PO; normeperidine is a toxic metabolite; routine use of this agent is not recommended
Butorphanol	–	1–2 q4h	Intranasal spray
Fentanyl	25–100 μg/h	–	72-h transdermal patch
Buprenorphine	5–20 μg/h		7-day tansdermal patch
Buprenorphine	0.3 q6-8h		Parenteral administration
Tramadol	–	50–100 q4-6h	Mixed opioid/adrenergic action

Ans. B

84. Food poisoning after eating mollusks is usually caused by:

A. Salmonella
B. Campylobacter
C. Shigella
D. Vibrio parahaemolyticus

Explanation:

Table: Bacterial food poisoning		
Incubation Period, Organism	**Symptoms**	**Common Food Sources**
1–6 h		
Staphylococcus aureus	Nausea, vomiting, diarrhea	Ham, poultry, potato or egg salad, mayonnaise, cream pastries
Bacillus cereus	Nausea, vomiting, diarrhea	Fried rice
8-16 h		
Clostridium perfringens	Abdominal cramps, diarrhea (vomiting rare)	Beef, poultry legumes, gravies
B. cereus	Abdominal cramps, diarrhea (vomiting rare)	Meats, vegetables, dried beans, cereals
>16 h		
Vibrio cholerae	Watery diarrhea	Shellfish, water
Enterotoxigenic *Escherichia coli*	Watery diarrhea	Salads, cheese, meats, water
Enterohemorrhagic *E.coli*	Bloody diarrhea	Ground beef, roast beef, salami, raw milk, raw vegetables, apple juice
Salmonella spp.	Inflammatory diarrhea	Beef, poultry, eggs, dairy products
Campylobacter jejuni	Inflammatory diarrhea	Poultry, raw milk
Shigella spp.	Dysentery	Potato or egg salad, lettuce, raw vegetables
Vibrio parahaemolyticus	Dysentery	Mollusks, crustaceans

Ans. D

85. All are first line antitubercular drugs except:

A. Streptomycin

B. Ethambutol

C. Isoniazid

D. Rifampicin

Explanation:

Table: Recommended dosage[a] for initial treatment of tuberculosis in adults and children		
Drug	**Daily Dose**	
	Adult	**Pediatric**
Isoniazid	5 mg/kg, max 300 mg	10 (7-15) mg/kg, max 300 mg
Rifampin	10 mg/kg, max 600 mg	15 (10-20) mg/kg, max 600 mg
Pyrazinamide	25 mg/kg, max 2 g	35 (30-40) mg/kg
Ethambutol[b]	15 mg/kg	20 (15-25) mg/kg

- Treatment regimen of choice for virtually all forms of drug susceptible TB in adults consists of a 2-month initial (intensive) phase of isoniazid, rifampin, pyrazinamide, and ethambutol followed by a 4-month continuation phase of isoniazid and rifampin.

Ans. A

86. Hyperinfection associated with enterococcal bacteremia in immunocompromised patients is:

A. Strongyloides

B. Ancylostoma

C. Schistosoma

D. Rodococcus

Explanation:

- Patients with enterococcal bacteremia usually have comorbidities and have been in the hospital for prolonged periods; they commonly have received several courses of antibiotics.
- Several studies indicate that the isolation of *E. faecium* from the blood may lead to worse outcomes and higher mortality rates than when other enterococcal species are isolated; this finding may be related to the higher prevalence of vancomycin and ampicillin resistance in *E. faecium* than in other enterococcal species, with consequent reduction of therapeutic options.
- In some cases (usually when gastrointestinal tract is the source), enterococcal bacteremia may be polymicrobial, with gram-negative organisms isolated at same time.
- Several cases have been documented in which enterococcal bacteremia was associated with Strongyloides stercoralis hyperinfection syndrome in immunocompromised patients.

Ans. A

87. All are true about hair examination except:

A. Brittle in Vitamin A deficiency
B. Color change in zinc deficiency
C. Corkscrew in Vitamin C deficiency
D. Dry in Vitamin E deficiency

Explanation:

Table: Physical examination data

Element	Notes
Body mass index (BMI)	BMI=weight in kg/(height in meters)^2 BMI <18.5 kg/m^2 proposed screen for malnutrition per National Institutes of Health guidelines. BMI $\leq$15 kg/m^2 or less is associated with increased mortality. Comparison with ideal body weight for stature can also be determined from reference tables. Note hydration status and edema at the time body weight is determined
Weight loss	Look for loss of muscle mass and subcutaneous fat Temporal and neck muscle wasting may be readily observed. Anthrompometrics inluding skin-folds and circumferences can be useful but require training to achieve reliability
Weakness/loss of strength	Decreased hand grip and leg extensor strength have been related to loss of muscle mass in malnurished states. Lower extremity weakness may be observed in thiamine deficiency
Peripheral edema	Peripheral edema may confound weight measurements and is often observed with reduced visceral proteins as well as inflammatory states. Edema may also be observed with thiamine deficiency
Hair examination	Hair findings are indicative of certain nutrient deficiences Loss: Portein, B_{12}, folate Brittle: Biotin Color change: Zinc Dry: Vitamins A and E Easy pluckability: Protein, biotin, zinc Coiled, corkscrew: Vitamins A and C Alopecia is common in severely malnourished persons Ask about excessive hair loss on pillow or when combing hair

Ans. A

88. Good evidence of benefit has emerged in patients undergoing elective gastrointestinal surgery and patients with traumatic brain injury with:

A. Polymer formulas with fibre
B. Standard polymeric formulas
C. Protein enriched formulas
D. Immune enhancing formulas

Explanation:

IMMUNE-ENHANCING FORMULAS

- In addition to providing macronutrients and conventional amounts of micronutrients, these products **(IEFs) contain large amounts of certain nutrients designed to favorably modulate immune response:** arginine and n-3 fatty acids especially, but also various combinations of glutamine, nucleotides, and antioxidants.
- It is difficult to evaluate IEFs because there are many different formulations on the market, and considerable heterogeneity in patient populations studied.
- Good evidence of benefit has emerged from clinical trials of perioperative IEFs in patients undergoing elective gastrointestinal surgery and patients with traumatic brain injury.
- EIFs have not yet demonstrated benefit in other kinds of critical illness

Ans. D

89. Late latent syphilis is defined as:

A. >6 months
B. >2 years
C. >1 years
D. >2 months

Explanation:

- Early latent syphilis is limited to the first year after infection, whereas late latent syphilis is defined as that of ≥1 year's duration (or of unknown duration).

Ans. C

90. Point mutation seen in:

A. FLT3
B. MDM2
C. MYC
D. CCND1

Explanation:

Table: Oncogenes commonly altered in human cancers

Oncogene	Function	Alteration in Cancer	Neoplasm
AKT1	Serine/threonine kinase	Point mutation	Skin
BRAF	Serine/threonine kinase	Point mutation	Melanoma, thyroid, colorectal
CCND1	Cell cycle progression	Amplification	Esophageal, head and neck
CTNNB1	Signal transduction	Point mutation	Colon, liver, uterine, melanoma
EGFR	Signal transduction	Point mutation	Lung
FLT3	Signal transduction	Point mutation	AML
IDH1	Chromatin modification	Point mutation	Glioma
MDM2	Inhibitor of p53	Amplification	Sarcoma, glioma
MDM4	Inhibitor of p53	Amplification	Breast
MYC	Transcription factor	Amplification	Prostate, ovarian, breast, liver, pancreatic
MYC1	Transcription factor	Amplification	Ovarian, bladder
MYCN	Transcription factor	Amplification	Neuroblastoma
PIK3CA	Phosphoinositol-3-kinase	Point mutation	Multiple caners
KRAS	GTPase	Point mutation	Pancreatic, colorectal, lung
NRAS	GTPase	Point mutation	Melanoma

Ans. A

91. Reactions frequently detected in blood banks are:

A. DHTR
B. TRALI
C. FNHTR
D. Allergic

Explanation:

- DHTRs are not completely preventable.
- These reactions occur in patients previously sensitized to RBC alloantigens who have a negative alloantibody screen due to low antibody levels.
- When the patient is transfused with antigen-positive blood, an anamnestic response results in the early production of alloantibody that binds donor RBCs.
- Alloantibody is detectable 1–2 weeks following the transfusion, and the post transfusion DAT may become positive due to circulating donor RBCs coated with antibody or complement.
- Transfused, alloantibody-coated erythrocytes are cleared by reticuloendothelial system.
- These reactions are detected most commonly in the blood bank when a subsequent patient sample reveals a positive alloantibody screen or a new alloantibody in a recently transfused recipient.
- No specific therapy is usually required, although additional RBC transfusions may be necessary.
- Delayed serologic transfusion reactions are similar to DHTR, as the DAT is positive and alloantibody is detected; however, RBC clearance is not increased

Ans. A

92. A 40 year old male who is rapidly desaturating due to covid-19 infection in nasal mask with 10 litres of oxygen. He was advised high flow nasal cannula (HFNC) for his hypoxemic respiratory failure. The range of oxygen delivery in HFNC is:

A. 5 to 50 L/minute
B. 5 to 60 L/minute
C. 5 to 70 L/minute
D. 5 to 100 L/minute

Explanation:

- Advantages of HFNC compared with conventional oxygen delivery systems include enhanced comfort, increased humidification of secretions to facilitate expectoration, washout of nasopharyngeal dead space to improve efficiency of ventilation, provision of a small positive airway pressure effect, and high flow rates to minimize the entrainment of room air for reliable delivery of fraction of inspired oxygen (FiO_2).
- Oxygen is delivered to the patient through wide bore nasal cannulae. We prefer to set the flow rate first, typically at 20 to 35 L/minute (range 5 to 60 L/minute). The FiO_2 (range 21 to 100 percent) is next set to target a desired peripheral oxygen saturation. Further adjustments of both settings can be made depending upon the initial clinical response. HFNC can be administered for prolonged periods (eg, days) and patients can be switched to conventional low-flow nasal cannulae once the flow rate reaches ≤20 L/minute and FiO_2 ≤50 percent.

Ans. B

93. A 65 year old male who is a known COPD patient was advised PPSV-23 pneumococcal vaccination. What is the duration of protection conferred by the vaccine?

A. 3 years
B. 5 years
C. 7 years
D. 10 years

Explanation:

- All persons ≥65 years old and those 2–64 years old who are at increased risk of pneumococcal disease should receive the 23-valent pneumococcal polysaccharide vaccine (PPSV23), which contains capsular polysaccharide from the 23 most prevalent serotypes of S. pneumoniae. – Persons >2 years old with continuing increased risk should be revaccinated every 5 years. – Persons whose only indication for vaccination is an age of ≥65 years do not need to be revaccinated.
- The efficacy of PPSV23 is controversial; it appears to be effective against invasive pneumococcal disease but less effective or ineffective against non-bacteremic pneumococcal pneumonia.
- The duration of protection conferred by PPSV23 is ~5 years.
- The poor response of infants and young children to pneumococcal polysaccharide vaccines prompted the development of pneumococcal conjugate vaccines. In the United States, the current recommendation is for infants to be routinely vaccinated with the conjugate vaccine PCV13, which contains the 13 serotypes most associated with disease. – Immunocompromised children and adults and all adults ≥65 years of age should receive PCV13 prior to receiving PPSV23. – Pneumococcal conjugate vaccines are highly effective at providing protection against vaccine-serotype invasive pneumococcal disease, pneumonia, otitis media, nasopharyngeal colonization, and all-cause mortality. – In the United States, there has been a >90% reduction in vaccine-serotype invasive pneumococcal disease among the whole population, including indirect protection of unvaccinated adults.

Ans. B

94. **Most common cause of Nontraumatic chylothorax is:**

A. Malignancy
B. Trauma
C. Developmental anomaly
D. Necrotizing infection

Explanation:

- Chylothorax refers to the presence of chyle in the pleural space. Malignancy (classically lymphoma) is the leading cause of nontraumatic chylothorax while inadvertent surgical injury to the thoracic duct is the major cause of traumatic chylothorax.
- The mechanisms involved include obstruction, direct involvement or tears, anatomic anomaly, or conduction deficit of the thoracic duct as well as excessive lymph production or transfer of chyle across the diaphragm from the abdomen.
- The initial diagnostic test for patients suspected to have chylothorax is analysis of pleural fluid for triglyceride and cholesterol levels.
- Pleural fluid is classically exudative with a high lymphocyte count (>70 percent), a normal glucose level, a low LDH, and a cholesterol level <200 mg/dL (<5.18 mmol/L).

Ans. A

95. **All are recommendations for respiratory support in septic shock patients except:**

A. A target tidal volume of 12 mL/kg of predicted body weight is recommended in sepsis-induced ARDS
B. Higher PEEP rather than lower PEEP is used in moderate to severe sepsis-induced ARDS
C. In severe ARDS (PaO2/FIO2, <150 mmHg), prone positioning is recommended
D. Routine use of a pulmonary artery catheter is not recommended

Explanation:

Table: Elements of care in sepsis and septic shock: Recommendations adapted from international consensus guidelines
Resuscitation
• Sepsis and septic shock constitute an emergency, and treatment should begin right away. • Resuscitation with IV crystalloid fluid (30 ml/kg) should begin within the first 3 hours. • Saline or balanced crystalloids are suggested for resuscitation. • If the clinical examination does not clearly identify the diagnosis, hemodynamic assessments (e.g., with focused cardiac ultrasound) can be considered. • In patients with elevated serum lactate levels, resuscitation should be guided towards normalizing these levels when possible. • In patients with septic shock requiring vasopressors, the recommended target mean arterial pressure in 65 mm Hg. • Hydroxyethyl starches and gelatins are not recommended. • Norepinephrine is recommended as the first choice vasopressor. • Vasopressin should be used with the intent of reducing the norepinephrine dose. • The use of dopamine should be avoided except in specific situations, e.g., in the those patients at highest risk of tacharrhythmias or relative bradycardia. • Dobutamine use is suggested when patients show persistent evidence of hypoperfusion despite adequate fluid loading and use of vasopressors. • Red blood cell transfusion is recommended only when the hemoglobin concentration decreases to <70 g/dl in the absence of acute myocardial infarction, severe hypoxemia, or acute hemorrhage.
Infection Control
• So long as no substantial delay is incurred, appropriate samples for microbiologic cultures should be obtained before antimicrobial therapy is started. • IV antibiotics should be initiated as soon as possible (within 1 hour); specifically, empirical broad-spectrum therapy should be used to cover all likely pathogens. • Antibiotic therapy should be narrowed once pathogens are identified and their sensitivities determined and/or once clinical improvement is evident. • If needed, source control should be undertaken as soon as is medically and logistically possible. • Daily assessment for de-esclation of antimicrobial therapy should be conducted.
Respiratory Support
• A target tidal volume of 6 ml/kg of predicted body weight (compared with 12 ml/kg in adult patients) is recommended in sepsis-induced ARDS. • A higher PEEP rather than a lower PEEP is used in moderate to severe sepsis-induced ARDS. • In severe ARDS (PaO_2/FIO_2, <150 mm Hg), prone positioning is recommended, and recruitment maneuvers and/or neuromuscular blocking agents for ≤ 48 hours are suggested. • A conservative fluid strategy should be used in sepsis-induced ARDS if there is no evidence of tissue hypoperfusion. • Routine use of a pulmonary artery catheter is not recommended. • Spontaneous breathing trials should be used in mechanically ventilated patients who are ready for earning.
General Supportive Care
• Patients requiring a vasopressor should have an arterial catheter placed as soon as is practical. • Hydrocortisone is not suggested in septic shock if adequate fluids and vasopressor therapy can restore hemodynamic stability. • Continuous or intermittent sedation should be minimized in mechanically ventilated sepsis patients, with titration targets used whenever possible. • A protocol-based approach to blood glucose management should be used in ICU patients with sepsis, with insulin dosing initiated when two consecutive blood glucose level are > 180 mg/dl. • Continuous or intermittent renal replacement therapy should be used in patients with sepsis and acute kidney injury. • Pharmacologic prophylaxis (unfractionated heparin or low-molecular-weight heparin) against venous thromboembolism should be used in the absence of contraindications. • Stress ulcer prophylaxis should be given to patients with risk factors for gastrointestinal bleeding. • The goals of care and prognosis should be discussed with patients and their families.

Ans. A

96. Spurling sign is positive in:

A. Traumatic spine injury
B. Cervical disk disease
C. Synovitis of the atlantoaxial joint
D. Cauda equina syndrome

Explanation:

- Herniated cervical disks are responsible for ~25% of cervical radiculopathies.
- **Extension and lateral rotation of the neck narrow the ipsilateral intervertebral foramen and may reproduce radicular symptoms (Spurling's sign).**
- In young adults, acute nerve root compression from a ruptured cervical disk is often due to trauma. Cervical disc herniation are usually posterolateral near the lateral recess.

Ans. B

97. Hyperpyrexia is:

A. More than 39°C
B. More than 40°C
C. More than 41°C
D. More than 41.5°C

Explanation:

- A fever of >41.5°C (>106.7°F) is called *hyperpyrexia*.
- This extraordinarily high fever can develop in patients with severe infections but most commonly occurs in patients with central nervous system (CNS) hemorrhages.
- In the pre antibiotic era, fever due to a variety of infectious diseases rarely exceeded 106°F, and there has been speculation that this natural "thermal ceiling" is mediated by neuropeptides functioning as central antipyretics

Ans. D

98. All can cause cancer except:

A. Silica
B. Asbestos
C. Coal dust
D. Beryllium

Explanation:

Table: Categories of occupational exposure and associated respiratory conditions

Occupational Exposures	Nature of Respiratory Responses	Comment
Inorganic Dusts		
Asbestos: Mining, processing, construction, ship repair	Fibrosis (asbestosis), pleural disease, cancer, mesothelioma	Virtually all new mining and construction with asbestos done in developing countries
Silica: Mining, stone cutting, sandblasting, quarrying	Fibrosis (silicosis), progressive massive fibrosis (PMF), cancer, tuberculosis, chronic obstructive pulmonary disease (COPD)	Improved protection in United States; persistent risk in developing countries
Coal dust: Mining	Fibrosis (coal worker's pneumoconiosis), PMF, COPD	Risk persists in certain areas of United States, increasing in countries where new mines open
Beryllium: Processing alloys for high-tech industries	Acute pneumonitis (rare), chronic granulomatous disease, lung cancer (high suspect)	Risk in high-tech industries persists

Contd.

Contd.

Other metals: Aluminium, chromium, cobalt, nickel, titanium, tungsten carbide, or 'hard metal' (contains cobalt)	Wide variety of conditions from acute pneumonitis to lung cancer and asthma	New diseases appear with new process development
Organic Dusts		
Cotton dust: Milling, processing	Byssinosis (an asthma-like syndrome), chronic bronchitis, COPD	Increasing risk in developing countries with drop in United States as job shift overseas
Grain dust: Elevator agents, dock workers milling bakers	Asthma, chronic bronchitis, COPD	Risk shifting more to migrant labor pool
Other agricultural dusts: Fungal spores, vegetable products, insect fragments, animal dander, bird and rodent feces, endotoxins, microorganisms, pollens	Hypersensitivity pneumonitis (farmers' lung), asthma, chronic bronchitis	Important in migrant labor pool but also resulting from in-home exposures
Toxic chemicals: Wide variety of industries; see Table 283-2	Asthma, chronic bronchitis, COPD, hypersensitivity pneumonitis, pneumoconiosis and cancer	Reduced risk with recognized hazards; increasing risk for developing countries where controlled labor practices are less stringent
Other Environmental Agents		
Uranium and radon daughters, secondhand tobacco smoke, polycyclic aromatic hydrocarbons (PAHs), biomass smoke, diesel exhaust, welding fumes, wood finishing	Occupational exposures estimated to contribute to up to 10% of all lung cancers; chronic bronchitis, COPD and fibrosis	In-home exposures important; in developing countries, biomass smoke is a major risk factor for COPD among women in these countries

Ans. C

99. A 40 year old male presents with non-productive cough and sub sternal discomfort. Sputum examination reveals charcot leyden crystals. Chest X-ray shows migratory, fleeting opacities. Which among the following does not cause this disease?

A. Ascariasis lumbricoides
B. Ancylostoma duodenale
C. Necator americanis
D. Paragonimus

Explanation:

- Three types of helminths, *Ascaris (A. lumbricoides*, *A. suum*), hookworms (*Ancylostoma duodenale*, *Necator americanus*), and *Strongyloides stercoralis*, have life cycles in which infecting larvae reach the lungs via the bloodstream, penetrate into alveoli, mature, and ascend the airways before descending the alimentary tract into the small bowel.
- The syndrome of transient pulmonary radiographic opacities and peripheral blood eosinophilia was originally described by Löffler; *Ascaris* infection acquired from the use of contaminated human night-soil as fertilizer was determined to be the cause. Subsequent investigations have confirmed that *Ascaris* is the most common cause of Löffler syndrome worldwide.

Ans. D

100. Orange discoloration of body fluids is seen with:

A. Vancomycin
B. Rifampin
C. Daptomycin
D. Fluoroquinolones

Explanation:

Table: Common adverse reactions to antibacterial agents		
Antibacterial(s)	**Potential Adverse Effects**	**Comments**
β-Lactams	Hypersensitivity reactions	Ranges from rash to anaphylaxis. Cross-reactivity among β-lactams is related to chemical structure and side chain similarity
	Neurotoxicity	More commonly described with cefepime and imipenem, but likely a class effects. Risk is increased in patients with history of seizures, renal impairment and advanced age
	Neutropenia/hematologic reactions	May be related to high doses and prolonged duration
Vancomycin	Nephrotoxicity	Risk increases with vancomycin trough levels > 20 μg/ml or concomitant administration with other potentially nephrotoxic agents. The effect is usually reversible
	"Red man syndrome"	Can be managed with a slower vancomycin infusion and pretreatment with antihistamine
Telavancin	QT prolongation	
	Interference with coagulation tests	May falsely affect INR, aPTT, apt Perform these tests before the next dose of telavancin (when serum drug levels are at their nadir)
	Taste disturbances	
	Nephrotoxicity	
Oritavancin	Interference with coagulation tests	May falsely affect INR, PT, aPTT. Perform these tests at least 24 hours after the dose is administered
	Gastrointestinal distress	
Dalbavancin	Gastrointestinal distress	
Deptomycin	Myopathy	Monitor CPK levels during therapy. Rhabdomyolysis has been reported but appears to be rare
	Eosinophilic pneumonia	
Aminoglycosides	Nephrotoxicity	Associated with prolonged use; usually reversible
	Ototoxicity	Can cause both vestibular and cochlear toxicity. Ototoxicity may be irreversible
Fluoroquinolones	QT_c prolongation	Moxifloxacin appears more likely than other quinolones to exert this effect. Risk of arrhythmia increases when these drugs are given concomitantly with other QT_c-prolonging agents
	Tendinitis	Risk is greater among the elderly and patients receiving steroids
	Dysglycemia	
	Exacerbation of myasthenia gravis	
Rifampin	Hepatotoxicity	Risk is greater when drug is given with other antituberculosis agents. When rifampin is given alone, LFT values may be transiently elevated without symptoms
	Orange discoloration of body fluids	
Tetracyclines and glycylcylines	Photosensitivity	
	Gastrointestinal distress	High incidence of diarrhea, nausea, vomiting
Macrolides	Gastrointestinal distress	Erythromycin is occasionally used as a therapeutic agent for some gastric motility disorders
	QT_c prolongation	Azithromycin use is associated with an increased risk of death from cardiovascular causes among patients at high baseline risk
Metronidazole	Peripheral neuropathy	Associated with prlonged use
Clindamycin	Diarrhea and pseudomembranous colitis	
Linezolid, tedizolid	Myelosuppression	Associated with prolonged use
	Optic and peripheral neuropathy	Associated with prolonged use
	Lactic acidosis	
TMP-SMX	Hypersensitivity reactions	Allergy usually associated with sulfonamide moiety
	Nephrotoxicity	Associated with high doses
	Hematologic effects	Associated with prolonged use

Contd.

Contd.

Nitrofurantoin	Pneumonitis and other pulmonary reactions	Associated with prolonged use
	Peripheral neuropathy	Associated with accumulation of nitrofurantoin in renal failure. Avoid use in renal impairment
Fosfomycin	Gastrointestinal effects	
Polymyxins	Nephrotoxicity	Associated with high dose
	Neurotoxicity	Neuromuscular blockade and muscle weakness are well described and usually reversible
Quinupristin-dalfopristin	Arthralgias and mylgias	
Chloramphenicol	Bone marrow suppression	Aplastic anemia or hematopoietic toxicity

Ans. B

101. Babes nodules and Negri body are seen in infection with:

A. Rabies
B. Rubella
C. Japanese encephalitis
D. Mumps

Explanation:

- Pathologic studies show mild inflammatory changes in the CNS in rabies, with mononuclear inflammatory infiltration in the leptomeninges, perivascular regions, and parenchyma, including microglial nodules called *Babes nodules*.
- Degenerative neuronal changes usually are not prominent, and there is little evidence of neuronal death; neuronophagia is observed occasionally.
- Pathologic changes are surprisingly mild in light of the clinical severity and fatal outcome of the disease.
- Most characteristic pathologic finding in rabies is the *Negri body.*
- Negri bodies are eosinophilic cytoplasmic inclusions in brain neurons that are composed of rabies virus proteins and viral RNA.
- These inclusions occur in a minority of infected neurons, are commonly observed in Purkinje cells of the cerebellum and in pyramidal neurons of the hippocampus, and are less frequently seen in cortical and brainstem neurons.
- Negri bodies are not observed in all cases of rabies.
- Lack of prominent degenerative neuronal changes has led to the concept that neuronal dysfunction—rather than neuronal death—is responsible for clinical disease in rabies.
- Basis for behavioral changes, including aggressive behavior of rabid animals, is not well understood but may be related to infection of serotonergic neurons in brainstem.

Ans. A

102. All the following act on RAF except:

A. Vemurafenib
B. Dabrafenib
C. Sorafenib
D. Trametinib

Explanation:

- *BRAF* V600E mutation has been detected in a notable fraction of melanomas, thyroid tumors, and hairy cell leukemia and preclinical models supported concept that *BRAF* V600E drives oncogenic signaling in these tumors.
- Vemurafenib and dabrafenib, with selective capacity to inhibit *BRAF* V600E serine kinase activity, were each shown to cause noteworthy responses in patients with *BRAF* V600E–mutated melanomas, although early relapse occurred in many patients treated with the drugs as single agents.

- Trametinib, acting downstream of *BRAF* V600E by directly inhibiting the MEK serine kinase by a non-ATP binding site mechanism, also displayed noteworthy responses in *BRAF* V600E–mutated melanomas, and the combination of trametinib and dabrafenib is even more active, by targeting *BRAF* V600E–driven pathway at two points in the pathway leading to gene activation.

Ans. D

103. Person-to-person spread (direct or indirect) is the primary transmission route for:

A. EPEC
B. EIEC
C. ETEC
D. EAEC

Explanation:

- Contaminated food and water are the primary transmission vehicles for ETEC, STEC/EHEC/ST-EAEC, EIEC, and EAEC, whereas person-to-person spread (direct or indirect) is the primary transmission route for EPEC and a secondary transmission route for STEC/EHEC/ ST-EAEC.
- Gastric acidity confers some protection against infection; therefore, persons with decreased stomach acid levels are especially susceptible.
- Humans are the major reservoir for such strains (except for STEC/EHEC, for which bovines are the main carriers); host range appears to be dictated by species-specific attachment factors.
- Although there is some overlap, each pathotype possesses a distinctive combination of virulence traits that results in a pathotype-specific pathogenic mechanism.
- With rare exceptions, these strains are largely incapable of causing disease outside the intestinal tract.
- Whereas disease due to STEC/EHEC/ST-EAEC occurs primarily in high-income countries, disease due to ETEC, EPEC, and EIEC occurs primarily in low- and middle-income countries in Asia, Africa, and Latin America, and disease due to EAEC occurs globally.

Ans. A

104. All salmonellae are motile except:

A. S.enterica
B. S.Typhimurium
C. S.bongori
D. S.gallinarum pullorum

Explanation:

- Salmonellae are gram-negative, non-spore-forming, facultatively anaerobic bacilli that measure 2–3 μm by 0.4–0.6 μm.
- Initial identification of salmonellae in the clinical microbiology laboratory is based on growth characteristics.
- Salmonellae, like other Enterobacteriaceae, produce acid on glucose fermentation, reduce nitrates, and do not produce cytochrome oxidase.
- In addition, all salmonellae except *Salmonella* Gallinarum-Pullorum are motile by means of peritrichous flagella, and all but *S.* Typhi produce gas (H2S) on sugar fermentation.
- Notably, only 1% of clinical isolates ferment lactose; a high level of suspicion must be maintained to detect these rare clinical lactose-fermenting isolates.

Ans. D

105. TLR localized to plasma membrane are all except:

A. TLR 3
B. TLR4
C. TLR5
D. TLR6

Explanation:

Table: Pattern recognition receptors (PRRs) and their ligands			
PRRs	**Localization**	**Ligand**	**Origin of the Ligand**
TLR			
• TLR1	Plasma membrane	Triacyl lipoprotein	Bacteria
• TLR2	Plasma membrane	Lipoprotein	Bacteria, viruses, parasite, self
• TLR3	Endolysosome	dsRNA	Virus
• TLR4	Plasma membrane	LPS	Bacteria, viruses, self
• TLR5	Plasma membrane	Flagellin	Bacteria
• TLR6	Plasma membrane	Diacyl lipoprotein	Bacteria, viruses
• TLR (human TLR8)	Endolysosome	ssRNA	Virus, bacteria, self
• TLR9	Endolysosome	CpG-DNA	Virus, bacteria, protozoa, self
• TLR10	Endolysosome	Unknown	Unknown
• TLR11	Plasma membrane	Profilin-like molecule	Protozoa
RLR			
• RIG-I	Cytoplasm	Short dsRNA, triphosphate dsRNA	RNA viruses, DNA virus
• MDA5	Cytoplasm	Long dsRNA	RNA viruses (picomaviridae)
• LPP2	Cytoplasm	Unknown	RNA viruses
NLR			
• NOD1	Cytoplasm	IE-DAP	Bacteria
• NOD2	Cytoplasm	MDP	Bacteria
CLR			
• Dectin-1	Plasma membrane	β^2-Glucan	Fungi
• Dectin-2	Plasma membrane	β^2-Glucan	Fungi
• MINCLE	Plasma membrane	SAP130	Self, fungi

Ans. A

106. C-X-C chemokines are similar to:

A. IL-4
B. IL-6
C. IL-8
D. IL-2

Explanation:

Table: Cytokine families grouped by structural similarity	
Hematopoietins	IL-2, IL-3, IL-4, IL-5, IL-6, IL-7, IL-9, IL-11, IL-12, IL-15, IL-16, IL-17, IL-21, IL-23, EPO, LIF, GM-CSF, G-CSF, OSM, CNTF, GH and TPO TNF-α, LT-α, LT-β, CD40L, CD30L, CD27L, 4-1BBL, OX40, OPG and FasL
IL-1	IL-1α, IL-1β, IL-1ra, IL-18, bFGF, aFGF and ECGF
PDGF	PDGF A, PDGF B and M-CSF
TGF-β	TGF-β and BMPs (1,2, 4 etc.)
C-X-C chemokines	IL-8, Gro-α/β/γ, NAP-2, ENA 78, GCP-2, PF4, CTAP-3, MIG and IP-10
C-C chemokines	MCP-1, MCP-2, MCP-3, MIP-1α, MIP-1β, RANTES

Ans. C

107. Clinical efficacy of triptans appears to be related more to:

A. Time to peak plasma level
B. Potency
C. Half-life
D. Bioavailability

Explanation:

- Each drug in the triptan class has similar pharmacologic properties but varies slightly in terms of clinical efficacy.
- Rizatriptan and eletriptan are, on a population basis, the most efficacious of the triptans currently available in the United States.
- Sumatriptan and zolmitriptan have similar rates of efficacy as well as time to onset, with an advantage of having multiple formulations, whereas almotriptan has a similar rate of efficacy to sumatriptan and is better tolerated, and frovatriptan and naratriptan are somewhat slower in onset and are also well tolerated.
- Clinical efficacy appears to be related more to the *t*max (time to peak plasma level) than to the potency, half-life, or bioavailability.
- This observation is consistent with a large body of data indicating that faster-acting analgesics are more effective than slower-acting agents.

Ans. A

108. Normal cell replication is arrested by all except:

A. IL-8
B. Rb
C. p16
D. p53

Explanation:

- Loss of replicative senescence: Normal cells stop dividing in vitro after 25–50 population doublings.
- **Arrest is mediated by the Rb, p16INK4a, and p53 pathways.**
- While most cells remain arrested, genetic and epigenetic changes in a subset of cells allows further replication leading to telomere loss, with crisis leading to death of many cells.
- Cells that survive often harbor gross chromosomal abnormalities and the ability to continue to proliferate.
- These cells express telomerase which maintains telomeres and is important for ongoing growth of these cells.
- Relevance to human in vivo cancer remains uncertain. Many human cancers express telomerase.

Ans. A

109. Anakinra is a:

A. Recombinant interleukin-1 (IL-1) receptor antagonist
B. Recombinant interleukin-2 (IL-2) receptor antagonist
C. Recombinant interleukin-3 (IL-3) receptor antagonist
D. Recombinant interleukin-4 (IL-4) receptor antagonist

Explanation:

- Anakinra is a recombinant interleukin-1 (IL-1) receptor antagonist that functions to block the biologic activity of naturally occurring IL-1.

Ans. A

110. Marker of mature B cells is:

A. IgG
B. IgM
C. IgA
D. IgD

Explanation:

Table: Physical, chemical and biologic properties of human immunoglobulins

Property	IgG	IgA	IgM	IgD	IgE
Usual molecular form	Monomer	Monomer, dimer	Pentamer, hexamer	Monomer	Monomer
Other chains	None	J chain, SC	J chain	None	None
Subclasses	G1, G2, G3, G4	A1, A2	None	None	None
Heavy chain allotypes	Gm (=30)	No A1, A2m (2)	None	None	None
Molecular mass, kDa	150	160, 400	950, 1150	175	190
Serum level in average adult, mg/ml	9.5-12.5	1.5-2.6	0.7-1.7	0.04	0.0003
Percentage of total serum Ig	75-85	7-15	5-10	0.3	0.019
Serum half-life, days	23	6	5	3	2.5
Synthesis rate, mg/kg per day	33	65	7	0.4	0.016
Antibody valence	2	2, 4	10,12	2	2
Classical complement activation	+(G1, 2?, 3)	–	++	–	–
Alternate complement activation	+(G4)	+	–	+	–
Binding cells via Fc	Macrophages, neutrophils, large granular lymphocytes	Lymphocytes	Lymphocytes	None	Mast cells, basophils, B cells
Biologic properties	Placental transfer, secondary Ab for most antipathogen responses	Secretory immunoglobulin	Primary Ab responses	Marker for mature B cells	Allergy, antiparasite responses

Ans. D

111. Most common organ affected in amyloidosis:

A. Heart
B. Kidney
C. Liver
D. Spleen

Explanation:

- Kidneys are the most common organ affected in amyloidosis (70-80 percent).
- Heart is affected next to kidneys (50-60 percent) and cardiac involvement is the leading cause of death in amyloidosis.
- Macroglossia which is a pathognomonic sign seen only in 10 percent of the patients.
- Splenomegaly also frequently seen.

Ans. B

112. Tuberculosis can cause which of the following?

A. Constrictive pericarditis
B. Subacute effusive constrictive pericarditis
C. Both A and B
D. None of the above

Explanation:

- Tuberculosis can cause pericardial effusion, constrictive pericarditis, and subacute effusive constrictive pericarditis.
- In developing nations tuberculosis is most common cause of chronic constrictive pericarditis.
- Clinical picture is that of chronic, systemic disease in a patient with pericardial effusion with clinical features of fever, weight loss, chest pain. ANTI tubercular treatment along with steroids are given.

Ans. C

113. Keshan's disease occurs due to deficiency of:

A. Carnitine
B. Magnesium
C. Selenium
D. Thiamine

Explanation:

- Keshan's disease is due to selenium deficiency causing dilated cardiomyopathy.
- It has been recently linked to coxsackie B virus. Lack of selenium causes more virulent strain of coxsackie B virus becoming dominant.
- Other manifestations in keshan's disease are cancers, HTN, stroke.
- Treated with selenium and vitamin E.
- Other deficiency conditions causing dilated cardiomyopathy are beriberi (thiamine def.).
- Carnitine deficiency, calcium deficiency, phosphate and magnesium deficiency.

Ans. C

114. All are true about FUO except:

A. Exercise-induced hyperthermia is characterized by an elevated CRP level or ESR
B. Factitious fever is fever artificially induced by the patient
C. In fraudulent fever, the patient is normothermic but manipulates the thermometer
D. Clue to fraudulent fever is dissociation between pulse rate and temperature

Explanation:

- *Exercise-induced hyperthermia* is characterized by an elevated body temperature that is associated with moderate to strenuous exercise lasting from half an hour up to several hours without an increase in CRP level or ESR; typically these patients sweat during temperature elevation.
- *Factitious fever* (fever artificially induced by patient—for example, by IV injection of contaminated water) should be considered in all patients but is more common among young women in health care professions.
- In *fraudulent fever*, the patient is normothermic but manipulates the thermometer. Simultaneous measurements at different body sites (rectum, ear, mouth) should rapidly identify this diagnosis. Another clue to fraudulent fever is a dissociation between pulse rate and temperature.

Ans. A

115. Most common infectious disease with FUO in elderly:

A. Tuberculosis
B. Pneumonia
C. Meningitis
D. Pharyngitis

Explanation:

- Tuberculosis is the most common infectious disease associated with FUO in elderly patients, occurring much more often than in younger patients.

Ans. A

116. 65 year old gentleman, known case of TB came to the hospital with complaints of confusion and 1 episode of seizure, nausea and abdominal pain. On patient had no signs of dehydration or volume overload. Routine investigations revealed sodium - 120meq/L. Potassium levels was elevated. 8 am serum cortisol was low. What is the treatment for this Euvolemic hyponatremia?

A. Desmopressin nasal spray
B. Tolvaptan
C. Demeclocyline
D. IV Hydrocortisone

Explanation:

- Euvolemic hyonatremia is due to expansion of total body water caused by excessive intake associated with failure to dilute the urine. It might be due to two causes – (1) cortisol deficiency, corrected by antiemetics or cortisol, (2) SIADH. Here since 8 am cortisol was low, euvolemic hyponatremia is due to cortisol deficiency.

Ans. D

117. Group A streptococcus causes all except:

A. Pharyngitis
B. Impetigo
C. Toxic shock syndrome
D. Meningitis

Explanation:

Table: Classification of streptococci

Lancefield Group	Representative Species	Hemolytic Pattern	Typical Infections
A	*S. pyogenes*	β	Pharyngitis, impetigo, cellulitis, scarlet fever
B	*S. agalactiae*	β	Neonatal sepsis and meningitis, puerperal infection, urinary tract infection, diabetic ulcer infection, endocarditis
C, G	*S. dysgalactiae subsp. equisimilis*	β	Cellulitis, bacteremia, endocarditis
D	Enterococci[a]: *E. faecalis, E. faecium*	Usually nonhemolytic	Urinary tract infection, nosocomial bacteremia, endocarditis
	Nonenterococci: S. *gallolyticus* (formerly *s. bovis)*	Usually nonhemolytic	Bacteremia, endocarditis
Variable or nongroupable	Viridans streptococci: *S. sanguis, S. mitis*	α	Endocarditis, dental abscess, brain abscess
	Intermedius or milleri group: *S. intermedius, S. anginosus, S. constellatus*	Variable	Brain abscess, visceral abscess
	Anaerobic streptococci[b]. *Peptostreptococcus magnus*	Usually nonhemolytic	Sinusitis, pneumonia, empyema, brain abscess, liver abscess

Ans. D

118. Botulinum toxin serotype causing most severe syndrome:

A. A
B. B
C. C
D. D

Explanation:

- All botulinum toxin serotypes have been demonstrated to cause botulism in nonhuman primates. Human cases associated with serotypes A, B, E and F are reported each year.
- **Serotype A produces most severe syndrome,** with the greatest proportion of patients requiring mechanical ventilation.
- **Serotype B causes milder disease.**
- Serotype E, most often associated with foods of aquatic origin (e.g., uneviscerated fish and seal oil), produces a syndrome of variable severity.
- Illnesses caused by toxin serotype F are infrequent and are characterized by rapid progression to quadriplegia and respiratory failure but also by relatively rapid recovery.

Ans. A

119. All are major components of innate immunity except:

A. TLRs
B. Macrophages
C. B lymphocytes
D. Cytokines

Explanation:

Table: Major components of the innate immune system	
Pattern recognition receptors (PRRs)	Toll-like receptors (TLRs), C-type lectin receptors (CLRs), retinoic acid-inducible gene (RIG)-1-like receptors (RLRs) and NOD-like receptors (NLRs)
Antimicrobial peptides	α-Defensins, β-defensins, cathelin, protegrin, granulysin, histatin, secretory leukoprotease inhibitor and probiotics
Cell	Macrophages, dendritic cells, NK cells, NK-T cells, neutrophils, eosinophils, mast cells, basophils and epithelial cells
Complement components	Classic and alternative complement pathway, and proteins that bind complement components
Cytokines	Autocrine, paracrine, endocrine cytokines that mediate host defense and inflammation, as well as recruit, direct, and regulate adaptive immune responses

Ans. C

120. Defective DNA Repair is seen in all except:

A. Fanconi anemia
B. Bloom syndrome
C. Kostmann syndrome
D. Ataxia telangiectasia

Explanation:

- Congenital neutropenia (Kostmann syndrome), due to mutations in the genes encoding the granulocyte colony-stimulating factor receptor and neutrophil elastase, is another disorder that may evolve into AML.
- Defective DNA repair (e.g., Fanconi anemia, Bloom syndrome, and ataxia-telangiectasia) are also associated with AML.

Ans. C

121. Sodoku is caused by:

A. Borrelia group
B. Spirillum minus
C. Trypanosoma
D. Ehrlichia

Explanation:

Disease	Etiology	Description	Group Affected/ Epidemiologic Factors	Clinical Syndrome
Rat-bite fever (sodoku)	*Spirillum minus*	Eschar at bite site; then blotchy violaceous or red-brown rash involving trunk and extremities	Rat bite; primarily found in Asia; rare in U.S.	Regional adeno-pathy; recurrent fevers if untreated
Relapsing fever	*Borrelia species*	Central rash at end of febrile episode; petechiae in some cases	Exposure to ticks or body lice	Recurrent fever, headache, myalgias, hepatosplenomegaly
Erythema margi-natum (rheumatic fever)	Group A *Streptococcus*	Erythematous annular papules and plaques occurring as polycyclic lesions in waves over trunk, proximal extremities; evolving and resolving within hours	Patients with rheumatic fever	Pharyngitis preceding polyarthritis, carditis, subcutaneous nodules, chorea

Ans. B

122. Ratio of drug concentration 300% in breast milk relative to serum is found with:

A. Lamotrigine
B. Valproate
C. Levetirecetam
D. Phenytoin

Explanation:

- Antiepileptic medications are excreted into breast milk to a variable degree. The ratio of drug concentration in breast milk relative to serum ranges from ~5% (valproic acid) to 300% (levetiracetam).
- Given the overall benefits of breast-feeding and the lack of evidence for long-term harm to the infant by being exposed to antiepileptic drugs, mother with epilepsy can be encouraged to breast-feed. This should be reconsidered, however, if there is any evidence of drug effects on the infant such as lethargy or poor feeding.

Ans. C

123. Not a component of HLA Class III is:

A. Complement C2
B. HSP 70
C. Beta 2 microglobulin
D. 21 alpha hydroxylase

Explanation:

- *HLA class III region* is a name given to a cluster of genes between the class I and class II complexes, which includes genes for the two closely related cytokines tumor necrosis factor (TNF-α) and lymphotoxin (TNF-α); the complement components C2, C4 and Bf; heat shock protein (HSP) 70; and the enzyme 21-hydroxylase.

Ans. C

124. Hepatic cytochrome P450 not inhibited by all below PPIs except:

A. Lansoprazole
B. Rabeprazole
C. Pantoprazole
D. Esomeprazole

Explanation:

- Hepatic cytochrome P450 can be inhibited by the earlier PPIs (omeprazole, lansoprazole). Rabeprazole, pantoprazole, and esomeprazole do not appear to interact significantly with drugs metabolized by the cytochrome P450 system.
- Overall clinical significance of this observation is not definitely established. Caution should be taken when using theophylline, warfarin, diazepam, atazanavir, and phenytoin concomitantly with PPIs.

Ans. A

125. All autoantigen autoimmune disease combination correct except:

A. Ri protein in Paraneoplastic cerebellar degeneration
B. βIV spectrin in Lower motor neuron syndrome
C. Synaptotagmin in Lambert-Eaton myasthenic syndrome
D. Voltage-gated calcium channels in Lambert-Eaton myasthenic syndrome

Explanation:

Table: Recombinant or purified autoantigens recognized by autoantibodies associated with human autoimmune disorders (Continued)

Autoantigen	Autoimmune Diseases
Cancer and Paraneoplastic Autoimmunity (Continued)	
Hu proteins	Paraneoplastic encephalomyelitis
Neuronal nicotinic acetylcholine receptor	Subacute autonomic neuropathy, cancer
p53	Cancer, systemic lupus erythematosus
p62 (IGF-II mRNA-binding protein)	Hepatocellular carcinoma (China)
Recoverin	Cancer-associated retinopathy
Ri protein	Paraneoplastic opsoclonus myoclonus ataxia
βIV spectrin	Lower motor neuron syndrome
Synaptotagmin	Lambert-Eaton myasthenic syndrome
Voltage-gated calcium channels	Lambert-Eaton myasthenic syndrome
Yo protein	Paraneoplastic cerebellar degeneration

Ans. A

126. All are mechanisms of autoimmunity except:

A. Peripheral anergy of autoreactive lymphocytes
B. Molecular mimicry
C. Superantigen stimulation
D. Loss of immunologic privilege

Explanation:

Table: Mechanism of autoimmunity
I. **Exogenous**
A. Molecular mimicry
B. Superantigenic stimulation
C. Microbial and tissue damage-associated adjuvanticity
II. **Endogenous**
A. Altered antigen presentation
1. Loss of immunologic privilege
2. Presentation of novel or cryptic epitopes (epitope spreading)
3. Alteration of self-antigen
4. Enhanced function of antigen-presenting cells
a. Costimulatory molecule expression
b. Cytokine production
B. Increased T cell help
1. Cytokine production
2. Costimulatory molecules
C. Increased B cell function
1. B cell activating factor
2. Costimulatory molecules
D. Apoptotic defects or defects in clearance of apoptotic material
E. Cytokine imbalance
F. Altered immunoregulation

Ans. A

127. Highly infectious among below:

A. HBsAg positive serum containing HBeAg

B. HBsAg positive serum containing HBeAg negative

C. HBsAg positive serum containing anti-HBe-positive serum

D. Anti HBsAg positive and anti-HBe-positive serum

Explanation:

- HBsAg-positive serum containing HBeAg is more likely to be highly infectious and to be associated with the presence of hepatitis B virions (and detectable HBV DNA) than HBeAg-negative or anti HBe-positive serum.
- For example, HBsAg-positive mothers who are HBeAg-positive almost invariably (>90%) transmit hepatitis B infection to their offspring, whereas HBsAg-positive mothers with anti-HBe rarely (10–15%) infect their offspring.

Ans. A

128. Most common isolates in sepsis include all except:

A. Proteus

B. E.coli

C. Klebsiella

D. Pseudomonas

Explanation:

- Sepsis can arise from both community-acquired and hospital-acquired infections.
- Of these infections, pneumonia is the most common source, accounting for about half of cases; next most common are intra-abdominal and genitourinary infections.

- Blood cultures are typically positive in only one-third of cases, while many cases are culture negative at all sites.
- ***Staphylococcus aureus*** **and** ***Streptococcus pneumoniae*** **are the most common gram-positive isolates, while** ***Escherichia coli, Klebsiella*** **species, and** ***Pseudomonas aeruginosa*** **are the most common gram-negative isolates.**
- In recent years, gram-positive infections have been reported more often than gram-negative infections, yet a 75-country point-prevalence study of 14,000 patients on intensive care units (ICUs) found that 62% of positive isolates were gram-negative bacteria, 47% were gram-positive bacteria, and 19% were fungi.

Ans. A

129. Criteria proposed for septic shock include all except:

A. Sepsis
B. Need for vasopressor therapy to elevate mean arterial pressure to ≥65 mmHg
C. A serum lactate concentration >2.0 mmol/L after adequate fluid resuscitation
D. A serum lactate concentration >5.0 mmol/L before fluid resuscitation

Explanation:

- Criteria are proposed for septic shock that include (1) sepsis plus (2) the need for vasopressor therapy to elevate mean arterial pressure to ≥65 mmHg, with (3) a serum lactate concentration >2.0 mmol/L after adequate fluid resuscitation.

Ans. D

130. All are possible treatment options for CML in pregnancy except:

A. Leukapheresis
B. Hydroxyurea
C. Imatinib
D. Interferon alpha

Explanation:

- Interferon α is considered in combination with TKIs (an investigational approach), sometimes after CML failure on TKIs, occasionally in patients during pregnancy, or as part of investigational strategies with TKIs to eradicate residual molecular disease.
- Women with CML who become pregnant should discontinue TKI therapy immediately.

Ans. C

131. Regarding psoriasis all are true except:

A. In 60-70% of cases psoriasis precedes joint disease
B. In 15-20% of cases, two manifestations appear within 1 year of each other
C. In 15-20% of cases, arthritis precedes the onset of psoriasis
D. It is more common in males compared to females

Explanation:

- In 60–70% of cases, psoriasis precedes joint disease.
- In 15–20% of cases, the two manifestations appear within 1 year of each other.
- In about 15–20% of cases, the arthritis precedes the onset of psoriasis and can present a diagnostic challenge.
- Frequency in men and women is almost equal, although the frequency of disease patterns differs somewhat in the two sexes.

- Disease can begin in childhood or late in life but typically begins in the fourth or fifth decade, at an average age of 37 years

Ans. D

132. Milan criteria is used for:

A. Staging of cancer
B. Basis for transplant eligibility
C. Extent of resection
D. All of the above

Explanation:

- Liver transplantation is the first treatment choice for cirrhotic patients with single tumors ≤5 cm and portal hypertension (including Child-Pugh's B and C) or with small multinodular tumors (≤3 nodules, each ≤3 cm).
- These so-called Milan criteria have been validated over the years and a meta-analysis reported 5-year and 10-year survival rates of ~70 and ~50%, respectively, similar to outcomes achieved in non-HCC transplantation indications

Ans. B

133. All are distributive shocks except:

A. Septic shock
B. Severe burns
C. Adrenal crisis
D. GI losses

Explanation:

Table: Pathophysiologic classification of shock
1. Distributive
a. Septic shock
b. Pancreatitis
c. Severe burns
d. Anaphylactic shock
e. Neurogenic shock
f. Endocrine shock
i. Adrenal crisis
2. Cardiogenic
a. Myocardial infarction
b. Myocarditis
c. Arrhythmia
d. Valvular
i. Severe aortic valve insufficiency
ii. Severe mitral valve insufficiency
3. Obstructive
a. Tension pneumothorax
b. Cardiac tamponade
c. Restrictive pericarditis
d. Pulmonary embolism
e. Aortic dissection
4. Hypovolemic
a. Hemorrhagic
b. GI losses
c. Burns
d. Polyuria
i. Diabetic ketoacidosis
ii. Diabetes insipidus

Ans. D

134. Chronic carriage of S. Typhi is associated with an increased risk of:

A. Pancreatic cancer
B. Stomach cancer
C. Liver cancer
D. Gallbladder cancer

Explanation:

- Up to 10% of untreated patients with typhoid fever excrete *S.* Typhi in the feces for up to 3 months, and 2–5% develop chronic asymptomatic carriage, shedding *S.* Typhi in either urine or stool for >1 year.
- Chronic carriage is more common among women, infants, and persons who have biliary abnormalities or concurrent bladder infection with *Schistosoma haematobium*.
- S. Typhi and other salmonellae are adapted to survive in the gallbladder environment by forming biofilms on gallstones and invading gallbladder epithelial cells.
- Chronic carriage is associated with an increased risk of gallbladder cancer, which is much more common in locales where *S.* Typhi is common, such as the Indian subcontinent.

Ans. D

135. Good evidence of benefit has emerged in patients undergoing elective gastrointestinal surgery and patients with traumatic brain injury with:

A. Polymer formulas with fibre
B. Standard polymeric formulas
C. Protein enriched formulas
D. Immune enhancing formulas

Explanation:

IMMUNE-ENHANCING FORMULAS

- In addition to providing macronutrients and conventional amounts of micronutrients, these products (IEFs) contain large amounts of certain nutrients designed to favorably modulate the immune response: arginine and n-3 fatty acids especially, but also various combinations of glutamine, nucleotides, and antioxidants.
- It is difficult to evaluate the IEFs because there are many different formulations on the market, and considerable heterogeneity in patient populations studied.
- Good evidence of benefit has emerged from clinical trials of perioperative IEFs in patients undergoing elective gastrointestinal surgery and patients with traumatic brain injury.
- EIFs have not yet demonstrated benefit in other kinds of critical illness.

Ans. D

136. 1 L of secretory diarrhea contains how much of zinc:

A. 4 mg
B. 8 mg
C. 12 mg
D. 16 mg

Explanation:

- It is insufficiently appreciated that 1 L of secretory diarrhea contains ~12 mg of zinc.
- Patients with intestinal fistulas or high volume chronic diarrhea require this amount of zinc in addition to their daily requirement of 15 mg to avoid zinc deficiency.
- Zinc may be provided parenterally or enterally (because of its low bioavailability, 12 mg parenteral zinc is equivalent to 30 mg oral elemental zinc).

Ans. C

137. All are absolute contraindications for renal transplant except:

A. Antibodies against the ABO blood group antigens
B. Antibodies against human leukocyte antigen (HLA) class I (A, B, C)

C. HIV infection

D. Antibodies against human leukocyte antigen (HLA) class class II (DR, DQ, DP) antigens

Explanation:

- All candidates must have a thorough risk-versus-benefit evaluation before being approved for transplantation.
- In particular, an aggressive approach to diagnosis of correctable coronary artery disease, presence of latent or indolent infection (HIV, hepatitis B or C, tuberculosis), and neoplasm should be a routine part of the candidate workup.
- Most transplant centers consider overt AIDS and active hepatitis absolute contraindications to transplantation because of the high risk of opportunistic infection.
- Some centers are now transplanting individuals with hepatitis and even HIV infection under strict protocols to determine whether the risks and benefits favor transplantation over dialysis.
- Over the last few years, new direct acting hepatitis C antiviral medications have been introduced and have been shown to be very effective therapies both pre- and post transplant. Those medications are reshaping our approach to patients with hepatitis C.

Ans. C

138. All are features of Cushing's syndrome except:

A. Obesity

B. Hypotension

C. Plethora

D. Glucose intolerance

Explanation:

- Patient with Cushing's syndrome may manifest specific findings, such as central fat redistribution, skin striae, and proximal muscle weakness, in addition to features seen commonly in the general population, such as obesity, plethora, hypertension, and glucose intolerance.
- Similarly, the insidious onset of hypothyroidism—with mental slowing, fatigue, dry skin, and other features—can be difficult to distinguish from similar, nonspecific findings in the general population.

Ans. B

139. All are major criteria for pathogenesis of autoimmune diseases except:

A. Presence of autoantibodies or evidence of cellular reactivity to self

B. Demonstration that relevant autoantibody or T cells can cause tissue pathology

C. Documentation of relevant autoantibody or lymphocytic infiltrate in the pathologic lesion

D. Beneficial effect from immunosuppressive agents

Explanation:

Table: Human autoimmune disease: Presumptive evidence for immunologic pathogenesis
Major Criteria
1. Presence of autoantibodies or evidence of cellular reactivity to self 2. Documentation of relevant autoantibody or lymphocytic infiltrate in the pathologic lesion 3. Demonstration that relevant autoantibody or T cells can cause tissue pathology a. Transplacental transmission b. Adaptive transfer into animals c. In vitro impact on cellular function
Supportive Evidence
1. Reasonable animal model 2. Beneficial effect from immunosuppressive agents 3. Association with other evidence of autoimmunity 4. No evidence of infection or other obvious cause

Ans. D

140. Most common cause of distributive shock is:

A. Sepsis
B. Pancreatitis
C. Anaphylactic shock
D. Adrenal crisis

Explanation:

- Distributive shock is the condition of reduced oxygen delivery where the primary physiologic disturbance is a reduction in SVR.
- It is unique among the types of shock in that there is a compensatory increase in CO
- Central venous pressure (CVP) and pulmonary capillary wedge pressure (PCWP) are usually reduced. **The most common cause of distributive shock is sepsis.**
- Sepsis has recently been redefined as the dysregulated host response to infection resulting in life-threatening organ dysfunction. When this process is accompanied by persistent hypotension requiring vasopressor support, it is classified as septic shock.

Ans. A

141. Mixed opioid/ adrenergic action is seen with:

A. Meperidine
B. Tramadol
C. Morphine
D. Codeine

Explanation:

Table: Narcotic analgesics: Usual doses and intervals			
Codeine	30-60 q4h	30-60 q4h	Nausea common
Oxycodone	–	5–10 q4–6h	Usually available with acetaminophen or aspirin
Morphine	5 q4h	30 q4h	
Morphine sustained release	–	15-60 bid to tid	Oral slow-release preparation
Hydromorphone	1–2 q4h	2–4 q4h	Shorter acting than morphine sulfate
Levorphanol	2 q6–8h	4 q6–8h	Longer acting than morphine sulfate; absorbed well PO
Methadone	5–10 q6–8h	5–20 q6–8h	Due to long half-life, respiratory depression and sedation may persist after analgesic effect subsides; therapy should not be initiated with > 40 mg/d, and dose escalation should be made no more frequently than every 3 days
Meperidine	50–100 q3–4h	300 q4h	Poorly absorbed PO; normeperidine is a toxic metabolite; routine use of this agent is not recommended
Butorphanol	–	1–2 q4h	Intranasal spray
Fentanyl	25–100 mg/h	–	72-hour tansdermal patch
Buprenorphine	5–20 mg/h		7-day transdermal patch
Buprenorphine	0.3 q6–8h		Parenteral administration
Tramadol	–	50–100 q4–6h	Mixed opioid/adrenergic action

Ans. B

142. All trigger asthma through mast cell activation except:

A. Irritant dust
B. Allergen
C. Exercise
D. Hyperventilation

Explanation:

- Most of the triggers for asthma symptoms appear to act indirectly, including allergens, exercise, hyperventilation, fog (via mast cell activation), irritant dusts, and sulfur dioxide (via cholinergic reflex).

Ans. A

143. All are anti IL-5 except:

A. Mepolizumab
B. Reslizumab
C. Benralizumab
D. Omalizumab

Explanation:

- Antibodies that block IL-5 (mepolizumab, reslizumab) or its receptor (benralizumab) markedly reduce blood and tissue eosinophils and reduce exacerbations in patients who have persistently increased sputum eosinophils despite maximal ICS therapy.

Ans. D

144. Differential diagnosis for Antiphospholipid syndrome include all except:

A. Thrombophilia
B. Coombs positive hemolytic anemia
C. Thrombocytopenia
D. Systemic monocytosis

Explanation:

Table: Clinical features of antiphospholipid syndrome

Manifestation	%
Venous Thrombosis and Related Consequences	
Deep vein thrombosis	39
Livedo reticularis	24
Pulmonary embolism	14
Superficial thrombophlebitis	12
Thrombosis in various other sites	11
Arterial Thrombosis and Related Consequences	
Stroke	20
Cardiac valve thickening/dysfunction and/or Libman-Sacks vegetations	14
Transient ischemic attack	11
Myocardial ischemia (infarction or angina) and coronary bypass graft thrombosis	10
Leg ulcers and/or digital gangrene	9
Arterial thrombosis in the extremites	7
Retinal artery thrombosis/amaurosis fugax	7
Ischemia of visceral organs or avascular necrosis of bone	6
Multi-infarct dementia	3
Neurologic Manifestations of Uncertain Etiology	
Migraine	20
Epilepsy	7
Chorea	1
Cerebellar ataxia	1
Transverse myelopathy	0.5
Renal Manifestations Due to Various Reasons (Renal Artery/Renal Vein/ Glomerular Thrombosis, Fibrous Intima Hyperplasia)	3
Musculoskeletal Manifestations	
Arthralgias	39
Arthritis	27
Obstetric Manifestations (Referred to the Number of Pregnancies)	
Preeclampsia	10
Eclampsia	4
Fetal Manifestations (Referred to the Number of Pregnancies)	
Early fetal loss (<10 weeks)	35
Late fetal loss (≥10 weeks)	17
Premature birth among the live births	11
Hematologic Manifestations	
Thrombocytopenia	30
Autoimmune hemolytic anemia	10

Ans. D

145. All are due to NALP3 gene mutation except:

A. Familial cold auto-inflammatory syndrome (FCAS)
B. Muckle-Wells syndrome (MWS)
C. Chronic infantile neurologic cutaneous and articular syndrome
D. Familial Mediterranean fever (FMF)

Explanation:

Table: Diseases associated with inflammasome activity

Disease	Clinical Features	Gene Mutated	Etiologic Agent	Inflammasome Involvement	Anakinra Response[a]
Familial cold autoinflammatory syndrome (FCAS)	Fever, arthralgia, cold-induced urticaria	*NALP3*		Overactive	Yes
Muckle-Wells syndrome (MWS)	Fever, arthralgia, urticaria, sensorineural deafness, amyloidosis	*NLRP3*		Overactive	Yes
Chronic infantile neurologic cutaneous and articular syndrome (CINCA, NOMID)	Fever, severe arthralgia, urticaria, neurologic problems, severe amyloidosis	*NALP3*		Overactive	Yes
Familial Mediterranean fever (FMF)	Fever, peritonitis, pleuritis, amyloidosis	Pyrin		Overactive	Partial
Pyogenic arthritis, pyoderma gangrenosum and acne syndrome (PAPA)	Pyogenic sterile arthritis	*PSTPIP1*		Overactive	Yes
Hyperimmunoglobulin D syndrome (HIDS)	Arthralgia, abdominal pain, lymphadenopathy	Mevalonate kinase		To be demonstrated	Yes
Tumor necrosis factor receptor-1-associated syndrome (TRAPS)	Fever, abdominal pain, skin lesions	*TNF-R1*		To be demonstrated	Yes
Systemic-Onset juvenile idiopathic arthritis (SOJIA)	Chronic joint inflammation		Unknown	To be demonstrated	Yes
Adult-Onset Still's disease (AOSD)	Arthralgia, fever		Unknown	To be demonstrated	Yes
Behçet's disease	Arhralgia, uveitis, ulcers		Unknown	To be demonstrated	Yes
Schnitzler's syndrome	Urticaria, fever, arthralgia		Unknown	To be demonstrated	Yes
Gout	Metabolic arthritis, pain		Uric acid (MSU)	Activated	Yes
Pseudogout	Arthritis		CPPD	Activated	Yes
Contact dermatitis	Urticaria		Irritants	Activated	Unknown
Fever syndrome	Fever	*NALP12*		Unknown	Unknown
Hydatidiform mole	Hydatid mole	*NALP7*		Unknown	Unknown
Vitiligo	Skin depigmentation, autoimmunity	*NLRP1*		Overactive	Unknown
Crohn's disease		*NLRP3*		Underactive	Unknown
Multiple sclerosis		*NLPR3*		Activated	Unknown
Psoriasitic arthritis		*NLRP3*		Activated	Yes

Ans. D

146. Carbapenems interact with:

A. Warfarin
B. Tacrlimus
C. Cyclosporine
D. Valproic acid

Explanation:

Antibacterial(s)	Interacting Agent(s)	Potential Effect and Management
Nafcillin	Warfarin, cyclosporine, tacrolimus	Decreased levels of warfarin, cyclosporine via CYP3A4 induction. Monitor levels of affected drug closely if drugs are given concomitantly
Ceftriaxone	Calcium-containing IV solutions	Concomitant use is contraindicated in neonates (<28 days); the combination can lead to precipitation of ceftriaxone-calcium particulate Ceftriaxone and calcium-containing solutions can be given to infants > 28 days of age provided they are given sequentially and the lines are thoroughly flushed between infusions.
Carbapenems	Valproic acid	Decreased levels of valproic acid. Monitor valproic acid levels closely if drugs are given concomitantly
Linezolid, tedizolid	Serotonergic and adrenergic agents (e.g., SSRIs, vasopressors)	Increased levels of serotonergic and adrenergic agents. Monitor for serotonin syndrome. Tedizolid may have less potential than linezolid to cause this drug interaction
Quinupristin-dalfopristin	Substrates of CYP3A4 (e.g., warfarin, ritonavir, cyclosporine, diazepam, verapamil)	Can result in increased levels of interacting drug
Fluoroquinolones	Theophylline[a]	Can result in theophylline toxicity
	Sucralfate; antacids containing aluminium, calcium, or magnesium; ferrouns sulfate- and zinc-containing multivitamins	Can result in subtherapeutic fluoroquinolone levels. Administer fluoroquinolone 2 hours before or 6 hours after interacting drug
	Tizanidine[a]	Can result in increased levels of tizanidine and hypotensive, sedative effects. Monitor for side effects if drugs are given concomitantly
Rifampin	Substrates of CYP3A4 (e.g., warfarin, ritonavir, cyclosporine, diazepam, verapamil, protease inhibitors, voriconazole	Can result in decreased levels of interacting drug. Avoid concomitant use if possible. If giving drugs concomitantly, monitor drug levels if possible
	Substrates of CYP2C19 (e.g., omeprazole, lansoprazole)	
	Substrates of CYP2C9 (e.g., warfarin, tolbutamide)	
	Substrates of CYP2C8 (e.g., repaglinide, rosiglitazone)	
	Substrates of CYP2B6 (e.g., efavirenz)	
	Hormone therapy (e.g., norethindrone)	Can result in decreased levels of hormone. If oral contraceptive and rifampin are given concomitantly, use alternative form of birth control

Ans. D

147. All are used for Post-exposure antimicrobial prophylaxis in plague except:

A. Levofloxacin
B. Ciprofloxacin
C. Doxycycline
D. Azithromycin

Explanation:

- Postexposure antimicrobial prophylaxis lasting 7 days is recommended following household, hospital, or other close contact with persons with untreated pneumonic plague.
- *Close contact* is defined as contact with a patient at <2 m.
- In animal aerosol-infection studies, levofloxacin and ciprofloxacin are associated with higher survival rates than doxycycline

Ans. D

148. Assessment of critically ill patient is done by all scores except:

A. APACHE
B. NYHANES
C. SOFA
D. SAPS

Explanation:

- Most commonly utilized scoring systems are the SOFA (Sequential Organ Failure Assessment), the

APACHE (Acute Physiology and Chronic Health Evaluation), and the SAPS (Simplified Acute Physiology Score) systems.

Ans. B

149. All are causes of Shock with cold, clammy extremities except:

A. Hypovolemic shock
B. Liver failure
C. Myocardial infarction
D. Adrenal crisis

Explanation:

Approach to Patient in Shock

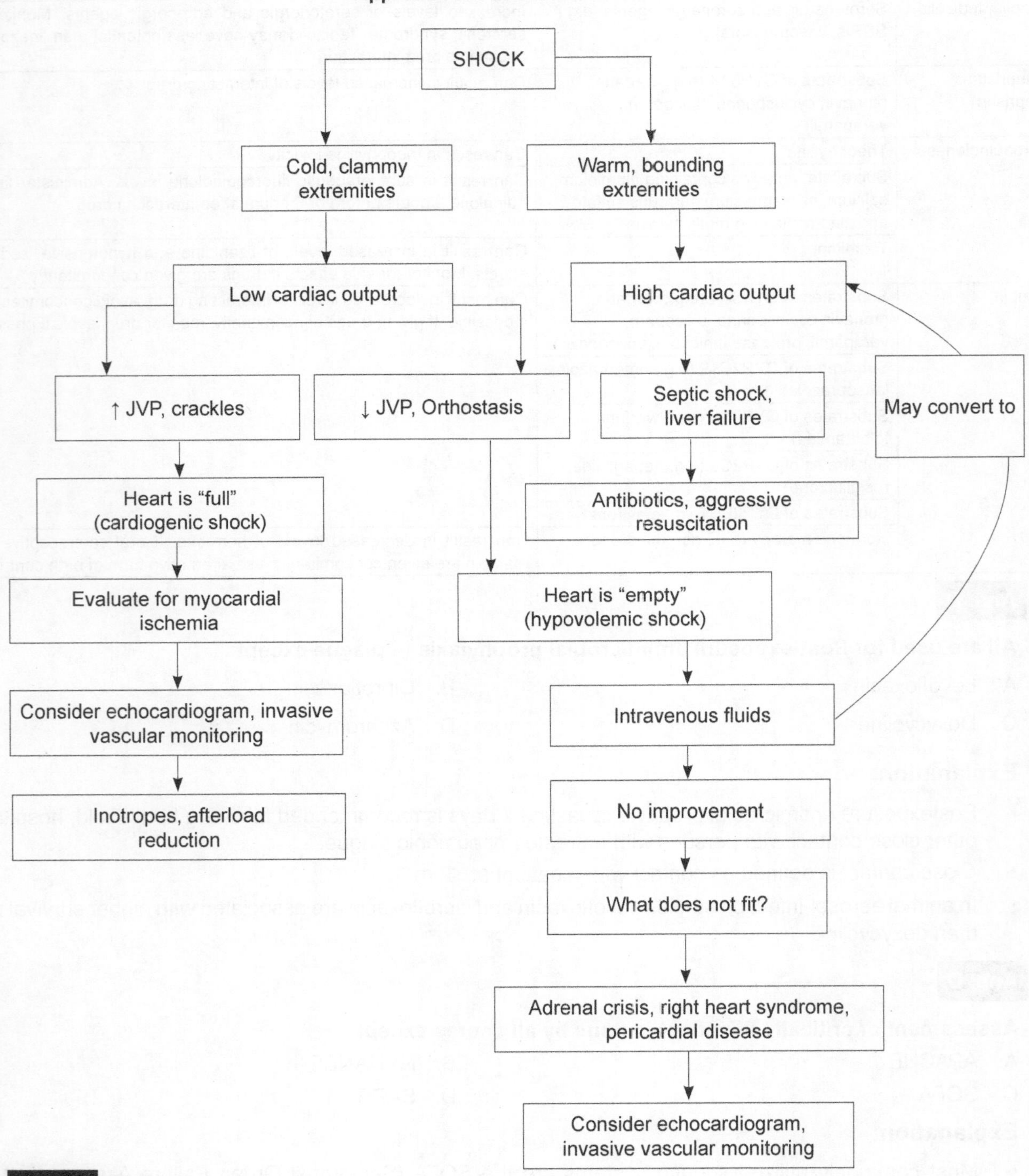

Ans. B

150. It is unlikely that the drug is the cause for FUO if fever persists even after stopping the drug for more than:

A. 24 hrs
B. 48 hrs
C. 72 hrs
D. 98 hrs

Explanation:

- If fever persists beyond 72 h after discontinuation of the suspected drug, it is unlikely that this drug is the cause.
- In patients without PDCs or with only misleading PDCs, funduscopy by an ophthalmologist may be useful in the early stage of diagnostic workup.

Ans. C

151. Intubation and mechanical ventilation is best needed for:

A. Type I respiratory failure
B. Type II respiratory failure
C. Type III respiratory failure
D. Type IV respiratory failure

Explanation:

TYPE IV RESPIRATORY FAILURE

- This form results from hypoperfusion of respiratory muscles in patients in shock. Normally, respiratory muscles consume <5% of total cardiac output and oxygen delivery.
- Patients in shock often experience respiratory distress due to pulmonary edema (e.g., in cardiogenic shock), lactic acidosis, and anemia.
- In this setting, up to 40% of cardiac output may be distributed to the respiratory muscles. Intubation and mechanical ventilation can allow redistribution of the cardiac output away from the respiratory muscles and back to vital organs while the shock is treated.

Ans. D

152. Most effective for DVT prophylaxis, those undergoing high risk orthopedic surgery is:

A. Aspirin
B. LMWH
C. Heparin
D. Fondaparinux

Explanation:

- Low-molecular-weight heparins such as enoxaparin are more effective than unfractionated heparin for DVT prophylaxis in high-risk patients (e.g., those undergoing orthopedic surgery) and are associated with a lower incidence of heparin-induced thrombocytopenia.
- Fondaparinux, a selective factor Xa inhibitor, is even more effective than enoxaparin in high-risk orthopedic patients.

Ans. D

153. CMV is associated with all except:

A. Glomerulopathy in kidney transplant recipients
B. Bronchiolitis obliterans in lung transplant recipients
C. Vanishing bile duct syndrome in liver transplant recipients
D. Aplastic crisis in bone marrow transplant recipients

Explanation:

- Most patients infected with CMV who undergo HSC transplantation excrete virus, with or without clinical findings. Serious CMV disease is much more common among allogeneic than autologous recipients and is often associated with GVHD.
- In addition to pneumonia and marrow suppression (and, less often, graft failure), manifestations of CMV disease in HSC transplant recipients include fever with or without arthralgias, myalgias, hepatitis, and esophagitis.
- CMV ulcerations occur in both the lower & upper gastrointestinal tract, and it may be difficult to distinguish diarrhea due to GVHD from that due to CMV infection.
- Finding of CMV in the liver of a patient with GVHD does not necessarily mean that CMV is responsible for hepatic enzyme abnormalities.
- It is interesting that ocular and neurologic manifestations of CMV infections are common in patients with AIDS but uncommon in patients who develop CMV disease after transplantation.

Table: Herpesvirus syndromes in transplant recipients

Virus	Reactivation Disease
Herpes simplex virus type 1	Oral lesions Esophageal lesions Pneumonia (Primarily HSC transplant recipients) Hepatitis (rare)
Herpes simplex virus type 2	Anogenital lesions Hepatitis (rare)
Varicella-zoster virus	Zoster (can disseminate)
Cytomegalovirus	Associated with graft rejection Fever and malaise Bone marrow failure Pneumonitis Gastrointestinal disease
Epstein-Barr virus	B cell lymphoproliferative disease/lymphoma Oral hairy leucoplakia (rare)
Human herpesvirus type 6	Fever Delayed monocyte/platelet engraftment Encephalitis (rare)
Human herpesvirus type 7	Undefined
Kaposi's sarcoma-associated virus (human herpesvirus type 8)	Kaposi's sarcoma Primary effusion lymphoma (rare) Multicentric Castleman's disease (rare) Marrow aplasia (rare)

Ans. D

154. Chronic pulmonary infections with systemic manifestations that mimic those of tuberculosis is seen with:

A. P. aeruginosa
B. B. cepacia
C. B. pseudomallei
D. S. maltophilia

Explanation:

- *B. pseudomallei* causes a wide spectrum of conditions, ranging from asymptomatic infection to abscesses, pneumonia, and disseminated disease.

- It is a significant cause of fatal community-acquired pneumonia and septicemia in endemic areas, with mortality rates as high as 44% reported in Thailand.
- Acute pulmonary infection is the most commonly diagnosed form of melioidosis.
- Pneumonia may be asymptomatic (with routine chest radiographs showing mainly upper-lobe infiltrates) or may present as severe necrotizing disease.
- *B. pseudomallei* also causes chronic pulmonary infections with systemic manifestations that mimic those of tuberculosis, including chronic cough, fever, hemoptysis, night sweats, and cavitary lung disease.
- Besides pneumonia, the other principal form of *B. pseudomallei* disease is skin ulceration with associated lymphangitis and regional lymphadenopathy.
- Spread from the lungs or skin, which is most often documented in debilitated individuals, gives rise to septicemic forms of melioidosis that carry a high mortality rate.

Ans. C

155. CCR2 receptor is connected to all below diseases except:

A. Atherosclerosis
B. Rheumatoid arthritis
C. Multiple sclerosis
D. Allergic asthma

Explanation:

Table: CC, CXC$_1$, CX$_3$, C$_1$ and XC families of chemokines and chemokine receptors

Chemokine Receptor	Chemokine Ligands	Cell Types	Disease Connection
CCR1	CCL3 (MIP-1α), CCL5 (RANTES), CCL7 (MCP-3), CCL14 (HCC1)	T cells, monocytes, eosinophils, basophils	Rheumatoid arthritis, multiple sclerosis
CCR2	CCL2 (MCP-1), CCL8 (MCP-2), CCL7 (MCP-3), CCL13 (MCP-4), CCL16 (HCC4)	Monocytes, dendritic cells (immature), memory T cells	Atherosclerosis, rheumatoid arthritis, multiple sclerosis, resistance to intracellular pathogens, type 2 diabetes mellitus
CCR3	CCL11 (eotaxin), CCL13 (eotaxin-2), CCL7 (MCP-3), CCL5 (RANTES), CCL8 (MCP-2), CCL13 (MCP-4)	Eosinophils, basophils, mast cells, T_H2, platelets	Allergic asthma and rhinitis
CCR4	CCL17 (TARC), CCL22 (MDC)	T cells (T_H2), dendritic cells (mature), basophils, macrophages, platelets	Parasitic infection, graft rejection, T cell homing to skin
CCR5	CCL3 (MIP-1α), CCL4 (MIP-1α), CCL5 (RANTES), CCL11 (eotaxin), CCL14 (HCC1), CCL16 (HCC4)	T cells, monocytes	HIV-1 co-receptor (T cell-tropic strains), transplant rejection
CCR6	CCL20 (MIP-3α, LARC)	T cells (T regulatory and memory), B cells, dendritic cells	Mucosal humoral immunity, allergic asthma, intestinal T cell homing
CCR7	CCL19 (ELC), CCL21 (SLC)	T cells, dendritic cells (mature)	Transport of T cells and dendritic cells to lymph nodes, antigen presentation and cellular immunity
CCR8	CCL1 (1309)	T cells (T_H2), monocytes, dendritic cells	Dendritic cell migration to lymph node, type 2 cellular immunity, granuloma formation
CCR9	CCL25 (TECK)	T cells, IgA+ plasma cells	Homing of T cells and IgA+ plasma cells to the intestine, inflammatory bowel disease
CCR10	CCL27 (CTACK), CCL28 (MEC)	T cells	T cell homing to intestine and skin

Contd.

Contd.

CXCR1	CXCL8 (interleukin-8), CXCL6 (GCP2)	Neutrophils, monocytes	Inflammatory lung disease, COPD
CXCR2	CXCL8, CXCL1 (GROα), CXCL2 (GROα), CXCL3 (GROα), CXCL5 (ENA-78), CXCL6	Neutrophils, monocytes, microvascular endothelial cells	Inflammatory lung disease, COPD, angiogenic for tumor growth
CXCR3-A	CXCL9 (MIG), CXCL10 (IP-10), CXCL11 (I-TAC)	Type 1 helper cells, mast cells, mesangial cells	Inflammatory skin disease, multiple sclerosis, transplant rejection
CXCR3-B	CXCL4 (PF4), CXCL9 (MIG), CXCL10 (IP-10) CXCL11 (I-TAC)	Microvascular endothelial cells, neoplastic cells	Angiostatic for tumor growth
CXCR4	CXCL12 (SDF-1)	Widely expressed	HIV-1 co-receptor (T cell-tropic), tumor metastases, hematopoiesis
CXCR5	CXCL13 (BCA-1)	B cells, follicular helper T cells	Formation of B cells follicles
CXCR6	CXCL16 (SR-PSOX)	CD8 + T cells, natural killer cells and memory CD4+ T cells	Inflammatory liver disease, atherosclerosis (CXCL16)
CX_3CR1	CX3CL1 (fractalkine)	Macrophages, endothelial cells, smooth-muscle cells	Atherosclerosis
XCR1	XCL1 (lymphotactin), XCL2	T cells, natural killer cells	Rheumatoid arthritis, IgA nephropathy, tumor response

Ans. D

156. NK cells express surface markers for all except:

A. CD 16
B. CD 56
C. CD 8
D. CD23

Explanation:

Table: Cells of the innate immune system and their major roles in triggering adaptive immunity

Cell Type	Major Role in Innate Immunity	Major Role in Adaptive Immunity
Macrophages	Phagocytose and kill bacteria; produce antimicrobial peptides; bind LPS; produce inflammatory cytokines	Produce IL- and TNF-α to upregulate lymphocyte adhesion molecules and chemokines to attract antigen-specific lymphocyte. Produce IL-12 to recruit T_H1 T helper cell responses; upregulate costi-mulatory and MHC molecules to facilitate T and B lymphocyte recognition and activation. Macrophages and dendritic cells, after LPS signalling, upregulate co-stimulatory molecules B7-1 (CD80) and B7-2 (CD86) that are required for activation of pathogen-specific T cells. There are also Toll-like proteins on B cells and dendritic cells that, after LPS ligation, induce CD80 and CD86 on these cells for T cell antigen presentation
Plasmacytoid dendritic cells (DCs) of lymphoid lineage	Produce large amounts of interferon-α (IFN-α), which has antitumor and antiviral activity, and are found in T cell zones of lymphoid organs; they circulate in blood	IFN-α is a potent activator of macrophage and mature DCs to phagocytose invading pathogens and present pathogen antigens to T and B cells

Contd.

Contd.

Myeloid dendritic cells are of two types: interstitial and Langerhans-derived	Interstitial DCs are strong producers of IL-12 and IL-10 and are located in T cell zones of lymphoid organs, circulate in blood, and are present in the interstices of lung, heart, and kidney; Langerhans DCs are strong producers of IL-12; are located in T cell zones of lymph nodes, skin epithelia, and the thymic medulla; and circulate in blood	Interstitial DCs are potent activators of macrophage and mature DCs to phagocytose invading pathogens and present pathogen antigens to T and B cells
Natural killer (NK) cells	Kill foreign and host cells that have low levels of MHC+ self-peptides. Express NK receptors that inhibit NK function in the presence of high expression of self-MHC	Produce TNF-α and IFN-γ, which recruit T_H1 helper T cell responses
NK-T cells	Lymphocytes with both T cell and NK surface markers that recognize lipid antigens of intracellular bacteria such as *Mycobacterium tuberculosis* by CD1 molecules and kill host cells infected with intracellular bacteria	Produce IL-4 to recruit T_H2 helper T cell responses, IgG1 and IGE production
Neutrophils	Phagocytose and kill bacteria, produce antimicrobial peptides	Produce nitric oxide synthase and nitric oxide, which inhibit apoptosis in lymphocytes and can prolong adaptive immune responses
Eosinophils	Kill invading parasites	Produce IL-5, which recruits Ig-specific antibody responses
Mast cells and basophils	Release TNF-α, IL-6 and IFN-γ in response to a variety of bacterial PAMPs	Produce IL-4, which recruits T_H2 helper T cell responses, and recruit IgG1- and IgE-specific antibody responses
Epithelial cells	Produce antimicrobial peptides; tissue-specific epithelia produce mediator of local innate immunity; e.g., lung epithelial cells produce surfactant proteins (proteins within the collectin family) that bind and promote clearance of lung-invading microbes	Produces TGF-β, which triggers IgA-specific antibody responses

Ans. D

157. All are true statements except:

A. Turner's syndrome associated with eosinophilic colitis

B. Hermansky pudlak syndrome associated with Granulomatous colitis

C. Wiskott Aldrich syndrome associated with thrombocytopenia

D. Glycogen storage disease associated with neutropenia

Explanation:

Table: Primary genetic disorders associated with IBD

Name	Genetic Association	Phenotype
Turner's syndrome	Loss of part of all of X chromosome	Associated with UC and colonic CD
Hermansky-Pudlak	Autosomal recessive chromosome 10q23	Granulomatous colitis, oculocutaneous albinism, platelet dysfunction, pulmonary fibrosis
Wiskott-Aldrich syndrome (WAS)	X-linked recessive disorder, loss of WAS protein function	Colitis, immunodeficiency, severely dysfunctional platelets and thrombocytopenia
Glycogen storage disease	Deficiency of the glucose-6-phosphate transport protein type B1	Granulomatous colitis, presents in infancy with hypoglycemia, growth failure, hepatomegaly and neutropenia
Immune dysregulation polyendocrinopathy, enteropathy X-linked (IPEX)	Loss of FoxP3 transcription factor and T regulatory cell function	UC-like autoimmune enteropathy, with endocrinopathy (neonatal type 1 diabetes or thyroiditis), dermatitis
Early-onset IBD	Deficient IL-10 and IL-10 receptor function	Severe, refractory IBD in early life

Ans. A

158. 40 year old presented to endocrinology OPD with history of increase in shoe size, and change in voice, occasional malena. On examination he was found to have coarsening of facial feature and increased hand, foot size. Fleshy nose +. Clinical diagnosis of acromegaly was made. GH acts via which of the membrane receptor?

A. GPCR
B. Tyrosine kinase
C. Serine threonine kinase
D. Cytokine receptor linked kinase

Explanation:

Table: Examples of membrane receptor families and signaling pathways

Receptors	Effectors	Signaling Pathways
G Protein–Coupled Seven-Transmembrane Receptor (GPCR)		
β-Adrenergic, LH, FSH, TSH	$G_s\alpha$, adenylate cyclase	Stimulation of cyclic AMP production, protein kinase A
Glucagon, PTH, PTHrP, ACTH, MSH, GHRH, CRH	Ca^{2+} channels	Calmodulin, Ca^{2+}-dependent kinases
α-Adrenergic, somatostatin	$G_i\alpha$	Inhibition of cyclic AMP production Activation of K^+, Ca^{2+} channels
TRH, GnRH	G_q, G_{11}	Phospholipase C, diacyl-glycerol, IP_3, protein kinase C, voltage-dependent Ca^{2+} channels
Receptor Tyrosine Kinase		
Insulin, IGF-I	Tyrosine kinases, IRS	MAP kinases, PI 3-kinase; AKT
EGF, NGF	Tyrosine kinases, ras	Raf, MAP kinases, RSK
Cytokine Receptor-Linked Kinase		
GH, PRL	JAK, tyrosine kinases	STAT, MAP kinase, PI 3-kinase, IRS-1
Serine Kinase		
Activin, TGF-β, MIS	Serine kinase	Smads

Ans. D

159. Hypertensive hemorrhage is uncommon in:

A. Putamen
B. Frontal lobe
C. Thalamus
D. Cerebellar hemisphere

Explanation:

Table: Causes of intracranial hemorrhage

Causes	Location	Comments
Head trauma	Intraparenchymal: Frontal lobes, anterior temporal lobes; subarachnoid; extra-axial (subdural, epidural)	Coup and contrecoup injury during brain deceleration
Hypertensive hemorrhage	Putamen, globus pallidus, thalamus, cerebellar hemisphere, pons	Chronic hypertension produces hemorrhage from small (~30-100 μm) vessels in these regions
Transformation of prior ischemic infarction	Basal ganglion, subcortical regions, lobar	Occur in 1-6% of ischemic strokes with predilection for large hemispheric infarctions
Metastatic brain tumor	Lobar	Lung, choriocarcinoma, melanoma, renal cell carcinoma, thyroid, atrial myxoma
Coagulopathy	Any	Risk for ongoing hematoma expansion
Drug	Any, lobar, subarachnoid	Cocaine, amphetamine
Arteriovenous malformation	Lobar, intraventricular, subarachnoid	Risk is ~2-3% per year for bleeding if previously unruptured
Aneurysm	Subarachnoid, intraparenchymal, rarely subdural	Mycotic and nonmycotic forms of aneurysms
Amyloid angiopathy	Lobar	Degenerative disease of intracranial vessels; associated with dementia, rare in patients < 60 years
Cavernous angioma	Intraparenchymal	Multiple cavernous angiomas linked to mutations in *KRIT1, CCM2* and *PDCD10 genes*
Dural arteriovenous fistula	Lobar, subarachnoid	Produces bleeding by venous hypertension
Capillary telangiectasias	Usually brainstem	Rare cause of hemorrhage

Ans. B

160. Most common neurologic cause of disability in the world is:

A. ICH
B. Cerebral tumor
C. Migraine
D. Hypertensive encephalopathy

Explanation:

- Migraine, the second most common cause of headache, and the most common headache-related, and indeed neurologic, cause of disability in the world, afflicts ~15% of women and 6% of men over a 1-year period.

Ans. C

161. All are enzyme inducing drugs except:

A. Valproate
B. Phenytoin
C. Carbamazepine
D. Phenobarbital

Explanation:

Table: Dosage and adverse effects of commonly used antiepileptic drugs								
Generic Name	Trade Name	Principal Uses	Typical Dose; Dose Interval	Half-Life	Therapeutic Range	Adverse Effects		Drug Interactions[a]
						Neurologic	Systemic	
Brivaracetam	Briviact	Focal-onset	100-200 mg/d; bid	7-10 h	Not established	Fatigue Dizziness Weakness Ataxia Mood changes	Gastrointestinal irritation	May increase carbamazepine-expoxide causing decreased tolerability May increase phenytoin
Carbamazepine	Tegretol[c]	Tonic-clonic Focal-onset	600-1800 mg/d (15-35 mg/kg, child); bid (capsules or tablets), tid-qid (oral suspension)	10-17 h (variable due to autoinduction; complete 3-5 weeks after initiation)	4-12 μg/ml	Ataxia Dizziness Diplopia Vertigo	Aplastic anemia Leuko-penia Gastrointestinal irritation Hepato-toxicity Hypo-natremia	Level decreased by enzyme-inducing drugs[b] Level increased by erythromycin, propoxyphene, isoniazid, cimetidine, fluoxetine
Clobazam	Onfi	Lennox-Gastaut syndrome	10-40 mg/d (5-20 mg/d for patients <30 kg body weight); bid	36-42 h (71-82 h for less active metabolite)	Not established	Fatigue Sedation Ataxia Aggression Insomnia	Constipation Anorexia Skin rash	Level increased by CYP2C19 inhibitors
Clonazepam	Klonopin	Absence Atypical absence Myoclonic	1-12 mg/d; qd-tid	24-48 h	10-70 ng/ml	Ataxia Sedation Lethargy	Anorexia	Level decreased by enzyme-inducing drugs[b]
Ethosuximide	Zarontin	Absence	750-1250 mg/d (20-40 mg/kg); qd-bid	60 h, adult 30 h, child	40-100 μg/ml	Ataxia Lethargy Headache	Gastrointestinal irritation Skin rash Bone marrow suppression	Level decreased by enzyme-inducing drugs[b] Level increased by valproic acid
Felbamate	Felbatol	Focal-onset Lennox-Gastaut syndrome Tonic-clonic	2400-3600 mg/d, tid-qid	16-22 h	30-60 μg/ml	Insomnia Dizziness Sedation Headache	Aplastic anemia Hepatic failure Weight loss Gastrointestinal irritation	Increases phenytoin, valproic acid, active carba-mazepine metabolite
Gabapentin	Neurontin	Focal-onset	900-2400 mg/d; tid-qid	5-9 h	2-20 μg/ml	Sedation Dizziness Ataxia Fatigue	Gastrointestinal irritation Weight gain Edema	No known significant interactions
Lacosamide	Vimpat	Focal-onset	200-400 mg/d; bid	13 h	Not established	Dizziness Ataxia Diplopia Vertigo	Gastrointestinal irritation Cardiac conduction (PR interval prolongation)	Level decreased by enzyme-inducing drugs[b]

Contd.

Contd.

Lamotrigine	Lamictal[c]	Focal-onset Tonic-clonic Atypical absence Myoclonic Lennox-Gastaut syndrome	150-500 mg/d; bid (immediate release), daily (extended release) (lower daily dose for regimens with valproic acid; higher daily dose for regimens with an enzyme inducer)	25 h 14 h (with enzyme-inducers), 59 h (with valproic acid)	2.5-20 μg/ml	Dizziness Diplopia Sedation Ataxia Headache	Skin rash Stevens-Johnson syndrome	Level decreased by enzyme-inducing drugs[b] and oral contraceptives Level increased by valproic acid
Levetiracetam	Keppra[c]	Focal-onset	1000-3000 mg/d; bid (immediate release), daily (extended release)	6-8 h	5-45 μg/ml	Sedation Fatigue Incoordination Mood changes	Anemia Leukopenia	No known significant interactions
Oxcarbazepine[c]	Trileptal	Focal-onset Tonic-clonic	900-2400 mg/d (30-45 mg/kg, child); bid	10-17 h (for active metabolite)	10-35 μg/ml	Fatigue Ataxia Dizziness Diplopia Vertigo Headache	See carbamazepine	Level decreased by enzyme-inducing drugs[b] May increase phenytoin

Ans. A

162. All come under loads due to reduced lung compliance except:

A. Alveolar edema
B. Atelectasis
C. Intrinsic positive end-expiratory pressure
D. Abdominal distension

Explanation:

- Overall load on the respiratory system can be sub classified into resistive loads (e.g., bronchospasm), loads due to reduced lung compliance (e.g., alveolar edema, atelectasis, intrinsic positive end-expiratory pressure loads due to reduced chest wall compliance (e.g., pneumothorax, pleural effusion, abdominal distention), and loads due to increased minute ventilation requirements (e.g., pulmonary embolus with increased dead-space fraction, sepsis).

Ans. D

163. Studies evaluating multifaceted, evidence-based strategies to decrease catheter-related bloodstream infections have shown improved outcomes with all below measures except:

A. Hand washing
B. Chlorhexidine skin preparation
C. Use of femoral site
D. Timely catheter removal

Explanation:

- Care bundles, which include measures such as frequent hand washing, are effective but underutilized strategies.
- Other components of care bundles, such as protective isolation of patients colonized or infected by drug-resistant organisms are also commonly used.
- Silver-coated endotracheal tubes reportedly reduce the incidence of ventilator-associated pneumonia.

- Studies evaluating multifaceted, evidence-based strategies to decrease catheter-related bloodstream infections have shown improved outcomes with strict adherence to measures such as hand washing, full-barrier precautions during catheter insertion, chlorhexidine skin preparation, avoidance of the femoral site, and timely catheter removal.

Ans. C

164. Nucleolar immunofluorescence pattern may indicate antibodies to all of the below except:

A. U3-RNP (fibrillarin)　　B. Th/To
C. PM/Scl　　D. RNA polymerase III

Explanation:

- Antinuclear autoantibodies are detected in almost all patients with SSc.
- Anti-topoisomerase I (Scl-70) and anti-centromere antibodies are mutually exclusive and each is highly specific for SSc.
- Topoisomerase I antibodies are associated with increased risk of ILD and poor outcomes.
- Anticentromere antibodies are associated with PAH, but only infrequently with significant cardiac, pulmonary, or renal involvement.
- Nucleolar immunofluorescence pattern may indicate antibodies to U3-RNP (fibrillarin), Th/To, or PM/Scl, whereas speckled immunofluorescence indicates antibodies to RNA polymerase III.

Ans. C

165. A 35 year old gentleman known hypertensive has come to the hospital for review as the blood pressure is difficult to control. Bloods reveal metabolic acidosis, hyperkalaemia and low renin and aldosterone levels. What is the most likely diagnosis?

A. Gordon syndrome　　B. Cushing's syndrome
C. Conn's syndrome　　D. Addison's disease

Explanation:

- Gordon syndrome is a rare familial renal tubular defect resulting in metabolic acidosis, low or normal renin, aldosterone and hyperkalemia. This differentiates it from Conns syndrome where aldosterone levels are elevated and there is hypokalemia. Addison disease does not lead to elevated blood pressure levels.

Ans. A

166. Iron absorption takes place in:

A. Stomach　　B. Proximal small intestine
C. Distal small intestine　　D. Large intestine

Explanation:

- Iron absorption mainly takes place in proximal small intestine under acidic conditions.
- Acidity favors conversion of ferric iron to ferrous form, which is then easily absorbed.

Ans. B

167. All are trials for Infliximab except:

A. GEMINI　　B. ACCENT II
C. PRECISE　　D. SONIC

Explanation:

- In the GEMINI I trial (A Phase 3, Randomized, Placebo-Controlled, Blinded, Multicenter Study of the Induction and Maintenance of Clinical Response and Remission by MLN002 in Patients With Moderate to Severe Ulcerative Colitis), 42% of UC patients treated every 8 weeks and 45% of those treated every 4 weeks were in clinical remission at week 52 compared with 16% placebo.
- In the GEMINI II trial, clinical remission rates for CD patients treated with vedolizumab were 36 to 39%, compared with 22% placebo at 52 weeks.

Ans. A

168. A 25 year old woman with meningococcal septicaemia treated with high dose IV ceftriaxone develops toe gangrene. She underwent amputation and postoperatively, she developed flank pain, drowsy. BP 90/50 mm Hg, Serum sodium – 118mEq/l, potassium – 6.5 mEq/L. Urine spot sodium is 30 mEq/l. What is the investigation of choice?

A. Overnight dexamethasone suppression test
B. High dose dexamethasone suppression test
C. CT abdomen
D. Cosyntropin test.

Explanation:

- Bilateral adrenal hemorrhage leads to this condition. This was due to meningococcaemia with disseminated intravascular coagulation (Waterhouse –Friderichsen syndrome), pseudomonas was the most common cause. Adrenal insufficiency results in mineralocorticoid deficiency, life threatening salt wasting and failure to excrete potassium. Diagnosis of adrenal insufficiency is established by Cosyntropin test.

Ans. D

169. All below matches are correct for donor kidney after death except:

A. I is brought in dead
B. II is awaiting cardiac arrest
C. IV is cardiac arrest after brainstem death
D. V is cardiac arrest in a hospital patient

Explanation:

Table: Definition of a non-heart-beating donor (donation after cardiac death[a] [DCD])	
I.	Brought in dead
II.	Unsuccessful resuscitation
III.	Awaiting cardiac arrest
IV.	Cardiac arrest after brainstem death
V.	Cardiac arrest in a hospital patient

Ans. B

170. Apo E4 associated with:

A. FTD
B. DLB
C. AD
D. All of the above

Explanation:

- *Apo* ε gene on chromosome 19 is involved in the pathogenesis of AD.
- Protein product, apolipoprotein E, participates in cholesterol transport and the gene has three alleles: ε2, ε3, and ε4.

- Apo ε4 allele confers increased risk of AD in the general population, including sporadic and late age-of-onset familial forms.
- Approximately 24–30% of the non-demented white population has at least one ε4 allele (12–15% allele frequency), and about 2% are ε4/ε4 homozygotes. Among patients with AD, 40–65% have at least one ε4 allele, highly significant elevation compared with controls.
- Increased risk associated with a single ε4 allele is especially prominent in women.
- Conversely, many patients with AD have no ε4 allele, and ε4 carriers may never develop AD. Therefore, ε4 is neither necessary nor sufficient to cause AD.

Ans. C

171. 35 year old male presented with history of severe headache and he was diagnosed to have accelerated hypertension. He was prescribed T. Telmisartan 40 mg 1-0-1. He was referred to tertiary centre for further management. For evaluation of young onset hypertension. He was ordered ARR to rule out primary hyperaldosteronism. How does telmesartan affects ARR?

A. Decrease
B. Increase
C. No effect
D. Any of the above

Explanation:

ARR

- Beta blocker causes an increase in aldosterone levels and decrease in renin levels leading to increased ARR.
- ACEI / ARB causes a decrease in aldosterone levels and increase in renin levels, leading to decreased ARR.
- CCB – No effect on ARR.

Ans. A

172. SQUID is used to measure:

A. Cardiac iron
B. Hepatic iron
C. Cardiac zinc
D. Hepatic zinc

Explanation:

- Patients who receive >100 units of packed RBCs usually develop hemosiderosis.
- Ferritin level rises, followed by early endocrine dysfunction (glucose intolerance and delayed puberty), cirrhosis and cardiomyopathy.
- Liver biopsy shows both parenchymal and reticuloendothelial iron.
- Superconducting quantum-interference device (SQUID) is accurate at measuring hepatic iron but not widely available.
- Cardiac toxicity is often insidious. Early development of pericarditis is followed by dysrhythmia and pump failure.
- Onset of heart failure is ominous, often presaging death within a year

Ans. B

173. Empirical addition of antifungal agents if fever and neutropenia persist without identification of an organism or site is after:

A. 3 days
B. 5 days
C. 7 days
D. 10 days

Explanation:

- Empirical addition of antifungal agents if fever and neutropenia persist for 7 days without identification of an adequately treated organism or site is frequent.

Ans. C

174. DD for nodular infiltrates in chest in immunocompromised patients include all except:

A. Aspergillus
B. Nocardia
C. Radiation pneumonitis
D. Recurrent tumor

Explanation:

Table: Differential diagnosis of chest infiltrates in immunocompromised patients

Infiltrate	Cause of Pneumonia	
	Infectious	**Noninfectious**
Localized	Bacteria (including *Legionella*, mycobacteria)	Local haemorrhage or embolism, tumor
Nodular	Fungi (e.g., *Aspergillus or Mucor*), *Nocardia*	Recurrent tumor
Diffuse	Viruses (especially cytomegalovirus), *Chlamydia, Pneumocystis, Toxoplasma gondii*, mycobacteria	Congestive heart failure, radiation pneumonitis, drug-induced lung injury, lymphangitic spread of cancer

Ans. C

175. Treatment of asymptomatic bacteria should be directed by urine culture report in:

A. Pregnant women
B. Neutropenic patients
C. Renal transplant recipients
D. All of the above

Explanation:

- Treatment of ASB does not decrease the frequency of symptomatic infections or complications except in pregnant women, persons undergoing urologic surgery, and perhaps neutropenic patients and renal transplant recipients.
- Treatment of ASB in pregnant women and patients undergoing urologic procedures should be directed by urine culture results. In all other populations, screening for and treatment of ASB are discouraged.
- Majority of cases of catheter-associated bacteriuria are asymptomatic and do not warrant antimicrobial therapy.

Ans. A

176. All are true except:

A. For posterior canal BPPV, the Epley maneuver is the most commonly used procedure
B. Vestibular migraine typically is treated with medications that are used for prophylaxis of migraine headaches
C. Glucocorticoids or gentamicin into the middle ear are typically the initial treatments for Meniere's disease
D. Bilateral vestibular hypofunction may be due to gentamicin or other aminoglycoside antibiotics

Explanation:

- Ménière's disease is thought to be due to excess fluid (endolymph) in the inner ear; hence the term *endolymphatic hydrops*.
- Patients suspected of having Ménière's disease should be referred to an otolaryngologist for further evaluation.
- Diuretics and sodium restriction are typically initial treatment.
- If attacks persist, injections of glucocorticoids or gentamicin into the middle ear may be considered.
- Non-ablative surgical options include decompression and shunting of the endolymphatic sac.
- Full ablative procedures (vestibular nerve section, labyrinthectomy) are seldom required.

Ans. C

177. All are true about Typhlitis except:

A. Fever with right lower quadrant tenderness
B. Plain films may reveal a right-lower-quadrant mass
C. CT with contrast gives more sensitive means of diagnosis
D. Surgery is the definitive means of treatment and early surgery is advised to decrease mortality

Explanation:

- Typhlitis (also referred to as necrotizing colitis, neutropenic colitis, necrotizing enteropathy, ileocecal syndrome, and cecitis) is a clinical syndrome of fever and right-lower-quadrant (or generalized abdominal) tenderness in an immunosuppressed host.
- This syndrome is classically seen in neutropenic patients after chemotherapy with cytotoxic drugs.
- It may be more common among children than among adults and appears to be much more common among patients with AML or ALL than among those with other types of cancer.
- Physical examination reveals right-lower-quadrant tenderness, with or without rebound tenderness.
- Associated diarrhea (often bloody) is common, and the diagnosis can be confirmed by the finding of thickened cecal wall on CT, MRI, or ultrasonography. Plain films may reveal a right-lower-quadrant mass, but CT with contrast or MRI is a much more sensitive means of diagnosis.
- Although surgery is sometimes attempted to avoid perforation from ischemia, most cases resolve with medical therapy alone.
- Disease is sometimes associated with positive blood cultures (which usually yield aerobic gram-negative bacilli), and therapy is recommended for a broad spectrum of bacteria (particularly gram-negative bacilli, which are likely to be found in the bowel flora).

Ans. D

178. Regarding Meniere's disease all are true except:

A. Episodic vertigo
B. High frequency hearing loss
C. Tinnitus
D. Aural fullness

Explanation:

- Ménière's disease is characterized by episodic vertigo, fluctuating sensorineural hearing loss, tinnitus, and aural fullness.
- Tinnitus and/or deafness may be absent during the initial attacks of vertigo, but it invariably appears as the disease progresses and increases in severity during acute attacks.

Ans. B

179. Clinical efficacy of triptans appears to be related more to:

A. Time to peak plasma level
B. Potency
C. Half-life
D. Bioavailability

Explanation:

- Each drug in the triptan class has similar pharmacologic properties but varies slightly in terms of clinical efficacy.
- Rizatriptan and eletriptan are, on a population basis, the most efficacious of the triptans currently available in United States.
- Sumatriptan and zolmitriptan have similar rates of efficacy as well as time to onset, with an advantage of having multiple formulations, whereas almotriptan has a similar rate of efficacy to sumatriptan and is better tolerated, and frovatriptan and naratriptan are somewhat slower in onset and are also well tolerated.
- Clinical efficacy appears to be related more to the *t* max (time to peak plasma level) than to the potency, half-life, or bioavailability.
- This observation is consistent with a large body of data indicating that faster-acting analgesics are more effective than slower-acting agents.

Ans. A

180. Chronic hyponatremia is hyponatremia for more than:

A. 12 hrs
B. 48 hrs
C. 72 hrs
D. 7 days

Explanation:

- Patients with acute hyponatremia present with symptoms that can range from headache, nausea, and/or vomiting, to seizures, obtundation, and central herniation; patients with chronic hyponatremia, present for >48 h, are less likely to have severe symptoms.
- Second, patients with chronic hyponatremia are at risk for ODS if plasma Na+ concentration is corrected by >8–10 m*M* within the first 24 h and/or by >18 m*M* within the first 48 h.
- Third, the response to interventions such as hypertonic saline, isotonic saline, or AVP antagonists can be highly unpredictable, such that frequent monitoring of plasma Na+ concentration during corrective therapy is imperative.

Ans. B

181. Patients with APS often have false positive serologic test for:

A. Herpes
B. EBV
C. Syphilis
D. CMV

Explanation:

Table: Classification and nomenclature of antiphospholipid antibodies

Name	Assay for their detection	Comments
Antibodies against cardiolipin (aCL)	Enzyme-linked immunosorbent assay (ELISA) using as antigen cardiolipin (CL), a negatively charged phospholipid	aCL from patients with APS recognize β2GPI existing in the human serum as well as in bovine serum, which is used to block the nonspecific binding sites on the ELISA plate. CL simply stabilizes β2GPI at high concentration on the polystyrene surface

Contd.

Contd.

Antibodies against β2GPI (anti-β2GPI)	ELISA using as antigen affinity purified or recombinant β2GPI in the absence of PL	Antibodies recognize β2GPI bound the the absence of CL to an oxidized polystyrene surface, where oxygen atoms in the moieties C-O or C=O were introduced by γ-irradiation
Lupus anticoagulant (LA)	Activated partial thromboplastin time (aPTT) Kaolin clotting time (KCT) Dilute Russel viper venom test (DRWT)	Antibodies recognize β2GPI or prothrombin (PT) and elongate aPTT, implying that they interfere with the generation or thrombin by prothrombin. Prolongation of the clotting times is an in vitro phenomenon, and LA induces thromboses in vivo

Ans. C

182. All are true regarding Clostridium difficile except:

A. Obligately aerobic
B. Gram positive
C. Spore forming bacillus
D. Clindamycin associated with CDI

Explanation:

- *C. difficile* is an obligately anaerobic, gram-positive, spore-forming bacillus whose spores are found widely in nature, particularly in environment of hospitals and chronic-care facilities.
- CDI occurs frequently in hospitals and nursing homes (or shortly after discharge from these facilities) where the level of antimicrobial use is high & environment is contaminated by *C. difficile* spores

Ans. A

183. All possible diagnosis and first test combinations are correct except:

A. Onset of severe liver disease in childhood or adolescence in conjunction with a family history of liver disease or neuropsychiatric disturbance should lead to investigation for Wilson's disease
B. A family history of cirrhosis, diabetes, or endocrine failure and the appearance of liver disease in adulthood should warrant genotyping of the HFE gene for the C282Y and H63D mutations typical of genetic hemochromatosis
C. In children and adolescents with iron overload, other non-HFE causes of hemochromatosis should be searched
D. A family history of emphysema should lead to investigation of α1 antitrypsin levels and, if levels are low, for protease inhibitor (Pi) genotype

Explanation:

- Abnormal iron studies in adult patients warrant genotyping of the *HFE* gene for the C282Y and H63D mutations typical of genetic hemochromatosis.
- In children and adolescents with iron overload, other non-*HFE* causes of hemochromatosis should be sought.
- A family history of emphysema should lead to investigation of α1 antitrypsin levels and, if levels are low, for protease inhibitor (Pi) genotype.

Ans. B

184. Most frequent metabolic complication of parenteral nutrition is:

A. Hyperglycemia
B. Hypoglycemia
C. Hyperkalemia
D. Hypokalemia

Explanation:

- Most frequent metabolic complication of PN is hyperglycemia in patients with insulin resistance due to noninsulin dependent diabetes mellitus, high-dose glucocorticoid therapy, or severe systemic inflammation; the problem is exacerbated by excessively high rates of glucose provision.
- Glucose concentrations are most easily kept at <140 mg/dl with the least risk of hypoglycemia by infusing hypocaloric amounts of glucose and, if necessary, meeting the patient's energy requirement with intravenous lipid.
- In ADM, the benefits of using the lowest insulin dose—minimal hyperinsulinemia and a reduced risk of hypoglycemia—almost always outweigh the doubtful goal of rapidly matching calorie provision to the patient's energy expenditure rate.

Ans. A

185. Weekly once used parenteral antibiotic for Staphylococcus infection is:

A. Tigecycline
B. Oritavancin
C. Ceftaroline
D. Tedizolid

Explanation:

- Dalbavancin and oritavancin are long-acting, parenterally administered lipoglycopeptides that have been used to treat complicated SSTIs.
- Because of their long half-lives, they can be administered on a weekly basis.
- Both have been used as single-dose regimens for treatment of SSTIs.
- Data on their use for the treatment of invasive staphylococcal infections are limited.

Ans. B

186. Disease which can be easily mistaken for botulism is:

A. Miller Fisher variant
B. Myasthenia gravis
C. Eaton-Lambert syndrome
D. Tick paralysis

Explanation:

- GBS, a rare autoimmune demyelinating polyneuropathy that often follows an acute infection, presents most often as an ascending paralysis.
- Case clusters are rare. Occasional GBS cases present as the Miller Fisher variant, which is a descending paralysis. The characteristic triad of ophthalmoplegia, ataxia, and are flexia in Miller Fisher variant GBS is easily mistaken for botulism.

Ans. A

187. Death from cholera is due to:

A. Septicemic shock
B. Hypovolemic shock
C. Cardiogenic shock
D. Renal failure

Explanation:

- Death from cholera is due to hypovolemic shock; thus treatment of individuals with cholera first and foremost requires fluid resuscitation and management.
- In light of the level of dehydration and the patient's age and weight, euvolemia should first be rapidly restored, and adequate hydration should then be maintained to replace ongoing fluid losses

Ans. B

188. All are ligands for LFA-2 except:

A. CD58 B. CD48

C. CD59 D. CD30

Explanation:

Table: Human leukocyte surface antigens--The CD classification of leukocyte differentiation antigens

Surface Antigen (Other Names)	Family	Molecular Mass, kDa	Distribution	Ligand(s)	Function
CD1a (T6, HTA-1)	Ig	49	CD, cortical thymocytes, Langerhans type of DCs	TCRγδ T cells	CD1 molecules present lipid antigens of intracellular bacteria such as Mycobacterium leprae and M. tuberculosis to TCR γδ T cells
CD1b	Ig	45	CD, cortical thymocytes, Langerhans type of DCs	TCRγδ T cells	
CD1c	Ig	43	DC, cortical thymocytes, subset of B cells, Langerhans type of DCs	TCRγδ T cells	
CD1d	Ig	37	Cortical thymocytes, intestinal epithelium, Langerhans type of DCs	TCRγδ T cells	
CD2 (T12, LFA-2)	Ig	50	T, NK	CD58, CD48, CD59, CD15	Alternative T cell activation, T cell anergy, T cell cytokine, T cell cytokine production, T-or NK-mediated cytolysis, T cell apoptosis, cell adhesion
CD3 (T3, Leu-4)	Ig	γ:25-28, δ:21-22, τ:20-25, η:21-22, ς:16	T	Associates with the TCR	T cell activation and function; ς is the signal transduction component of the CD3 complex
CD4 (T4, Leu-3)	Ig	55	T, myeloid	MHC-II, HIV, gp120, IL-16, SABP	T cell selection, T cell activation, signal transduction with p56lck, primary receptor for HIV
CD7 (3A1, Leu-9)	Ig	40	T, NK	K-12 (CD7L)	T and NK cell signal transduction and regulation of IFN-γ, TNF-α production
CD8 (T8, Leu-2)	Ig	34	T	MHC-I	T cell selection, T cell activation, signal transduction with P56lck
CD14 (LPS-receptor)	LRG	53–55	M, G (weak), not by myeloid progenitors	Endotoxin (lipopolysaccharide), lipoteichoic acid, PI	TLR4 mediates with LPS and other PAMP activation of innate immunity

Contd.

Contd.

CD16a (FcγRIIia)	Ig	50−80	NK, Macrophages neutrophils	Fc portion of IgG	Mediates phagocytosis and ADCC
CD19 B4	Ig	95	B (except plasma cells), FDC	Not known	Associates with CD21 and CD81 to form a complex involved in signal transduction in B cell development, activation and differentiation
CD20 (B1)	Unassigned	33-37	B (except plasma cells)	Not known	Cell signaling, may be important for B cell activation and proliferation
CD21 (B2, CR2, EBV-R, C3dR)	RCA	145	Mature B, FDC, subset of thymocytes	C3d, C3dg, iC3b, CD23, EBV	Associated with CD19 and CD81 to form a complex involved in signal transduction in B cell development, activation and differentiation; Epstein-Barr virus receptor
CD22 (BL-CAM)	Ig	130-140	Mature B	CDw 75	Cell adhesion, signalling through association with p72sky, p53/56lyn P13 kinase, SHP1, fLCγ
CD23 (FcεRII, B6, Leu-20, BLAST-2)	C-type lectin	45	B, M, FDC	IgE, CD21, CD11b, CD11c	Regulated IgE synthesis, cytokine release by monocytes
CD28	Ig	44	T, plasma cells	CD80, CD86	Co-stimulatory for T cell activation; involved in the decision between T cell activation and anergy
CD32a (FcγRIIa)	Ig	40	NK, macrophages, neutrophils	Fc portion of IgG	Mediates phagocytosis and ADCC
CD40	TNFR	48−50	B, DC, EC, thymic epithelium, MP, cancers	CD154	B cell activation, proliferation and differentiation; formation of GCs; isotype switching; rescue from apoptosis
CD45 (LCA, T200, B220)	PTP	180, 200, 210, 220	All leukocytes	Galectin-1, CD2, CD3, CD4	T and B activation thymocyte development, signal transduction, apoptosis
CD45RA	PTP	210, 220	Subset T, medullary thymocytes, "naïve" T	Galectin-1, CD2, CD3, CD4	Isoforms of CD45 containing exon4 (A), restricted to a subset of T cells
CD45RB	PTP	200, 210, 220	All leukocytes	Galectin-1, CD2, CD3, CD4	Isoforms of CD45 containing exon 5 (B)
CD45RC	PTP	210, 220	Subset T, medullary thymocytes, "naïve" T	Galectin-1, CD2,CD3, CD4	Isoforms of CD45 containing exon 6 (C), restricted to a subset of T cells
CD45RO	PTP	180	Subset T, cortical thymocytes, "memory" T	Galectin-1, CD2, CD3, CD4	Isoforms of CD45 containing no differentially spliced exons, restricted to a subset of T cells

Ans. D

189. Phagocytosis and ADCC (antibody-dependent cell-mediated cytotoxicity) of IgA-coated pathogens is mediated by:

A. CD16a
B. CD32a
C. CD64
D. CD89

Explanation:

Table: Human leukocyte surface antigens–The CD classification of leukocyte differentiation antigens (Continued)					
Surface Antigen (Other Names)	**Family**	**Molecular Mass, kDa**	**Distribution**	**Ligand(s)**	**Function**
CD64 (FcγRI)	Ig	45–55	Macrophages and monocytes	Fc portion of IgG	Mediates phagocytosis and ADCC
CD80 (B7-1 BB1)	Ig	60	Activated B and T, MP, DC	CD28, CD152	Co-regulator of T cells activation; signalling through CD28 stimulates and through CD152 inhibits T cell activation
CD86 (B7-2, B70)	Ig	80	Subset B, DC, EC, activated T, thymic epithelium	CD28, CD152	Co-regulator of T cell activation; signalling through CD28 stimulates and through CD152 inhibits T cell activation
CD89 (FCαR)	Ig	55-100	Neutrophils, esoinophils, monocytes and MP	Fc portion of IgG	Mediates phagocytosis and ADCC of IgA-coated pathogens
CD95 (APO-1, Fas)	TNFR	43	Activated T and B	Fas ligand	Mediates apoptosis
CD152 (CTLA-4)	Ig	30-33	Activated T	CD80, CD86	Inhibits T cell proliferation
CD154 (CD 40L)	TNF	33	Activated CD4+ T, subset CD8+ T, NK, M, basophil	CD40	Co-stimulatory for T cell activation, B cell proliferation and differentiation
CD279 (PD-1)	Ig	50–55	B, T, TfH	PD-L1, PD-L2	Inhibits T cells proliferation

Ans. D

190. 26 year old female presented with history of weight gain and menstrual irregularity. On examination abdominal obesity + broad purple striae + > 1 cm, easy bruisability +, history of taking medication for generalized body pain+. A probable diagnosis of Cushing syndrome was made. The hormone excess in this condition acts on which receptor?

A. GPCR
B. Tyrosine kinase
C. Intracellular receptor
D. JAK STAT

Explanation:

- Steroids, thyroid hormones, vitamin D, and retinoids are lipid-soluble and interact with intracellular nuclear receptors.

Ans. C

191. Warm antibody AIHA is seen in all except:

A. HIV
B. EBV
C. SLE
D. CLL

Explanation:

Table: Classification of acquired immune hemolytic anemias

	Type of Antibody	
Clinical Setting	**Cold, Mostly IgM, Optimal Temperature 4°C–30°C**	**Warm, Mostly IgG, Optimal Temperature 37°C; or Mixed**
Primary	CAD	AIHA (idiopathic)
Secondary to viral infection	EBV CMV Other	HIV Viral vaccines
Secondary to other infection	Mycoplasma infection: Paroxysmal cold hemoglobinuria	
Secondary to/associated with other disease	CAD in: Waldenstrom's disease Lymphoma	AIHA in: SLE CLL Other malignancy Chronic inflammatory disorders (e.g., IBD) After allogeneic HSCT After immune check-point modulating drugs
Secondary to drugs: Drug-induced immune hemolytic anemia	Small minority (e.g., with lenalidomide)	**Majority:** Currently most common culprit drugs are cefotetan, ceftriaxone, piperacillin
	Drug-dependent: Antibody destroys red cells only when drug present (e.g., rarely penicillin)	
	Drug-independent: Antibody can destroy red cells even when drug no longer present (e.g., methyldopa)	

Ans. B

192. Wiscott Aldrich syndrome is characterized by all except:

A. X-linked disease with clinical manifestations like recurrent bacterial infections, eczema, bleeding caused by thrombocytopenia
B. Null mutations predispose affected individuals to severe eczema & autoimmune manifestations
C. Thrombocytopenia can be severe & compounded by peripheral destruction of platelets associated with autoimmune disorders
D. Typical feature is increased size of platelets on blood smear

Explanation:

- WAS is a complex, recessive, X-linked disease with an incidence of ~1 in 200,000 live births. It is caused by mutations in the *WASP* gene that affect not only T lymphocytes but also the other lymphocyte subsets, dendritic cells, and platelets.
- WAS is typically characterized by the following clinical manifestations: recurrent bacterial infections, eczema, and bleeding caused by thrombocytopenia.
- However, these manifestations are highly variable—mostly as a consequence of the many different *WASP* mutations that have been observed.

- Null mutations predispose affected individuals to invasive and bronchopulmonary infections, viral infections, severe eczema, and autoimmune manifestations.
- Latter include autoantibody-mediated blood cytopenia, glomerulonephritis, skin and visceral vasculitis (including brain vasculitis), erythema nodosum, and arthritis.
- Another possible consequence of WAS is lymphoma, which may be virally induced (e.g., by EBV or Kaposi's sarcoma–associated herpesvirus).
- Thrombocytopenia can be severe and compounded by the peripheral destruction of platelets associated with autoimmune disorders.
- Hypomorphic mutations usually lead to milder outcomes that are generally limited to thrombocytopenia.
- It is noteworthy that even patients with "isolated" X-linked thrombocytopenia can develop severe autoimmune disease or lymphoma later in life.
- Immunologic workup is not very informative; there can be a relative CD8+ T cell deficiency, frequently accompanied by low serum IgM levels and decreased antigen-specific antibody responses.
- A typical feature is reduced-sized platelets on a blood smear. Diagnosis is based on intracellular immunofluorescence analysis of WAS protein (WASp) expression in blood cells.
- WASp regulates the actin cytoskeleton and thus plays an important role in many lymphocyte functions, including cell adhesion and migration and the formation of synapses between antigen-presenting and target cells.
- Predisposition to autoimmune disorders is in part related to defective regulatory T cells.
- Treatment of WAS should match the severity of disease expression.
- Prophylactic antibiotics, immunoglobulin G (IgG) supplementation, and careful topical treatment of eczema are indicated.
- Although splenectomy improves platelet count in a majority of cases, this intervention is associated with a significant risk of infection (both before and after HSCT).
- Allogeneic HSCT is curative, with fairly good results overall.
- Gene therapy trials are also under way. A similar condition has been reported in a girl with a deficiency in the Wiskott-Aldrich interacting protein.

Ans. D

193. Which of the following is considered as recipient or donor high risk factor?

A. Donor cold ischemia time >12 hrs
B. Donor age >50 yrs
C. Donor age >40 yrs with hypertension
D. Donor kidney biopsy >20% glomerulosclerosis

Explanation:

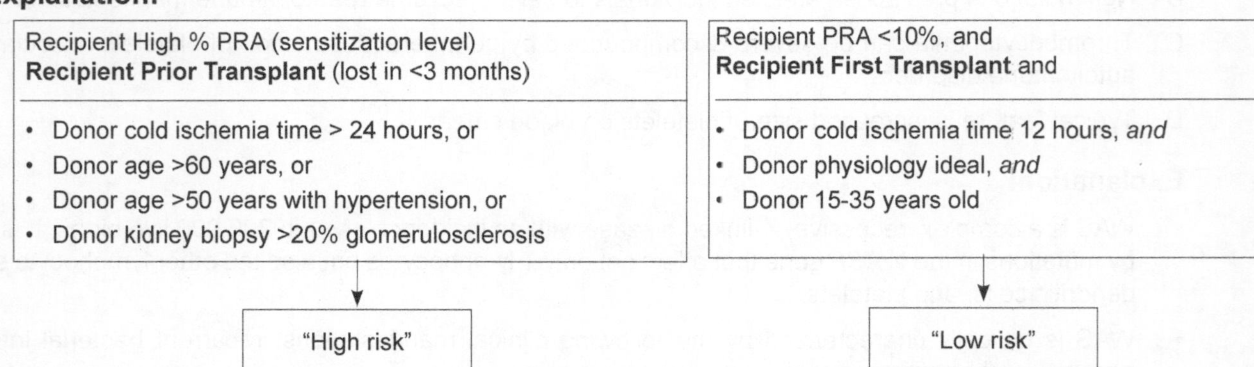

Ans. D

194. Autoantigen associated with cancer associated neuropathy is:

A. Hu
B. p53
C. p62
D. Recoverin

Explanation:

Table: Recombinant or purified autoantigens recognized by autoantibodies associated with human autoimmune disorders	
Autoantigen	**Autoimmune Disease**
Hu proteins	Paraneoplastic encephalomyelitis
Neuronal nicotinic acetylcholine receptor	Subacute autonomic neuropathy, cancer
p53	Cancer, systemic lupus erythematosus
p62 (IGF-II mRNA-binding protein)	Hepatocellular carcinoma (China)
Recoverin	Cancer-associated retinopathy
Ri protein	Paraneoplastic opsoclonus myoclonus ataxia
βIV spectrin	Lower motor neuron syndrome
Synaptotagmin	Lambert-Eaton myasthenic syndrome
Voltage-gated calcium channels	Lambert-Eaton myasthenic syndrome
Yo protein	Paraneoplastic cerebellar degeneration

Ans. D

195. 42 year old male presented with history of cough with expectoration and occasional hemoptysis. On examination no pedal edema. On routine evaluation found to have low sodium. True about euvolemic hyponatremia are a/e:

A. Creatinine will be low
B. Uric acid will be high
C. Cortisol deficiency may be present
D. Urine sodium will be high

Explanation:

- In euvolemic hyponatremia: Uric acid will be low.

Table: Differential diagnosis of hyponatremia based on clinical assessment of extracellular fluid volume (ECFV)				
Clinical Findings	**Type I, Hypervolemic**	**Type II, Hypovolemic**	**Type III, Euvolemic**	**SIADH and SIAD Euvolemic**
History				
• CHF, cirrhosis or nephrosis	Yes	No	No	No
• Salt and water loss	No	Yes	No	No
• ACTH-cortisol deficiency and/or nausea and vomiting	No	No	Yes	No
Physical examination				
• Generalized edema, ascites	Yes	No	No	No
• Postural hypotension	Maybe	Maybe	Maybe[a]	No
Laboratory				
• BUN, Creatinine	High-normal	High-normal	Low-normal	Low-normal
• Uric acid	High-normal	High-normal	Low-normal	Low-normal
• Serum potassium	Low-normal	Low-normal[b]	Normal[c]	Normal

Contd.

Contd.

Laboratory				
• Serum urate	High	High	Low	Low
• Serum albumin	Low-normal	High-normal	Normal	Normal
• Serum cortisol	Normal-high	Normal-high[d]	Low[e]	Normal
• Plasma renin activity	High	High	Low[f]	Low
• Urinary sodium (meq per unit of time)[g]	Low	Low[h]	High[i]	High[j]

Ans. B

196. Which of the following is a part of alternate complement pathway?

A. C1q
B. Factor D
C. C5-C8
D. C1r

Explanation:

- Complement system is composed of a complex cascade of plasma proteins that leads to the deposition of C3b fragments on the surface of particles and the formation of immune complexes that can culminate in the activation of a lytic complex at the bacterial surface.
- C3 cleavage can be mediated via three pathways: the classic, alternate, and lectin pathways.
- C3b coats particles as part of opsonization process that facilitates phagocytosis following binding to cognate receptors.
- Deficiency in any component of the classic pathway (c1q, c1r, c1s, C4, and C2) can predispose an individual to bacterial infections that are tissue-invasive or that occur in the respiratory tract.
- Likewise, a C3 deficiency or a deficiency in factor I (a protein that regulates C3 consumption, thus leading to a C3 deficiency due to its absence) also results in the same type of vulnerability to infection.
- It has recently been reported that a very rare deficiency in ficolin-3 predisposes affected individuals to bacterial infections.
- Deficiencies in the alternative pathway (factors D and properdin) are associated with the occurrence of invasive *Neisseria* infections.

Ans. B

197. ACE elevations of >50% of upper limit of normal are seen in all except:

A. Sarcoidosis
B. Leprosy
C. Pulmonary tuberculosis
D. Hyperthyroidism

Explanation:

- Serum levels of angiotensin-converting enzyme (ACE) can be helpful in the diagnosis of sarcoidosis. However, the test has somewhat low sensitivity and specificity.
- Elevated levels of ACE are reported in 60% of patients with acute disease and only 20% of patients with chronic disease.
- Although there are several causes for mild elevation of ACE, including diabetes, elevations of >50% of the upper limit of normal are seen in only a few conditions including sarcoidosis, leprosy, Gaucher's disease, hyperthyroidism, and disseminated granulomatous infections such as miliary tuberculosis.
- Because the ACE level is determined by a biologic assay, the concurrent use of an ACE inhibitor such as lisinopril will lead to a very low ACE level.

Ans. C

198. Infant with features mental retardation, enteropathy, neuropathy, deafness, ichthyosis. A diagnosis of MEDNIK syndrome was made.

Gene associated with above mentioned syndrome is:

A. APISI mutation

B. ATP7A mutation

C. ATP7B mutation

D. AIRE mutation

Explanation:

Of copper metabolism with features of both Menke's and Wilson's diseases has been reported. It is termed the MEDNIK (mental retardation, enteropathy, deafness, neuropathy, ichthyosis, keratodermia) syndrome and is caused by mutations in the AP1S1 gene, which encodes an adaptor protein necessary for intracellular trafficking of copper pump proteins ATP7A (Menke's disease) and ATP7B (Wilson's disease).

Ans. A

199. A 60 year old male was brought to the ER with complaints of sudden onset of breathlessness following a RTA. BLUE protocol was followed to assess the patient. Ultrasound chest can detect all of the following except:

A. Pneumothorax

B. Pleural effusion

C. Pulmonary edema

D. Pulmonary hypertension

Explanation:

- Diagnostic Ultrasound is not useful for assessing the pulmonary parenchyma or pulmonary vasculature, but it can detect and localize pleural abnormalities such as pleural effusion and pneumothorax.

Ans. D

200. 59 year old female presented to causality with history of fall in home and sustained left femur fracture. She was operated for the same. Post op she was evaluated for osteoporosis. She was treated with antiosteoporotic drug. ACTIVE trial is on:

A. Abaloparatide

B. Romosozumab

C. Denosumab

D. Odanacatib

Explanation:

Analogues for what appeared to be an optimized anabolic profile. In the Phase 3 Abaloparatide Comparator Trial in Vertebral Endpoints (ACTIVE) study, 2463 postmenopausal women with osteoporosis were randomized to blinded daily subcutaneous abaloparatide.

Ans. A

201. A 52 year old male presented to the OPD with complaints of cough, breathlessness and right sided pleuritic chest pain. Chest X-ray shows ellis curve on the right lung suggestive of right sided pleural effusion. Which among the following statements regarding chest X-ray is false?

A. Postero-anterior and lateral views are most often used to diagnose respiratory symptoms

B. Antero-posterior view is routinely taken in bed-ridden patients

C. Lateral decubitus view can be used to estimate the size of freely flowing pleural effusion

D. None of the above

Explanation:

- Chest X-ray (CXR), generally including both posteroanterior and lateral views, is often the first diagnostic study in pts presenting with respiratory symptoms. With diffuse lung disease, CXR can detect an alveolar, interstitial, or nodular pattern. CXR can also detect pleural effusion and pneumothorax, as well as abnormalities in the hila and mediastinum. Lateral decubitus views can be used to estimate the size of freely flowing pleural effusions.

Ans. D

202. A 40 year old male was diagnosed with smatter triad of aspirin sensitivity, nasal polyposis and asthma. Intrinsic asthma is associated with:

A. Atopic dermatitis
B. Allergic rhinitis
C. Allergic conjunctivitis
D. All of the above

Explanation:

- Majority of asthmatics have childhood-onset disease. Most asthmatics have atopy, and they often have atopic dermatitis (eczema) and/or allergic rhinitis. This phenotype is known as extrinsic asthma. A minority of asthmatic pts do not have atopy (negative skin prick tests to common allergens and normal serum total IgE levels). These individuals, occasionally referred to as intrinsic asthmatics, often have adult-onset disease.

Ans. D

203. Largest mammalian lymphoid organ system is:

A. MALT
B. Thoracic duct
C. GALT
D. Sympathetic duct

Explanation:

- In the healthy adult, mucosa-associated lymphoid tissue (MALT) contains 80% of all immune cells within the body and constitutes the largest mammalian lymphoid organ system.

Ans. A

204. A 50 year old male with 40 pack years of smoking was advised smoking cessation and pneumococcal vaccination. Match the following smoking cessation drugs:

A. Vernicillin	1. Inhibits the re uptake of nor epinephrine and dopamine
B. Bupropion	2. Partial agonists for nicotinic ACH receptors
C. Nicotin	3. Banned in India.
D. E-cigarettes	4. Binds selectively to nicotinic cholinergic receptors

A. A2, B1, C4, D3
B. A2, B4, C1, D3
C. A3, B4, C2, D1
D. A3, B1, C4, D2

Explanation:

- Elimination of tobacco smoking has been convincingly shown to reduce decline in pulmonary function and to prolong survival in pts with COPD; complete smoking cessation is essential for all COPD patients.
- Although lung function does not typically improve substantially after smoking cessation, the rate of decline in FEV1 often reverts to that of nonsmokers.
- Pharmacologic treatment to assist with smoking cessation is often beneficial. Use of nicotine replacement therapy (available as a transdermal patch, gum, lozenge, nasal spray, and oral inhaler) can increase rates

of smoking cessation; oral bupropion also produces significant benefit and can be combined successfully with nicotine replacement.

- Varenicline, a partial agonist for nicotinic acetylcholine receptors, also can promote smoking cessation. All adult, nonpregnant smokers without specific contraindications should be offered pharmacologic treatment to assist with smoking cessation.

Ans. A

205. A 65 year old male presented to the OPD with acute exacerbation of COPD with symptoms of cough with mucopurulent sputum, breathlessness and fever for 2 days duration. Common pathogens associated with COPD exacerbation include all except:

A. Moraxella catarrhalis
B. Streptococcus pneumonia
C. Staphylococcus aureus
D. Hemophilus influenza

Explanation:

- Because bacterial infections often trigger COPD exacerbations, antibiotic therapy should be strongly considered, especially with increased sputum volume or change in sputum color. Common pathogens include Streptococcus pneumoniae, Haemophilus influenzae, and Moraxella catarrhalis.
- Antibiotic choice should depend on the local antibiotic sensitivity patterns and the severity of disease.

Ans. C

206. A 30-year-old female in the third trimester of pregnancy, presents to the causality with progressive dyspnoea for the past 2 days. On examination, breath sounds are diminished on both the lung bases. The HR is 120 beats per minute and BP-100/70mmHg. Baseline blood investigations were found to be normal. Chest X-ray is normal. Which of the following is the next diagnostic procedure?

A. D-dimer
B. CT pulmonary angiography
C. Lower limb Doppler
D. Lung perfusion scintigraphy

Explanation:

- D dimers are typically elevated during pregnancy and therefore are not useful in this patient.
- CT pulmonary angiography and lung perfusion scintigraphy are both associated with ionizing radiation and hence should be used with caution in pregnancy.
- Hence lower limb Doppler would be the ideal first diagnostic procedure in this scenario to detect deep vein thrombosis.
- If this is positive, pulmonary embolism can be assumed and treated with heparin.

Ans. C

207. All are true about lower back pain except:

A. ALBP is defined as pain of <3 months in duration
B. There is good evidence to support the use of opioid analgesics or tramadol as first-line therapy for ALBP
C. Back pain is the most frequent reason for seeking complementary and alternative treatments
D. Term sciatica is used when the leg pain radiates posteriorly in a sciatic or L5/S1 distribution

Explanation:

- There is no good evidence to support the use of opioid analgesics or tramadol as first-line therapy for ALBP.
- Their use is best reserved for patients who cannot tolerate acetaminophen or NSAIDs and for those with severe refractory pain.
- As with muscle relaxants, these drugs are often sedating, so it may be useful to prescribe them at night time only.

- Side effects of short-term opioid use include nausea, constipation, and pruritus; risks of long-term opioid use include hypersensitivity to pain, hypogonadism, and dependency.
- Falls, fractures, driving accidents, and fecal impaction are other risks.
- Clinical efficacy of opioids for chronic pain beyond 16 weeks of use is unproven.

Ans. B

208. 48 year old male married recently came to OPD to enquire regarding the effect of having a child at this age. As a physician you advised him that there are increased incidence of disease associated with increased paternal age. Disease which increases with increase in paternal age:

A. Achondroplasia
B. Marfan's syndrome
C. Apert syndrome
D. All of the above

Explanation:

Disease which increases with advanced paternal age:

- Achondroplasia
- Marfan's syndrome
- Apert syndrome
- Schizophrenia
- Autism
- Polyposis coli

The frequency of chromosomal aneuploidy is increased in the sperm of older men. However, the **incidence of autosomal dominant diseases, such as achondroplasia, polyposis coli, Marfan syndrome, and Apert syndrome, increase in the offspring of men who are advanced in age, consistent with transmission of sporadic missense mutations.** Advanced paternal age **may be associated with increased rates of de novo mutations, which may contribute to an increased risk of neurodevelopmental diseases such as schizophrenia and autism.**

Ans. D

209. Clutton's joint is seen in:

A. Congenital syphilis
B. Primary syphilis
C. Secondary syphilis
D. Tertiary syphilis

Explanation:

- In early congenital syphilis, periarticular swelling and immobilization of involved limbs (*Parrot's pseudoparalysis*) complicate osteochondritis of long bones.
- *Clutton's joint*, a late manifestation of congenital syphilis that typically develops between ages 8 and 15 years, is caused by chronic painless synovitis with effusions of large joints, particularly knees and elbows.
- Secondary syphilis may be associated with arthralgias, with symmetric arthritis of the knees and ankles and occasionally of the shoulders and wrists, and with sacroiliitis.
- Arthritis follows subacute to chronic course with a mixed mononuclear and neutrophilic synovial-fluid pleocytosis (typical cell counts, 5000–15,000/μL).
- Immunologic mechanisms may contribute to the arthritis, and symptoms usually improve rapidly with penicillin therapy.
- In tertiary syphilis, Charcot joint results from sensory loss due to tabes dorsalis.

Ans. A

210. Agents causing community acquired pneumonia in outpatients include all except:

A. Streptococcus pneumonia
B. Mycoplasma pneumonia
C. C.pneumoniae
D. Staphylococcus aureus

Explanation:

Table: Microbial causes of community-acquired pneumonia by site of care

Outpatients	Hospitalized patients	
	Non-ICU	ICU
Streptococcus pneumoniae	*S. pneumoniae*	*S. pneumoniae*
Mycoplasma pneumoniae	*M. pneumoniae*	*Staphylococcus aureus*
Haemophilus influenzae	*Chlamydia pneumoniae*	*Legionella spp.*
C. pneumoniae	*H. influenzae*	Gram-negative bacilli
Respiratory viruses[a]	*Legionella* spp.	*H. influenzae*
	Respiratory viruses[a]	Respiratory viruses

Ans. D

211. Coxiella burnetti transmitted through all except:

A. Sheep
B. Birds
C. Cats
D. Goats

Explanation:

Table: Epidemiologic factors suggesting possible causes of community-acquired pneumonia

Factor	Possible Pathogen(s)
Alcoholism	*Streptococcus pneumoniae*, oral anaerobes, *Klebsiella, pneumoniae, Acinetobacter* spp., *Mycobacterium tuberculosis*
COPD and/or smoking	*Haemophilus influenzae, Pseudomonas aeruginosa, Legionella spp.*, S. pneumoniae, *Moraxella catarrhalis, Chlamydia pneumoniae*
Structural lung disease (e.g., bronchiectasis)	*P. aeruginosa, Burkholderia cepacia, Staphylococcus aureus*
Dementia, stroke, decreased level of consciousness	Oral anaerobes, gram-negative enteric bacteria
Lung abscess	CA-MRSA, oral anaerobes, endemic fungi, *M. tuberculosis*, atypical mycobacteria
Travel to Ohio or St. Lawrence river valley	*Histoplasma capsulatum*
Travel to southwestem United States	Hantavirus, *Coccidioides* spp.
Travel to Southeast Asia	*Burkholderia pseudomallei*, avian influenza virus
Stay in hotel or on cruise ship in previous 2 weeks	*Legionella* spp.
Local influenza activity	Influenza virus, *S. pneumoniae, S. aureus*
Exposure to bats or birds	*H. capsulatum*
Exposure to birds	*Chlamydia psittaci*
Exposure to rabbits	*Francisella tularensis*
Exposure to sheep, goats, parturient cats	*Coxiella burnetii*

Ans. B

212. 32 year old female presented with features of tetany, tremor, seizures and found to have normal calcium. On further evaluation found to Have serum Mg+2 levels of 0.9mg/dl which is low. History of drug intake+. Which of the drug causes hypomagnesemia?

A. Rituximab
B. Cetuximab
C. Infliximab
D. Romososumab

Explanation:

Table: Causes of hypomagnesemia	
I. Impaired intestinal absorption A. Hypomagnesemia with secondary hypocalcemia (TRPM6 mutations) B. Malabsorption syndromes C. Vitamin D deficiency D. Proton pump inhibitors II. Increased intestinal losses A. Protracted vomiting/diarrhea B. Intestinal drainage, fistulas III. Impaired renal tubular reabsorption A. Genetic magnesium-wasting syndromes 1. Gitelman's syndrome 2. Bartter's syndrome 3. Claudin 16 or 19 mutations 4. Potassium channel mutations (KV1.1, Kir 4.1) 5. Na^+, K^+-ATPase γ-subunit mutations (FXYD2) B. Acquired renal disease 1. Tubulointerstitial disease 2. Postobstruction, ATN (diuretic phase) 3. Renal transplantation C. Drugs and toxins 1. Ethanol 2. Diuretics (loop, thiazide, osmotic) 3. Cisplatin 4. Pentamidine, foscarnet 5. Cyclosporine 6. Aminoglycosides, amphotericin B 7. Cetuximab	D. Other 1. Extracellular fluid volume expansion 2. Hyperaldosteronism 3. SIADH 4. Diabetes mellitus 5. Hypercalcemia 6. Phosphate depletion 7. Metabolic acidosis 8. Hyperthyroidism IV. Rapid shifts from extracellular fluid A. Intracellular redistribution 1. Recovery from diabetic ketoacidosis 2. Refeeding syndrome 3. Correction of respiratory acidosis 4. Catecholamines B. Accelerated bone formation 1. Post-parathyroidectomy 2. Treatment of vitamin D deficiency 3. Osteoblastic metastases C. Other 1. Pancreatitis, burns, excessive sweating 2. Pregnancy (third trimester) and lactation

Drug causing hypomagnesemia:

- Cetuximab
- Aminoglycosides
- PPI
- Foscarnet
- Pentamidine
- Cyclosporine
- Cisplatin
- Diuretics
- Ethanol
- Amphotericin B

Ans. B

213. Osmolarity of parenteral nutrition solution is:

A. >1500 mOsm/L
B. >1200 mOsm/L
C. >500 mOsm/L
D. >1000 mOsm/L

Explanation:

- PN delivers a complete nutritional regimen directly into the bloodstream in the form of crystalline amino acids, dextrose, triglyceride emulsions, minerals (calcium, phosphate, magnesium, and zinc), electrolytes, and micronutrients.
- Because of its high osmolarity (>1200 mOsm/L) and often large volume, PN is infused into a central vein in adults.
- Ready-to-use PN admixtures typically containing 4–7% hydrous amino acids and 20–25% dextrose (with or without electrolytes) are available in 2-chamber (amino acids and dextrose) or 3-chamber (amino acids, dextrose, and lipid) bags that are intermixed and vitamins, trace minerals and additional electrolytes added just prior to infusion.

Ans. B

214. Continuous EN is the only option with:

A. Oral feeding
B. Nasogastric feeding
C. Intragastric feeding
D. Jejunal feeding

Explanation:

- Debilitated patients with delayed gastric emptying, impaired gag reflex, and ineffective cough are at high risk of aspiration pneumonia.
- Aspiration is particularly common in mechanically ventilated patients. Ventilator-associated pneumonia is mostly caused by aspiration of microbial pathogens in the mouth and throat past the cuffs of endotracheal or tracheostomy tubes, but tracheal suctioning induces coughing and gastric regurgitation.
- Measures to prevent ventilator-associated pneumonia include elevation of head of bed, mouth hygiene and gastrointestinal decontamination, nurse-directed algorithms for formula advancement and, sometimes, post–pyloric feeding.
- EN does not have to be held for gastric residual volumes less than 300 to 400 mL in the absence of other signs of gastrointestinal intolerance (nausea, vomiting, severe abdominal pain, abdominal distention).
- Continuous EN is often tolerated better than bolus feeding, and it is the only option with jejunal feeding.

Ans. D

215. All antigen are localized to cytoplasm except:

A. HDV
B. HCV
C. HEV
D. HAV

Explanation:

- HBcAg predominates in the nucleus, but, occasionally, scant amounts are also seen in the cytoplasm and on the cell membrane. HDV antigen is localized to the hepatocyte nucleus, whereas HAV, HCV, and HEV antigens are localized to the cytoplasm.

Ans. A

216. A female patient weighs ~60 kg. Calculate free water deficit in this patient with serum sodium of 150 meq/l.

A. 3.11L
B. 2.14L
C. 5.21L
D. 6.44L

Explanation:

- Free water deficit = $\frac{\text{TBW} \times (\text{S. Na+} - 140)}{140}$
- TBW : 0.6 × body weight (kg) in Males
  : 0.5 × body weight (kg) in females

Ans. B

217. All are seen in Cushing's syndrome except:

A. DVT/PE
B. Increased WBC
C. Eosinophilia
D. Increased susceptibility to infections

Explanation:

- Patient with Cushing's syndrome may manifest specific findings, such as central fat redistribution, skin striae, and proximal muscle weakness, in addition to features seen commonly in the general population, such as obesity, plethora, hypertension, and glucose intolerance.
- Similarly, the insidious onset of hypothyroidism—with mental slowing, fatigue, dry skin, and other features—can be difficult to distinguish from similar, nonspecific findings in the general population.
- Typical features of chronic cortisol excess include thin skin, central obesity, hypertension, plethoric moon facies, purple striae and easy bruisability, glucose intolerance or diabetes mellitus, gonadal dysfunction, osteoporosis, proximal muscle weakness, signs of hyperandrogenism (acne, hirsutism), and psychological disturbances (depression, mania, and psychoses).
- Hematopoietic features of hypercortisolism include leukocytosis, lymphopenia and eosinopenia.
- Immune suppression includes delayed hypersensitivity and infection propensity.

Ans. C

218. Most common side effect of inhibitors of VEGF is:

A. Hypertension
B. Vomiting
C. Hemorrhage
D. Inhibition of wound healing

Explanation:

- Hypertension is the most common side effect of inhibitors of VEGF (or its receptors), but can be treated with antihypertensive agents and uncommonly requires discontinuation of therapy.
- Rare but serious potential risks include arterial thromboembolic events, including stroke and myocardial infarction, hemorrhage, bowel perforation, and inhibition of wound healing.

Ans. A

219. All are true about opioids except:

A. Normeperidine accumulation is increased in patients with renal failure
B. Synergistic respiratory depression is common when opioids are administered with other CNS depressants, most commonly the benzodiazepines

C. Methylnaltrexone has proven effective for relief of opioid-induced constipation

D. Alvimopan is given subcutaneously and has proven effective in lowering the respiratory depression caused by opioids

Explanation:

- Alvimopan is available as an orally administered agent that is restricted to the intestinal lumen by limited absorption; methyl naltrexone is available in a subcutaneously administered form that has virtually no penetration into the CNS.
- Both agents act by binding to peripheral μ-receptors, thereby inhibiting or reversing the effects of opioids at these peripheral sites.
- Action of both agents is restricted to receptor sites outside of the CNS; thus, these drugs can reverse adverse effects of opioid analgesics that are mediated through their peripheral receptors without reversing their analgesic effects.
- Alvimopan has proven effective in lowering the duration of persistent ileus following abdominal surgery in patients receiving opioid analgesics for postop pain control.
- Methyl naltrexone has proven effective for relief of opioid-induced constipation in patients taking opioid analgesics on a chronic basis.

Ans. D

220. SIRS criteria include all of the following except:

A. Fever
B. Hypotension
C. Tachycardia
D. Tachypnea

Explanation:

Table: Definitions and criteria for sepsis and septic shock

Condition	Definition	Common Clinical Features	Criteria in 1991/2003 ("Sepsis-1"/ "Sepsis-2")	Criteria in 2016 ("Sepsis-3")
Sepsis	A life-threatening organ dysfunction caused by a dysregulated host response to infection	Include signs of infection, with organ dysfunction, plus altered mentation; tachypnea; hypotension; hepatic, renal or hematologic dysfunction	Suspected (or documented) infection plus ≥ 2 systemic in inflammatory response syndrome (SIRS) criteria[a]	Suspected (or documented) infection and an acute increase in ≥ 22 sepsis-related organ failure assessment (SOFA) points[b]
Septic shock	A subset of sepsis in which underlying circulatory and cellular/metabolic abnormalities lead to substantially increased mortality risk	Signs of infection, plus altered mentation, oliguria, cool peripheries, hyperlactemia	Suspected (or documented) infection plus persistent arterial hypotension (systolic arterial pressure, < 90 mm Hg; mean arterial pressure, < 60 mm Hg; or change in systolic by > 40 mm Hg from baseline	Suspected (or documented) infection plus vasopressor therapy needed to maintain mean arterial pressure at ≥ 65 mm Hg and serum loctate > 2.0 mmol/l; despite adequate fluid resuscitation

[a] SIRS criteria include 1 point for each of the following (score range, 0.4: fever >38°C (>100.4°F) or < 36°C (< 96.8°F); tachypnea with > 20 breaths per min; tachycardia with heart rate > 90 beats per min; leucocytosis with white blood cell count >12,000/ml; leukopenia (< 4000/μl) or > 10% bands.

[b] SOFA score is a 24-point measure of organ dysfunction that uses six organ systems (renal, cardiovascular, pulmonary, hepatic, neurologic, hematologic), where 0-4 points are assigned per organ system.

Ans. B

221. All true about exposure and infection except:

A. Raw meat with Toxoplasma gondii
B. Unpasteurized milk with M.bovis
C. Unpurified water with Norovirus
D. Raw seafood with Vibrio

Explanation:

- As certain pathogens are associated with specific dietary habits, inquiring about a patient's diet can provide insight into possible exposures.
- For example, Shiga toxin–producing strains of *Escherichia coli* and *Toxoplasma gondii* are associated with consumption of raw or undercooked meat; *Salmonella typhimurium*, *Listeria monocytogenes*, and *Mycobacterium bovis* with unpasteurized milk; *Leptospira* species, parasites, and enteric bacteria with unpurified water; and *Vibrio* species, norovirus, helminths, and protozoa with raw seafood.

Ans. C

222. Most common infection caused by Enterococci is:

A. Nosocomial UTI
B. Meningitis
C. Peritonitis
D. Pneumonia

Explanation:

- Enterococci are well-known causes of nosocomial UTI—the most common infection caused by these organisms. Enterococcal UTIs are usually associated with indwelling catheterization, instrumentation, or anatomic abnormalities of the genitourinary tract, and it is often challenging to differentiate between true infection and colonization (particularly in patients with chronic indwelling catheters).
- Presence of leukocytes in the urine in conjunction with systemic manifestations (e.g., fever) or local signs and symptoms of infection with no other explanation and a positive urine culture (≥105 CFU/mL) suggests the diagnosis.

Ans. A

223. Most common side effects of β2- agonists when given by inhalation is:

A. Muscle tremors
B. Myositis
C. Nausea
D. Headache

Explanation:

- Adverse effects are not usually a problem with β2-agonists when given by inhalation.
- Most common side effects are muscle tremor and palpitations, which are seen more commonly in elderly patients. There is a small fall in plasma potassium due to increased uptake by skeletal muscle cells, but this effect does not usually cause any clinical problem.

Ans. A

224. Relative bradycardia occurs in which of the following fever?

A. Typhoid
B. Brucellosis
C. Leptospirosis
D. All of the above

Explanation:

Fever associated with relative bradycardia

- Typhoid

- Brucellosis
- Leptospirosis
- Drug induced fever
- Factitious fever

Ans. D

225. In malaria fever is characterized by certain patterns, fever during third day is caused by:

A. P.vivax
B. P.ovale
C. P.Falciparum
D. P.Malaria

Explanation:

Fever Pattern

- P. vivax- Fever every third day
- P. malaria- Fever every fourth day

Ans. A

226. Which of the following painful conditions won't respond to tricyclic anti-depressants?

A. Fibromyalgia
B. Migraine
C. Myocardial infarction
D. Post herpetic Neuralgia

Explanation:

Painful conditions that respond to tricyclic anti-depressants

- Post herpetic Neuralgia
- Diabetic Neuropathy
- Fibromyalgia
- Tension Headache
- Migraine Headache
- Rheumatoid arthritis
- Cancer
- Chronic low back pain
- Central post stroke pain

Ans. C

227. Eschar is seen in which of the following fever:

A. Rickettsial pox
B. Chronic meningococcemia
C. Viral Haemorrhagic fever
D. Bacillary Angiomatosis

Explanation:

Eschar is seen in

- Scrub typhus
- Rat bite fever
- Rickettsial pox
- Tularemia
- Ecthyma Gangrenosum

Ans. A

228. Forschheimer spots are seen in:

A. Rubella
B. Measles
C. HIV
D. Scrub typhus fever

Explanation:

- Forschheimer spots are special rashes seen in Rubella infection.

Ans. A

229. Treatment of choice for hypovolemic hyponatremia is:

A. Fluid restriction
B. Tolvaptan
C. Conivaptan
D. Normal saline

Explanation:

- In hypovolemic hyponatremia, the imbalance can be corrected easily and quickly by stopping the loss of sodium and water and/or replacing the deficits by mouth or IV infusion of normal or hypertonic saline.
- As with the treatment of other forms of hyponatremia, care must be taken to ensure that plasma sodium does not increase too rapidly or too far.
- Fluid restriction and administration of AVP antagonists are contraindicated in type II hyponatremia because they would only aggravate the underlying volume depletion and could result in hemodynamic collapse.

Ans. D

230. Drug of choice for SIADH due to V2 receptor gene mutation:

A. Tolvaptan
B. Urea
C. Fludrocortisone
D. Demeclocycline

Explanation:

- In SIADH due to an activating mutation of the V2 receptor, the V2 antagonists may not block the antidiuresis or raise plasma osmolarity/sodium. In that condition, use of an osmotic diuretic such as urea is reported to be effective in preventing or correcting hyponatremia.
- However, some vaptans may be effective in patients with a different type of activating mutation so the response to this therapy may be neither predictable nor diagnostic.

Ans. B

231. SIADH is caused by all except:

A. Pneumonia
B. Stroke
C. NSIAD
D. Cortisol

Explanation:

- Euvolemic hyponatremia, however, is due mainly to expansion of total body water caused by excessive intake in the face of a failure to dilute the urine in response to excessive water intake.
- Impaired dilution is usually caused by a defect in the osmotic suppression of AVP that can have either of two causes.
- One is a nonhemodynamic stimulus such as nausea or a cortisol deficiency, which can be corrected quickly by treatment with antiemetics or cortisol.
- Other is a primary defect in osmoregulation caused by another disorder such as malignancy, stroke, or pneumonia that cannot be easily or quickly corrected.

- Latter is commonly known as the syndrome of inappropriate antidiuretic hormone (SIADH).
- Much less often, euvolemic hyponatremia can also result from AVP-independent activation of renal V2 receptors, a variant known as nephrogenic inappropriate antidiuresis or NSIAD.

Ans. D

232. Assertion(A): Primary polydipsia causes hyponatremia.
Reason(R): Increase in fluid intake causes reduces plasma sodium concentration.

A. Both (A) and (R) are correct and (R) explains (A)

B. Both (A) and (R) are correct but (R) doesn't explain (A)

C. (R) is correct But (A) is false

D. (A) is correct But (R) is false

Explanation:

- In primary polydipsia, the pathogenesis of the polydipsia and poly-uria is the reverse of that in pituitary, nephrogenic, and gestational DI.
- In primary polydipsia, an abnormality in cognition or thirst causes excessive intake of fluids and an increase in body water that reduces plasma osmolarity/sodium, AVP secretion, and urinary concentration.
- Dilution of the urine, in turn, results in a compensatory increase in urinary free-water excretion that usually offsets the increase in intake and stabilizes plasma osmolarity/sodium at a level only 1–2% below basal.
- Thus, hyponatremia or clinically appreciable over hydration is uncommon unless the polydipsia is very severe or the compensatory water diuresis is impaired by a drug or disease that stimulates or mimics the antiduretic effect of endogenous AVP.

Ans. C

233. A 40 year old patient came with vertigo and tinnitus. His examination showed peripheral nystagmus. Which of the following findings is not suggestive of peripheral nystagmus?

A. Direction changes with gaze

B. Mixed vertical and torsional nystagmus

C. Inhibited by visual fixation

D. Normal head impulse test

Explanation:

- Nystagmus from an acute peripheral lesion is unidirectional, with fast phases beating away from the ear with the lesion. Nystagmus that changes direction with gaze is due to a central lesion.
- Transient mixed vertical-torsional nystagmus occurs in benign paroxysmal positional vertigo (BPPV), but pure vertical or pure torsional nystagmus is a central sign
- Nystagmus from a peripheral lesion may be inhibited by visual fixation, whereas central nystagmus is not suppressed.
- Absence of a head impulse sign in a patient with acute prolonged vertigo should suggest a central cause.
- Unilateral hearing loss suggests peripheral vertigo. Findings such as diplopia, dysarthria, and limb ataxia suggest a central disorder.

Ans. A

234. Which of the following drug is neprilysin inhibitor?

A. Seralaxin

B. Nesiritide

C. Sacubitril – Valsartan

D. Levosimendan

Explanation:

- Sacubitril is an endopeptidase inhibitor and valsartan is an angiotensin receptor blocker has been now a days prescribed in heart failure with reduced ejection fraction.
- It is an neprilysin inhibitor. This combination is called as ARNI (Angiotensin receptor – neprilysin inhibitor)
- Seralaxin is an is recombinant human relaxin 2 that causes vasodilatation and decreases the effect of vasoconstrictors. It is approved in Russia for acute heart failure.
- Nesiritide is an is an recombinant type of human B type natriuretic peptide which is normally produced by ventricular myocardium. It causes counter regulation of the renin angiotensin aldosterone system, stimulating cyclic guanosine monophosphate causing smooth muscle relaxation.
- Levosimendan is an calcium sensitizer it increases sensitivity of heart to calcium causing increase in cardiac contractility, used as an ionotropic agent in case of cardiogenic shock. It is an longer acting.

Ans. C

235. Liddles syndrome occurs due to mutation in which channel?

A. Sodium
B. Potassium
C. Calcium
D. Magnesium

Explanation:

Liddles syndrome

- It is an Autosomal dominant hereditary disorder of sodium channel mutation (SCNN1 B and SCNN1 C genes) causing hypertension.
- It is associated with low renin, low potassium, metabolic alkalosis, low aldosterone
- It occurs due to dysregulation of sodium channel in epithelial cells of kidney causing more reabsorption of sodium and excretion of potassium. Thus more sodium reabsorption causes more retention of water in body causing hypertension.
- As more extravascular volume is present so there is low aldosterone in liddles syndrome.
- It is treated with low sodium diet & potassium sparing diuretics (amiloride, triamterene).

Ans. A

236. Fever is typically absent in TSS caused by:

A. C.sordellii
B. Staph. Aureus
C. Streptococcus
D. Staph. Epidermidis

Explanation:

- TSS caused by *Clostridium sordellii* is associated with childbirth or with skin injection of black-tar heroin.
- Diagnosis of TSS is defined by the clinical criteria of fever, rash, hypotension, and multiorgan involvement. (Of note, fever is typically absent when TSS is caused by *C. sordellii*).
- Mortality rate is 5% for menstruation associated TSS, 10–15% for nonmenstrual TSS, 30–70% for streptococcal TSS, and up to 90% for obstetric *C. sordellii* TSS.
- Clindamycin improves outcomes when included in the treatment regimen.
- Some studies have shown that use of IV immunoglobulin is associated with improved survival as well.

Ans. A

237. Live virus vaccines are contraindicated in:

A. Pregnancy
B. Breast feeding
C. Both of the above
D. None of the above

Explanation:

- Live-virus vaccines are contraindicated during pregnancy because of the hypothetical risk that vaccine virus replication will cause congenital infection or have other adverse effects on the fetus.
- Most live-virus vaccines, including varicella vaccine, are not secreted in breast milk; therefore, breast-feeding is not a contraindication for live-virus or other vaccines.
- Pregnancy is not a contraindication to administration of inactivated vaccines, but most are avoided during pregnancy because relevant safety data are limited.

Ans. A

238. All are true about fulminant malaria except:

A. Fulminant malaria is caused by Plasmodium falciparum

B. By definition, any patient with a change in mental status or repeated seizure in the setting of fulminant malaria has cerebral malaria

C. Nuchal rigidity and photophobia are common

D. Symmetric encephalopathy is typical, and upper motor neuron dysfunction with decorticate and decerebrate posturing can be seen in advanced disease

Explanation:

- Cerebral malaria should be urgently considered if patients who have recently travelled to areas endemic for malaria present with a febrile illness and lethargy or other neurologic signs.
- Fulminant malaria is caused by *Plasmodium falciparum* and is associated with temperatures of >40°C (>104°F), hypotension, jaundice, acute respiratory distress syndrome, and bleeding.
- By definition, any patient with a change in mental status or repeated seizure in the setting of fulminant malaria has cerebral malaria.
- In adults, this nonspecific febrile illness progresses to coma over several days; occasionally, coma occurs within hours and death within 24 h.
- **Nuchal rigidity and photophobia are rare.**
- On physical examination, symmetric encephalopathy is typical, and upper motor neuron dysfunction with decorticate and decerebrate posturing can be seen in advanced disease.
- Unrecognized infection results in a 20–30% mortality rate.

Ans. C

239. Regarding Rhinocerebral mucormycosis all are true except:

A. High grade fever

B. Dull sinus pain

C. Diplopia

D. Proptosis

Explanation:

- Individuals with diabetes or immunocompromising conditions such as solid organ transplants or hematologic malignancies are at risk for invasive rhinocerebral mucormycosis.
- Patients present with low-grade fever, dull sinus pain, diplopia, decreased mental status, decreased ocular motion, chemosis, proptosis, dusky or necrotic nasal turbinates, and necrotic hard-palate lesions that respect the midline.
- Without rapid recognition and intervention, the process continues on an inexorable invasive course, with mortality rates of 50–85% or greater.
- Uncontrolled diabetes and increasing age are negative prognostic factors.

Ans. A

240. Infants are the target for this vaccination:

A. Zoster
B. Hepatitis B
C. Tetanus
D. Rotavirus

Explanation:

Table: Disease preventable with vaccines routinely administered in the United States to children and/or adults	
Condition	**Target Populations(s) for Routine Use**
Pertussis	Children, adolescents, adults
Diphtheria	Children, adolescents, adults
Tetanus	Children, adolescents, adults
Poliomyelitis	Children
Measles	Children
Mumps	Children
Rubella, congenital rubella syndrome	Children
Hepatitis B	Children and high-risk adults
Hemophilus influenzae type b infection	Children
Hepatitis A	Children
Influenza	Children, adolescents, adults
Varicella	Children
Pneumococcal disease	Children, older adults
Meningococcal disease	Adolescents and high-risk adults
Rotavirus infection	Infants
Human papillomavirus infection, cervical and anogenital cancers	Adolescents and young adults
Zoster	Older adults

Ans. D

241. All are risk factors for resistance to usual therapy for community acquired MRSA except:

A. Summer month onset
B. Neutropenia
C. Elderly, with comorbidities
D. Erythematous rash

Explanation:

Table: Risk factors for pathogens resistant to usual therapy for community-acquired pneumonia[a]		
Multidrug-Resistant Gram-Negative Bacteria and MRSA	**Nosocomial MRSA**	**Community-Acquired MRSA**
Hospitalization ≥ 2 days in previous 90 days	Hospitalization ≥ 2 days in previous 90 days	Cavitary infiltrate or necrosis
Use of antibiotics in previous 90 days	Use of antibiotics in previous 90 days	Gross hemoptysis
Immunosuppression	Chronic hemodialysis in previous 30 days	Neutropenia
Nonambulatory status	Documented prior MRSA colonization	Erythematous rash
Tube feedings	Congestive heart failure	Concurrent influenza
Gastric acid suppression	Gastric acid suppression	Young, previously healthy status
Severe COPD or bronchiectasis[b]		Summer-month onset

Ans. C

242. Most of the activated KRAS alleles contain point mutations in following codons except:

A. 12
B. 13
C. 14
D. 61

Explanation:

- Point mutation (alternatively known as single nucleotide substitution) is a common mechanism of oncogene activation.
- For example, mutations in *KRAS* are present in > 95% of pancreatic cancers and 40% of colon cancers but are less common in other cancer types, although they can occur at significant frequencies in leukemia, lung, and thyroid cancers.
- Remarkably—and in contrast to diversity of mutations found in tumor-suppressor genes—most of the activated *K*RAS alleles contain point mutations in codons 12, 13, or 61.
- These mutations reduce RAS GTPase activity, leading to constitutive activation of the mutant RAS protein.
- Restricted pattern of mutations observed in oncogenes compared to that of tumor-suppressor genes reflects fact that gain-of-function mutations must occur at specific sites, while a broad variety of mutations can lead to loss of activity.

Ans. C

243. Which of the following is true regarding Tietze's syndrome?

A. Cervical radiculitis
B. Costochondritis
C. Tendinits
D. Zoster Herpes

Explanation:

- Chest discomfort can be produced by any musculoskeletal disorder involving the chest wall or the nerves of the chest wall, neck, or upper limbs.
- Costochondritis causing tenderness of the costochondral junctions (*Tietze's syndrome*) is relatively common.
- Cervical radiculitis may manifest as a prolonged or constant aching discomfort in the upper chest and limbs. Pain may be exacerbated by motion of the neck.
- Occasionally, chest pain can be caused by compression of the brachial plexus by the cervical ribs, and tendinitis or bursitis involving the left shoulder may mimic the radiation of angina. Pain in a dermatomal distribution can also be caused by cramping of intercostal muscles or by herpes zoster

Ans. B

244. Primary diagnostic test for CNS infections caused by CMV, EBV, HHV6 and enterovirus is:

A. Intrathecal antibody
B. Virus specific IgM
C. CSF PCR
D. Brain biopsy

Explanation:

- CSF PCR has become the primary diagnostic test for CNS infections caused by CMV, EBV, HHV-6, and enteroviruses. In the case of VZV CNS infection, CSF PCR and detection of virus-specific IgM or intrathecal antibody synthesis both provide important aids to diagnosis.
- Sensitivity and specificity of CSF PCRs vary with the virus being tested. The sensitivity (~96%) and specificity (~99%) of HSV CSF PCR are equivalent to or exceed those of brain biopsy. It is important to recognize that HSV CSF PCR results need to be interpreted after considering the likelihood of disease in the patient being tested, the timing of the test in relationship to onset of symptoms, and the prior use of antiviral therapy.
- A negative HSV CSF PCR test performed by a qualified laboratory at the appropriate time during illness in a patient with a high likelihood of HSV encephalitis based on clinical and laboratory abnormalities significantly reduces the likelihood of HSV encephalitis but does not exclude it.

- For example, in a patient with a pretest probability of 35% of having HSV encephalitis, a negative HSV CSF PCR reduces the posttest probability to ~2%, and for a patient with a pretest probability of 60%, a negative test reduces the posttest probability to ~6%. In both situations, a positive test makes the diagnosis almost certain (98–99%).

Ans. C

245. Coxiella burnetti transmitted through all except:

A. Sheep
B. Birds
C. Cats
D. Goats

Explanation:

Table: Epidemiologic factors suggesting possible causes of community-acquired pneumonia	
Factor	**Possible Pathogen(s)**
Alcoholism	*Streptococcus pneumoniae, oral anaerobes, Klebsiella pneumoniae, Acinetobacter spp., Mycobacterium tuberculosis*
COPD and/or smoking	*Haemophilus influenzae, Pseudomonas aeruginosa, Legionella spp., S. pneumoniae, Moraxella catarrhalis, Chlamydia pneumoniae*
Structural lung disease (e.g., bronchiectasis)	*P. aeruginosa, Burkholderia cepacia, Staphylococcus aureus*
Dementia, stroke, decreased level of consciousness	Oral anaerobes, gram-negative enteric bacteria
Lung abscess	CA-MRSA, oral anaerobes, endemic fungi, *M. tuberculosis*, atypical mycobacteria
Travel to Ohio or St. Lawrence river valley	*Histoplasma capsulatum*
Travel to southwestern United States	Hantavirus, *Coccidioides* spp.
Travel to Southeast Asia	*Burkholderia pseudomallei*, avian influenza virus
Stay in hotel or on cruise ship in previous 2 weeks	*Legionella* spp.
Local influenza activity	Influenza virus, *S. pneumoniae, S. aureus*
Exposure to bats or birds	*H. capsulatum*
Exposure to birds	*Chlamydia psittaci*
Exposure to rabbits	*Francisella tularensis*
Exposure to sheep, goats, parturient cats	*Coxiella burnetii*

Ans. B

246. CMV is associated with all except:

A. Glomerulopathy in kidney transplant recipients
B. Bronchiolitis obliterans in lung transplant recipients
C. Vanishing bile duct syndrome in liver transplant recipients
D. Aplastic crisis in bone marrow transplant recipients

Explanation:

- During the early period (<1 month after transplantation), infections are most commonly caused by extracellular bacteria (staphylococci, streptococci, enterococci, and *E. coli* and other gram-negative organisms, including nosocomial organisms with broad antibiotic resistance), which often originate in surgical-wound or anastomotic sites.

- Type of transplant largely determines the spectrum of infection. In subsequent weeks, the consequences of the administration of agents that suppress cell-mediated immunity become apparent, and acquisition—or, more commonly, reactivation—of viruses, mycobacteria, endemic fungi, and parasites (from the recipient or from the transplanted organ) can occur.
- CMV infection is often a problem, particularly in the first 6 months after transplantation, and may present as severe systemic disease or as infection of the transplanted organ.
- HHV-6 reactivation (assessed by plasma PCR) occurs within the first 2–4 weeks after transplantation and may be associated with fever, leukopenia, and very rare cases of encephalitis. Data suggest that replication of HHV-6 and HHV-7 may exacerbate CMV-induced disease. CMV is associated not only with generalized immunosuppression but also with organ-specific, rejection-related syndromes: glomerulopathy in kidney transplant recipients, bronchiolitis obliterans in lung transplant recipients, vasculopathy in heart transplant recipients, and vanishing bile duct syndrome in liver transplant recipients. A complex interplay between increased CMV replication and enhanced graft rejection is well established: elevated immunosuppression leads to increased CMV replication, which is associated with graft rejection.
- For this reason, considerable attention has been focused on the diagnosis, prophylaxis, and treatment of CMV infection in SOT recipients. Early transmission of WNV to transplant recipients from a donated organ or transfused blood has been reported; however, the risk of WNV acquisition has been reduced by implementation of screening procedures. In rare instances, rabies virus and lymphocytic choriomeningitis virus also have been acutely transmitted in this setting; although accompanied by distinct clinical syndromes, both viral infections have resulted in fatal encephalitis. As screening for unusual viruses is not routine, only vigilant assessment of the prospective donor is likely to prevent the use of an infected organ.

Ans. D

247. Carbapenems interact with:

A. Warfarin
B. Tacrlimus
C. Cyclosporine
D. Valproic acid

Explanation:

Table: Significant antibacterial drug interactions		
Antibacterial(s)	**Interacting Agent(s)**	**Potential Effects and Management**
Nafcillin	Warfarin, cyclosporine, tacrolimus	Decreased levels of warfarin, cyclosporine, via CYP3A4 induction. Monitor levels of affected drug closely if drugs are given concomitantly
Ceftriaxone	Calcium-containing IV solutions	Concomitant use is contraindicated in neonates (< 28 days); the combination can lead to precipitation of ceftriaxone-calcium particulate Ceftriaxone and calcium-containing solutions can be given to infants > 28 days of age provided they are given sequentially and the lines are thoroughly flushed between infusions
Carbapenems	Valproic acid	Decreased levels of valproic acid. Monitor valproic acid levels closely if drugs are given concomitantly.
Linezolid, tedizolid	Serotonergic and adrenergic agents (e.g., SSRIs, vasopressors)	Increased levels of serotonergic and adrenergic agents. Monitor for serotonin syndrome. Tedizolid may have less potential than linezolid to cause this drug interaction

Contd.

Contd.

Quinupristin-dalfopristin	Substrates of CYP3A4 (e.g., warfarin, ritonavir, cyclosporine, diazepam, verapamil)	Can result in increased level of interacting drug
Fluoroquinolones	Theophylline[a]	Can result in theophylline toxicity
	Sucralfate; antacids containing aluminium, calcium, or magnesium; ferrous sulfate- and zinc-containing multivitamins	Can result in subtherapeutic fluoroquinolone levels. Administer fluoroquinolone 2 hours before or 6 hours after interacting drug
	Tizanidine[a]	Can result in increased levels of tizanidine and hypotensive, sedative effects. Monitor for side effects if drugs are given concomitantly

Ans. D

248. About daptomycin all are true except:

A. Active against gram positive organisms
B. Not active against enterococci
C. Side effect is elevation of CPK
D. May cause reversible Eosinophilic pneumonia

Explanation:

- Daptomycin is a lipopeptide antibiotic with activity against a broad range of gram-positive organisms. This drug is active against staphylococci (including MRSA and coagulase-negative staphylococci), streptococci, and enterococci.
- Daptomycin remains active against enterococci that are resistant to vancomycin. In addition, it exhibits activity against Bacillus, Corynebacterium, Peptostreptococcus, and Clostridium species.
- Daptomycin's pharmacodynamic parameter for efficacy is concentration-dependent killing.
- Resistance to daptomycin is rare, but MICs may be higher for VISA strains.
- Daptomycin can be used in skin and soft tissue infections, bacteremia, endocarditis, and osteomyelitis. It is an important alternative for MRSA and other gram-positive infections when bactericidal therapy is needed and vancomycin cannot be used.
- Daptomycin is generally well tolerated, and its main toxicity consists of elevation of creatine phosphokinase (CPK) levels and myopathy.

Ans. D

249. Regarding COX-2 selective drugs, all are true except:

A. Same analgesic potency as non-selective agents
B. Less gastric irritation
C. Lower risk of kidney injury
D. Better in acute post-operative pain

Explanation:

- COX- 2-selective drugs have similar analgesic potency and produce less gastric irritation than the nonselective COX inhibitors.
- Use of COX-2-selective drugs does not appear to lower the risk of nephrotoxicity compared to nonselective NSAIDs.

Ans. C

250. Anaerobic/aerobic ratio in all these anatomic sites is 1:1 except:

A. Tooth surface
B. Stomach
C. Ileum
D. Colon

Explanation:

Table: The anaerobic human microbiota: An overview			
Anatomic Site	**Total Bacteria**[a]	**Anaerobic/Aerobic ratio**	**Potential Pathogen(s)**
Nose	10^3–10^4	2:1	*Peptostreptococcus* spp., *Prevotella* spp.
Oral Cavity			
Saliva	10^8–10^9	10:1	*Fusobacterium nucleatum, Prevotella melaninogenica, Prevotella oralis group, Bacteroides ureolyticus* group, *Peptostreptococcus* spp.
Tooth surface	10^{10}–10^{11}	1:1	
Gingival crevices	10^{11}–10^{12}	10^3:1	
Gastrointestinal Tract			
Stomach	0–10^5	1:1	*Bacteroides* spp. (principally members of the *B. fragilis* group), *Prevotella* spp., *Clostridium* spp., *Peptostreptococcus* spp.
Jejunum/ileum	10^4–10^7	1:1	
Cecum and colon	10^{11}–10^{12}	10^3:1	
Female genital tract	10^7–10^9	10:1	*Peptostreptococcus* spp., *Bacteroides* spp., Prevotella bivia
Skin	10^4–10^5	100:1	*Cutibacterium acnes*

Ans. D

251. All are mechanisms for preventing autoimmunity except:

A. Molecular mimicry
B. Idiotype network
C. Regulatory T cells
D. Sequestration of self-antigens

Explanation:

Table: Mechanisms preventing autoimmunity

1. Sequestration of self-antigens
2. Generation and maintenance of tolerance
   a. Central deletion of autoreactive lymphocytes
   b. Peripheral anergy of autoreactive lymphocytes
   c. Receptor replacement in autoreactive lymphoctyes
3. Regulatory mechanisms
   a. Regulatory T cells
   b. Regulatory B cells
   c. Regulatory mesenchymal cells
   d. Regulatory cytokines
   e. Idiotype network

Ans. A

252. Stimulation of autoantibody is the mechanism of tissue damage in all the below except:

A. Graves' disease
B. Goodpasture's syndrome
C. Granulomatosis with polyangiitis
D. Pemphigus vulgaris

Explanation:

Table: Mechanisms of tissue damage in autoimmune disease

Effector	Mechanism	Target	Disease
Autoantibody	Blocking or inactivation	α Chain of the nicotinic acetylcholine receptor	Myasthenia gravis
		Phospholipid– β_2-glycoprotein I complex	Antiphospholipid syndrome
		Insulin receptor	Insulin-resistant diabetes mellitus
		Instrinsic factor	Pernicious anemia
	Stimulation	TSH receptor (LATS)	Graves' disease
		Proteinase-3 (ANCA)	Granulomatosis with polyangiitis
		Epidermal cadherin	Pemphigus vulgaris
		Desmoglein 3	
	Complement activation	α_3 Chain of collagen IV	Goodpasture's syndrome
	Immune complex formation	Double-stranded DNA	Systemic lupus erythematosus
		Immunoglobulin	Rheumatoid arthritis
	Opsonization	Platelet GIIb:IIIa	Autoimmune thrombocytopenic purpura
			Autoimmune haemolytic anemia
	Antibody-dependent cellular cytotoxicity	Rh antigens, I antigen	Hashimoto's thyroiditis
		Thyroid peroxidase, thyroglobulin	
T cells	Cytokine production		Rheumatoid arthritis, multiple sclerosis, type 1 diabetes mellitus
	Cellular cytotoxicity		Type 1 diabetes mellitus

Ans. B

253. Transplant elbow is usually caused by:

A. Listeria

B. Klebsiella

C. S.aureus

D. Aspergillus

Explanation:

- "Transplant elbow", a recurrent bacterial infection in and around the elbow that is thought to result from a combination of poor tensile strength of the skin of steroid-treated patients and steroid-induced proximal myopathy, requires patients to push themselves up with their elbows to get out of chairs.
- Bouts of cellulitis (usually caused by *S. aureus*) recur until patients are provided with elbow protection.

Ans. C

254. UTIs in young women appears to be caused by:

A. S. epidermidis

B. Staphylococcus lugdunensis

C. Staphylococcus schleiferi

D. S. saprophyticus

Explanation:

- Capacity of *S. saprophyticus* to cause UTIs in young women appears to be related to its enhanced capacity to adhere to uroepithelial cells.
- A 160-kDa hemagglutinin/adhesin may contribute to this affinity.

Ans. D

255. After Heart transplantation some prophylaxis is always warranted for infection with:

A. T. gondii
B. CMV
C. Aspergillus
D. L. monocytogenes

Explanation:

- T. gondii residing in heart of a seropositive donor may be transmitted to a seronegative recipient.
- Thus serologic screening for T. gondii infection is important before and in the months after cardiac transplantation.
- Rarely, active disease can be introduced at the time of transplantation.
- Overall incidence of toxoplasmosis is so high in the setting of heart transplantation that some prophylaxis is always warranted.
- Although alternatives are available, the most frequently used agent is TMP-SMX, which prevents infection with Pneumocystis as well as with Nocardia and several other bacterial pathogens.
- CMV also has been transmitted by heart transplantation.
- Toxoplasma, Nocardia, and Aspergillus can cause CNS infections.
- **L. monocytogenes meningitis should be considered in heart transplant recipients with fever and headache.**

Ans. A

256. All prolong QTc except:

A. Arsenic trioxide
B. Carfilzomib
C. Osimertinib
D. Pazopanib

Explanation:

Drug	Target	Adverse Events	Notes
Diagnostically Guided Protein Kinase Antagonists			
Imatinib	Bcr-Abl fusion protein (CML/ ALL); D-kit mutants, PDFR variants (GI stromal tumor; eosinophilic syndromes)	Nausea Periorbital edema Rare CHF QTc prolongation	Myelosuppression not frequent in solid tumor indications
Nilotinib	Bcr-Abl fusion protein (CML) and some imatinib-reistant variants	Interaction with CYP3A4-metabolized drugs CHF Hepatotoxicity Hypothyroidism	Chronic phase and in patients resistant to imtinib
Dasatinib	Bcr-Abl fusion protein (CML/ ALL); wild-type and imatinib-reistant mutants	Myelosuppression (bleeding, infection) Pulmonary hypertension CHF Fluid retention QTc prolongation	Chronic phase and imatinib or nilotinib resistant
Bosutinib	Bcr-Abl fusion protein (CML); wild-type and imatinib-resistant mutants	Myelosuppression Hepatic QTc prolongation	Chronic phase and imatinib or nilotinib resistant

Contd.

Contd.

Ponatinib	T3151 mutation of Bcr-Abl fusion protein (CML)	Clotting Hepatic CHF Pancreatitis Neuropathy Rash	
Gefitinib	First-line treatment of NSCLC with ATP site mutation of EGFR	Diarrhea Interstitial pneumonitis	In the United States, only with prior documented benefit in second-line treatment of NSCLC
Erlotinib	First-line treatment of NSCLC with ATP site mutation of EGFR; second-line treatment of wild-type EGFR NSCLC	Rash Diarrhea Rare interstitial pneumonitis	1 hour before, 2 hours after meals
Afatinib	First-line treatment of NSCLC with ATP site mutation of EGFR	Diarrhea Cutaneous	Interacts with Pgp inhibitors
Crizotinib	EML 4-Alk fusion protein	Interstitial pneumonitis Hepatic QTc prolongation Bradycardia	
Vemurafenib	*BRAF* V600E in melanoma	Nausea Rash Cutaneous Second cutaneous neoplasms	
Dabrafenib	*BRAF* V600E in melanoma	Cutaneous Second cutaneous neoplasms	
Trametinib	*BRAF* V600E in melanoma (both as single agent and in combination with dabrafenib)	Rash Diarrhea Lymphedema	In combination with dabrafenib, second neoplasms, hemorrhage, venous thrombosis, CHF, ocular, hyperglycemia
Drug	**Indication**	**Adverse Events**	**Notes**
Diagnostically Guided Retinoid			
Tretinoin	APL t(15,17)	Teratogenic Cutaneous	APL differentiation syndrome: Pulmonary dysfunction/infiltrate, pleural/pericardial effusion, fever
Multikinase Inhibitors			
Sorafenib	Renal cell, hepatocellular, differentiated thyroid carcinoma	Diarrhea Hand-foot syndrome Other rash Hypertension CHF	Targets c-raf, VEGFR

Contd.

Contd.

Pazopanib	Renal cell carcinoma, soft tissue sarcoma	Fatigue Diarrhea/GI Hypertension Thromboses QTc	Target VEGFR, c-kit PGDFR
Regorafenib	Second-line colorectal cancer; GI stromal tumor	Hypertension Hand-foot syndrome Thromboses Perforations	VEGFR/TIE2
Sunitinib	Renal cell carcinoma, pancreatic neuroendocrine tumor, GI stromal tumor	Fatigue Diarrhea Neutropenia	Target VEGFR
Vandetanib	Medullary thyroid cancer	Diarrhea Rash Hypertension Prolonged QTc Thromboses	Target VEGFR, ret, EGFR
Cabozantinib	Medullary thyroid cancer	Hypertension Wound healing Fistulas Osteonecrosis Proteinuria	Target VEGFR, c-met
Axitinib	Renal cell carcoinoma, second line	Diarrhea/other GI Fatigue Hand-foot syndrome	Target VEGFR, PDGFR, c-kit
Osimertinib	Non-small cell lung cancer, EGFR T790M mutation	Interstitial lung disease QTc prolongation Cardiomyopathy	
Proteasome Inhibitors			
Bortezomib	Multiple myeloma, mantle cell lymphoma	Neuropathy Thrombocytopenia GI	
Carfilzomib	Multiple myeloma, second line	Infusion reaction CHF Thrombocytopenia Pulmonary Tumor lysis	
Histone Deacetylase Inhibitors			
Vorinostat	Cutaneous T-cell lymphoma, second line	Fatigue Diarrhea Thrombocytopenia Embolism	

Contd.

Contd.

Romidepsin	Cutaneous T-cell lymphoma, second line	Nausea Vomiting Cytopenias Cardiac conduction	
mTOR Inhibitors			
Temsirolimus	Renal cell carcinoma, second line or poor prognosis	Stomatitis Thrombocytopenia Nausea Anorexia, fatigue Metabolic (glucose, lipid)	
Everolimus	Renal cell carcinoma, advanced; subependymal giant-cell astrocytoma; breast cancer; hormone receptor positive, resistant to antiestrogen; pancreatic neuroendocrine	Stomatitis Fatigue	

Miscellaneous			
Arsenic trioxide	APL	↑QT_c	APL differentiation syndrome (see under tretinoin)
Vismodegib	Metastatic basal cell carcinoma	GI Hair loss Fatigue Muscle spasm Dysgeusia	Target smoothened receptor in hedgehog pathway

Ans. B

257. Diagnosis of complement deficiency of classical pathway is done by:

A. CD4/CD8 ratio
B. CH50 test
C. AP50 test
D. None of the above

Explanation:

- Diagnosis of a complement deficiency relies primarily on testing the status of the classic and alternate pathway via functional assays, that is, the CH50 and AP50 tests, respectively.
- When either pathway is profoundly impaired, determination of the status of the relevant components in that pathway enables a precise diagnosis.
- Appropriate vaccinations and daily administration of oral penicillin are efficient means of preventing recurrent infections. It is noteworthy that several complement deficiencies (in the classic pathway and the lytic phase) may also predispose affected individuals to autoimmune diseases (notably systemic lupus erythematosus.

Ans. B

258. Adipocytes secrete all except:

A. Retinol binding protein 4
B. Leptin
C. TNF beta
D. IL-6

Explanation:

- Obesity accompanying type 2 DM, particularly in a central or visceral location, is thought to be part of the pathogenic process. In addition to these white fat depots, humans now are recognized to have brown fat, which has much greater thermogenic capacity. Efforts are under way to increase the activity or quantity of brown fat.
- Increased adipocyte mass leads to increased levels of circulating free fatty acids and other fat cell products. **For example, adipocytes secrete a number of biologic products (nonesterified free fatty acids, retinol-binding protein 4, leptin, TNF-α, resistin, IL-6 and adiponectin).** In addition to regulating body weight, appetite, and energy expenditure, adipokines also modulate insulin sensitivity.
- Increased production of free fatty acids and some adipokines may cause insulin resistance in skeletal muscle and liver.
- Venous drainage of the visceral adipose beds is the portal circulation and this likely contributes to hepatic dysfunction.
- Free fatty acids also impair glucose utilization in skeletal muscle, promote glucose production by the liver, and impair beta cell function.
- In contrast, production by adipocytes of adiponectin, an insulin-sensitizing peptide, is reduced in obesity, and this may contribute to hepatic insulin resistance.
- Adipocyte products and adipokines also produce an inflammatory state and may explain why markers of inflammation such as IL-6 and C-reactive protein are often elevated in type 2 DM.
- In addition, inflammatory cells have been found infiltrating adipose tissue.

Ans. C

259. Complete resolution of pain with indomethacin is seen in:

A. Hemicrania continua
B. Paroxysmal hemicranias
C. SUNCT
D. SUNA

Explanation:

- Essential features of hemicrania continua are moderate and continuous unilateral pain associated with fluctuations of severe pain; **complete resolution of pain with indomethacin;** and exacerbations that may be associated with autonomic features, including conjunctival injection, lacrimation, and photophobia on affected side.
- Age of onset ranges from 10 to 70 years; women are affected twice as often as men. The cause is unknown.

Ans. A

260. Feature of paralytic rabies is:

A. Hyperexcitability
B. Hydrophobia
C. Quadriceps & facial weakness
D. Aerophobia

Explanation:

- About 20% of patients have paralytic rabies in which muscle weakness predominates and cardinal features of encephalitic rabies (hyperexcitability, hydrophobia, and aerophobia) are lacking.
- There is early and prominent flaccid muscle weakness, often beginning in the bitten extremity and spreading to produce quadriparesis and facial weakness.
- Sphincter involvement is common, sensory involvement is usually mild, and these cases are commonly misdiagnosed as Guillain-Barré syndrome.
- Patients with paralytic rabies generally survive a few days longer than those with encephalitic rabies, but multiple-organ failure nevertheless ensues.

Ans. C

261. A 10 year old with hereditary ataxia showed low VLDL and vitamin E deficiency and was diagnosed as Abetalipoproteinemia. He shows mutation in which gene?

A. Microsomal triglyceride transfer protein (MTP)

B. Mutation on alpha TTP (Tocopherol transfer protein)

C. Frataxin gene

D. Huntingtin gene

Explanation:

- Abetalipoproteinemia
  - Microsomal triglyceride transfer protein (MTP)
  - Impairment of formation and secretion of VLDL in liver
  - Deficiency of delivery of vitamin E and other fat soluble vitamins
  - Form of hereditary ataxia

Ans. A

262. Not true about maintenance immunosuppressive drugs in kidney transplantation is:

A. Azathioprine- Marrow suppression (Platelets > RBC > WBC)

B. Belatacept- Post transplant lymphoproliferative disease

C. Mycophenolate mofetil/sodium- Diarrhea, cramps, dose related liver & marrow suppression is uncommon

D. Sirolimus/Everolimus- Hyperlipidemia & thrombocytopenia

Explanation:

Table: Maintenance immunosuppressive drugs

Agent	Pharmacology	Mechanisms	Side Effects
Glucocorticoids	Increased bioavailability with hypoalbuminemia and liver disease; prednisone/prednisolone generally used	Binds cytosolic receptors and heat shock proteins. Blocks transcription of IL–1, –2, –3, –6, TNF-α and IFN-γ	Hypertension, glucose intolerance, dyslipidemia, osteoporosis
Cyclosporine (CsA)	Lipid-soluble polypeptide, variable absorption, microemulsion more predictable	Trimolecular complex with cyclophilin and calcineurin$\rightarrow$block in cytokine (e.g., IL-2) production; however. stimulates TGF-β production	Similar to CsA, but hirsutism/ hyperplasia of gums unusual and diabetes more likely
Tacrolimus	Macrolide, well absorbed	Trimolecular complex with FKBP-12 and calcineurin $\rightarrow$block in cytokine (e.g., IL-2) production; may stimulate TGF-β production	Similar to CsA, but hirsutism/ hyperplasia of gums unusual and diabetes more likely
Azathioprine	Mercaptopurine analogue	Hepatic metabolites inhibit purine synthesis	Marrow suppression (WBC > RBC > platelets)
Mycophenolate mofetil/sodium	Mtabolized to mycophenolic acid	Inhibits purine synthesis via inosine monophosphate dehydrogenase	Diarrhea/cramps; dose-related liver and marrow suppression is uncommon

Contd.

Contd.

Sirolimus/Everolimus	Macrolide, poor oral bioavailability	Complexes with FKBP-12 and then blocks p70- S6 kinase in the IL-2 receptor pathway for proliferation	Hyperlipidemia, thrombocytopenia
Belatacept	Fusion protein, intravenous injections	Binds CD80 and CD86, prevents CD28 binding and T cell activation	Post-transplant Lymphoproliferative Disease (PTLD)

Ans. A

263. A patient with ATM gene mutation presents with ataxia, myoclonus and telangiectasia. Which is false regarding his disease?

A. Thymic hypoplasia
B. Neoplasms common
C. Frequent pulmonary infections
D. Decrease alpha feto protein

Explanation:

Ataxia Telangiectasia

- ATM gene–Defective DNA repair
- Ataxia, dysarthria, extensor plantar responses, myoclonic jerks, areflexia, and distal sensory deficits
- Telangiectasia–conjunctiva, extensor surfaces
- Recurrent pulmonary infections
- Neoplasms–Hodgkin's disease, acute T cell leukemias and breast cancer

Ans. D

264. HIV doesn't increase risk of autoimmune disease of:

A. RA
B. APLA
C. Sjögren syndrome
D. All of the above

Explanation:

- HIV infection shares many similarities with a variety of autoimmune diseases, including a substantial polyclonal B cell activation that is associated with a high incidence of antiphospholipid antibodies, such as anticardiolipin antibodies, VDRL antibodies, and lupus-like anticoagulants.
- In addition, HIV-infected individuals have an increased incidence of antinuclear antibodies.
- Despite these serologic findings, there is no evidence that HIV-infected individuals have an increase in two of the more common autoimmune diseases, i.e., systemic lupus erythematosus and rheumatoid arthritis. In fact, it has been observed that these diseases may be somewhat ameliorated by the concomitant presence of HIV infection, suggesting that an intact CD4+ T cell limb of the immune response plays an integral role in the pathogenesis of these conditions.

Ans. A

265. Molecular defects associated with EBV include all except:

A. RFXANK
B. IL2 inducible T cell kinase deficiency
C. DOCK2 deficiency
D. RORC deficiency

Explanation:

- Defective expression of HLA class II molecules is hallmark of a group of four recessive genetic defects all of which affect molecules (RFX5, RFXAP, RFXANK, and CIITA) involved in transactivation of the genes coding for HLA class II.

- As a result, low but variable CD4+ T cell counts are observed in addition to defective antigen-specific T and B cell responses. These patients are particularly susceptible to herpesvirus, adenovirus, and enterovirus infections and chronic gut/liver *Cryptosporidium* infections.

Ans. A

266. All are true about Ataxia telangiectasia except:

A. Autosomal dominant disorder
B. Causes B cell defects
C. Associated with T cell immunodeficiency
D. Hallmark features are telengiectasia and cerebellar ataxia

Explanation:

- Autosomal recessive disorder *ataxia-telangiectasia* (AT) is the most frequently encountered condition in this group. It has an incidence of 1:40,000 live births and causes B cell defects (low IgA, IgG2 deficiency, and low antibody production), which often require immunoglobulin replacement.
- AT is associated with a progressive T cell immunodeficiency.
- As the name suggests, the hallmark features of AT are telangiectasia and cerebellar ataxia. The latter manifestations may not be detectable before the age of 3–4 years, so that AT should be considered in young children with IgA deficiency and recurrent and problematic infections.
- Diagnosis is based on a cytogenetic analysis showing excessive chromosomal rearrangements (mostly affecting chromosomes 7 and 14) in lymphocytes.
- AT is caused by a mutation in the gene encoding the ATM protein—a kinase that plays an important role in the detection and repair of DNA lesions (or cell death if the lesions are too numerous) by triggering several different pathways. Overall, AT is a progressive disease that carries a very high risk of lymphoma, leukemia, and (during adulthood) carcinomas. A variant of AT ("AT-like disease") is caused by mutation in the *MRE11* gene.

Ans. A

267. Erythropoietin is increased by:

A. Estrogen
B. Castration
C. Testosterone
D. PTH

Explanation:

- Difference in the levels of hemoglobin between men and women is related to the effects of androgen and estrogen on erythropoiesis.
- Testosterone and anabolic steroids augment erythropoiesis; castration and estrogen administration to males decrease erythropoiesis.
- Patients who are hypothyroid or have deficits in pituitary hormones also may develop a mild anemia.
- Pathogenesis may be complicated by other nutritional deficiencies because iron and folic acid absorption can be affected by these disorders.
- Usually, correction of the hormone deficiency reverses the anemia.

Ans. C

268. APACHE II score includes all except:

A. Acute physiology score
B. Glasgow coma score
C. Age
D. Acute health points

Explanation:

- APACHE II system is the most commonly used SOI scoring system in North America.
- Age, type of ICU admission (after elective surgery vs nonsurgical or after emergency surgery), chronic health problems, and 12 physiologic variables (the worst values for each in the first 24 h after ICU admission) are used to derive a score.
- Predicted hospital mortality rate is derived from a formula that takes into account APACHE II score, the need for emergency surgery, and a weighted, disease-specific diagnostic category.

Ans. B

269. A person presented to OPD with swelling and pain of upper limb. History of road traffic accident is present and was diagnosed as chronic regional pain syndrome type 1. He doesn't show which of the following features?

A. Mostly affects one limb
B. Occurs only after severe injury
C. Symptoms are unrelated to severity of initial injury
D. Symptoms not confined to peripheral nerve distribution

Explanation:

CRPS type 1

- Commonly affects one limb
- Not related to severity of injury
- Pain not confined to single peripheral nerve

CRPS type 2

- After specific injury to peripheral nerve
- Confined to single peripheral nerve. Can spread later

Ans. B

270. Not true about Anagrelide is:

A. Phosphodiesterase inhibitor
B. Can reduce platelet count
C. Protective in venous thrombosis
D. Has marrow toxicity

Explanation:

- Anagrelide, a phosphodiesterase inhibitor, can reduce platelet count and, if tolerated, is preferable to hydroxyurea because it lacks marrow toxicity and is also protective against venous thrombosis while hydroxyurea is not.
- A reduction in platelet number may be necessary for the treatment of erythromelalgia or ocular migraine if salicylates are not effective or if the platelet count is sufficiently high to increase the risk of hemorrhage, but only to the degree that symptoms are alleviated.

Ans. D

271. Antigen related to CAD (Coronary Artery Disease) is:

A. Desmin
B. Desmoglein 1
C. Desmoglein 3
D. F-actin

Explanation:

Autoantigen	**Autoimmune Diseases**
Cell- or Organ-Specific Autoimmunity	
Acetylcholine receptor	Myasthenia gravis
Actin	Chronic active hepatitis, primary biliary cirrhosis
Adenine nucleotide translator (ANT)	Dilated cardiomyopathy, myocarditis
β-Adrenoreceptor	Dilated cardiomyopathy
Aromatic L-amino acid decarboxylase	Autoimmune polyendocrine syndrome type 1 (APS-1)
Asialoglycoprotein receptor	Autoimmune hepatitis
Bactericidal/permeability-increasing protein (Bpi)	Cystic fibrosis vasculitides
Calcium-sensing receptor	Acquired hypoparathyroidism
Cholesterol side-chain cleavage enzyme (CYP11a)	Autoimmune polyglandular syndrome-1
Collagen type IV-α-3-chain	Goodpasture's syndrome
Cytochrome P450 2D6 (CYP2D6)	Autoimmune hepatitis
Desmin	Crohn's disease, coronary artery disease
Desmoglein 1	Pemphigus foliaceus
Desmoglein 3	Pemphigus vulgaris
F-actin	Autoimmune hepatitis
GM gangliosides	Guillain-Barré syndrome
Glutamate decarboxylase (GAD65)	Type 1 diabetes, stiff-person syndrome
Glutamate receptor (GLUR)	Rasmussen encephalitis
H/K ATPase	Autoimmune gastritis
17-α-Hydroxylase (CYP17)	Autoimmune polyglandular syndrome-1
21-Hydroxylase (CYP21)	Addison's disease
IA-2 (ICA512)	Type 1 diabetes
Insulin	Type 1 diabetes, insulin hypoglycemic syndrome (Hirata's disease)
Insulin receptor	Type B insulin resistance, acanthosis, systemic lupus erythematosus (SLE)
Aminoacyl-tRNA synthetase (several)	Polymyositis, dermatomyositis
Cardiolipin	Systemic lupus erythematosus, antiphospholipid syndrome
Carbonic anhydrase II	Systemic lupus erythematosus, Sjögren's syndrome, systemic sclerosis
Collagen (multiple types)	Rheumatoid arthritis, systemic lupus erythematosus, progressive systemic sclerosis
Centromere-associated proteins	Systemic sclerosis
DNA-dependent nucleoside-stimulated ATPase	Dermatomyositis
Fibrillarin	Scleroderma
Fibronectin	Systemic lupus erythematosus, rheumatoid arthritis, morphea
Glucose-6-phosphate isomerase	Rheumatoid arthritis
β2-Glycoprotein 1 (B2-GPI)	Primary antiphospholipid syndrome
Golgin (95, 97, 160, 180) Heat shock protein	Sjögren's syndrome, systemic lupus erythematosus, rheumatoid arthritis Various immune-related disorders

Contd.

Contd.

Hemidesmosomal protein 180	Bullous pemphigoid, herpes gestationis, cicatricial pemphigoid
Histone H2A-H2B-DNA	Systemic lupus erythematosus
IgE receptor	Chronic idiopathic urticaria
Keratin	Rheumatoid arthritis
Ku-DNA-protein kinase	Systemic lupus erythematosus
Ku-nucleoprotein La phosphoprotein (La 55-B)	Connective tissue syndrome, Sjögren's sydrome
Myeloperoxidase	Necrotizing and crescentic glomerulonephritis (NCGN), systemic vasculitis
Proteinase 3 (PR3)	Granulomatosis with polyangiitis (Wegener's), Churg-Strauss syndrome
RNA polymerase I-III (RNP)	Systemic sclerosis, systemic lupus erythematosus

Ans. A

272. Antigen related to Pemphigus foliacues is:

A. Desmin
B. Desmoglein 1
C. Desmoglein 3
D. F-actin

Explanation:

Autoantigen	Autoimmune Diseases
Acetylcholine receptor	Myasthenia gravis
Actin	Chronic active hepatitis, primary biliary cirrhosis
Adenine nucleotide translator (ANT)	Dilated cardiomyopathy, myocarditis
β-Adrenoreceptor	Dilated cardiomyopathy
Aromatic L-amino acid decarboxylase	Autoimmune polyendocrine syndrome type 1 (APS-1)
Asialoglycoprotein receptor	Autoimmune hepatitis
Bactericidal/permeability-increasing protein (Bpi)	Cystic fibrosis vasculitides
Calcium-sensing receptor	Acquired hypoparathyroidism
Cholesterol side-chain cleavage enzyme (CYP11a)	Autoimmune polyglandular syndrome-1
Collagen type IV-α-3-chain	Goodpasture's syndrome
Cytochrome P450 2D6 (CYP2D6)	Autoimmune hepatitis
Desmin	Crohn's disease, coronary artery disease
Desmoglein 1	Pemphigus foliaceus
Desmoglein 3	Pemphigus vulgaris
F-actin	Autoimmune hepatitis
GM gangliosides	Guillain-Barré syndrome
Glutamate decarboxylase (GAD65)	Type 1 diabetes, stiff-person syndrome
Glutamate receptor (GLUR)	Rasmussen encephalitis
H/K ATPase	Autoimmune gastritis
17-α-Hydroxylase (CYP17)	Autoimmune polyglandular syndrome-1
21-Hydroxylase (CYP21)	Addison's disease
IA-2 (ICA512)	Type 1 diabetes

Contd.

Contd.

Insulin	Type 1 diabetes, insulin hypoglycemic syndrome (Hirata's disease)
Insulin receptor	Type B insulin resistance, acanthosis, systemic lupus erythematosus (SLE)
Aminoacyl-tRNA synthetase (several)	Polymyositis, dermatomyositis
Cardiolipin	Systemic lupus erythematosus, antiphospholipid syndrome
Carbonic anhydrase II	Systemic lupus erythematosus, Sjögren's syndrome, systemic sclerosis
Collagen (multiple types)	Rheumatoid arthritis, systemic lupus erythematosus, progressive systemic sclerosis
Centromere-associated proteins	Systemic sclerosis
DNA-dependent nucleoside-stimulated ATPase	Dermatomyositis
Fibrillarin	Scleroderma
Fibronectin	Systemic lupus erythematosus, rheumatoid arthritis, morphea
Glucose-6-phosphate isomerase	Rheumatoid arthritis
β2-Glycoprotein 1 (B2-GPI)	Primary antiphospholipid syndrome
Golgin (95, 97, 160, 180) Heat shock protein	Sjögren's syndrome, systemic lupus erythematosus, rheumatoid arthritis Various immune-related disorders
Hemidesmosomal protein 180	Bullous pemphigoid, herpes gestationis, cicatricial pemphigoid
Histone H2A-H2B-DNA	Systemic lupus erythematosus
IgE receptor	Chronic idiopathic urticaria
Keratin	Rheumatoid arthritis
Ku-DNA-protein kinase	Systemic lupus erythematosus
Ku-nucleoprotein La phosphoprotein (La 55-B)	Connective tissue syndrome, Sjögren's sydrome
Myeloperoxidase	Necrotizing and crescentic glomerulonephritis (NCGN), systemic vasculitis
Proteinase 3 (PR3)	Granulomatosis with polyangiitis (Wegener's), Churg-Strauss syndrome
RNA polymerase I-III (RNP)	Systemic sclerosis, systemic lupus erythematosus

Ans. B

273. A 18 year old male presented with delayed puberty with absent secondary sexual characteristics and micropenis. On evaluation patient was found to have colour blindness, anosmia and synkinesia. Genetic mutation associated with it:

A. KAL 1

B. FGFR1

C. CHD7

D. All of the above

Explanation:

- X-linked KAL gene, mutations of which impair embryonic migration of GnRH neurons from the hypothalamic olfactory placode to the hypothalamus.
- Other : Autosomal recessive (i.e., GPR54, KISS1)
- Dominant (i.e., FGFR1) modes of transmission have been described
- Other genes : GNRH1, PROK2, PROKR2, CHD7, PCSK1, FGF8, NELF, WDR11, TAC3, TACR3, and SEMA3E.

Ans. D

274. Matrix assisted laser description/ionization/time of flight (MALDI-TOF)mass spectrometry used to identify species of:

A. Burkholderia
B. Bartonella
C. Nocardia
D. Campylobacter

Explanation:

- Species are definitively determined by molecular techniques. In recent comparisons, the results were similar for species identification by molecular testing and matrix-assisted laser desorption/ionization/time-of-flight (MALDI-TOF) mass spectrometry. MALDI-TOF is much more practical for clinical laboratories and is becoming common in laboratories in high-resource countries.

Ans. C

275. All are DNA repair defects except:

A. Nijmegen breakage syndrome
B. Ataxia telangiectasia
C. Dyskeratosis congenita
D. SCID

Explanation:

- **T Cell Primary Immunodeficiency's with DNA Repair Defects** This is a group of PIDs characterized by a combination of T and B cell defects of variable intensity, together with a number of nonimmunologic features resulting from DNA fragility. The autosomal recessive disorder *ataxia-telangiectasia* (AT) is the most frequently encountered condition in this group. It has an incidence of 1:40,000 live births and causes B cell defects (low IgA, IgG2 deficiency, and low antibody production), which often require immunoglobulin replacement. AT is associated with a progressive T cell immunodeficiency. As the name suggests, the hallmark features of AT are telangiectasia and cerebellar ataxia. The latter manifestations may not be detectable before the age of 3–4 years, so that AT should be considered in young children with IgA deficiency and recurrent and problematic infections. Diagnosis is based on a cytogenetic analysis showing excessive chromosomal rearrangements (mostly affecting chromosomes 7 and 14) in lymphocytes. AT is caused by a mutation in the gene encoding the ATM protein—a kinase that plays an important role in the detection and repair of DNA lesions (or cell death if the lesions are too numerous) by triggering several different pathways. Overall, AT is a progressive disease that carries a very high risk of lymphoma, leukemia, and (during adulthood) carcinomas. A variant of AT ("AT-like disease") is caused by mutation in the *MRE11* gene.
- *Nijmegen breakage syndrome* (NBS) is a less common condition that also results from chromosome instability (with the same cytogenetic abnormalities as in AT). NBS is characterized by a severe T and B cell combined immune deficiency with autosomal recessive inheritance. Individuals with NBS exhibit microcephaly and a bird-like face, but have neither ataxia nor telangiectasia. The risk of malignancies is very high. NBS results from a deficiency in nibrin (NBSI, a protein associated with MRE11 and Rad50 that is involved in checking DNA lesions) caused by hypomorphic mutations.
- Severe forms of *dyskeratosis congenita* (also known as Hoyeraal-hreidarsson syndrome) combine a progressive immunodeficiency that can also include an absence of B and NK lymphocytes, progressive bone marrow failure, microcephaly, in utero growth retardation, and gastrointestinal disease. The disease can be X-linked or, more rarely, autosomal recessive. It is caused by the mutation of genes encoding telomere maintenance proteins, including dyskerin (DKC1).
- Finally, *immunodeficiency with centromeric and facial anomalies* (ICF) is a complex syndrome of autosomal recessive inheritance that variably combines a mild T cell immune deficiency with a more severe B cell immune deficiency, coarse face, digestive disease, and mild mental retardation. A diagnostic feature is the detection by cytogenetic analysis of multiradial aspects in multiple chromosomes (most frequently 1, 9, and 16) corresponding to an abnormal DNA structure secondary to defective DNA methylation. It is the consequence of a deficiency in most cases in the DNA methyltransferase DNMT3B, ZBTB24, CDCA7, or HELLS.

Ans. D

276. Sodium level is associated with convulsion include:

A. <135 mmol/L
B. <130 mmol/L
C. <125 mmol/L
D. <119 mmol/L

Explanation:

- Sodium levels <125 mmol/L induce confusion, and levels <119 mmol/L are typically associated with coma and convulsions, especially when these levels are achieved quickly. In hyperosmolar coma, the serum osmolarity is generally >350 mosmol/L.

Ans. D

277. Which of the following feature is seen in both neurogenic & cardiogenic syncope?

A. Proximal & distal myoclonus
B. Pupils are usually dilated
C. Roving eye movements can occur
D. Urinary incontinence can occur

Explanation:

- During syncopal event, proximal and distal myoclonus (typically arrhythmic and multifocal) may occur, raising the possibility of epilepsy.
- Eyes typically remain open and usually deviate upward.
- Pupils are usually dilated.
- Roving eye movements may occur.
- Grunting, moaning, snorting and stertorous breathing may be present.
- Urinary incontinence may occur. Fecal incontinence is very rare.
- Postictal confusion is also rare, although visual and auditory hallucinations and near death and out-of-body experiences are sometimes reported.

Ans. A

278. Drug group D1 of MDR-TB is:

A. Bedaquiline
B. Delamanid
C. Ethambutol
D. Meropenem

Explanation:

Table: General steps in designing a longer regimen for the treatment of multidrug-resistant tuberculosis (MDR-TB)[a]

Step	Drug group	Options
1. Add *one* later-generation fluoroquinolone	A[b]	Levofloxacin Moxifloxacin Gatifloxacin
2. Add *one* second-line injectable agent	B	Amikacin Capreomycin Kanamycin (Streptomycin[c])
3. Add *two or more* second-line agents	C[b]	Ethionamide/prothionamide Cycloserine/terizidone Linezolid Clofazimine

Contd.

Contd.

4. Add pyrazinamide and any other first-line agent if they can help strengthen the regimen	D1	Pyrazinamide Ethambutol High-dose isoniazid
5. Add bedaquiline or delamanid[d]	D2	Bedaquiline Delamanid
6. Add any of these agents if the regimen cannot be composed otherwise	D3	*p*-Aminosalicylic acid Imipenem-cilastatin[e] Meropenem[e] Amoxicillin-clavulanate[a] (Thioacetazone[f])

Ans. C

279. Drug used in Muckle Wells syndrome is:

A. Anakinara
B. Abatacept
C. Rituximab
D. Tocilizumab

Explanation:

- Anakinra is the recombinant form of the naturally occurring IL-1 receptor antagonist.
- Although anakinra has seen limited use for the treatment of RA, it has enjoyed a resurgence of late as an effective therapy of some rare inherited syndromes dependent on IL-1 production, including neonatal-onset inflammatory disease, Muckle-Wells syndrome, and familial cold urticaria, as well as systemic juvenile-onset inflammatory arthritis and adult-onset Still's disease.
- Anakinra should not be combined with an anti-TNF drug due to the high rate of serious infections observed with this regimen in a clinical trial.

Ans. A

280. Reduced anion gap is seen with:

A. Hypoalbuminemia
B. Ileostomy fluid loss
C. Recovery from DKA
D. Lactic acidosis

Explanation:

- Reduced anion gap is seen with Hypoalbuminemia, Plasma cell dyscrasia, Monoclonal protein & Bromide intoxication (normal variant).

Ans. A

281. Which proteolytic enzyme is exopeptidase?

A. Amylase
B. Chymotrypsin
C. Aminopeptidase
D. Trypsin

Explanation:

- *Proteolytic enzymes* include endopeptidases (trypsin, chymotrypsin), which act on internal peptide bonds of proteins and polypeptides; exopeptidases (carboxypeptidases, aminopeptidases), which act on the free carboxyl- and amino-terminal ends of peptides, respectively; and elastase.
- *Proteolytic enzymes* are secreted as inactive zymogen precursors.
- Ribonucleases (deoxyribonucleases, ribonuclease) are also secreted.

Ans. C

282. CMT1A is caused due to:

A. PMP22 duplication
B. PMP22 deletion
C. MFN2 duplication
D. MFN2 deletion

Ans. A

283. A 18-year-old male presents to OPD with a 2-day history of persistent fever, abdominal pain, and right knee pain. During the past year, he has had 4 similar episodes, each lasting 2 to 3 days. He feels well between episodes. He takes no medications. On physical examination, temperature is 38.3°C (101.0°F), blood pressure is 150/86 mm Hg, pulse rate is 102/min, and respiration rate is 18/min. There is diffuse abdominal tenderness without rebound and no evidence of hepatosplenomegaly or lymphadenopathy. Right knee has an effusion A well-demarcated, raised, erythematous, warm, and painful rash is noted on the right lower extremity overlying the shin. Laboratory studies reveal an erythrocyte sedimentation rate of 42 mm/h and a normal serum ferritin level; antinuclear antibody test results are negative. Urinalysis reveals 1+ protein with no cells or casts. Which of the following is the most likely diagnosis?

A. Adult-onset Still disease
B. Crohn disease
C. Familial Mediterranean fever
D. Reactive arthritis

Explanation:

Table: The hereditary recurrent fever syndromes

	FMF	TRAPS	HIDS	MWS	FCAS	NOMID
Ethnicity	Jewish, Arab, Turkish, Armenian, Italian	Any ethnic group	Predominantly Dutch, northern European	Any ethnic group	Any ethnic group	Any ethnic group
Inheritance	Recessive[a]	Dominant	Recessive	Dominant	Dominant	Most commonly de novo mutations; somatic mosaicism in a significant minority
Gene/ chromosome	*MEFV*/16p13.3	*TNFRSF1A*/12p13	*MVK*/12q24	*NLRP3*/1q44	*NLRP3*/1q44	*NLRP3*/1q44
Protein	Pyrin	p55 TNF receptor	Mevalonate kinase	NLRP3 (cryopyrin)	NLRP3 (cryopyrin)	NLRP3 (cryopyrin)
Attack length	1-3 days	Often > 7 days	3-7 days	1-2 days	Minutes–3 days	Continuous, with flares
Serosa	Pleurisy, peritonitis; asymptomatic pericardial effusions	Pleurisy, peritonitis, pericarditis	Abdominal pain, but seldom peritonitis; pleurisy, pericarditis uncommon	Abdominal pain; pleurisy, pericarditis rare	Rare	Rare
Skin	Erysipeloid erythema	Centrifugally migrating erythema	Diffuse maculopapular rash; oral ulcers	Diffuse urticaria-like rash	Cold-induced urticaria-like rash	Diffuse urticaria-like rash
Joints	Acute monoarthritis; chronic hip arthritis (rare)	Acute monoarthritis, arthralgia	Arthralgia, oligoarthritis	Arthralgia, large joint oligoarthritis	Polyarthralgia	Epiphyseal, patellar overgrowth, clubbing
Muscle	Exercise-induced myalgia common; protracted febrile myalgia rare	Migratory myalgia	Uncommon	Myalgia common	Sometimes myalgia	Sometimes myalgia
Eyes, ears	Uncommon	Periorbital edema, conjunctivitis, rarely uveitis	Uncommon	Conjunctivitis, episcleritis, optic disc edema; sensorineural hearing loss	Conjunctivitis	Conjunctivitis, uveitis, optic disc edema, blindness, sensorineural hearing loss

Contd.

Contd.

CNS	Aseptic meningitis rare	Headache	Headache	Headache	Headache	Aseptic meningitis seizures
Amyloidosis	Most common in M694V homozygotes	~15% of cases, most often cysteine mutations, T50M	Uncommon	~25% of cases	Uncommon	Late complication
Treatment	Oral colchicine prophylaxis, IL-1 inhibitors for refractory cases	Glucocorticoids, etanercept, IL-1 inhibitors	NSAIDs for fever; IL-1 inhibitors	Anakinra, rilonacept, canakinumab	Anakinra, rilonacept, canakinumab	Anakinra

Ans. C

284. A 30 year old patient suffering from retroviral disease is on ART. He presented with symptoms of neuropathy. Which of the following drugs are not responsible for his symptoms?

A. Zidovudine
B. Stavudine
C. Lamivudine
D. Didanosine

Ans. A

285. A patient who works in an industry suffered from lead poisoning. Which of the following is false regarding the patient?

A. Most common presentation is encephalopathy
B. Causes sensory motor neuropathy
C. RBC show basophilic stippling
D. Treated with EDTA, BAL, Penicillamine

Explanation:

- The most common presentation of lead poisoning is an encephalopathy
- Motor neuropathy can also occur
- Laboratory investigation can reveal a microcytic hypochromic anemia with basophilic stippling of erythrocytes
- Chelation therapy with calcium disodium ethylene-diaminetetraacetic acid (EDTA), British anti-Lewisite (BAL), and penicillamine also demonstrates variable efficacy.

Ans. B

286. A patient multiple teeth caries has undergone procedure with denture cream containing zinc. He can develop all of the following symptoms except:

A. Neutropenia
B. Myelopathy
C. Neuropathy
D. Macrocytic anemia

Explanation:

- Excess zinc is an established cause of copper deficiency. Zinc upregulates enterocyte production of metallothionine, which results in decreased absorption of copper
- Hematologic abnormalities of copper deficiency- microcytic anemia, neutropenia, and occasionally Pancytopenia
- Myeloneuropathy can occur

Ans. D

287. Usually vitamin deficiencies causes neuropathy. However, which of the following vitamins cause neuropathy in deficiency as well as in excess doses?

A. Thiamine
B. Riboflavin
C. Pyridoxine
D. Cobalamine

Ans. C

288. Drug used for chemoprophylaxis for leptospirosis during pregnancy is:

A. Doxycycline B. Azithromycin

C. Ampicillin D. Amoxicillin

Explanation:

Table: Treatment and chemoprophylaxis of leptospirosis in adults[a]

Indication	Regimen
Treatment	
Mild leptospirosis	Doxycycline[b] (100 mg PO bid) *or* Amoxicillin (500 mg PO tid) *or* Ampicillin (500 mg PO tid)
Moderate/severe leptospirosis	Penicillin (1.5 million units IV or IM q6h) *or* Ceftriaxone (2 g/d IV) *or* Cefotaxime (1 g IV q6h) *or* Doxycycline[b] (loading dose of 200 mg IV, then 100 mg IV q12h)
Chemoprophylaxis[c]	
	Doxycycline[b] (200 mg PO once a week) *or* Azithromycin (250 mg PO once or twice a week)

[a] All regiments are given for 7 days.

[b] Doxycycline should not be given to pregnant women or children.

[c] The efficacy of doxycycline prophylaxis in endemic of epidemic settings remains unclear. Experiments in animal models and a cost-effectiveness model indicate that azithromycin has a number of characteristics that may make it efficacious in treatment and prophylaxis.

Ans. B

289. Gold standard method for diagnosis of Leigonella infection is:

A. Culture B. Direct Fluorescent antibody staining of sputum

C. Urinary antigen testing D. Antibody serology

Explanation:

- "Gold-standard" method for diagnosis of *Legionella* infection is isolation of organism from respiratory secretions, although culture for 3–5 days—and sometimes up to 2 weeks for non *pneumophila* species—is required.
- Antibiotics added to the medium suppress the growth of competing flora from nonsterile sites, and dyes color the colonies and assist in identification.

Table: Utility of special laboratory tests for the diagnosis of legionnaries' disease

Test	Sensitivity, %	Specificity, %
Culture		
• Sputum[a]	80	100
• Transtracheal aspirate	90	100
Direct fluorescent antibody staining of sputum	50-70	96-99
Urinary antigen testing[b]	70	100
Antibody serology[c]	40-60	96-99

[a] Use of multiple selective media with dyes.

[b] Reliable only for *L. pneumophila* serogroup 1.

[c] IgG and IgM testing of both acute- and convalescent-phase sera. A single titer of $\geq$1:256 is considered presumptive, while a fourfold rise in titer between the acute and convalescent phases is considered definitive. Titers peak at 3 months.

Ans. A

290. An unresponsive 3-year-old boy is brought into the ED by his parents after he was rescued from their swimming pool. The parents were hosting a midsummer barbecue when they heard screaming kids and found their son face-down in the swimming pool. Vital signs at admission to the ED were heart rate 40 beats/min, blood pressure 50/20 mm Hg, SatO2 88%, and body temperature 33° C. What are the next best steps?

A. Bronchoscopy lavage

B. Prone positioning

C. Mechanical ventilation as in all ARDS patients

D. Pediatrics Advance Cardiac Life Support (ACLS)

Explanation:

- Pediatric near drowning should be treated as an emergency with standard pediatric ACLS.
- However, immediately after recovery, should focus on pulmonary toilette by body positioning, suctioning, and titration of the ventilator in anticipation of impending respiratory complications; refractory hypoxemia; and ARDS.

Ans. D

291. A 65 year old male patient who is known case of chronic kidney disease has come to ER with c/o breathlessness for the past 2 days. Patient is disoriented. He has no recent blood reports. On auscultation bilateral rales are present. Hemodynamic parameters include hr-102/min, spo2-90% with face mask, O2 at 6l/min, Bp-180/96 mmHg, RR-30/min. Arterial blood gas shows reductions in both PaO2 and PaCo2. Further management includes:

A. Positive pressure ventilation is contraindicated

B. Beta blockers must be used to control the blood pressure

C. Patient must be in Supine position

D. Preload must be reduced

Explanation:

- In case of acute pulmonary edema administer supplemental oxygen to achieve O2 saturation ≥92%; if inadequate, use positive-pressure ventilation by face or nasal mask, and if necessary, endotracheal intubation.
- Early arterial blood gases show reductions of both PaO2 and PaCO2. With progressive respiratory failure, hypercapnia develops with acidemia.
- Reduce preload:
  a. Seat pt upright to reduce venous return, if not hypotensive.
  b. Intravenous loop diuretic (e.g., furosemide, initially 0.5–1.0 mg/kg); use lower dose if patient does not take diuretics chronically.
  c. Nitroglycerin (sublingual 0.4 mg × 3 q5min) followed by 5–20 μg/min IV if needed.
  d. Morphine 2–4 mg IV acts as a venodilator and may relieve dyspnea and anxiety; use with caution and assess frequently for hypotension or respiratory depression; naloxone should be available to reverse effects if necessary.
  e. Consider ACE inhibitor if pt is hypertensive, or in setting of acute MI with heart failure.
  f. Consider nesiritide (recombinant brain natriuretic peptide; 2-μg/kg bolus IV followed by 0.01 μg/kg per min) for refractory symptoms—do not use in acute MI or cardiogenic shock.
- Inotropic agents are indicated in cardiogenic pulmonary edema and severe LV dysfunction: dopamine, dobutamine, milrinone.

- Precipitating cause of cardiogenic pulmonary edema should be sought and treated, particularly acute arrhythmias or infection. For refractory pulmonary edema associated with persistent cardiac ischemia, early coronary revascularization may be life-saving.

Ans. D

292. A 65-year-old male is involved in a motor vehicle accident and is brought to the emergency department for evaluation. He is drowsy, with headache, nausea and emesis with significant facial swelling, hyphema right eye, fracture right radius, broken ribs 4-6 on the left with flail chest. Which of the following drug combinations would be preferred for induction and paralysis during intubation?

A. Propofol and scoline
B. Ketamine and atracurium
C. Etomidate and rocuronium
D. Ketamine and rocuronium

Explanation:

- Hyphaema suggests intracranial involvement (most likely bleed), with headache, nausea, emesis hence drugs which increase intracranial pressure cannot be used like ketamine and scoline.
- In order to not affect existing hemodynamics the best combination would be etomidate and rocuronium for induction and paralysis.

Ans. C

293. Most common clinical manifestation of Clostridium difficile infection?

A. Diarrhea
B. Fever
C. Abdominal pain
D. Leukocytosis

Explanation:

- Diarrhea is the most common manifestation caused by C. difficile. Stools are almost never grossly bloody and range from soft and unformed to watery or mucoid in consistency, with a characteristic odor.
- Clinical and laboratory findings include fever in 28% of cases, abdominal pain in 22%, and leukocytosis in 50%.
- When adynamic ileus (which is seen on X-ray in ~20% of cases) results in cessation of stool passage, the diagnosis of CDI is frequently overlooked.
- A clue to the presence of unsuspected CDI in these patients is unexplained leukocytosis, with ≥15,000 white blood cells (WBCs)/μL. Such patients are at high risk for complications of C. difficile infection, particularly toxic megacolon and sepsis.

Ans. A

294. Not associated with Orthopnea among following:

A. Abdominal Obesity
B. Abdominal Ascites
C. Diaphragmatic weakness
D. Hepatopulmonary syndrome

Explanation:

- Orthopnea– Dyspnea occurring in recumbent position & usually a feature of heart failure than exertional dyspnea.
- Relieved by sitting upright or sleeping with additional support.
- Orthopnea can also occur with abdominal obesity, ascites & pulmonary disease patients.

Hepatopulmonary syndrome

- Leads to Orthodeoxia→ Hypoxia in upright position.
- Leads to Platypnea→ Sensation of shortness of breath when upright.

Ans. D

295. Identify the fundus image:

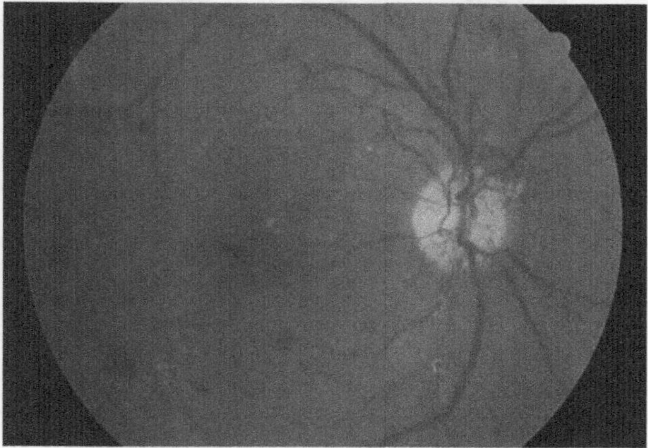

A. Diabetic retinopathy
B. Retinitis pigmentosa
C. Central retinal vein occlusion
D. Leukemia

Explanation:

- Neovascularization of vessels proliferating from optic disc, microaneurysm and blot hemorrhages are seen in Diabetic retinopathy.
- In retinitis pigmentosa jet black bony spicule lesions seen.

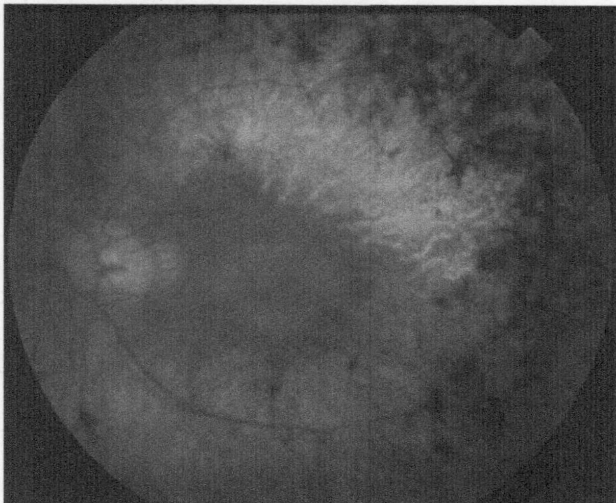

- In Central retinal vein occlusion splashed tomato appearance seen.

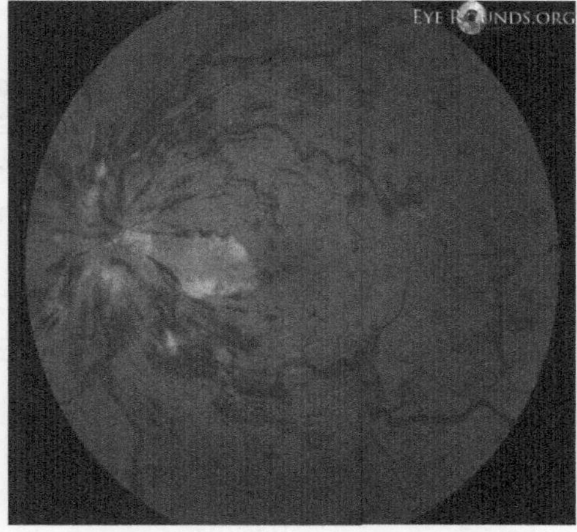

- In leukemia roth spots are seen.

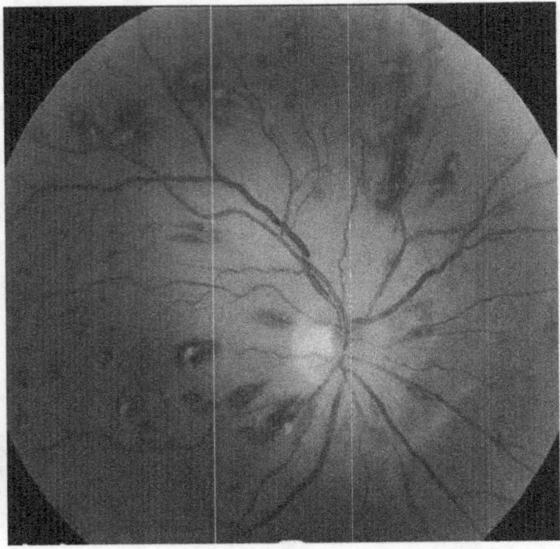

Ans. A

296. A 40 year old woman known hypertensive on calcium channel blockers, betablockers, ARBs, diuretics came to the hospital with complaints of headache. Her BP was 160/100 mm Hg. Routine investigations reveal hypokalemia. What is the next step in controlling her blood pressure?

A. Add alphablockers
B. Add ACE Inhibitors
C. To do aldosterone renin ratio
D. To stop diuretics due to hypokalemia.

Explanation:

- In patients with hypertension, not controlled by more than 3 drugs including a diuretic or hypokalemia or adrenal mass or a family history of early onset hypertension, mineralocorticoid excess should be suspected.

Ans. C

297. A 32 year male presented to ER with signs of severe hemodynamic instability BP- 80/40 mm Hg, HR- 120/mt, RR- 24/mt , SPO2- 95 room air- with history of chronic alcoholism, USG shows flat Jugular veins, this condition is seen in:

A. Pancreatitis
B. Cardiac tamponade
C. Tension pneumothorax
D. Superior vena cava syndrome

Explanation:

- Jugular veins are flat in oligemic or distributive (septic) shock; jugular venous distention (JVD) is typical in cardiogenic shock; JVD in presence of paradoxical pulse suggests cardiac tamponade.

CATEGORIES OF SHOCK

- **Distributive shock (profound decrease in systemic vascular tone:** Sepsis, Pancreatitis, Anaphylaxis, Neurogenic (e.g., spinal cord injury) & Endocrine-related (Addison's disease, myxedema)
- **Cardiogenic shock:** Myopathic (acute MI, fulminant myocarditis), Mechanical (acute severe mitral regurgitation, acute severe aortic insufficiency [e.g., aortic dissection], severe aortic stenosis, acute VSD), Arrhythmic
- **Obstructive shock:** Pericardial tamponade, Massive pulmonary embolism, Tension pneumothorax
- **Hypovolemic shock:** Hemorrhage, GI losses (vomiting, diarrhea), Burns, Polyuria (diabetic ketoacidosis, diabetes insipidus).

Ans. A

298. A 30 year old patient who is a known case of Kearn Sayre syndrome and his mother suffering from similar illness presents with all of the following except:

A. Progressive external ophthalmoplegia
B. Retinitis pigmentosa
C. Heart block
D. Autosomal transmission

Explanation:

- **Kearn-Sayre Syndrome (KSS)**–defined triad of clinical findings: onset before age 20, CPEO, and pigmentary retinopathy, plus one or more of the following features: complete heart block, cerebrospinal fluid (CSF) protein >1 g/L (100 mg/dL), or cerebellar ataxia
- It occurs due to mitochondrial DNA deletion and maternal inheritance

Ans. D

CHAPTER 2

RESPIRATORY SYSTEM

1. All belong to obstructive lung diseases except:

A. Myasthenia gravis

B. Asthma

C. Bronchiectasis

D. Bronchiolitis

Explanation:

Table: Categories of respiratory disease	
Category	**Examples**
Obstructive lung disease	Asthma Chronic obstructive pulmonary disease (COPD) Bronchiectasis Bronchiolitis
Restrictive pathophysiology–parenchymal disease	Idiopathic pulmonary fibrosis (IPF) Asbestosis Desquamative interstitial pneumonitis (DIP) Sarcoidosis
Restrictive pathophysiology–neuromuscular weakness	Amyotrophic lateral sclerosis (ALS) Guillain-Barré syndrome Myasthenia gravis
Restrictive pathophysiology–chest wall/pleural disease	Kyphoscoliosis Ankylosing spondylitis Chronic pleural effusions
Pulmonary vascular disease	Pulmonary embolism Pulmonary arterial hypertension (PAH) Pulmonary venoocclusive disease Vasculitis
Malignancy	Bronchogenic carcinoma (non-small-cell and small-cell lung cancer) Metastatic disease
Infectious diseases	Pneumonia Bronchitis Tracheitis

Ans. A

2. **A 24-year-old woman is seen for a complaint of shortness of breath and wheezing. She notes the symptoms to be worse when she has exercised outdoors and is around cats. She has had allergic rhinitis in the spring and summer for many years and suffered from eczema as a child. On physical examination, she is noted to have expiratory wheezing. Her pulmonary function tests demonstrate an FEV1 of 2.67 (79% predicted), FVC of 3.81 L (97% predicted), and an FEV1/FVC ratio of 70% (86% predicted). After administration of albuterol, the FEV1 increases to 3.0 L (12.4%). Which of the following statements regarding the patient's disease process is true?**

A. Confirmation of the diagnosis will require methacholine challenge testing

B. Mortality due to the disease has been increasing over the past decade

C. Most common risk factor in individuals with the disorder is genetic predisposition

D. Severity of the disease does not vary significantly within a given patient with disease

Explanation:

- Patient in this clinical scenario presents with symptoms typical of asthma, including shortness of breath and wheezing.
- She also manifests evidence of atopy, the most common risk factor for developing asthma, with sensitivity to outdoor allergens and cats. In addition, the patient has a history of allergic rhinitis and eczema, both of which are commonly seen in individuals with asthma. Indeed, over 80% of asthma patients have a concomitant diagnosis of allergic rhinitis. Atopy is present in 40%–50% of the population of affluent countries, but only a small proportion of these individuals develop asthma.
- Many studies have shown a genetic predisposition via family history and recent genome-wide screens, but no single genetic profile has shown high positive predictive value. Overall, the prevalence of asthma in developed countries has increased over the past 30 years, but recently has leveled off, with a prevalence of about 15% in children and 10%–12% in adults.
- Asthma deaths remain rare and have decreased in recent decades. In the 1960s, asthma deaths did increase with an overuse of short-acting β-agonist medications.
- However, since the introduction of inhaled corticosteroids as maintenance therapy, deaths have declined.
- Risk factors for fatal asthma include frequent use of rescue inhalers, lack of therapy with inhaled corticosteroids, and prior hospitalizations for asthma.
- Interestingly, the overall disease severity does not vary significantly within a given patient over the course of the disease. Individuals who have mild asthma typically continue to have mild asthma, whereas those with severe disease present with severe disease.
- Diagnosis of asthma can be made by demonstrating airflow obstruction with significant reversibility on bronchodilator administration.
- In this case, the FEV1/FVC ratio is decreased to 70%, which is low. In addition, the FEV1 increases by 12.4% and 230 mL.
- This meets criteria for bronchodilator reversibility of increases of at least 200 mL and 12%.
- Bronchoprovocation testing with methacholine can be considered in individuals who have suspected asthma but have normal pulmonary function tests.

Ans. D

3. **Hypertrophic osteoarthropathy (HOA) is uncommon in:**

A. Sarcoidosis

B. Bronchiectasis

C. Pulmonary TB

D. Mesothelioma

Explanation:

- HOA was initially called as HPOA. No more we use the word HPOA (Hypertrophic pulmonary osteoarthropathy).
- HOA occurs in patients with intrathoracic malignancies, most common being bronchogenic carcinoma and pleural tumors.

- Lung metastases infrequently cause HOA. HOA is also seen in patients with intrathoracic infections, including lung abscesses, empyema, and bronchiectasis, but is uncommon in pulmonary tuberculosis.
- Lung metastasis and Tuberculosis are uncommon to cause HOA.
- Most common cause of HOA is Malignancy (Ca Lung)*

Ans. C

4. All of the following are indications for lung Transplantation in COPD patients except:

A. BODE index ≥7

B. FEV1 < 15–20%

C. Severe PHT

D. Two or more severe exacerbations in preceding year

Explanation:

Disease-Specific Guidelines for Referral and Transplantation Chronic Obstructive Pulmonary Disease (COPD)

Listing for Transplantation

1. BODE index ≥7
2. FEV1 <15–20%
3. Moderate to severe pulmonary hypertension
4. **Three or more severe exacerbations in preceding year**
5. One severe exacerbation with acute hypercapnic respiratory failure

Table: Disease-specific guidelines for referral and transplantation
Chronic Obstructive Pulmonary Disease
Referral for Evaluation • Progressive despite medications, oxygen and pulmonary rehabilitation • FEV_1 < 25% • PaO_2 < 60 mm Hg or $PaCO_2$ > 50 mm Hg • BODE index 5-6 **Listing for Transplantation** • BODE index ≥ 7 • FEV_1 <15-20% • Moderate to severe pulmonary hypertension • Three or more severe exacerbations in preceding year • One severe exacerbation with acute hypercapnic respiratory failure

Ans. D

5. Most common organism causing community acquired pneumonia is:

A. Streptococcus pneumonia

B. Methicillin sensitive staphylococcus aureus

C. Mycoplasma pneumonia

D. Klebsiella pneumonia

Explanation:

- Most common organism causing community acquired pneumonia is Streptococcus pneumonia

Ans. A

6. Abnormalities in multiple molecular pathways & genes for PAH are all except?

A. Decreased expression of voltage regulated potassium channel

B. Decreased tissue factor expression

C. Mutation in bone morphogenic protein receptor 2

D. Overactivation of serotonin transporter

Explanation:

- Abnormalities in multiple molecular pathways and genes that regulate the pulmonary vascular endothelial and smooth muscle cells have been identified.
- These abnormalities include decreased expression of the voltage-regulated potassium channel, mutations in bone morphogenetic protein receptor-2, increased tissue factor expression, overactivation of serotonin transporter, hypoxia induced activation of hypoxia-inducible factor-1α, and activation of nuclear factor of activated T cells.
- As a result, there is a decrease in apoptosis of smooth muscle cells and the emergence of apoptosis resistant endothelial cells that promote their accumulation and can obliterate the vascular lumen.
- In addition, thrombin deposition in pulmonary vasculature from prothrombotic state that develops as an independent abnormality or as a result of endothelial dysfunction may amplify obliterative arteriopathy.

Table: Molecular determinants of the pathogenesis of pulmonary arterial hypertension
Alterations in regulators of proliferation
• Growth factors
– PDGF
– FGF
– VEGF
– EGF
• TGF-β
• BMP
• Transcription factors
• MMPs
• Cytokines
• Chemokines
• Mitochondria
Alterations in inflammatory mediators
• Altered T-cell subsets
• Monocytes and macrophages
• IL-1β
• IL-β
• MCP-1
• RANTES
• Fractalkine
Alterations in vascular tone
• Endothelin
• Nitric oxide
• Serotonin
• Prostaglandin
• K^+ channels
• Ca^{2+} channels

Hypoxia induced remodelling
• HIF-1α
• ROS
• Mitochondria
Alterations in TGF-β signalling pathways
• BMPR2
• ALK1
• Endoglin
• Smad9
• TGF-β1

Ans. B

7. **All are true regarding Type 4 respiratory failure except:**
   A. Due to hypoperfusion od respiratory muscles in shock patients
   B. Normally respiratory muscles consume <5% of total cardiac output & oxygen delivery
   C. In type 4 respiratory failure, upto 40% of cardiac output is distributed to respiratory muscle
   D. Non invasive positive pressure ventilation is used for treatment

Explanation:

- Results from hypoperfusion of respiratory muscles in patients in shock.
- Normally, respiratory muscles consume <5% of total cardiac output and oxygen delivery.
- Patients in shock often experience respiratory distress due to pulmonary edema (e.g., in cardiogenic shock), lactic acidosis, and anemia.
- In this setting, up to 40% of cardiac output may be distributed to the respiratory muscles.
- Intubation and mechanical ventilation can allow redistribution of cardiac output away from the respiratory muscles and back to vital organs while the shock is treated.

Ans. D

8. **Below Flow volume loop indicates:**

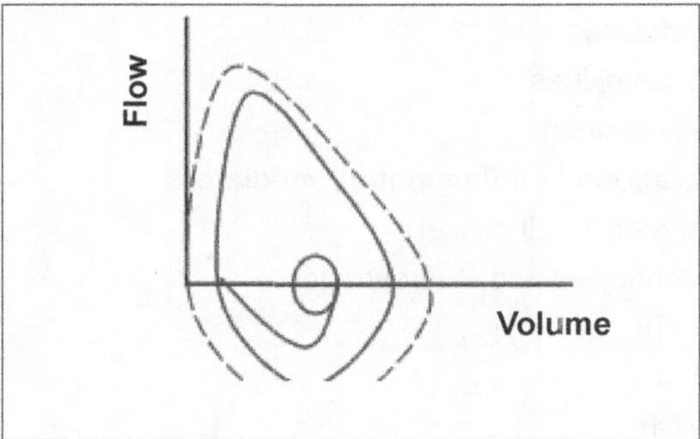

   A. Restriction due to increased lung elastic recoil
   B. Restriction due to chest wall abnormality
   C. Restriction due to respiratory muscle weakness
   D. Obstruction due to airway narrowing

Explanation:

	Restriction due to increased lung elastic recoil (pulmonary fibrosis)	Restriction due to chest wall abnormality (moderate obesity)	Restriction due to respiratory muscle weakness (myasthenia gravis)	Obstruction due to airway narrowing (acute asthma)	Obstruction due to decreased elastic recoil (severe emphysema)
TLC	60%	95%	75%	100%	130%
FRC	60%	65%	100%	104%	220%
RV	60%	100%	120%	120%	310%
FVC	60%	92%	60%	90%	60%
FEV_1	75%	92%	60%	35% pre-b.d. 75% post-b.d.	35% pre-b.d. 38% post-b.d.
R_{aw}	1.0	1.0	1.0	2.5	1.5
D_{Lco}	60%	95%	80%	120%	40%

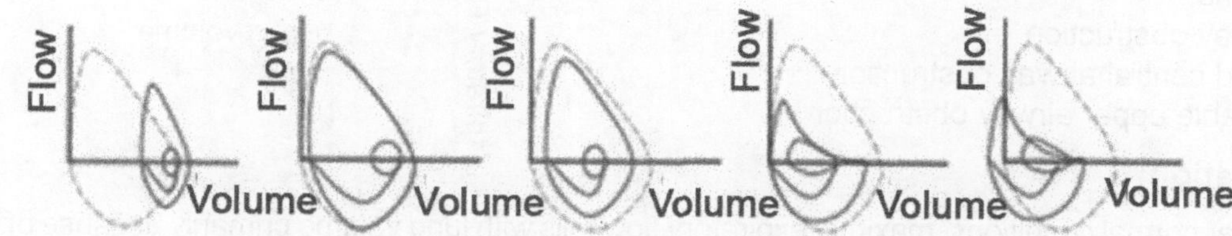

Ans. C

9. Spontaneous breathing trial is declared a failure & stopped if:

A. Respiratory rate <30/min for >5 min
B. Heart rate >120/min
C. SBP<100 mm Hg
D. Increased anxiety or diaphoresis

Explanation:

Spontaneous breathing trial is declared a failure and stopped if *any* of the following occur:

1. Respiratory rate >35/min for >5 min
2. O2 saturation <90%
3. Heart rate >140/min or a 20% increase or decrease from baseline
4. Systolic blood pressure <90 mmHg or >180 mmHg, or
5. Increased anxiety or diaphoresis
   - If, at the end of the spontaneous breathing trial, none of the above events has occurred and the ratio of the respiratory rate and tidal volume in liters (f/VT) is <105, patient can be extubated

Ans. B & D

10. Not true about airway resistance is:

A. Total resistance of pulmonary & upper airways is measured in same body plethysmograph used to measure FRC
B. In healthy, Raw is very low (<2cm H2O/L/sec & half of detected resistance resides within upper airway
C. In lung, most resistance originates in peripheral airways
D. Airways resistance measurement tends to be insensitive to peripheral airflow obstruction

Explanation:

- Total resistance of the pulmonary and upper airways is measured in the same body plethysmograph used to measure FRC.
- Patient is asked once again to pant, but this time against a closed and then opened shutter.
- Panting against the closed shutter reveals the thoracic gas volume as described above.
- When the shutter is opened, flow is directed to and from the body box, so that volume fluctuations in the box reveal the extent of thoracic gas compression, which in turn reveals the pressure fluctuations driving flow.
- Simultaneous measurement of flow allows the calculation of lung resistance (as flow divided by pressure). In health, Raw is very low (<2 cmH2O/L/s), and half of the detected resistance resides within the upper airway.
- In lung, most resistance originates in the central airways.

Ans. C

11. What does this flow volume loop indicate?

A. Normal
B. Airway obstruction
C. Fixed central airway obstruction
D. Variable upper airway obstruction

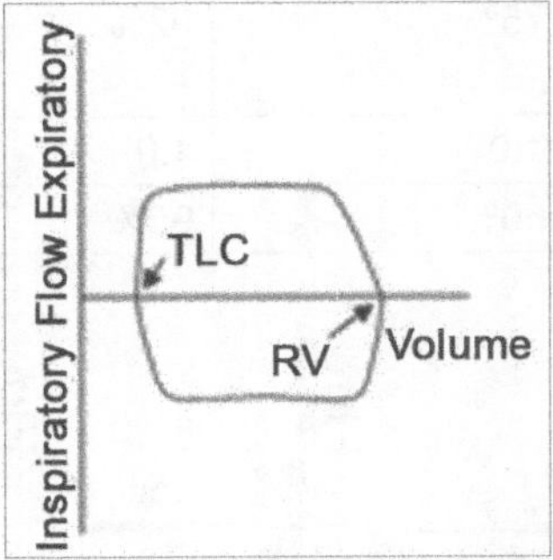

Explanation:

- Under normal conditions, maximal expiratory flow falls with lung volume primarily because of the dependence of lung recoil pressure on lung volume. In pulmonary fibrosis, lung recoil pressure is increased at any lung volume, and thus the maximal expiratory flow is elevated when considered in relation to lung volume. Conversely, in emphysema, lung recoil pressure is reduced; this reduction is a principal mechanism by which maximal expiratory flows fall.
- Diseases that narrow the airway lumen at any transmural pressure (e.g., asthma or chronic bronchitis) or that cause excessive airway collapsibility (e.g., tracheomalacia) also reduce maximal expiratory flow.

Ans. C

12. DLco is increased in:

A. Pulmonary fibrosis
B. Moderate obesity
C. Myasthenia gravis
D. Acute asthma

Explanation:

	Restriction due to increased lung elastic recoil (pulmonary fibrosis)	**Restriction due to chest wall abnormality (moderate obesity)**	**Restriction due to respiratory muscle weakness (myasthenia gravis)**	**Obstruction due to airway narrowing (acute asthma)**	**Obstruction due to decreased elastic recoil (severe emphysema)**
TLC	60%	95%	75%	100%	130%
FRC	60%	65%	100%	104%	220%
RV	60%	100%	120%	120%	310%
FVC	60%	92%	60%	90%	60%
FEV_1	75%	92%	60%	35% pre-b.d. 75% post-b.d.	35% pre-b.d. 38% post-b.d.
R_{aw}	1.0	1.0	1.0	2.5	1.5
D_{Lco}	60%	95%	80%	120%	40%

Ans. D

13. **A 66 year old male who is a known COPD patient presents with complaints of weight gain and decreased visual acuity. Which among the following drugs has contributed to this complication?**

A. Albuterol
B. Prednisolone
C. Roflumilast
D. Ipratropium bromide

Explanation:

- Although inhaled bronchodilator medications have not been proven to increase longevity in COPD, they may significantly reduce respiratory symptoms and exacerbations. Short- and long-acting β-adrenergic agonists, short- and longacting anticholinergics, and theophylline derivatives all may be used. Inhaled bronchodilator medications generally have fewer side effects than oral bronchodilator medications. Pts with mild symptoms and infrequent exacerbations can usually be managed with an inhaled short-acting anticholinergic such as ipratropium or a short-acting β agonist such as albuterol. Combination therapy with long-acting β agonists and/or long-acting anticholinergics should be added in pts with significant respiratory symptoms and/or frequent exacerbations.
- Chronic systemic corticosteroid treatment is not recommended in COPD pts due to the risk of multiple complications, including osteoporosis, weight gain, cataracts, and glucose intolerance.
- Roflumilast reduces exacerbation frequency in severe COPD pts with chronic bronchitis and a prior history of exacerbations; however, side effects including nausea often limit its use.

Ans. B

14. **A 60 year old COPD patient develops new onset pedal oedema. On examination JVP is raised and loud second heart sound is heard. Which among the following contributing factors is the most important for the development of this complication?**

A. Hypoxia
B. Hypercapnia
C. Secondary infection
D. Respiratory alkalosis

Explanation:

- One of the long-term complications of COPD is cor pulmonale. Cor pulmonale is the impairment of right ventricular function due to hypoxia in COPD patients. It comes under group 3 of pulmonary hypertension seen in chronic lung diseases such as COPD.

Ans. A

15. **A 40 year old male comes to the OPD with complaints of fever, chills, cough, pleuritic chest pain and breathlessness. Chest xr ay shows infective pattern on lung parenchyma. Which among the following is true regarding the CURB 65 score which is used to assess this patient?**

A. Urea >8 mmol/L
B. Respiratory rate >20/min
C. Blood pressure, Systolic <90 mm Hg or Diastolic <60 mm Hg
D. Age >65 years

Explanation:

- Two sets of criteria identify pts who will benefit from hospital care. It is not clear which set is superior, and application of each tool should be tempered by a consideration of factors relevant to the individual pt. – Pneumonia Severity Index (PSI): Points are given for 20 variables, including age, coexisting illness, and abnormal physical and laboratory findings. On this basis, pts are assigned to one of five classes of mortality risk. – CURB-65: Five variables are included: confusion (C); urea >7 mmol/L (U); respiratory rate ≥30/min (R); blood pressure, systolic ≤90 mmHg or diastolic ≤60 mmHg (B); and age ≥65 years (65). Pts with a score of 0 can be treated at home, pts with a score of 1 or 2 (not counting any point given for age ≥65 years) should be hospitalized, and pts with a score of ≥3 may require management in the ICU.

Ans. C

16. **Identify the flow-volume loops image:**

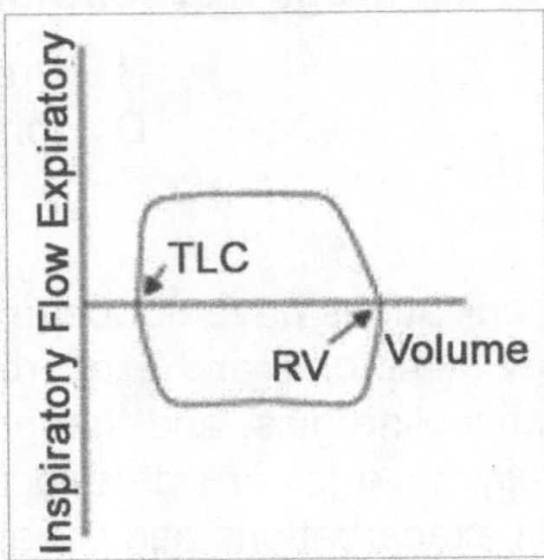

A. Normal
B. Variable upper airway obstruction
C. Variable lower airway obstruction
D. Fixed central airway obstruction

Explanation:

- Image shows abnormality both during inspiration and expiration seen in fixed central airway obstruction as in tracheal stenosis such as Guillain barre syndrome and prolonged intubation greater than 2weeks.

Other options:

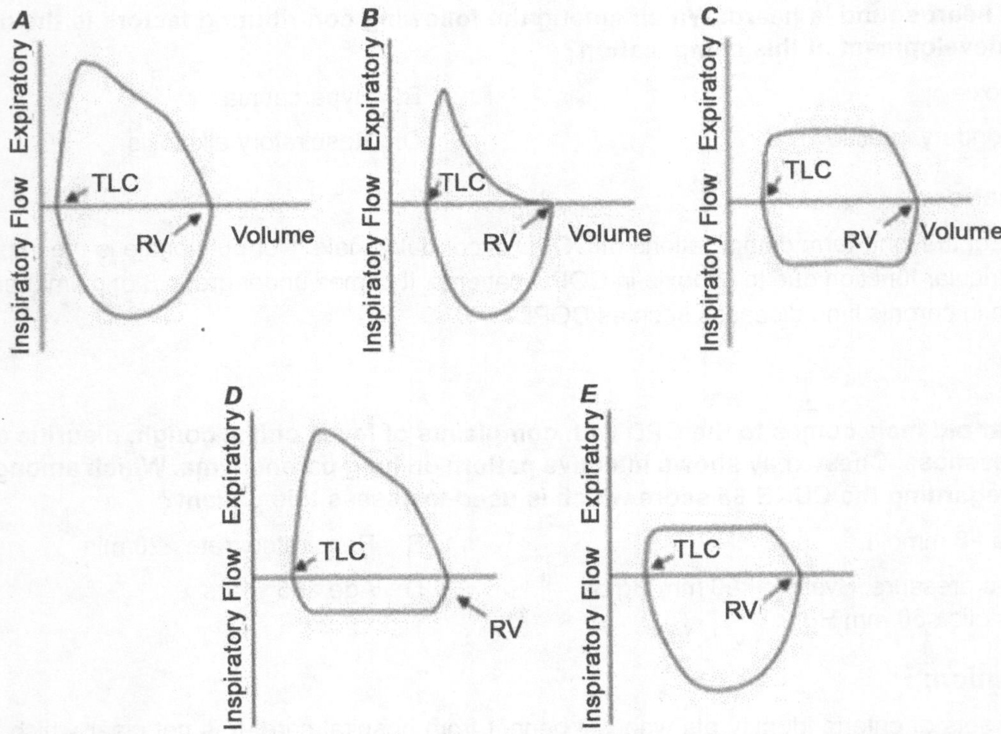

Figure: Flow-volume loops. *A.* Normal *B.* Airflow obstruction. *C.* Fixed central airway obstruction (either above or below the thoracic inlet). *D.* Variable upper airway obstruction (above the thoracic inlet). *E.* Variable lower airwary obstruction (below the thoracic inlet); RV, residual volume; TLC, total lung capacity.

Ans. D

17. A 55 year old obese male comes to the OPD with complaints of day time somnolence and nocturnal breathing. A polysomnography reveals a AHI (apnoea-hypopnea index) of 15. Which among the following is the treatment of choice for this patient?

A. Modafinil
B. CPAP
C. Tracheostomy
D. Psychotherapy

Explanation:

- In pts with OSAHS, efforts to reduce weight in obese pts, limit alcohol use, optimize sleep duration, regulate sleep schedules, treat nasal allergies, and carefully withdraw sedative medications should be pursued. The primary therapy for OSAHS is continuous positive airway pressure (CPAP), delivered through a nasal or nasal-oral mask. Selecting a comfortable mask delivery system and titrating the appropriate amount of CPAP are essential. Airway drying related to CPAP can be reduced by including a heated humidification component in the CPAP system. Alternative OSAHS therapies include mandibular repositioning splints (oral devices), which hold the jaw and tongue forward to widen the pharyngeal airway. These devices are typically used for mild OSAHS pts or pts who do not tolerate CPAP. Several types of surgical procedures have been used in OSAHS, including bariatric surgery in obese pts, tonsillectomy, and pharyngeal surgery. Tracheostomy is curative since it bypasses the upper airway obstruction site, but it is rarely used. No drugs have been proven to reduce apneic events. Treatment of CSA is challenging; it involves managing any predisposing conditions, such as congestive heart failure.

Ans. B

18. Ultrasound scan of a 55 year old male showed right sided pleural effusion and ascites. Which among the following is false regarding hepatic hydrothorax?

A. Transjugular intrahepatic portosystemic shunt is helpful (TIPS).
B. It occurs in approximately 5-15% patients with liver cirrhosis.
C. Pathophysiology is due to the passage of ascites from the peritoneal cavity into the pleural cavity through small diaphragmatic defects.
D. Liver transplantation is contraindicated.

Explanation:

- The diagnosis in hepatic hydrothorax refers to the presence of transudative pleural effusion with the exclusion of other alternative causes. Patient often has signs of ascites as well as other findings associated with cirrhosis. Pleural effusion is predominantly seen on the right side. Treatment options include salt restricted diet, diuretics, serial thoracenteses, TIPS, pleurodesis, thoracoscopic surgery for diaphragmatic repair and liver transplantation.

Ans. D

19. A 30 year old male presents with complaints of chronic cough and breathlessness. HRCT reveals bronchiectasis more pronounced in the upper lung fields. What is the diagnosis?

A. Chronic recurrent aspiration
B. Cystic fibrosis
C. Non tuberculous mycobacteria
D. ILD

Explanation:

- Bronchiectasis is an irreversible airway dilation that involves the lung in either a focal (due to obstruction) or a diffuse (due to a systemic or infectious process) manner. The most widely cited mechanism of infectious bronchiectasis is the "vicious cycle hypothesis," in which susceptibility to infection and poor mucociliary clearance result in microbial colonization of the bronchial tree. Cystic fibrosis and post tuberculosis related bronchiectasis are most commonly seen in the upper lobes. Non tubercular mycobacteria predominantly involves middle lobe. In ILD and post aspiration, bronchiectasis is seen in the lower lobes.

Ans. B

20. A 78-year-old woman is admitted to the medical intensive care unit (ICU) with multilobar pneumonia. On initial presentation to the emergency department, her initial oxygen saturation was 60% on room air and only increased to 82% on a non-rebreather face mask. She was in marked respiratory distress and intubated in the emergency department. Upon admission to the ICU, she was sedated and paralyzed. The ventilator is set in the assist control mode with a respiratory rate of 24 breaths/min, tidal volume of 6 mL/kg, FiO2 of 1.0, and positive end-expiratory pressure of 12 cmH2O. An arterial blood gas measurement is performed on these settings; the results are pH of 7.20, PCO2 of 32 mmHg, and PO2 of 54 mmHg. What is the cause of the hypoxemia?

A. Hypoventilation alone

B. Hypoventilation and ventilation-perfusion mismatch

C. Shunt

D. Ventilation-perfusion mismatch

Explanation:

- In this patient presenting with multilobar pneumonia, hypoxemia is present that does not correct with increasing concentration of inspired oxygen.
- Inability to overcome hypoxemia or the lack of a notable increase in partial pressure of arterial oxygen (PaO2) or oxygen saturation (SaO2) with increasing fraction of inspired oxygen physiologically defines a shunt. A shunt occurs when deoxygenated blood is transported to the left heart and systemic circulation without having the capability of becoming oxygenated.
- Causes of shunt include alveolar collapse (atelectasis), intra-alveolar filling processes, intrapulmonary vascular malformations, or structural cardiac disease leading to right-to-left shunt. In this case, the patient has multilobar pneumonia leading to alveoli that are being perfused but unable to participate in gas exchange because they are filled with pus and inflammatory exudates.
- Acute respiratory distress syndrome is another common cause of shunt physiology. V/Q mismatch is the most common cause of hypoxemia and results when there are some alveolar units with low ratios (low ventilation to perfusion) that fail to fully oxygenate perfused blood.
- When blood is returned to the left heart, the poorly oxygenated blood admixes with blood from normal alveolar units.
- Resultant hypoxemia is less severe than with shunt and can be corrected with increasing the inspired oxygen concentration. Hypoventilation with or without other causes of hypoxemia is not present in this case, as the PCO2 <40 mmHg indicates hyperventilation.
- Acidosis present in this case is of a metabolic rather than a pulmonary source. Because the patient is paralyzed, she is unable to increase her respiratory rate above the set rate to compensate for the metabolic acidosis.

Ans. C

21. An 18-year-old female has complaints of early nocturnal cough and breathlessness. She has signs of atopy and raised IgE levels. Which among the following drugs can worsen the symptoms in this disease?

A. Aspirin

B. Indomethacin

C. Propranolol

D. All of the above

Explanation:

- The majority of asthmatics have childhood-onset disease. Most asthmatics have atopy, and they often have atopic dermatitis (eczema) and/or allergic rhinitis. β-Adrenergic blocking medications can markedly worsen asthma symptoms and should typically be avoided in asthmatics. Approximately 1–5% of asthmatics have sensitivity to aspirin and other cyclooxygenase inhibitors.

Ans. D

22. A 70 year old male presents to the OPD with complaints of exertional dyspnoea and dry cough. On examination patient has bilateral basilar fine velcro crackles. Which among the following is false in this disease?

A. Reduction in FEC
B. A positive bronchodilator reversibility
C. Reduction in compliance
D. Reduction in diffusion capacity

Explanation:

- Bibasilar end-inspiratory crackles are commonly observed in interstitial lung disease. Interstitial lung diseases (ILDs) are a group of >200 disease entities characterized by diffuse lung parenchymal abnormalities: Lung function measurements can assess the extent of pulmonary involvement in pts with ILD. Most ILDs produce a restrictive ventilatory defect with reduced total lung capacity. The forced expiratory volume in 1 s (FEV1) and forced vital capacity (FVC) are typically reduced, but the ratio of FEV1 /FVC is usually normal to increased. Reduction in the diffusing capacity of the lung for carbon monoxide (DLCO) is commonly observed. Positive bronchodilator reversibility is seen in bronchial asthma.

Ans. B

23. Identify the marked structure in the CT image shown:

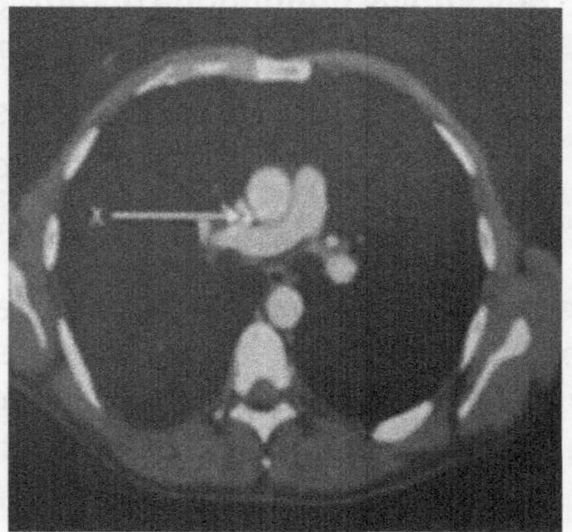

A. Ascending aorta
B. Descending aorta
C. Superior vena cava
D. Inferior vena cava

Explanation:

Normal anatomical structures seen in CT scan are:

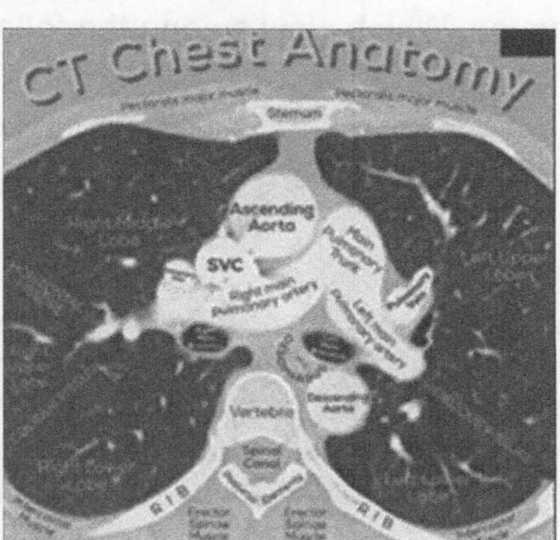

Ans. C

24. Most common cause for Chylothorax?

A. Mediastinal tumors
B. Surgical trauma
C. Idiopathic
D. Tuberculosis

Explanation:

- Chylothorax occurs when the thoracic duct is disrupted and chyle accumulates in pleural space.
- Most common cause of chylothorax is trauma (most frequently thoracic surgery), but it also may result from tumors in the mediastinum.
- Patients with chylothorax present with dyspnea, and a large pleural effusion is present on the chest radiograph.
- Thoracentesis reveals milky fluid, and bio-chemical analysis reveals a triglyceride level that exceeds 1.2 mmol/L (110 mg/dL).
- Patients with chylothorax & no obvious trauma should have lymphangiogram and a mediastinal CT scan to assess mediastinum for lymph nodes.
- Treatment of choice for most chylothoraxes is insertion of a chest tube plus administration of octreotide.

Ans. B

25. Chest radiograph of a 15 year old boy shows continuous diaphragm sign and naclerio's V sign. Physical examination reveals Hamman's sign. This is seen in which type of emphysema?

A. Pan acinar
B. Mediastinal
C. Centrilobular
D. None of the above

Explanation:

- Pneumomediastinum is a mediastinal abnormality that can result from alveolar rupture, esophageal perforation, or dissection of air from the neck or abdomen. Diagnosed by chest radiography, pneumomediastinum typically does not require specific treatment.
- Hamman's sign is a crunching sound, synchronous with the heart beat, heard over the precardium mainly during systole.
- The continuous diaphragm sign is seen in chest x ray as a thin lucent line outlining the superior surface of the diaphragm and separating it from the heart.
- Naclerio's V sign : The gas outlines the lateral margin of the descending aorta and extends laterally over left hemidiaphragm.

Ans. B

26. A 40 year old male presents to the OPD with sudden onset breathing difficulty. Chest X-ray reveals minimal right sided pleural effusion. Which view among the following X-rays is best to diagnose this disease?

A. AP view
B. Lateral view
C. PA view
D. Lateral decubitus view

Explanation:

- The chest X-ray (CXR), generally including both posteroanterior and lateral views, is often the first diagnostic study in pts presenting with respiratory symptoms. With some exceptions (e.g., pneumothorax), the CXR pattern is usually not sufficiently specific to establish a diagnosis; instead, the CXR serves to detect disease, assess magnitude, and guide further diagnostic investigation. With diffuse lung disease, CXR can detect an alveolar, interstitial, or nodular pattern. CXR can also detect pleural effusion and pneumothorax, as well as abnormalities in the hila and mediastinum. Lateral decubitus views can be used to estimate the size of freely flowing pleural effusions.

Ans. D

27. A 40 year old male presents to the ER with acute onset of hypoxemia and respiratory distress. Chest imaging shows patchy bilateral ground glass opacities and dependant air space consolidation. Which among the following is the most likely etiology?

A. Hamman rich syndrome
B. IPF (Idiopathic pulmonary fibrosis)
C. NSIP (Non specific interstitial pneumonitis)
D. Sarcoidosis

Explanation:

- **Acute interstitial pneumonia:** Characterized by acute onset of hypoxemia and respiratory distress, AIP (Hamman-Rich syndrome) has high mortality with frequent recurrences among survivors. Chest imaging frequently shows patchy bilateral ground glass opacities and dependent air-space consolidation. Treatment is supportive and usually includes mechanical ventilation.
- IPF, NSIP and Sarcoidosis have insidious onset of breathlessness.

Ans. A

28. A 20 year old male with complaints of chronic chough and chest radiograph showing pneumatoceles. Which of the following pathogens is most commonly associated with this presentation?

A. Staphylococcus aureus
B. Streptococcus pyogens
C. Legionella pneumonia
D. Hemopilus influenza

Explanation:

- Pneumatoceles are thin walled, air containing cysts of the lungs. They are classically associated with staphylococcus aureus. Pneumatoceles frequently occur in association with empyema. In most cases they resolve spontaneously. However on occasion pneumatoceles can result in pneumothorax.

Ans. A

29. A 30 year old male presents to the OPD with pharyngitis, tracheobronchitis and wheezing. He was found to be infected with eaton's agent. Which among the following is the most sensitive investigation of choice for this disease?

A. PCR analysis
B. Sputum culture
C. Serological testing for IgG and IgM antibodies
D, Cold agglutinin titers

Explanation:

- Eaton's agent refers to mycoplasma pneumoniae. Clinical findings, nonmicrobiologic laboratory tests, and CXR are not useful in distinguishing M. pneumoniae pneumonia from pneumonia of other etiologies. Acute M. pneumoniae infection can be diagnosed by PCR analysis of respiratory tract secretions, which is 65–90% sensitive and 90–100% specific. M. pneumoniae culture (which requires special medium) is not recommended for routine diagnosis because its sensitivity is ≤60% and growth of the organism can take weeks. Serologic testing for IgM and IgG antibodies to M. pneumoniae requires acute and convalescent-phase samples and is therefore less useful for diagnosis of active infections. Moreover, IgM antibodies to M. pneumoniae can persist for up to 1 year after acute infection. Measurement of cold agglutinin titers is no longer recommended for the diagnosis of M. pneumoniae infection because the findings are nonspecific.

Ans. A

30. A 20 year old female has diarrhoea, confusion, high grade fever with bilateral pneumonitis. What is the diagnosis?

A. Legionella
B. Neisseria meningitis
C. Streptococcus pneumonia
D. Klebsiella pneumonia

Explanation:

- Legionellosis manifests as either an acute, febrile, self-limited illness (Pontiac fever) or pneumonia (Legionnaires' disease). Pontiac fever is a flulike illness with a 24- to 48-h incubation period. Malaise, fatigue, and myalgias occur in 97% of cases. Fever, chills, and headaches are also very common, but pneumonia does not develop. The disease is selflimited and does not require antimicrobial treatment. Recovery takes place in a few days. Legionnaires' disease is more severe than other atypical pneumonias and is more likely to result in ICU admission.
- After a usual incubation period of 2–10 days, nonspecific symptoms (e.g., fever, malaise, fatigue, headache, anorexia) develop and are followed by a cough that is usually mild and only slightly productive. Chest pain and GI difficulties can be prominent.
- Radiologic findings are nonspecific, but pleural effusions are present in 28–63% of pts on hospital admission
- Legionnaires' disease is not readily distinguishable from pneumonia of other etiologies on the basis of clinical manifestations, but diarrhea, confusion, temperatures >39°C (>102.2°F), hyponatremia, increased aminotransferase levels, hematuria, hypophosphatemia, and elevated CPK levels are documented more frequently than in other pneumonias.
- Extrapulmonary infection results from hematogenous dissemination and most commonly affects the heart (e.g., myocarditis, pericarditis).

Ans. A

31. A 30 year old male presents to the OPD with chronic cough, breathlessness and evening rise of temperature. Sputum gene expert shows MTB detected and rifampicin resistance not detected. Which among the following statements is false?

A. Rifampicin turns body fluids red-orange

B. Isoniazid is used to treat active and latent TB

C. Ethambutol causes peripheral scotoma

D. The usual dosage of pyrazinamide is 15-30mg/kg daily.

Explanation:

- Rifampicin distributes well throughout body tissues, including inflamed meninges. It turns body fluids (e.g., urine, saliva, tears) red-orange and is excreted through bile and the enterohepatic circulation.
- Isoniazid is a critical drug for active and latent TB disease. The usual adult dosage is 300 mg/d or 900 mg twice per week.
- Ethambutol can cause dose-dependent optic neuritis, producing central scotoma and impairing both visual acuity and the ability to see green.
- The usual dosage is 15–30 mg/kg daily (maximum, 2 g/d). The drug distributes well throughout the body, including the CSF.

Ans. C

32. A 15 year old male presents to the ER with sudden onset breathlessness. On examination there was tachypnoea, tachycardia, absent breath sounds in the left hemi thorax. On percussion there was hyper resonant notes throughout the left hemithorax. Which among the following is false regarding the disease?

A. COPD Is the most common cause of secondary spontaneous pneumothorax

B. Simple aspiration may be adequate for initial primary spontaneous pneumothorax

C. Pleurodesis should be considered in secondary spontaneous pneumothorax

D. Tension pneumothorax can be treated conservatively with observation of vitals

Explanation:

- Pneumothorax (Ptx) is defined as gas in the pleural space. Spontaneous Ptx occurs without trauma to the thorax. Primary spontaneous Ptx occurs in the absence of underlying lung disease and typically results from apical pleural blebs. Simple aspiration may be adequate treatment for an initial primary spontaneous Ptx, but recurrence typically requires thoracoscopic intervention. Secondary spontaneous Ptx occurs in the setting of underlying lung disease, most commonly chronic obstructive pulmonary disease. Chest tube placement is typically required for secondary spontaneous Ptx; thoracoscopy and/or pleurodesis (with pleural abrasion or a sclerosing agent) should also be considered. Traumatic Ptx, resulting from either penetrating or nonpenetrating chest trauma, usually requires chest tube placement. Iatrogenic Ptx can occur from transthoracic needle biopsy, thoracentesis, placement of a central venous catheter, or transbronchial biopsy. Treatment with supplemental O2 or aspiration is often adequate for iatrogenic Ptx, but chest tube placement may be required. Tension Ptx can result from trauma or mechanical ventilation. Positive pleural pressure in mechanical ventilation can rapidly lead to a tension Ptx with reduced cardiac output. Urgent treatment is required, either with a chest tube or, if not immediately available, with a large-bore needle inserted into the pleural space through the second anterior intercostal space.

Ans. D

33. A 46 year old male presents with cough, breathlessness, fever and haemoptysis for the past 3 weeks. On evaluation it was found haemoptysis was due to Rasmussen's aneurysm. Which among the following is the most common aetiology for this complication?

A. Tuberculosis
B. Sarcoidosis
C. A V fistula
D. Asbestos inhalation

Explanation:

- Rasmussen's aneurysm is a relatively uncommon cause of haemoptysis. It refers to the formation of an aneurysm in the setting of cavitary infection that extends into the adventitia and media of bronchial arteries, resulting in inflammation and thinning of the vessel wall. This aneurysm subsequently ruptures into the cavity, producing massive haemoptysis.

Ans. A

34. A 40 year old female has defaulted ATT after 3 months of treatment for pulmonary tuberculosis 3 years ago. Her present sputum investigations are as follows :

Sputum AFB is 3+

Sputum CBNAAT shown MTB detected, rifampicin resistance detected

First line LPA (line probe assay) shows MTB detected, resistance to isoniazid & rifampicin

Second line LPA shows resistance to fluoroquinolones and aminoglycosides.

What is the diagnosis?

A. MDR TB
B. Pre XDR TB
C. XDR TB
D. INH mono resistant TB

Explanation:

- MDR TB – Multi drug resistant TB. Resistance to isoniazid and rifampicin
- Pre XDR TB – Resistance to isoniazid and rifampicin along with a resistance to **either** aminoglycosides **or** fluoroquinolones.
- XDR TB – Extensively drug resistant TB. Resistance to isoniazid and rifampicin and also to **both** fluoroquinolones **and** aminoglycosides.

Ans. C

35. A 55 year old known coronary artery disease patient presented with acute onset cough and pink frothy sputum. His NT PRO BNP was raised and chest radiograph showed kerley B lines. Kerley B lines are predominantly seen in chest radiograph in which zone?

A. Upper zone
B. Mid zone
C. Lower zone
D. Both A and B

Explanation:

- Kerley B lines results from thickening of the sub pleural interstitia. They have a predilection for the lower lung zones abutting a pleural surface. These lines are particularly well seen in chronic left ventricular failure, mitral valve disease, asbestosis and viral pneumonia.
- Kerley A lines radiate from the hilum into the lung periphery preferentially towards the upper lobes. They are most commonly seen in acute left ventricular failure and pulmonary oedema. Pink frothy sputum is pathogonomic of pulmonary edema.

Ans. C

36. A 40 years old female comes to the OPD with complaints of cough and breathlessness for a duration of 1 month. Breathlessness is aggravated in supine position. Chest radiograph revealed bilateral pleural effusion. Pleural fluid analysis revealed transudative pleural effusion. Which among the following is the most common cause?

A. Liver cirrhosis
B. Tuberculosis
C. Congestive heart failure
D. Nephrotic syndrome

Explanation:

- Pleural effusion is defined as excess fluid accumulation in the pleural space. Pleural effusions are typically detected by chest imaging (radiograph or CT); chest ultrasound can guide thoracentesis procedures. The two major classes of pleural effusions are transudates, which are caused by systemic influences on pleural fluid formation or resorption, and exudates, which are caused by local influences on pleural fluid formation and resorption.
- Common causes of transudative effusions are left ventricular heart failure, cirrhosis, and nephrotic syndrome. Among the transudative effusion, congestive heart failure is the most common.
- Common causes of exudative effusions are bacterial pneumonia, malignancy, viral infection, and pulmonary embolism.
- Light's criteria : Exudates fulfill at least one of the following three criteria: high pleural fluid/ serum protein ratio (>0.5), pleural fluid lactate dehydrogenase (LDH) greater than two-thirds of the laboratory normal upper limit for serum LDH, or pleural/ serum LDH ratio >0.6.

Ans. C

37. A 50 year old male comes to the OPD with right sided pleuritic chest pain and breathlessness. Chest radiograph reveals right sided moderate pleural effusion. Pleural fluid analysis reveals glucose of 30mg/dL. Which of the following is the most likely diagnosis?

A. SLE
B. Sarcoidosis
C. Rheumatoid pleuritis
D. Pulmonary hypertension

Explanation:

- In case of low glucose in pleural fluid one must consider a differential diagnosis of malignancy, rheumatoid pleuritis and bacterial infections. Rheumatoid pleuritis is the most common cause.
- The cause for low glucose in Rheumatoid pleuritis is due to defective glucose transport.

Ans. C

38. A 60 year old male is on long term treatment for respiratory failure. He has progressive breathlessness and worsening lung function despite medical treatment. He was advised lung transplant for his condition. Which among the following diseases is not an indication for lung transplantation?

A. COPD
B. Interstitial lung disease
C. Idiopathic pulmonary artery hypertension
D. Bronchial asthma

Explanation:

- The most common diseases that lead to lung transplantation are COPD, interstitial lung disease, idiopathic pulmonary artery hypertension, cystic fibrosis and alpha 1 antitrypsin deficiency.
- Types of lung transplant:
  1. Single lung transplant
  2. Double lung transplant
  3. Heart lung transplant

Ans. D

39. Most common cause of pleural effusion is:

A. Left ventricular failure
B. ARDS
C. Liver cirrhosis
D. Malignancy

Explanation:

- Most common cause of pleural effusion is left ventricular failure.
- Effusion occurs because the increased amounts of fluid in lung interstitial spaces exit in part across the visceral pleura; this overwhelms capacity of the lymphatics in the parietal pleura to remove fluid.
- In patients with heart failure, diagnostic thoracentesis should be performed if the effusions are not bilateral and comparable in size, if patient is febrile, or if the patient has pleuritic chest pain to verify that the patient has a transudative effusion.

Ans. A

40. A 50 year old male presents to the OPD with progressive breathlessness, chronic cough and recurrent bronchopulmonary infections. He has infertility and had 2 operations for nasal polyposis and recurrent sinusitis. CT chest shows bilateral bronchiectatic changes. Which one of the following is the most likely diagnosis?

A. Sarcoidosis
B. Allergic bronchopulmonary aspergillosis
C. Primary ciliary dyskinesia
D. Non tubercular mycobacterium

Explanation:

- Primary ciliary dyskinesia is also called immotile cilia syndrome. It is an autosomal recessive disorder. Clinical features include sinusitis, nasal polyposis and infertility. Cells lining the nasopharynx, middle ear, paranasal sinuses, the lower respiratory tract and the reproductive tract contain cilia and are generally affected in this disease.

Ans. C

41. A known HIV patient presents to the ER with sudden onset of fever, breathlessness and non-productive cough. Chest X-ray reveals bilateral diffuse perihilar interstitial infiltrates. Which of the following is the most likely diagnosis?

A. Tuberculosis
B. Kaposi sarcoma
C. Pneumocystis pneumonia
D. Pulmonary edema

Explanation:

- Pneumocystis, an opportunistic fungal pulmonary pathogen, is an important cause of pneumonia in immunocompromised hosts.
- The organisms are inhaled into the alveolar space, where they proliferate, provoking a mononuclear cell response. Alveoli become filled with and are damaged by proteinaceous material, with consequently increased alveolar– capillary injury and surfactant abnormalities. On histology, alveoli are seen to be filled with foamy, vacuolated exudates.
- CXR classically reveals bilateral diffuse interstitial infiltrates that are perihilar and symmetrical, although this finding is not specific for PCP. Cysts and pneumothoraces are common CXR findings, especially in HIV-infected pts. Chest CT shows diffuse ground-glass opacities in virtually all pts with PCP, and a normal chest CT essentially rules out the diagnosis.

Ans. C

42. A 28 year old male presents to the ER with sudden onset of breathing difficulty fever, generalized myalgia and loss smell and taste sensation. RTPCR for covid-19 infection was positive and CORADS score was 5 on CT scan. He was treated with dexamethasone 6mg for 10 days. This was based on which of the following trials?

A. Solidarity trial
B. Recovery trial
C. ACTT trial
D. MIST trial

Explanation:

- The outcome of recovery trial is that in hospital patients with covid-19, the use of dexamethasone 6mg once daily resulted in lower 28th day mortality among those who were receiving either invasive mechanical ventilation or oxygen alone but not among those receiving no respiratory support.
- The ACTT trial showed remdesivir was superior to placebo and shortening the time to recovery in adults who were hospitalized with covid-19 infection.
- On the contrary, in solidarity trial there was no proven benefit with remdisivir in covid-19 infection.
- MIST trial showed treatment of para pneumonic effusion improved with intra-pleural instillation of tissue plasminogen activator and DNase.

Ans. B

43. A 60 year old male with ischaemic heart disease is admitted with an episode of acute pulmonary oedema. His vitals are SpO2 – 86%, BP-160/90mmHg and PR-110 beats/min. He was treated with CPAP therapy. Which of the following is an indication for CPAP?

A. Acute exacerbation of COPD
B. Pneumocystis pneumonia
C. Acute cardiogenic pulmonary edema
D. All of the above

Explanation:

The main indications for NIV (non invasive ventilation) are:

- Acute exacerbation of COPD
- Pneumocystis pneumonia
- Acute cardiogenic pulmonary edema.

Other conditions where NIV maybe initiated but data to confirm its efficacy are less include:

- Acute respiratory failure due to bronchial asthma exacerbation
- Acute hypoxemic non-hypercapnic respiratory failure
- Post extubation, post-operative or chest trauma induced acute respiratory failure.

Ans. D

44. A 30 year old male presents to the ER with spontaneous pneumothorax. Which of the following is the most common cause?

A. Lung abscess
B. Bronchiectasis
C. Rupture of apical bleb
D. Malignancy

Explanation:

- Pneumothorax (Ptx) is defined as gas in the pleural space. Spontaneous Ptx occurs without trauma to the thorax. Primary spontaneous Ptx occurs in the absence of underlying lung disease and typically results from apical pleural blebs. Simple aspiration may be adequate treatment for an initial primary spontaneous Ptx, but recurrence typically requires thoracoscopic intervention. Secondary spontaneous Ptx occurs in the setting of underlying lung disease, most commonly chronic obstructive pulmonary disease. Chest tube placement is typically required for secondary spontaneous Ptx; thoracoscopy and/or pleurodesis (with pleural abrasion or a sclerosing agent) should also be considered.

Ans. C

45. A 50 year old male presents to the OPD with exertional dyspnoea and non productive cough. Physical examination reveals clubbing and fine inspiratory crackles at the lung bases. Which of the following statement regarding ILD is false?

A. Lung biopsy is usually required to confirm the diagnosis
B. Antifibrotic treatment can slow the decline of pulmonary function in idiopathic pulmonary fibrosis
C. Desquamative interstitial pneumonia and respiratory bronchiolitis associated ILD are exclusively seen in smokers
D. Shrinking lung syndrome is seen in rheumatoid arthritis

Explanation:

- IPF, which typically includes a pathologic pattern known as usual interstitial pneumonia (UIP), is the most common idiopathic interstitial pneumonia. Cigarette smoking is a risk factor for IPF. Common respiratory symptoms include exertional dyspnea and a nonproductive cough. Physical examination is notable for inspiratory crackles at the lung bases. Clubbing may occur. High-resolution chest CT scans show subpleural reticular opacities predominantly in the lower lung fields, which are associated with honeycombing and traction bronchiectasis in advanced disease. Surgical lung biopsy is usually required to confirm the diagnosis, although pts with classic UIP patterns on CT scan may not require a biopsy. IPF can include acute exacerbations characterized by accelerated clinical deterioration over days to weeks; these exacerbations are associated with high mortality. Antifibrotic treatment with pirfenidone and nintedanib can slow the decline of pulmonary function in IPF, but immunosuppressive therapies are not effective.
- Page 762. Desquamative interstitial pneumonia (DIP) includes extensive macrophage accumulation in intraalveolar spaces with minimal fibrosis. It is seen almost exclusively in cigarette smokers and improves with smoking cessation. Respiratory bronchiolitis-associated ILD is a subset of DIP that includes central bronchial wall thickening, ground-glass opacities, and air trapping on HRCT; it also resolves in most pts after smoking cessation.
- Shrinking lung syndrome is a rare complication of SLE. It is characterized by unexplained dyspnoea, restrictive pattern on PFT and an elevated hemidiaphragm.

Ans. D

46. A 50 year old male has a road traffic accident (fall from bike). On examination the chest wall exhibits paradoxical motion. CT chest shows fracture of the right 4th, 5th and the 6th ribs each in 2 places. What is the diagnosis?

A. Flail chest
B. Rupture of diaphragm
C. Pulmonary contusion
D. Haemothorax

Explanation:

- Flail chest occurs when three or more adjacent ribs are each fractured in two places, creating one floating segment comprised of several rib sections and soft tissues between them. This unstable section of the chest wall exhibits paradoxical motion with breathing. Treatment options include stabilization of the flail chest segment, oxygen supplementation, NIV or mechanical ventilation depending upon the severity of the disease.

Ans. A

47. A 60 year old male presents to the OPD with chronic cough and exertional dyspnoea. He is a chronic smoker with a smoking index of 30 pack years. All the following conditions are aggravated due to smoking except:

A. Squamous cell lung carcinoma
B. Respiratory bronchiolitis related ILD
C. Hypersensitivity pneumonitis
D. Langerhans cell histiocytosis

Explanation:

- Desquamative interstitial pneumonia (DIP) includes extensive macrophage accumulation in intra alveolar spaces with minimal fibrosis. It is seen almost exclusively in cigarette smokers and improves with smoking cessation. Respiratory bronchiolitis-associated ILD is a subset of DIP that includes central bronchial wall thickening, ground-glass opacities, and air trapping on HRCT; it also resolves in most pts after smoking cessation.
- Cigarette smoking is associated with a decreased risk of developing hypersensitivity pneumonitis. As examples smoking appears to diminish the risk of developing farmer's lung and pigeon breeders disease.

Ans. C

48. A 50 year old male presents to the OPD with exertional dyspnoea, fatigue, syncope and peripheral oedema. On examination JVP is raised and a loud P2. ECHO shows right atrial and right ventricular enlargement with a mean pulmonary artery pressure of 30mmHg. Which of the following is false regarding this disease?

A. Diuretics are given to reduce peripheral edema
B. Oxygen supplementation is given if PO2 is reduced
C. For patients with persistent right heart failure lung transplantation maybe considered
D. Pulmonary artery hypertension is more common in males

Explanation:

- Elevation of pulmonary artery (PA) pressure (i.e., mean PA pressure >22 mmHg) due to pulmonary vascular or parenchymal disease, increased left heart filling pressures, or a combination. Symptoms include exertional dyspnea, fatigue, angina (due to RV ischemia), syncope, peripheral edema.
- Most pts with idiopathic PAH present in fourth and fifth decades, female > male predominance; may be familial. Major symptom is dyspnea, often with insidious onset. Right heart catheterization demonstrates a mean pulmonary artery pressure ≥25 mmHg, pulmonary vascular resistance >240 dyne-s/cm5 , with a mean pulmonary capillary wedge pressure ≤15 mmHg. Mean survival of PAH is 5–6 years, even with therapy.
- Treatment includes limitation of physical activities, use diuretics for peripheral edema, O2 supplementation if PO2 reduced.

Ans. D

49. A 13 year old female presents to the OPD with complaints of breathing difficulty and haemoptysis. CT chest reveals an anterior mediastinal mass of 8 × 5 cms. Which among the following is the most likely diagnosis?

A. Lymphoma
B. Neurofibroma
C. Pheochromocytoma
D. Oesophageal tumor

Explanation:

Differential diagnosis for:

(A) Anterior Mediastinal Mass

- Thymic malignancy
- Lymphoma
- Thyroid malignancy
- Germ cell tumours– Teratoma, seminoma

(B) Middle Mediastinal Mass

- Bronchogenic cyst
- Pericardial cyst
- Oesophageal tumors

(C) Posterior Mediastinal Mass

- Neurogenic tumours– Neurofibroma, neurosarcoma, pheochromocytoma
- Meningocele

Ans. A

50. A known COPD patient develops pulmonary hypertension. He was given an oral soluble guanylyl cyclase stimulator. Which among the following is the drug that was given?

A. Selexipag
B. Riociguat
C. Treprostinil
D. Macitentan

Explanation:

- **Treatment of PAH:** Limit physical activities, use diuretics for peripheral edema, O2 supplementation if PO2 reduced. If short-acting vasodilators are beneficial during right heart catheterization, pt may benefit from high-dose calcium channel blocker (e.g., nifedipine, up to 240 mg/d, or amlodipine up to 20 mg/d); monitor for hypotension or worsening of right heart failure during such therapy.
- Page 729 & 730 Additional approved therapies for PAH include:
  1. Endothelin receptor antagonists: bosentan (62.5 mg PO bid × 1 month, then 125 mg PO bid), macitentan (10 mg once daily) and ambrisentan (5–10 mg daily) significantly improve pulmonary vascular resistance and exercise tolerance.
  2. Phosphodiesterase type 5 inhibitors: sildenafil (20–80 mg PO tid) and tadalafil (40 mg daily) also improve exercise tolerance in PAH. Do not prescribe concurrently with nitrates; the combination could result in marked hypotension.
  3. Prostaglandins (iloprost by inhalation, epoprostenol by continuous IV infusion, and treprostinil by IV, SC, or inhalation routes) improve symptoms, exercise tolerance, and, in the case of epoprostenol, survival. The most common side effect is flushing.
  4. The oral soluble guanylyl cyclase stimulator riociguat has been shown to improve exertional capacity in pts with PAH.
  5. The oral prostaglandin I2 receptor selexipag reduces the frequency of hospitalization and disease progression in pts being treated with an endothelin receptor antagonist, sildenafil, or both. For selected pts with persistent right heart failure, lung transplantation may be considered.

Ans. B

51. A 50 year old male comes to the OPD with complaints of dry cough and episodic haemoptysis. He gives a past history of tuberculous infection before 10 years for which he completed 6 months of treatment with ATT. With the help of CT chest he was diagnosed to have bronchiectasis sicca. In which lobe of the lung is this most commonly seen?

A. Upper lobe
B. Lower lobe
C. Middle lobe
D. Lingula

Explanation:

- Bronchiectasis is an irreversible airway dilation that involves the lung in either a focal (due to obstruction) or a diffuse (due to a systemic or infectious process) manner. Bronchiectasis can arise from infectious or non-infectious causes :
  - The epidemiology varies greatly with the underlying etiology; in general, the incidence of bronchiectasis increases with age and is higher among women than among men.
  - Of pts with bronchiectasis, 25–50% have idiopathic disease.
- A rare variant known as bronchiectasis sicca manifests as episodic haemoptysis with little to no sputum production. Dry bronchiectasis is usually a sequela of tuberculosis and is found in the upper lobe of the lung.

Ans. A

52. A 40 year old female presents to the OPD with complaints of chronic cough and copious amount of sputum production. On examination there is clubbing of fingers and coarse crackles are heard over both the lungs. Which of the following is false regarding the treatment of the disease?

A. Acute exacerbations should be treated with 7-10 days course of antibiotics
B. Hypertonic saline and chest physiotherapy helps in the early resolution of the disease
C. For patients with 2 or more recurrences per year suppressive antibiotic treatment is advised
D. Lung transplantation should be considered in patients with worsening in medical therapy

Explanation:

- Treatment of infectious bronchiectasis is directed at the control of active infection and at improvements in secretion clearance and bronchial hygiene.
- Acute exacerbations should be treated with a 7- to 10-day course of antibiotics targeting the causative or presumptive pathogen; H. influenzae and P. aeruginosa are isolated commonly.
- Hydration and mucolytic administration, aerosolization of bronchodilators and hyperosmolar agents (e.g., hypertonic saline), and chest physiotherapy can be used to enhance secretion clearance.
- For pts with three or more recurrences per year, suppressive antibiotic treatment to minimize the microbial load and reduce the frequency of exacerbations has been proposed.
- In select cases, surgery (including lung transplantation) should be considered.

Ans. C

53. A 70 year old male develops bronchiectasis as a result of damage to the bronchial wall and parenchymal distortion secondary to idiopathic pulmonary fibrosis. Which of the following is not a radiological feature of this disease?

A. Tram track appearance
B. Bilateral hyper inflated lung
C. Signet ring sign
D. Lack of bronchial tapering

Explanation:

- The diagnosis of bronchiectasis is based on clinical presentation with consistent CXR findings, such as parallel "tram tracks", a "signet-ring sign" (a cross sectional area of the airway with a diameter at least 1.5

times that of the adjacent vessel), lack of bronchial tapering, bronchial wall thickening, or cysts emanating from the bronchial wall.

- Bilateral hyper inflated lungs is seen in COPD.

Ans. B

54. Chest X-ray of Sarcoidosis patient suggests which stage?

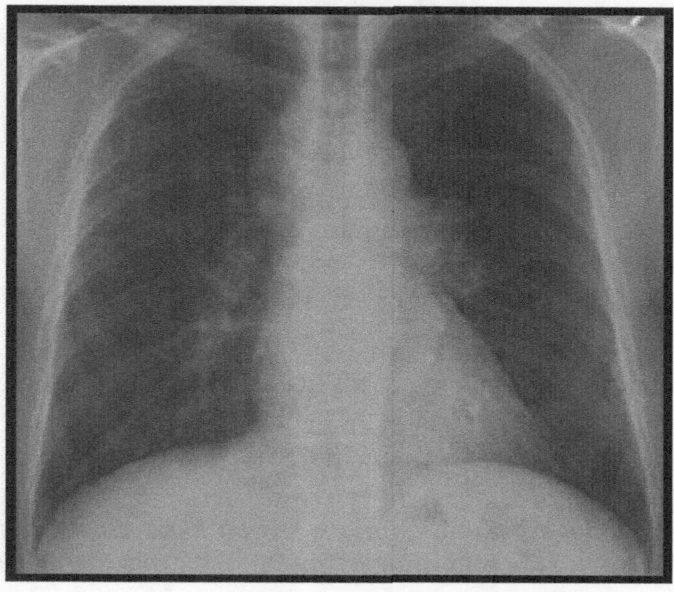

A. Stage 1
B. Stage 2
C. Stage 3
D. Stage 4

Explanation:

- CT scan is more sensitive, the standard scoring system described by Scadding in 1961 for chest roentgenograms remains preferred method of characterizing the chest involvement.
- Stage 1 is hilar adenopathy alone often with right paratracheal.
- Stage 2 is a combination of adenopathy plus infiltrates, whereas stage 3 reveals infiltrates alone. Stage 4 consists of fibrosis.

Ans. A

55. An infant has a positive new born screening test for cystic fibrosis. What cut off of sweat chloride confirms the diagnosis?

A. Sweat chloride >30 mmol/L
B. Sweat chloride >40 mmol/L
C. Sweat chloride >50 mmol/L
D. Sweat chloride >60 mmol/L

Explanation:

- Cystic fibrosis is caused by mutations in the cystic fibrosis trans membrane conductance regulator protein(CFTR). Deranged chloride transport leads to thick viscous secretions in the lungs, pancreas, liver, intestine and reproductive tract. The diagnosis of cystic fibrosis requires clinical symptoms consistent with cystic fibrosis in atleast one organ system and evidence of CFTR dysfunction (elevated sweat chloride >60mmol/L, presence of two disease causing mutations in the CFTR gene or abnormal nasal potential difference).

Ans. D

56. A patient presents with breathing difficulty, cough and fever for 1 month duration. CT chest reveals military mottling. All the following can cause this radiological pattern except:

A. Silicosis
B. Hemosiderosis
C. Tuberculosis
D. Aspergillosis

Explanation:

The differential diagnosis for miliary mottling include:

- Miliary tuberculosis
- Milary metastasis
- Sarcoidosis
- Pneumoconiosis(silicosis)
- Hemosiderosis
- Hypersensitivity pneumonitis
- Langerhan's cell histiocytosis
- Pulmonary alveolar proteinosis

The term military opacities refers to innumerable small pulmonary nodules of size 1mm to 3 mm scattered throughout the lung.

Ans. D

57. A 50 year old morbidly obese patient who is a known hypertensive was diagnosed with obesity hypoventilation syndrome. All the following are required for this diagnosis except:

A. Sleep disordered breathing
B. Hypertension
C. BMI > 30 kg/sq.m
D. PaCO2 > 45 mm Hg

Explanation:

- Chronic hypoventilation can result from parenchymal lung diseases, chest wall abnormalities (e.g., severe kyphoscoliosis), sleep-disordered breathing, neuromuscular diseases, and abnormal respiratory drive. Obesity-hypoventilation syndrome (OHS) is diagnosed by body mass index ≥30 kg/m2 and PaCO2 >45 mmHg in the absence of other causes of hypercapnia. Sleep-disordered breathing, typically obstructive sleep apnea, is seen in most OHS pts. Central hypoventilation syndrome is a rare disorder that includes a failure of the normal respiratory response to hypoxemia and/or hypercapnia.

Ans. B

58. Brochiectesis in a adult male is seen in:

A. Cystic fibrosis
B. Previous Mycoplasma infection
C. Previous Bordetella pertussis infection
D. All of the above

Explanation:

- Most widely cited mechanism of infectious bronchiectasis is "vicious cycle hypothesis," in which susceptibility to infection and poor mucociliary clearance result in microbial colonization of the bronchial tree.
- Some organisms, such as Pseudomonas aeruginosa, exhibit a particular propensity for colonizing damaged airways and evading host defense mechanisms.
- Impaired mucociliary clearance can result from inherited conditions such as CF or dyskinetic cilia syndrome, and it has been proposed that a single severe infection (e.g., pneumonia caused by Bordetella pertussis or Mycoplasma pneumoniae) can result in significant airway damage and poor secretion clearance.

- Presence of the microbes incites continued chronic inflammation, with consequent damage to the airway wall, continued impairment of secretions and microbial clearance, and ongoing propagation of the infectious/ inflammatory cycle.

Ans. D

59. A 70 year old male was diagnosed to have interstitial lung disease based on surgical lung biopsy. All the following parameters are decreased in this patient except:

A. FEV1
B. Diffusion capacity
C. FEV1/FVC
D. FVC

Explanation:

- Interstitial lung disease is a type of restrictive lung disease. In restrictive lung diseases both FEV1 and FVC are reduced and hence the ratio is of FEV1/FCV is normal.
- DLCO is also reduced in interstitial lung diseases.

Ans. C

60. A 20 year old male to the ER with sudden onset breathlessness and chest pain in the right mammary region. Chest X-ray reveals right sided pneumothorax. He is tachycardic, tachypnoeic and rapidly desaturating. Which among the following is the first line of management in this patient?

A. Emergency thoracotomy
B. CT chest
C. Needle in the second intercostal space
D. ICD tube in the 5th intercostal space

Explanation:

- Pneumothorax (Ptx) is defined as gas in the pleural space. Spontaneous Ptx occurs without trauma to the thorax. Primary spontaneous Ptx occurs in the absence of underlying lung disease and typically results from apical pleural blebs. Simple aspiration may be adequate treatment for an initial primary spontaneous Ptx, but recurrence typically requires thoracoscopic intervention. Secondary spontaneous Ptx occurs in the setting of underlying lung disease, most commonly chronic obstructive pulmonary disease. Chest tube placement is typically required for secondary spontaneous Ptx; thoracoscopy and/or pleurodesis (with pleural abrasion or a sclerosing agent) should also be considered.

Ans. C

61. A patient presents with malignant pleural effusion one the right side. She was advised to undergo chemical pleurodesis. Which among the following antibiotic is commonly used for chemical pleurodesis?

A. Amoxicillin
B. Azithromycin
C. Rifampicin
D. Doxycycline

Explanation:

- Pleurodesis is a procedure that obliterates the pleural space to prevent recurrent pleural effusion or recurrent pneumothorax. It is commonly performed by inducing intra pleural inflammation and fibrosis by either instilling a chemical irritant or performing mechanical abrasion. Common indications include malignant pleural effusion, recurrent pneumothorax. The chemical irritants that are used to induce pleurodesis are talc, tetracycline, minocycline, doxycycline, silver nitrate, povidone iodine, bleomycin and corny bacterium parvum with parenteral methyl prednisolone acetate.

Ans. D

62. A 40 year old known asthmatic comes to the OPD with complaints of fever, malaise, expectoration of brownish mucous plugs and occasional haemoptysis. On further evaluation he was diagnosed to have allergic bronchopulmonary aspergillosis (ABPA). Which of the following is false regarding this disease?

A. Distal bronchiectasis
B. Peripheral eosinophilia
C. Past history of bronchial asthma
D. Raised IgE levels

Explanation:

- ABPA is a complex hypersensitivity reaction of the airways that occurs when bronchi become colonized by aspergillus species. It is most commonly seen in patients with either asthma or cystic fibrosis. Both total IgE and total eosinophil count are raised. Imaging features include central bronchiectasis and high attenuation mucus.

Ans. A

63. A 50 year old male with smoking index of 30 presents to the OPD with chronic cough, breathlessness and expiratory wheeze. PFT reveals FEV1/FVC ratio of 0.6 and FEV1 68%. He was diagnosed to have moderate COPD according to GOLD criteria. Which of the following statements is false regarding this disease?

A. Reid index is <0.4
B. Barrel shaped chest
C. Associated with osteoporosis
D. Roflumilast is one of the drugs used to treat this disease

Explanation:

- Reid index is a ratio between the thickness of the submucosal glands and the thickness between the epithelium and cartilage that covers the bronchi. A normal reid index is less than 0.4.In a COPD patient reid index is >0.4.
- All other features are consistent with COPD.

Ans. A

64. A 50 year old male patient's chest radiograph shows rapid development of multiple peripheral basilar nodules in association with mild airflow obstruction. He has worked in coal industry for the past 20 years. On evaluation he was found to have Caplan's syndrome. This syndrome is associated with:

A. SLE
B. Systemic sclerosis
C. Sjögren's syndrome
D. Rheumatoid arthritis

Explanation:

- Caplan's syndrome occurs only in patients with both rheumatoid arthritis and pneumoconiosis (coal, asbestos, silica). Histologically Caplan's syndrome's nodules are similar to rheumatoid nodules, except that the Caplan nodules typically have a layer of black dust surrounding a central necrotic area.

Ans. D

65. A 50 year old male with complaints of cough and feeling of chest tightness which is aggravated especially on the first day of the week when they return to work after a weekend. What is the diagnosis?

A. Berylliosis
B. Byssinosis
C. Bagosis
D. Asbestosis

Explanation:

- Cotton dust exposures occur in the production of yarns for textiles and rope making. At the early stages of byssinosis, chest tightness occurs near the end of the first day of the workweek. In progressive cases, symptoms are present throughout the workweek. After at least 10 years of exposure, chronic airflow obstruction can develop. In symptomatic individuals, limiting further exposure is essential.
- Beryllium exposure may occur in the manufacturing of alloys, ceramics, and electronic devices. Although acute beryllium exposure can rarely produce acute pneumonitis, a chronic granulomatous disease very similar to sarcoidosis is much more common.

Ans. B

66. A 60 year old covid-19 patient develops sudden onset breathlessness and pleuritic chest pain. His D dimer levels are elevated and CT pulmonary angiography shows pulmonary embolism. Which among the following ECG findings is most commonly seen in acute pulmonary embolism:

A. S1 Q3 T3
B. P pulmonale
C. Sinus tachycardia
D. Right axis deviation

Explanation:

- Normal d-dimer level essentially rules out PE in pts with low-to-moderate likelihood of PE, although hospitalized pts often have elevated d-dimer levels due to other disease processes. Although hypoxemia and an increased alveolar-arterial O2 gradient may be observed in PE, arterial blood gases are rarely useful in diagnosing PE. Elevated serum troponin, plasma heart-type fatty acid-binding protein, and brain natriuretic peptide levels can be seen in PE. The electrocardiogram can show an S1Q3T3 sign in PE, but that finding is not frequently observed.
- Sinus tachycardia is the most commonly observed feature in pulmonary embolism.

Ans. C

67. A 60 year old male presents with acute onset chest pain and dyspnoea post medial sternotomy done for cardiac surgery. He was diagnosed to have acute mediastinitis based on mediastinal needle aspiration from the wound discharge. The most common cause of acute mediastinitis is:

A. Tracheal rupture
B. Tuberculosis
C. Oesophageal perforation
D. Idiopathic

Explanation:

- Mediastinitis can be an acute or chronic process. Acute mediastinitis can result from esophageal perforation, following cardiac surgery with median sternotomy, or from infections in the neck, oral cavity, or face. Esophageal perforation can occur spontaneously or iatrogenically; surgical exploration of the mediastinum, repair of the esophageal perforation, and drainage of the pleural space and mediastinum are required. Mediastinitis after median sternotomy typically presents with wound drainage and is diagnosed by mediastinal needle aspiration. Treatment requires immediate drainage, debridement, and IV antibiotics. Chronic mediastinitis can range from granulomatous lymph node inflammation to fibrosing mediastinitis. Most cases are due to tuberculosis or histoplasmosis.

Ans. C

68. Chest radiograph of a 40 year old female who is being evaluated for solitary pulmonary nodule shows popcorn type of calcification. Which among the following is the most likely diagnosis?

A. Tuberculoma
B. Hamartoma
C. Rheumatoid nodule
D. Bronchial adenoma

Explanation:

- A pulmonary nodule is defined on imaging as a small (less than 3 cm), well defined lesion completely surrounded by lung parenchyma.
- Lesions more than 3 cm on imaging are considered as lung masses.
- A nodule with popcorn type of calcification is suggestive of Pulmonary Hamartoma.
- A solitary pulmonary nodule is defined as a discrete, well-marginated, rounded opacity less than or equal to 3 cm in diameter that is completely surrounded by lung parenchyma, does not touch the hilum or mediastinum, and is not associated with adenopathy, atelectasis, or pleural effusion.
- Common causes of a malignant nodule include primary lung cancer, lung metastases, and carcinoid tumors.
- Common causes of a benign pulmonary nodule include infectious granulomas (Tuberculoma) and benign tumors such as a pulmonary hamartoma.

Ans. B

69. A 40 year old with symptoms of URI and acute bronchitis was microbiologically confirmed to have Mycoplasma pneumoniae pneumonia. Which among the following is the drug of choice in this patient?

A. Penicillin
B. Cefuroxime
C. Erythromycin
D. Clindamycin

Explanation:

- Mycoplasma pneumoniae is among the most common bacterial causes of upper respiratory tract infection (URI), acute bronchitis, and community-acquired pneumonia (CAP) in adults and children.
- Mycoplasma pneumoniae lacks a cell wall and is one of the smallest free-living organisms. Because it lacks a cell well, it is not visible on Gram stain and is not susceptible to antibiotics that inhibit cell wall synthesis, such as penicillins.
- These features designate M. pneumoniae as an "atypical" pathogen.
- The drug of choice is macrolides (Azithromycin, Erythromycin).
- Other treatment options include Tetracyclines and fluoroquincne.

Ans. C

70. X-ray of an 43 year old female diagnosed with sarcoidosis staged as:

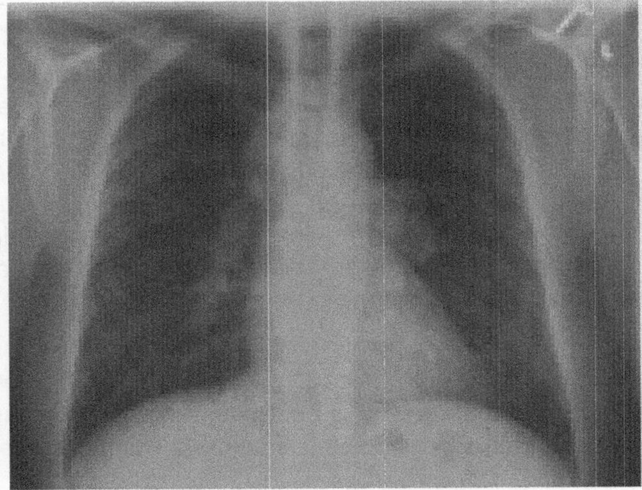

A. Stage 1
B. Stage 2
C. Stage 3
D. Stage 4

Explanation:

Scadding scoring based on X-ray findings:

- Stage 1: Hilar adenopathy alone, as shown in X-ray bilateral hilar adenopathy
- Stage 2: Adenopathy plus infiltrates
- Stage 3: Infiltrates alone
- Stage 4: Fibrosis.

Ans. A

71. A 50 year old male with Chest radiograph showing right sided Ellis curve. He has history of contact with sputum positive pulmonary TB patient. All the following are characteristic of Tuberculous pleural effusion except:

A. ADA 20 units/L
B. Pleural fluid CBNAAT positive for MTB
C. High interferon gamma level in pleural fluid
D. Cytology showing lymphocytic effusion

Explanation:

- Patients with tuberculous pleural effusion usually have an acute febrile illness with nonproductive cough and pleuritic chest pain. Night sweats, chills, weakness, dyspnea, and weight loss can also occur.
- The diagnosis of tuberculous pleural effusion may be definitively established via demonstration of *Mycobacterium tuberculosis* in pleural fluid or a pleural biopsy specimen. In the setting of high clinical suspicion for tuberculosis, a presumptive diagnosis of tuberculous pleural effusion may be established in the setting of pleural fluid analysis with lymphocytic-to-neutrophil ratio >0.75 and adenosine deaminase (ADA) >40 units/L or by demonstration of one or more caseating granulomas on pleural biopsy.
- Tuberculous pleural effusion is characterized by exudative effusion, high interferon gamma levels in pleural fluid and cytology showing lymphocytic effusion. The sensitivity of pleural fluid CBNAAT/GENEXPERT to detect TB is low but is highly specific.
- ADA < 40 units/L should raise the suspicion of alternative diagnosis other than Tubercular etiology.

Ans. A

72. A 62 year old male presents to the OPD with complaints of breathlessness and left sided pleuritic chest pain. On examination trachea is shifted to the right, with stony dull note on percussion in the left hemithorax. Which of the following condition is not an etiology for this type of clinical presentation?

A. Pancreatitis
B. Thoracic duct involvement above T5 level
C. Esophageal rupture
D. Amoebic liver abscess

Explanation:

- Clinical presentation is consistent with left sided pleural effusion. The common causes of left sided pleural effusion are pancreatitis, Thoracic duct involvement above T5 level, Esophageal rupture, left sided subdiaphragmatic abscess and post CABG surgery.
- The common causes of right sided pleural effusion are amoebic liver abscess, meig syndrome and thoracic duct involvement below T5 level.
- The thoracic duct ascends through the aortic hiatus of the diaphragm entering the posterior mediastinum, still to the right of the vertebral column. It courses posterior to the esophagus at the T7 level and crosses over the midline to the left side of the thorax around the T5 vertebral level. So any lesion above T5 causes left sided effusion while lesions below T5 cause right sided effusion.

Ans. D

73. A 78-year-old woman is admitted to the medical intensive care unit (ICU) with multilobar pneumonia. On initial presentation to the emergency department, her initial oxygen saturation was 60% on room air and only increased to 82% on a non-rebreather face mask. She was in marked respiratory distress and intubated in the emergency department. Upon admission to the ICU, she was sedated and paralyzed. The ventilator is set in the assist-control mode with a respiratory rate of 24 breaths/min, tidal volume of 6 mL/kg, FiO2 of 1.0, and positive end-expiratory pressure of 12 cmH2O. An arterial blood gas measurement is performed on these settings; the results are pH of 7.20, PCO2 of 32 mmHg, and PO2 of 54 mmHg. What is the cause of the hypoxemia?

A. Hypoventilation alone

B. Hypoventilation and ventilation-perfusion mismatch

C. Shunt

D. Ventilation-perfusion mismatch

Explanation:

- In this patient presenting with multilobar pneumonia, hypoxemia is present that does not correct with increasing the concentration of inspired oxygen.
- Inability to overcome hypoxemia or the lack of a notable increase in partial pressure of arterial oxygen (PaO2) or oxygen saturation (SaO2) with increasing fraction of inspired oxygen physiologically defines a shunt.
- A shunt occurs when deoxygenated blood is transported to the left heart and systemic circulation without having the capability of becoming oxygenated.
- Causes of shunt include alveolar collapse (atelectasis), intra-alveolar filling processes, intrapulmonary vascular malformations, or structural cardiac disease leading to right-to-left shunt. In this case, the patient has multilobar pneumonia leading to alveoli that are being perfused but unable to participate in gas exchange because they are filled with pus and inflammatory exudates.
- Acute respiratory distress syndrome is another common cause of shunt physiology. V/Q mismatch is the most common cause of hypoxemia and results when there are some alveolar units with low ratios (low ventilation to perfusion) that fail to fully oxygenate perfused blood.
- When blood is returned to the left heart, the poorly oxygenated blood admixes with blood from normal alveolar units.
- Resultant hypoxemia is less severe than with shunt and can be corrected with increasing the inspired oxygen concentration.
- Hypoventilation with or without other causes of hypoxemia is not present in this case, as the PCO2 <40 mmHg indicates hyperventilation.
- Acidosis present in this case is of a metabolic rather than a pulmonary source. Because patient is paralyzed, she is unable to increase her respiratory rate above the set rate to compensate for the metabolic acidosis.

Ans. C

74. A patient with left sided pleural effusion presents with raised pleural fluid amylase levels. All the following diseases presents with raised pleural fluid amylase except:

A. Acute and chronic pancreatitis

B. Esophageal rupture

C. Malignancy

D. Rheumatoid arthritis

Explanation:

- Although not routinely tested in pleural fluid samples, amylase measurements can assist when pancreatic or esophageal etiologies of an effusion appear possible. The finding of an amylase-rich pleural effusion, defined as either a pleural fluid amylase greater than the upper limits of normal for serum amylase or a pleural fluid to serum amylase ratio greater than 1, narrows the differential diagnosis of an exudative effusion to the following major possibilities:

– Acute pancreatitis
– Chronic pancreatic pleural effusion
– Esophageal rupture
– Malignancy

Ans. D

75. A 65-year-old man is evaluated for progressive dyspnea on exertion and dry cough that have worsened over the course of 6 months. He has not had dyspnea at rest and denies wheezing. He has not experienced chest pain. He has a history of coronary artery disease and atrial fibrillation and previously underwent a coronary artery bypass surgery 12 years previously. His medications include metoprolol, aspirin, warfarin, and enalapril. He previously smoked 1 pack of cigarettes daily for 40 years, quitting 5 years previously. His vital signs are as follows: blood pressure 122/68 mmHg, heart rate 68 bpm, respiratory rate 18 breaths/min, and oxygen saturation 92% on room air. His chest examination demonstrates bibasilar crackles present about one-third of way up bilaterally. No wheezing is heard. He has an irregularly irregular rhythm with a II/VI holosystolic murmur at the apex. The jugular venous pressure is not elevated. No edema is present, but clubbing is noted. Pulmonary function testing reveals an FEV1 of 65% predicted, FVC of 67% predicted, FEV1/FVC ratio of 74%, TLC of 68% predicted, and diffusion capacity for carbon monoxide (DLCO) of 62% predicted. Which test is most likely to determine the etiology of the patient's dyspnea?

A. Bronchoscopy with transbronchial lung biopsy
B. CT pulmonary angiography
C. Echocardiography
D. HRCT scan of the chest

Explanation:

- This patient presents with a slowly progressive illness manifested by dyspnea on exertion, dry cough, clubbing, and the presence of crackles on examination. In addition, pulmonary function tests demonstrate restrictive lung disease.
- This scenario is characteristic of an individual with interstitial lung disease, most commonly idiopathic pulmonary fibrosis in individuals at this age.
- A more thorough history should be obtained to determine if there are any other exposures or symptoms that could identify other causes of interstitial lung disease.
- Next step in the evaluation of this patient is to perform a high-resolution CT scan (HRCT) chest. HRCT employs thinner cross-sectional images at approximately 1–2 mm rather than the usual 7–10 mm.
- This creates more visible details and is particularly useful for recognizing subtle changes of the interstitium and small airways including interstitial lung disease, bronchiolitis, and bronchiectasis. Bronchoscopy with transbronchial biopsy typically does not provide detail required to adequately diagnose interstitial lung disease.
- It may be considered if there are specific features on HRCT that would suggest an alternative diagnosis. However, in most instances, the pathologic diagnosis of interstitial lung disease requires a surgical lung biopsy to provide definitive diagnosis.
- This patient's symptoms do not suggest coronary artery disease/congestive heart failure. Thus, echocardiography & nuclear stress testing are not indicated. CT scanning has evolved over the years to offer several different techniques that are useful in a variety of circumstances.
- Standard CT imaging is most useful for the evaluation and staging of lung masses. Helical CT scanning requires only a single breath hold and provides continuous collection of data with improved contrast enhancement and thinner collimation.
- Once the data are obtained, the images can be reconstructed into other views including sagittal and coronal planes as well as three-dimensional volumetric representations. A recent use of this technology is employed in the setting of virtual bronchoscopy to aid in the planning and performance of bronchoscopy.

- Multidectector CT scans can obtain multiple slices in a single rotation that are thinner than the usual cuts. Multidetector CT scanners are used in the performance of the CT pulmonary angiogram.

Ans. D

76. A 38-year-old woman is brought to the emergency department for status asthmaticus. She rapidly deteriorates and dies of her disease. All of the following pathologic findings would likely be seen in this individual except:

A. Infiltration of the airway mucosa with eosinophils and activated T lymphocytes
B. Infiltration of the alveolar spaces with eosinophils and neutrophils
C. Occlusion of the airway lumen by mucous plugs
D. Thickening and edema of the airway wall

Explanation:

- Pathology of asthma has largely been determined by examining bronchial biopsies of patients with asthma as well as the lungs of individuals who die from asthma.
- These pathologic changes are centered around airways with sparing of alveolar spaces.
- Airways are infiltrated by eosinophils, activated T lymphocytes, and activated mucosal mast cells.
- However, the degree of inflammation does not correlate with the severity of asthma.
- Another common finding in all asthmatics and individuals with eosinophilic bronchitis is thickening of the basement membrane due to collagen deposition in the subepithelium.
- Airway smooth muscle is hypertrophied as well. Overall, this leads to thickening of airway wall, which may also exhibit edematous fluid, particularly in those with fatal asthma.
- In cases of fatal asthma, it is also common to find multiple airways that are occluded by mucus plugs.
- However, the disease is limited to the airways, and infiltration of the alveolar spaces by inflammatory cells is not seen.

Ans. B

77. A 60 year old male has underwent bilateral lung transplant for ILD. Post surgery patient develops breathlessness, fever and dry cough. Chest radiograph shows bilateral, perihilar symmetrical infiltrates. His serum LDH and serum beta-D-glucan levels are raised:

Which among the following is the drug of choice for this disease?

A. Cotrimoxazole
B. Doxycycline
C. Azithromycin
D. Amoxycillin

Explanation:

- The clinical features and lab investigations are suggestive of pneumocystis pneumonia.
- Pneumocystis pneumonia (PCP) is a potentially life-threatening infection that occurs in immunocompromised individuals, especially in those with HIV but also in hematopoietic cell and solid organ transplant recipients; those with cancer (particularly hematologic malignancies); and those receiving glucocorticoids, chemotherapeutic agents, and other immunosuppressive medications.
- The drug of choice for both prophylaxis and treatment is cotrimoxazole.
- The alternative treatment options include atovaquone, clindamycin plus primaquine, dapsone, clindamycin and IV pentamidine.

Ans. A

78. Which of the following patients is appropriately diagnosed with asthma?

A. A 24-year-old woman treated with inhaled corticosteroids for cough and wheezing that has persisted for 6 weeks following a viral upper respiratory infection

B. A 26-year-old man who coughs and occasionally wheezes following exercise in cold weather

C. A 34-year-old woman evaluated for chronic cough with an FEV1/FVC ratio of 68% with an FEV1 that increases from 1.68 L (52% predicted) to 1.98 L (61% predicted) after albuterol (18% change in FEV1)

D. A 44-year-old man who works as a technician caring for the mice in a medical research laboratory and complains of wheezing, shortness of breath, and cough that are most severe at the end of the week

Explanation:

- Preferred method for diagnosing asthma is demonstration of airflow obstruction on spirometry that is at least partially reversible.
- This is demonstrated in option C, with a decreased FEV1/FVC ratio, decreased FEV 1, and a significant increase in FEV1 following administration of albuterol. For an individual to be considered responsive to a bronchodilator, the individual should experience an increase in either FEV1 or FVC of at least 200 mL and 12%.
- Option A describes someone with postviral cough syndrome, which can persist for several weeks following a viral upper respiratory infection.
- Option B describes someone with exercise-induced bronchoconstriction (EIB), which, in absence of other symptoms to suggest asthma, should not be diagnosed as asthma. Isolated EIB lacks the characteristic airway inflammation of asthma and does not progress to asthma. Although it is estimated that 80%–90% of individuals with asthma experience EIB, many individuals who have EIB do not also have asthma. EIB is caused by hyperventilation with inhalation of cool dry air that leads to bronchospasm.
- Option D describes someone with occupational asthma that has occurred after working with animals in the medical laboratory for many years. Symptoms that are characteristic of occupational asthma are symptoms only while at work that improve on the weekends and during holidays. Option D describes someone with COPD. In COPD, 25%–48% of individuals can demonstrate bronchial hyper-responsive in response to methacholine.

Ans. C

79. A 10 year old female presents to the ER with complaints of wheezing. She is a known asthmatic on treatment with bronchodilators and corticosteroids. Her PFT shows Bronchodilator reversibility. Which among the following is not used in the treatment of this patient?

A. Zileuton
B. Nedocromil
C. Montelukast
D. Roflumilast

Explanation:

The treatment options for bronchial asthma include:

- Beta agonists: Salbutamol, formoterol, salmeterol
- Steroids: Budesonide, fluticasone
- Anti IgE: Omalizumab
- Mast cell stabilizers: Nedocromil, sodium cromoglycate

Ans. D

80. A 70 year old male presents with complaints of breathlessness and wheezing for the past 1 year. PFT is suggestive of obstructive airway disease and chest radiograph shows hyperinflation. Which among the following is false in this disease?

A. Reduced FEV1
B. Positive bronchodilator reversibility
C. Reduction in DLCO
D. Barrel shaped chest

Explanation

- Diagnosis for the clinical scenario is COPD. COPD is confirmed when a patient with compatible symptoms is found to have irreversible airflow limitation (i.e., a post bronchodilator forced expiratory volume in one second [FEV_1]/forced vital capacity [FVC] ratio less than 0.7. Reduction in DLCO correlates to the degree of disease severity in COPD.
- Barrel shaped chest is produced due to lung hyperinflation. Positive bronchodilator response is seen in bronchial asthma.

Ans. B

81. Chest radiograph of a 50 year old male shows egg shell calcification and progressive massive fibrosis. He gives a history of working in a stone quarry for 30 years. Due to his occupational exposure he is at risk of developing all the following diseases except:

A. Tuberculosis
B. Fungal infection
C. Atypical mycobacterial infection
D. Sarcoidosis

Explanation:

- Silicosis results from exposure to free silica (crystalline quartz), which occurs in mining, stone cutting, sand blasting, abrasive industries (e.g., glass and cement manufacturing), foundry work, and quarrying. Heavy exposures over relatively brief time periods (as little as 10 months) can cause acute silicosis—which is pathologically similar to pulmonary alveolar proteinosis and associated with a characteristic chest CT pattern known as "crazy paving". Acute silicosis can be severe and progressive; whole lung lavage may be of some therapeutic benefit. Longer-term exposures can result in simple silicosis, with small rounded opacities in the upper lobes of the lungs. Calcification of hilar lymph nodes can give a characteristic "eggshell" appearance on radiographic studies. Progressive nodular fibrosis can result in masses >1 cm in diameter in complicated silicosis. When such masses become very large, the term progressive massive fibrosis is used to describe the condition. Due to impaired cell-mediated immunity, silicosis pts are at increased risk of tuberculosis, atypical mycobacterial infections, and fungal infections. Silica may also be a lung carcinogen.

Ans. D

82. A 45 year old man was advises bronchoscopy for evaluation of non resolving pneumonia. Which among the following is the most common complication of this procedure?

A. Hemorrhage
B. Infection
C. Hypoxemia
D. Pneumothorax

Explanation

- Bronchoscopy is a procedure that provides direct visualization of the tracheobronchial tree, typically to the subsegmental level. The fiberoptic bronchoscope is used in most cases, but rigid bronchoscopy is valuable in specific circumstances, including massive hemorrhage and foreign body removal. Flexible fiberoptic bronchoscopy allows visualization of the airways; identification of endobronchial abnormalities, including tumors and sites of bleeding; and collection of diagnostic specimens by washing, brushing, biopsy, or lavage. Washing involves instilling sterile saline through the bronchoscope channel onto the surface of a lesion; part of the saline is suctioned back through the bronchoscope and processed for cytology and microorganisms. Bronchial brushings can be obtained from the surface of an endobronchial lesion or from a more distal mass or infiltrate (potentially with fluoroscopic guidance) for cytologic and microbiologic studies. Biopsy forceps can be used to obtain biopsies of endobronchial lesions or passed into peribronchial alveolar tissue (often with fluoroscopic guidance) to obtain transbronchial biopsies of more distal lung tissue. Transbronchial biopsy is particularly useful in diagnosing diffuse infectious processes, lymphangitic spread of cancer, and granulomatous diseases. Complications of transbronchial biopsy include hemorrhage and pneumothorax.

Ans. C

83. A 10 year old female demonstrates bronchodilator reversibility with an increase in FEV1 by ≥200 mL and ≥12% from baseline FEV1 15 min after a short-acting β agonist (often albuterol metered-dose inhaler two puffs or 180 µg) in pulmonary function testing. Which among the following is not used in diagnosis of this disease?

A. RAST
B. Allergic skin testing
C. Ventilation perfusion scanning
D. FeNO (Fractional exhaled nitric oxide)

Explanation:

- The diagnosis is bronchial asthma since bronchodilator reversibility is positive. Airway hyperresponsiveness is characteristic of asthma; it can be assessed by exposure to direct bronchoconstrictors such as methacholine or histamine. Greater airway responsiveness is associated with increased asthmatic symptoms. The peak expiratory flow rate (PEFR) can be used by the pt to track asthma control objectively at home. Measurement of lung volumes is not typically performed, but increases in total lung capacity and residual volume may be observed. The diffusing capacity for carbon monoxide is usually normal. Blood tests are usually not helpful. Specific IgE measurements for inhaled allergens (radioallergosorbent test [RAST]) or allergy skin testing may assist in determining allergic triggers. Total serum IgE is markedly elevated in bronchopulmonary aspergillosis (BPA). Exhaled nitric oxide levels can provide an assessment of eosinophilic airway inflammation.
- Ventilation perfusion scanning is used to diagnose pulmonary embolism.

Ans. C

84. A 40 year old male develops panacinar emphysema, panniculitis of the skin and unexplained liver failure. He was diagnosed to have alpha 1 antitrypsin deficiency. All the following are true in this disease except?

A. Apical bulla in the lung
B. Serum level of alpha 1 antitrypsin < 11 micromol/L
C. Genotyping and phenotyping helps in the diagnosis
D. During the first four decades of life, liver dysfunction is the major threat to the health

Explanation:

- Alpha-1 antitrypsin is a member of the serpin family of protease inhibitors. It protects the lower airways from damage caused by proteolytic enzymes, such as elastase. The normal alpha-1 antitrypsin (AAT) allele is the M allele. Over 150 allelic variants have been described, of which the most common severely deficient variant is the Z allele. Clinical manifestations of severe deficiency of AAT typically involve the lung (eg, early onset emphysema), liver (eg, cirrhosis), and, rarely, the skin (e.g., panniculitis).
- Pulmonary function testing typically demonstrates development of airflow limitation, consistent with COPD. Among middle-aged adults with AATD associated with a homozygous Z allele (PI*ZZ), the mean forced expiratory volume in one second (FEV_1) of predicted is moderately to severely reduced. Emphysema associated with AATD often shows a characteristic radiographic pattern, in which bullous changes are more prominent at the lung bases than at the apices. Beyond the four decades of life, patients with severe deficiency of AAT have an accelerated rate of lung function decline, especially with cigarette smoking and some occupational exposures.

Ans. A

85. In lung diseases CT is particularly useful in all except:

A. Assessing hilar and mediastinal disease
B. In identifying and characterizing disease adjacent to chest wall/spine
C. In identifying areas of fat density or calcification in pulmonary nodules
D. To distinguish tumor from post-stenotic atelectasis

Explanation:

- CT is particularly valuable in assessing hilar and mediastinal disease (often poorly characterized by plain radiography), in identifying and characterizing disease adjacent to the chest wall or spine (including pleural disease), and in identifying areas of fat density or calcification in pulmonary nodules. Its utility in the assessment of mediastinal disease has made CT an important tool in the staging of lung cancer. With the additional use of contrast material, CT also makes it possible to distinguish vascular from nonvascular structures, which is particularly important in distinguishing lymph nodes and masses from vascular structures primarily in the mediastinum, and vascular disorders such as pulmonary embolism.

Ans. D

86. Causes of Loffler Syndrome include all except:

A. Ascariasis B. Cysticercosis

C. Hookworm D. Schistosomiasis

Explanation:

Table: Infectious causes of pulmonary eosinophilia
Loffler Syndrome
Ascaris Hookworm Schistosomiasis
Heavy Parasite Burden
Strongyloidiasis
Direct Pulmonary Penetration
Paragonimiasis Visceral larval migrans
Immunologic Response to Organisms in Lungs
Filariasis Dirofilariasis
Cystic Disease
Echinococcus Cysticercosis
Other Nonparasitic
Coccidioidomycosis Basidiobolomycosis Paracoccidioidomycosis Tuberculosis

Ans. B

87. A 60 year old male was advised CPAP (CONTINUOUS POSITIVE AIRWAY PRESSURE) as he was desaturating with nasal oxygen delivered via face mask. All the following are contraindications to CPAP except:

A. Cardiovascular instability B. Facial burns

C. Conscious patient D. Copious secretions

Explanation:

- Numerous studies suggest that noninvasive mask ventilation (noninvasive ventilation [NIV]) can improve outcomes in acute COPD exacerbations with respiratory failure (PaCO2 >45 mmHg). Contraindications to NIV include cardiovascular instability, impaired mental status, inability to cooperate, copious secretions, craniofacial abnormalities or facial trauma, extreme obesity, or significant burns. Progressive hypercarbia, refractory hypoxemia, or alterations in mental status that compromise ability to comply with NIV therapy, hemodynamic instability, and respiratory arrest may necessitate endotracheal intubation for mechanical ventilation. Sufficient expiratory time during mechanical ventilatory support is required to avoid the development of auto-PEEP.

Ans. C

88. A 50 year male develops primary lung abscess. The sputum is purulent in consistency and is foul smelling. Which among the following is the drug of choice in this patient?

A. Clindamycin
B. Doxycycline
C. Erythromycin
D. Levofloxacin

Explanation:

- Lung abscess—necrosis and cavitation of the lung following microbial infection— can be categorized as primary (~80% of cases) or secondary lung abscess.
- Primary lung abscesses usually arise from aspiration in the absence of an underlying pulmonary or systemic condition, are often polymicrobial (primarily including anaerobic organisms and microaerophilic streptococci), and occur preferentially in dependent segments (posterior upper and superior lower lobes) of the right lung.
- Secondary lung abscesses arise in the setting of an underlying condition (e.g., a postobstructive process, an immunocompromising condition) and can be due to a number of different organisms, among which P. aeruginosa and other gram-negative rods are most common.
- For primary lung abscesses, the recommended regimens are clindamycin (600 mg IV tid) or an IV-administered β-lactam/β-lactamase combination. After clinical improvement, the pt can be transitioned to an oral regimen (clindamycin, 300 mg qid; or amoxicillin/clavulanate).
- In secondary lung abscesses, antibiotic coverage should be directed at the identified pathogen. Continuation of oral treatment is recommended until imaging shows that the lung abscess has cleared or regressed to a small scar.

Ans. A

89. A 50 year old female with prior history of pulmonary tuberculosis comes with complaints of chronic and breathlessness for 3 months duration. Sputum examination reveals triple layer sputum. Which of the following disease is most characteristic of this presentation?

A. COPD
B. Community acquired pneumonia
C. Bronchiectasis
D. ABPA

Explanation:

- Bronchiectasis is characterized by postural cough and expectoration of **large quantities of foul smelling sputum** with **three characteristic layers**. Fowl smell is due to anaerobic infection. The three layers are purulant sediment, clear middle liquid and top foamy layer.

Ans. C

90. A 10 year old boy presents to the OPD with 3 day history of cough and fever. Chest radiograph reveals round pneumonia. Which among the following is the most common bacterial etiology for this condition?

A. H. influenza
B. Staph aureus
C. Streptococcus pneumoniae
D. Mycoplasma pneumonia

Explanation:

- Pulmonary consolidation in young children sometimes appears to be spherical (ie, "round pneumonia"). Round pneumonias tend to be >3 cm, solitary, and posteriorly located. The most common bacterial etiology for round pneumonia is *S. pneumoniae*; additional bacterial causes include other streptococci, *Haemophilus influenzae*, *S. aureus*, and *M. pneumoniae*.
- The pathophysiology of round pneumonia is the development of inter alveolar communication and collateral airways known as pores of kohn and canals of lambert.

Ans. C

91. A 40 year old female develops lobar pneumonia due to streptococcus pneumoniae. All the following are phases are seen in the alveoli except:

A. Red hepatization
B. Resolution
C. Hyalinization
D. Grey hepatization

Explanation:

- Classic pneumonia (typified by that due to Streptococcus pneumoniae) presents as a lobar pattern and evolves through four phases characterized by changes in the alveoli:
  - **Edema**: Proteinaceous exudates are present in the alveoli.
  - **Red hepatization**: Erythrocytes and neutrophils are present in the intraalveolar exudate.
  - **Gray hepatization**: Neutrophils and fibrin deposition are abundant.
  - **Resolution**: Macrophages are the dominant cell type.

Ans. C

92. A 70 year old male presents to the OPD with chronic cough for 2 months duration. On auscultation cavernous type of breath sounds is heard in the left hemithorax. Which of the following is the most probable diagnosis?

A. Pleural effusion
B. Tuberculous cavity
C. Consolidation
D. Pleurisy

Explanation:

Auscultatory findings:

1. **Tubular breath sounds** (High pitched bronchial breath sounds) –seen in consolidation, above the level of pleural effusion, complete collapse(atelectasis) with patent bronchus, mass interposed between chest wall and the large airways.
2. **Cavernous breath sounds** (Low pitched bronchial breath sounds) – seen in cavity.
3. **Amphoric breath sounds** (low pitched bronchial breath sounds with metallic overtones) – seen in broncho pleural fistula, Tension pneumothorax and superficial large cavity.

Ans. B

93. A 40 year old male develops sudden onset respiratory distress and cyanosis 2 hours following cardiac surgery under general anaesthesia. H was diagnosed to have Mendelson syndrome. Which among the following best describes the condition?

A. Chemical aspiration pneumonitis
B. Bacterial aspiration pneumonitis
C. Pulmonary embolism
D. Air embolism

Explanation:

- The best studied clinical example of chemical pneumonitis is that associated with the aspiration of gastric acid first described by Mendelson in 1946 and sometimes referred to as mendelson syndrome. Chemical aspiration pneumonitis also occurs perioperatively, most often during intubation or extubation for anesthesia or during procedures like laryngoscopy.
- Mendelson's original series included 61 obstetrical patients who aspirated gastric contents during ether anesthesia. Respiratory distress and cyanosis rapidly followed, usually within two hours of a witnessed aspiration. Chest radiographs showed opacities that were usually located in one or both lower lobes. Despite the initial severity of the illness, all 61 patients had a rapid clinical recovery within 24 to 36 hours, with radiographic resolution within four to seven days without the use of antimicrobial therapy.

Ans. A

94. A 40 year old male presents with upper lobe bronchiectasis, sinusitis and sweat chloride levels >60mmol/L. This genetic disorder is due to mutation in a single large gene on chromosome no:

A. 5 B. 6

C. 7 D. 8

Explanation:

- The diagnosis is Cystic fibrosis. Cystic fibrosis (CF) is caused by mutations in the cystic fibrosis transmembrane conductance regulator (CFTR) protein. Deranged chloride transport leads to thick, viscous secretions in the lungs, pancreas, liver, intestine, and reproductive tract. Most patients develop multisystem disease involving several or all of these organs.
- The diagnosis of CF requires clinical symptoms consistent with CF in at least one organ system and evidence of CFTR dysfunction (elevated sweat chloride, presence of two disease-causing mutations in the *CFTR* gene, or abnormal nasal potential difference [NPD].
- CF is caused by pathogenic mutations in a single large gene on chromosome 7 that encodes the cystic fibrosis transmembrane conductance regulator (CFTR) protein.

Ans. C

95. All are true about response to hypoxia except:

A. During hypoxia, systemic arterioles dilate

B. In pulmonary vascular smooth-muscle cells, inhibition of K+ channels causes depolarization which, in turn, activates voltage-gated Ca2+ channels raising the cytosolic [Ca2+] and causing smooth-muscle cell contraction

C. Hypoxia-induced pulmonary arterial constriction shunts blood away from poorly ventilated portions toward better ventilated portions of the lung

D. Hypoxia-induced pulmonary arterial constriction, increases pulmonary vascular resistance and right ventricular preload

Explanation:

- Decreased O2 availability to cells results in an inhibition of oxidative phosphorylation and increased anaerobic glycolysis.
- This switch from aerobic to anaerobic metabolism, Pasteur effect, reduces the rate of adenosine 5′-triphosphate (ATP) production.
- In severe hypoxia, when ATP production is inadequate to meet the energy requirements of ionic and osmotic equilibrium, cell membrane depolarization leads to uncontrolled Ca2+ influx and activation of Ca2+-dependent phospholipases and proteases.
- These events, in turn, cause cell swelling, activation of apoptotic pathways, and, ultimately, cell death.

- Adaptations to hypoxia are mediated, in part, by the upregulation of genes encoding a variety of proteins, including glycolytic enzymes, such as phosphoglycerate kinase and phosphofructokinase, as well as the glucose transporters Glut-1 and Glut-2; and by growth factors, such as vascular endothelial growth factor and erythropoietin, which enhance erythrocyte production.
- Hypoxia-induced increase in expression of these key proteins is governed by the hypoxiasensitive transcription factor, hypoxia-inducible factor-1 (HIF-1).
- During hypoxia, systemic arterioles dilate, at least in part, by opening of KATP channels in vascular smooth-muscle cells due to hypoxia-induced reduction in ATP concentration.
- By contrast, in pulmonary vascular smooth-muscle cells, inhibition of K+ channels causes depolarization which, in turn, activates voltage-gated Ca2+ channels raising the cytosolic [Ca2+] and causing smooth-muscle cell contraction.
- Hypoxia-induced pulmonary arterial constriction shunts blood away from poorly ventilated portions toward better ventilated portions of the lung; however, it also increases pulmonary vascular resistance and right ventricular afterload.

Ans. D

96. A 50 year old male presented with right sided exudative pleural effusion. Patient gives history of taking native medicines for knee joint pain. All the following drugs can cause pleural effusion except:

A. Nitrofurantoin
B. Amiodarone
C. Dantrolene
D. Spironolactone

Explanation:

- Drug-induced pleural disease:
  a. Nitrofurantoin
  b. Dantrolene
  c. Methysergide
  d. Bromocriptine
  e. Procarbazine
  f. Amiodarone
  g. Dasatinib

Ans. D

97. A 65 year old COPD patient ABG shows the following values:

pH – 7.36

PCO2 – 55 mm Hg

PO2 – 40 mm Hg

Bicarbonate – 30.6 mmol/L

Which of the following best describes his acid-base status?

A. Compensated respiratory acidosis
B. Uncompensated respiratory acidosis
C. Compensated respiratory alkalosis
D. Uncompensated respiratory alkalosis

Explanation:

- Since PCO2 is raised it comes under type 2 respiratory failure. The pH here is normal while the bicarbonate levels are increased in response to raised PCO2. Hence this is a compensated respiratory acidosis.

Ans. A

98. A 10 year old child presents to the ER with acute exacerbation of bronchial asthma. Among the following which is the most omnious sign?

A. Cyanosis
B. Feeble breath sounds and absent wheezing
C. Pulsus paradoxus
D. Usage of accessory muscles of chest

Explanation:

- The signs of severe exacerbation include tachypnoea, tachycardia, usage of accessory of the chest, diaphoresis and pulsus paradoxus.
- Feeble breath sounds and wheezing is a sign of impending respiratory failure.

Ans. D

99. A 18 year old male presented to the OPD with cough and breathlessness that was aggravated during night time. His PFT showed bronchodilator reversibility and his blood eosinophil levels were raised. All the following are differential diagnosis for asthma except:

A. Eosinophilic pneumonia
B. Churg Strauss syndrome
C. Vocal cord dysfunction
D. Sarcoidosis

Explanation:

- The differential diagnosis of asthma includes other disorders that can cause wheezing and dyspnea. Upper airway obstruction by tumor or laryngeal edema can mimic asthma, but stridor in the large airways is typically noted on physical examination. Localized wheezing in the chest may indicate an endobronchial tumor or foreign body. Congestive heart failure can cause wheezing but is typically accompanied by bibasilar crackles. Eosinophilic pneumonias and Churg-Strauss syndrome (eosinophilic granulomatosis with polyangiitis) may present with wheezing. Vocal cord dysfunction can mimic severe asthma and may require direct laryngoscopy to assess. When asthma involves chronic airflow obstruction, distinguishing it from chronic obstructive pulmonary disease (COPD) can be very difficult, and some pts have both asthma and COPD (asthma-COPD overlap syndrome).

Ans. D

100. A patient was advised biological treatment for bronchial asthma since he had poor symptom control with beta 2 adrenergic agonist and steroids. Which among the following drugs does not block the IL 5 pathway?

A. Benralizumab
B. Omalizumab
C. Mepolizumab
D. Reslizumab

Explanation:

- Omalizumab is a blocking antibody that neutralizes IgE; with SC injection every 2–4 weeks, it appears to reduce acute asthma exacerbation frequency in severe asthmatics. However, it is expensive and considered only for highly selected pts with elevated total serum IgE levels and refractory asthma symptoms despite maximal inhaled bronchodilator and ICS therapy. Antibodies that block IL-5 (mepolizumab, reslizumab) or its receptor (benralizumab) markedly reduce blood and tissue eosinophils and reduce exacerbations in pts who have persistently increased sputum eosinophils despite maximal ICS therapy.

Ans. B

101. A known COPD patient with frequent exacerbations and poor symptom control with medical treatment was offered long term supplemental oxygen therapy (LTOT). All the following are Indications for LTOT except:

A. PaO2 <55 mm Hg
B. SpO2 <88%
C. PaO2 56-59 mmHg with signs of cor pulmonale
D. None of the above

Explanation:

- Long-term supplemental oxygen therapy has been shown to reduce symptoms and improve survival in COPD pts who are chronically hypoxemic. Documentation of the need for O2 requires a measurement of PaO2 or oxygen saturation (SaO2) after a period of stability. Pts with a PaO2 ≤55 mmHg or SaO2 ≤88% should receive O2 to raise the SaO2 to ≥90%. O2 is also indicated for pts with PaO2 of 56–59 mmHg or SaO2 <90% if associated with signs and symptoms of pulmonary hypertension or cor pulmonale.

Ans. D

102. A 40 year old male presented with chronic cough and breathlessness. He had mucopurulent expectoration. On examination he had clubbing and bilateral coarse crackles. The apex beat was felt in the right 5th intercoastal space in the midclavicular line. Which of the following is not a feature of kartagener's syndrome?

A. Bronchiectasis
B. Pancreatic insufficiency
C. Sinusitis
D. Situs inversus

Explanation:

- Kartagener's syndrome is a triad of: bronchiectasis, sinusitis and situs inversus. It is a sub group of primary ciliary dyskinesia. Situs inversus generally occurs as a complete reversal of the circulatory system and viscera known as situs inversus totalis.

Ans. B

103. A patient with unilateral diaphragmatic paralysis undergoes sniff test. Which of the following is false regarding this procedure?

A. Diaphragmatic movement is observed fluoroscopically while the patient sniffs
B. A positive test shows paradoxical elevation of the paralysed hemi diaphragm with inspiration
C. M mode ultrasonography may substitute the fluoroscopic exam
D. No role of sniff test in diaphragmatic eventration

Explanation:

- A frontal, upright chest radiograph that shows an elevated hemidiaphragm is sensitive, but not specific for the diagnosis of unilateral diaphragmatic paralysis. The diagnosis can be easily confirmed with a fluoroscopic "sniff" test, in which diaphragmatic movement is observed fluoroscopically while the patient sniffs forcefully. The sniff test shows paradoxical elevation of the paralyzed hemidiaphragm with inspiration compared with the rapid descent of the normal hemidiaphragm. The sniff test is positive in over 90 percent of patients. The use of M-mode ultrasonography may substitute the fluoroscopic exam as it will detect the paradoxical motion of the afflicted hemi-diaphragm during the "sniff" maneuver.
- Eventration of the diaphragm is a disorder in which all or part of the diaphragmatic muscle is replaced by fibroelastic tissue, leading to a thinned and pliable central portion of the diaphragm.
- Fluoroscopy with sniff testing of a diaphragmatic eventration typically shows normal or slightly reduced diaphragmatic motion on the affected side. When the eventration is large, the hemidiaphragm may appear immobile on sniff testing.

Ans. D

104. A 40 year old male was found to be infected with mycobacterium avium complex based on bronchoscopic wash culture. Which among the following is not used in the treatment of this disease?

A. Isoniazid
B. Rifamycin
C. Clarithromycin
D. Ethambutol

Explanation:

- The American Thoracic Society has published guidelines for the diagnosis of pulmonary NTM disease that require the growth of NTM from two of three sputum samples, a positive bronchoalveolar lavage sample, or a pulmonary parenchyma biopsy sample with granulomatous inflammation or mycobacteria found on section and NTM in culture. Although these guidelines are specific to MAC, M. abscessus, and M. kansasii, they probably apply to other NTM as well.
- MAC infection requires multidrug therapy with a macrolide (clarithromycin or azithromycin), ethambutol, and a rifamycin (rifampin or rifabutin). Therapy is prolonged, generally continuing for 12 months after culture conversion; typically, a course lasts for at least 18 months.
- M. kansasii lung disease is similar to TB in many ways and is also effectively treated with isoniazid (300 mg/d), rifampin (600 mg/d), and ethambutol (15 mg/kg per day). Treatment should continue until cultures have been negative for at least 1 year.

Ans. A

105. Increased mortality prediction in ARDS is done by:

A. Severity as by Berlin definition
B. PEEP
C. Respiratory system compliance
D. Extent of alveolar infiltrates on chest radiography

Explanation:

- Increasing severity of ARDS, as defined by consensus Berlin definition, predicts increased mortality. Surprisingly, there is little additional value in predicting ARDS mortality from other parameters of lung injury, including the level of PEEP (≥10 cm H2O), respiratory system compliance (≤40 mL/cm H2O), extent of alveolar infiltrates on chest radiography, and the corrected expired volume per minute (≥10 L/min) (as a surrogate measure of dead space).

Ans. A

106. A 50 year old male with complaints of breathlessness was found to have raised JVP, loud P2 and pedal oedema. Chest X-ray shows enlarged central pulmonary artery. Which among the following is the gold standard to establish the diagnosis of pulmonary hypertension?

A. DLCO
B. CT chest
C. Right heart catheterization
D. ECHO

Explanation:

- CXR shows enlarged central PA; may demonstrate vascular "pruning." ECG typically indicates RV hypertrophy and RA enlargement. Echocardiogram shows RV and RA enlargement, RV hypertrophy; RV systolic pressure can be estimated from Doppler velocity of tricuspid regurgitation; echo "bubble study" identifies right-to-left intracardiac shunts that can cause Group 1 PH. Pulmonary function tests (PFTs) identify underlying obstructive or restrictive lung disease; impaired CO diffusion capacity is common. Chest CT identifies contributing interstitial lung disease or pulmonary thromboembolic disease (note that ventilation perfusion [V/Q] scan is more sensitive for detection of chronic thromboembolism as cause of Group 4 PH). ANA titer, rheumatoid factor, anti-Scl-70 antibodies are elevated in specific collagen vascular conditions that can result in PH. HIV testing should be performed in individuals at risk. Cardiopulmonary exercise testing can differentiate pulmonary from cardiac contributions to dyspnea. Right heart catheterization assesses PA pressures, cardiac output, and pulmonary vascular resistance, quantifies underlying congenital vascular shunts, and distinguishes left-sided heart disease from pulmonary causes of PH; during procedure, response to short-acting vasodilators can be tested.

Ans. C

107. A known ILD patient develops pulmonary hypertension due to hypoxia. He comes under which group of pulmonary hypertension?

A. Group 1 B. Group 2
C. Group 3 D. Group 4

Explanation:

1. **Pulmonary Arterial Hypertension**
   - Idiopathic
   - Heritable (mutations/familial cases)
   - Collagen vascular diseases (e.g., scleroderma, SLE, rheumatoid arthritis)
   - Congenital systemic to pulmonary shunts (e.g., ventricular septal defect, patent ductus arteriosus, atrial septal defect)
   - Portal hypertension HIV infection Drugs or toxins (e.g., fenfluramine)
2. **Pulmonary Hypertension Due to Left Heart Disease**
   - LV systolic or diastolic dysfunction
   - Left-sided valvular disease
3. **Pulmonary Hypertension Due to Lung Disease or Hypoxia**
   - Chronic obstructive lung disease
   - Interstitial lung disease
   - Sleep-disordered breathing
   - Chronic hypoventilation
4. **Chronic Pulmonary Thromboembolic Disease**
   - Chronic pulmonary embolism

Ans. C

108. A 50 year old female develops COPD secondary to biomass fuel cooking. Which among the following particle size is considered to be most dangerous?

A. 15 micro meter B. 10 micro meter
C. 5 micro meter D. 2 micro meter

Explanation:

- The susceptibility to develop many pulmonary diseases is influenced by environmental factors. This chapter will focus on occupational and toxic chemical exposures. However, a variety of nonoccupational indoor exposures such as environmental tobacco smoke exposure (lung cancer), radon gas (lung cancer), and biomass fuel cooking (chronic obstructive pulmonary disease [COPD]) also should be considered. Particle size is an important determinant of the impact of inhaled environmental exposures on the respiratory system. Particles >10 μm in diameter typically are captured by the upper airway. Particles 2.5–10 μm in diameter will likely deposit in the upper tracheobronchial tree, while smaller particles (including nanoparticles) will reach the alveoli.

Ans. D

109. A 20 year old male presented to the OPD with chronic cough and breathlessness. On examination he had features consistent with SVC syndrome (facial puffiness which exacerbated on bending down)

He was diagnosed as a case of mediastinal fibrosis based on CECT chest and biopsy.

The organism most frequently related to mediastinal fibrosis is:

A. Histoplasma
B. Staphylococcus
C. Streptococcus
D. Actinomyces

Explanation:

- Mediastinitis can be an acute or chronic process. Acute mediastinitis can result from esophageal perforation, following cardiac surgery with median sternotomy, or from infections in the neck, oral cavity, or face. Esophageal perforation can occur spontaneously or iatrogenically; surgical exploration of the mediastinum, repair of the esophageal perforation, and drainage of the pleural space and mediastinum are required. Mediastinitis after median sternotomy typically presents with wound drainage and is diagnosed by mediastinal needle aspiration. Treatment requires immediate drainage, debridement, and IV antibiotics. Chronic mediastinitis can range from granulomatous lymph node inflammation to fibrosing mediastinitis. Most cases are due to tuberculosis or histoplasmosis.

Ans. A

110. Most common cause of URI is:

A. Influenza virus
B. Adenovirus
C. Rhinovirus
D. Coronavirus

Explanation:

- There are at least 100 immunotypes of rhinovirus, the most common cause of URI (~30–40% of cases); other causes include influenza virus (three immunotypes; as well as parainfluenza virus (four immunotypes), coronavirus (at least three immunotypes), and adenovirus (47 immunotypes).
- Respiratory syncytial virus (RSV), a well-established pathogen in pediatric populations, is also a recognized cause of significant disease in elderly and immunocompromised individuals.

Ans. C

111. A 50 year old male presented to the OPD with progressive cough and breathlessness. On examination he had bilateral fine Velcro crackles in the lower lung fields. His PFT showed restrictive pattern and his DLCO was reduced. He was diagnosed as a case of ILD based on HRCT chest. All the following are granulomatous ILD except?

A. Sarcoidosis
B. Hypersensitivity pneumonitis
C. Churg strauss syndrome
D. Desquamated interstitial pneumonia.

Explanation:

- Common granulomatous ILDs include sarcoidosis and HP. HP is an inflammatory lung disorder caused by repeated inhalation of an organic antigen in a susceptible individual. Treatment involves avoiding exposure to the causative antigen; systemic corticosteroids may be required in subacute or chronic HP. Granulomatous vasculitides include inflammatory infiltrates of blood vessels with associated granulomas. Hemoptysis is frequently observed. Granulomatosis with polyangiitis (Wegener's disease) commonly affects the lungs; chest imaging abnormalities include lung nodules, patchy ground glass opacities, hilar lymphadenopathy, and consolidative opacities. Eosinophilic GPA (Churg Strauss syndrome) frequently includes asthma, peripheral blood eosinophilia, and chronic sinusitis; common chest imaging abnormalities include consolidative opacities and small pleural effusions.

Ans. D

112. DD for nodular infiltrates in chest in immunocompromised patients include all except:

A. Aspergillus
B. Nocardia
C. Radiation pneumonitis
D. Recurrent tumor

Explanation:

Table: Differential diagnosis of chest infiltrates in immunocompromised patients

Infiltrate	Cause of Pneumonia	
	Infectious	**Noninfectious**
Localized	Bacterial (including *Legionella,* mycobacteria)	Local haemorrhage or embolism, tumor
Nodular	Fungi (e.g., *Aspergillus or Mucor*), Nocardia	Recurrent tumor
Diffuse	Viruses (especially cytomegalovirus), *Chlamydia, Pneumocystis, Toxoplasma gondii,* mycobacteria	Congestive heart failure, radiation pneumonitis, drug-induced lung injury, lymphangitic spread of cancer

Ans. C

113. A 42 year old female had complaints of cough with mild hemoptysis for 3 days duration. Chest x ray was suggestive of bronchopneumonia. Pseudo haemoptysis is seen in:

A. Streptococcus pneumoniae
B. Pseudomonas aeruginosa
C. E. coli
D. Serratia marcescens

Explanation:

- Pseudo haemoptysis has appearance of red coloured sputum without the presence of RBCs. This phenomenon is seen in Serratia marcescens due to the production of the red pigment prodigiosin.

Ans. D

114. Factors indicating requirement for thoracentesis are all except:

A. Pleural fluid pH <7.2
B. Loculated pleural effusion
C. Pleural fluid glucose >60 mg/dl
D. Gross pus in the pleural space

Explanation:

- Possibility of a parapneumonic effusion should be considered whenever a patient with bacterial pneumonia is initially evaluated.
- Presence of free pleural fluid can be demonstrated with a lateral decubitus radiograph, computed tomography (ct) of chest, or ultrasound.
- If the free fluid separates the lung from the chest wall by >10 mm, a therapeutic thoracentesis should be performed.

Factors indicating the likely need for procedure more invasive than a thoracentesis (in increasing order of importance) include following:

1. Loculated pleural fluid
2. Pleural fluid ph <7.20
3. Pleural fluid glucose <3.3 mmol/l (<60 mg/dl)
4. Positive gram stain or culture of the pleural fluid
5. Presence of gross pus in the pleural space

Ans. C

115. A 50 year old female presented to the OPD with loss of weight and hemoptysis. She had undergone mastectomy for Breast carcinoma before 2 years. What is the diagnosis of this chest radiograph?

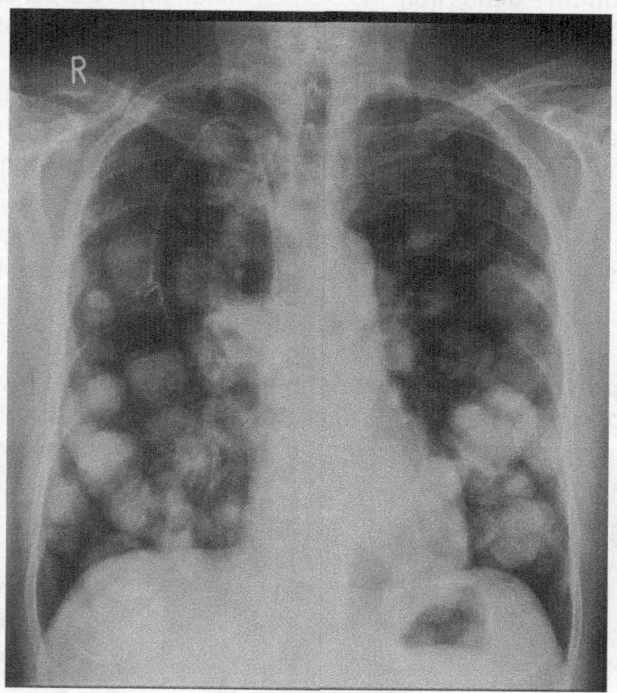

A. Nodular ILD
B. Cannonball metastasis
C. Sarcoidosis
D. TB

Explanation:

- Large, round, circumscribed lesions are seen in the right and left para cardiac borders indicating the presence of cannon ball metastasis. Most common primary for lung metastases are breast carcinoma, malignant melanoma, sarcoma, colon carcinoma and testicular carcinoma.

Ans. B

116. Wheezing is uncommon in most forms of ILD but can be present in below conditions except:

A. Sarcoidosis
B. Hypersensitive pneumonitis
C. Eosinophilic GPA
D. Idiopathic pulmonary fibrosis

Explanation:

- End-inspiratory fine crackles, or rales, noted at the lung bases are found in most patients with IPF and may be one of the earliest signs of the disease.
- However, rales are nonspecific and can be found in many forms of ILD and other disorders.
- **Wheezing is uncommon in most forms of ILD but can be present in some disorders, such as sarcoidosis, HP, and eosinophilic GPA.**
- Signs of advanced disease include cyanosis, digital clubbing, and cor pulmonale.

Ans. D

117. Posterior mediastinum includes all except:

A. Descending thoracic aorta
B. Pulmonary artery
C. Esophagus
D. Thoracic duct

Explanation:

- **Anterior mediastinum** extends from the sternum anteriorly to the pericardium and brachiocephalic vessels posteriorly. It contains the thymus gland, the anterior mediastinal lymph nodes, and the internal mammary arteries and veins.
- **Middle mediastinum** lies between the anterior and posterior mediastina and contains the heart; the ascending and transverse arches of the aorta; the venae cavae; the brachiocephalic arteries and veins; phrenic nerves; trachea, main bronchi, and their contiguous lymph nodes; & pulmonary arteries and veins.
- Posterior mediastinum is bounded by the pericardium and trachea anteriorly and the vertebral column posteriorly. It contains the descending thoracic aorta, the esophagus, the thoracic duct, the azygos and hemiazygos veins, and the posterior group of mediastinal lymph nodes.

Ans. B

118. A 45 year old male presented to the fever clinic with acute onset fever and breathlessness. He gives history of loose stools and myalgia for 2 days. What is the probable diagnosis for this CT chest image?

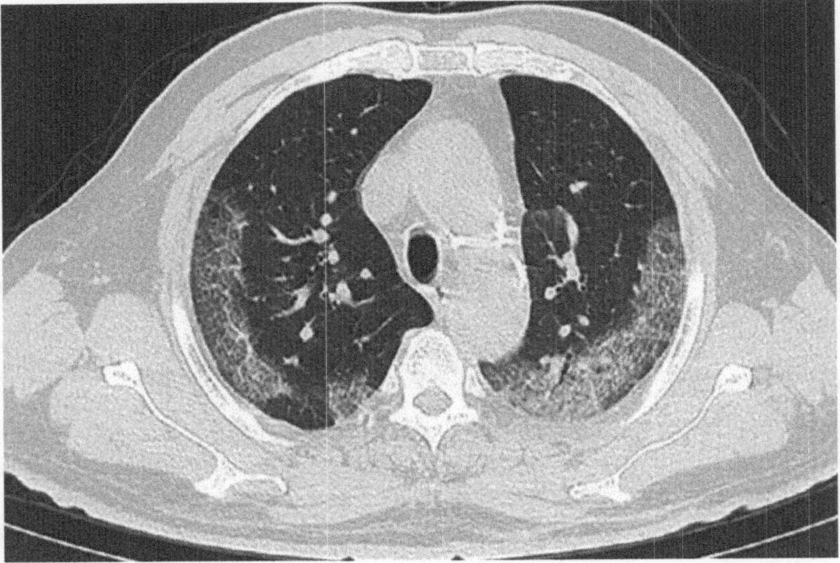

A. Pulmonary edema
B. Covid-19
C. PCP pneumonia
D. Pulmonary haemorrhage

Explanation:

- Bilateral peripheral ground glass opacities on CT chest should raise a suspicion of covid-19 infection.
- Peri hilar, central ground glass opacities are seen in pulmonary edema, PCP pneumonia and pulmonary haemorrhage.

Ans. B

119. Improvements in ventilation-perfusion matching and short- and long-term survival advantage in patients with acute lung injury and refractory hypoxemia has been shown by:

A. ECMO
B. Proportional assist ventilation
C. Prone positioning
D. Neurally adjusted ventilatory-assist ventilation

Explanation:

- Several nonconventional strategies have been evaluated for their ability to improve gas exchange and survival rates in severe hypoxemic respiratory failure.

- These strategies include high-frequency oscillatory ventilation (HFOV), airway pressure release ventilation (APRV), partial liquid ventilation (PLV) using perfluorocarbons and the administration of nitric oxide gas delivered through the airways.
- Although case reports and small uncontrolled cohort studies have shown benefit, randomized controlled trials have failed to demonstrate consistent improvements in outcome with these strategies.
- Some "salvage" techniques have gained acceptance given recent positive clinical outcomes. A randomized trial of extracorporeal membrane oxygenation (ECMO) documented positive outcomes, although older studies had failed to document positive results.
- However, with the popularity of venous-venous access, and encouraging reports in small series and uncontrolled trials, use of ECMO has increased world-wide.
- Guidelines for ECMO centers have been published, and if considered in patients with severe respiratory failure refractory to conventional therapy, the patient should be referred to a center familiar with the procedure.
- Second of these techniques, prone positioning, should be available in all units caring for these patients.
- Several multi-center randomized trials in patients with acute lung injury and refractory hypoxemia have shown that prone positioning improves ventilation-perfusion matching and provides short- and long-term survival advantage.

Ans. C

120. A 60 year old female has bilateral lower lobe bronchiectasis in her CT chest film. She is a known case of pulmonary Tuberculosis treated before 2 years. Suppressive antibiotics which can be given for bronchiectasis are all except:

A. Nebulized tobramycin
B. Azithromycin
C. Clindamycin
D. Inhaled colistin

Explanation:

- Long-term suppressive antibiotics are given in case of bronchiectasis with more than 3 exacerbations per year. The antibiotics given are azithromycin or erythromycin, inhaled gentamycin, inhaled tobramycin, inhaled colistin.

Ans. C

121. A 50 year old male present with chronic progressive breathlessness. On examination his JVP is elevated, there is loud 2nd heart sound and bilateral pedal edema. Right heart catheterization reveals pulmonary Hypertension. Pre capillary pulmonary hypertension is defined as:

A. PAP >15 mm Hg, PCWP >15 mm Hg
B. PAP >25 mm Hg, PCWP <15 mm Hg
C. PAP >15 mm Hg, PCWP >25 mm Hg
D. PAP <25 mm Hg, PCWP <15 mm Hg

Explanation:

- Most pts with idiopathic PAH present in fourth and fifth decades, female > male predominance; may be familial. Major symptom is dyspnea, often with insidious onset. Right heart catheterization demonstrates a mean pulmonary artery pressure ≥ 25 mm Hg, pulmonary vascular resistance >240 dyne-s/cm5, with a mean pulmonary capillary wedge pressure ≤15 mm Hg. Mean survival of PAH is 5–6 years, even with therapy.

Ans. B

122. A known asthmatic patient presents with mono neuritis multiplex. He also has chronic rhino sinusitis and peripheral blood eosinophilia. What is the diagnosis?

A. ABPA
B. Cystic fibrosis
C. ChurgStrauss syndrome
D. None of the above

Explanation:

- Churg-Strauss syndrome (CSS) or allergic granulomatosis and angiitis, is a multisystem disorder characterized by chronic rhinosinusitis, asthma, and prominent peripheral blood eosinophilia (≥ 1500 cells/microL and/or >10 percent eosinophils on differential leukocyte count). The exact etiology of EGPA is unknown.
- A peripheral neuropathy, usually mononeuritis multiplex, is seen in up to 75 percent of patients with EGPA. Central nervous system manifestations may include subarachnoid and cerebral hemorrhage, cerebral infarction, cranial nerve palsies and loss of visual acuity.
- Two-thirds of EGPA patients have skin involvement; findings include palpable purpura, subcutaneous nodules, and macular or papular erythematous rashes. Skin biopsy is often helpful for confirming the diagnosis.
- Antineutrophil cytoplasmic antibodies (ANCAs) are noted in 30 to 60 percent of EGPA patients. The majority of ANCAs associated with EGPA are directed against myeloperoxidase with a perinuclear staining pattern (called MPO-ANCA or P-ANCA).

Ans. C

123. Treatment of chylothorax include all except:

A. Octreotide
B. Percutaneous transabdominal thoracic duct blockage
C. Thoracic duct ligation
D. Prolonged tube thoracostomy with chest tube drainage

Explanation:

- Chylothorax occurs when thoracic duct is disrupted and chyle accumulates in pleural space.
- Most common cause of chylothorax is trauma (most frequently thoracic surgery), but it also may result from tumors in the mediastinum.
- Patients with chylothorax present with dyspnea, and a large pleural effusion is present on the chest radiograph.
- Thoracentesis reveals milky fluid, and biochemical analysis reveals a triglyceride level that exceeds 1.2 mmol/L (110 mg/dL).
- Patients with chylothorax and no obvious trauma should have a lymphangiogram and a mediastinal CT scan to assess the mediastinum for lymph nodes.
- Treatment of choice for most chylothoraxes is insertion of a chest tube plus the administration of octreotide.
- If these modalities fail, percutaneous transabdominal thoracic duct blockage effectively controls most chylothoraces.
- An alternative treatment is ligation of the thoracic duct.
- Patients with chylothoraxes should not undergo prolonged tube thoracostomy with chest tube drainage because this will lead to malnutrition and immunologic incompetence.

Ans. D

124. A 50 year old male develops acute breathlessness after 4 days of admission in the hospital for pneumonia infection. His initial chest radiograph showed only infiltrates in the right upper zone which progressed to bilateral diffuse infiltrates in both the lung fields in the chest radiograph taken after 3 days. All the following predispose to ARDS except?

A. Fat embolism
B. Septicemia
C. Multiple blood transfusions
D. Status asthmaticus

Explanation:

- Acute respiratory distress syndrome (ARDS) develops rapidly and includes severe dyspnea, diffuse pulmonary infiltrates, and hypoxemia; it typically causes respiratory failure. Key diagnostic criteria for ARDS include (1) diffuse bilateral pulmonary infiltrates on CXR; (2) PaO2 (arterial partial pressure of oxygen in mmHg)/FIO2 (inspired O2 fraction) ≤300 mmHg; (3) absence of elevated left atrial pressure; and (4) acute onset within 1 week of a clinical insult or new or worsening respiratory symptoms. Although many medical and surgical conditions can cause ARDS, most cases (>80%) result from sepsis, pneumonia, trauma, multiple blood transfusions, gastric acid aspiration and drug overdose.

Ans. D

125. A 50 year old male presents to ER with severe breathing difficulty and diaphoresis. On examination he is tachypneic, tachycardic and cyanosed. Chest radiograph shows peri hilar butterfly appearance. Which among the following drugs is not used in the treatment for this disease?

A. Positive pressure ventilation
B. Furosemide
C. Morphine
D. Prednisolone

Explanation:

- In acute pulmonary edema, pt appears severely ill, often diaphoretic, sitting bolt upright, tachypneic, and cyanosis may be present. Bilateral pulmonary rales; third heart sound may be present. Frothy, blood-tinged sputum may occur.
- Immediate, aggressive therapy is mandatory for survival. The following measures should be instituted as simultaneously as possible for cardiogenic pulmonary edema: 1. Administer supplemental oxygen to achieve O2 saturation ≥92%; if inadequate, use positive-pressure ventilation by face or nasal mask, and if necessary, endotracheal intubation. 2. Reduce preload: a. Seat pt upright to reduce venous return, if not hypotensive. b. Intravenous loop diuretic (e.g., furosemide, initially 0.5–1.0 mg/kg); use lower dose if pt does not take diuretics chronically c. Nitroglycerin (sublingual 0.4 mg × 3 q5min) followed by 5–20 μg/min IV if needed. d. Morphine 2–4 mg IV acts as a venodilator and may relieve dyspnea and anxiety; use with caution and assess frequently for hypotension or respiratory depression; naloxone should be available to reverse effects if necessary. e. Consider ACE inhibitor if pt is hypertensive, or in setting of acute MI with heart failure. f. Consider nesiritide (recombinant brain natriuretic peptide; 2-μg/kg bolus IV followed by 0.01 μg/kg per min) for refractory symptoms—do not use in acute MI or cardiogenic shock. 3. Inotropic agents are indicated in cardiogenic pulmonary edema and severe LV dysfunction: dopamine, dobutamine, milrinone (Chap. 12). 4. The precipitating cause of cardiogenic pulmonary edema (Table 15-1) should be sought and treated, particularly acute arrhythmias or infection. For refractory pulmonary edema associated with persistent cardiac ischemia, early coronary revascularization may be life-saving. For noncardiac pulmonary edema, identify and treat/remove cause.

Ans. D

126. Regarding Birt-Hogg-Dubé syndrome all are true except:

A. Autosomal dominant
B. Hemangioma
C. Fibrofolliculomas
D. Pulmonary cysts

Explanation:

- Birt-Hogg-Dubé syndrome is a rare human autosomal dominant genetic disorder characterized by fibrofolliculomas (benign tumors arising in hair follicles), pulmonary cysts, and kidney tumors.

- Renal tumors are usually of the chromophobe type, but they can exist as hybrids with other cell types.
- This disorder is associated with mutations in the *FLCN* gene, which codes for folliculin.

Ans. B

127. A 40 year old female was advised chest radiograph for evaluation of her cough. Chest radiograph showed bilateral ectatic changes and CT chest showed central bronchiectasis. Central bronchiectasis is seen in:

A. ABPA
B. Post tubercular bronchiectasis
C. Cystic adenoid malformation
D. Non tuberculous mycobacterium

Explanation:

- Central bronchiectasis is seen in ABPA, cystic fibrosis, William Campbell syndrome and Mounier Kuhn syndrome. Upper lobe predominant bronchiectasis is seen in cystic fibrosis and post tubercular bronchiectasis. Lower lobe bronchiectasis is seen in post aspiration and other infective conditions.

Ans. A

128. Major health effects from exposure to asbestos include all except:

A. Pleural fibrosis
B. Peritoneal mesothelioma
C. Hepatic fibrosis
D. Pulmonary fibrosis

Explanation:

- Major health effects from exposure to asbestos are pleural and pulmonary fibrosis, cancers of the respiratory tract, and pleural and peritoneal mesothelioma.
- Asbestosis is a diffuse interstitial fibrosing disease of the lung that is directly related to the intensity and duration of exposure.
- Disease resembles other forms of diffuse interstitial fibrosis
- Usually, exposure has taken place for at least 10 years before the disease becomes manifest.
- Mechanisms by which asbestos fibers induce lung fibrosis are not completely understood but are known to involve oxidative injury due to generation of reactive oxygen species by transition metals on surface of fibers as well as from cells engaged in phagocytosis.

Ans. C

129. Most common pulmonary manifestation of SSc is:

A. ILD
B. Pulmonary hypertension
C. Pleural effusion
D. Pleural thickening

Explanation:

- ILD is most common pulmonary manifestation of SSc.
- ILD occurs in about 50% of SSc patients with diffuse disease and in about 30% of patients with limited disease.
- Pulmonary hypertension can occur separately or concomitantly with ILD and is more frequent in patients with limited SSc.

Ans. A

130. A 40 year old male presents with acute onset of breathlessness. His SpO2 is 80%, pulse rate is 130 bpm and blood pressure is 90/60 mmHg. His ABG shows PaO2 of 40mmHg, PCO2 of 40 mmHg and Ph of 7.20. he was diagnosed to have Type 3 respiratory failure. This is seen in which of the following condition?

A. Kyphoscoliosis
B. Flail chest
C. Pulmonary fibrosis
D. Post-operative atelectasis

Explanation:

- **Type 1 Respiratory Failure:** Respiratory failure is defined as inadequate gas exchange due to malfunction of one or more components of the respiratory system. There are two main types of acute respiratory failure: hypoxemic and hypercarbic. Hypoxemic respiratory failure is defined by arterial O2 saturation.
- **Type 2 Respiratory Failure:** Hypercarbic respiratory failure is characterized by alveolar hypoventilation and respiratory acidosis. Hypercarbic respiratory failure results from decreased minute ventilation and/or increased physiologic dead space.
- **Type 3 Respiratory Failure:** Perioperative respiratory failure related to lung atelectasis, which can be treated with physiotherapy, positional changes, and/or non-invasive positive-pressure ventilation.
- **Type 4 Respiratory Failure:** Hypoperfusion of respiratory muscles related to shock, which typically improves with intubation and mechanical ventilation.

Ans. D

131. A 40 year man came to the ER with acute onset breathlessness. Chest radiograph revealed right upper lobe pneumonia. His SpO2 was 90%, pulse rate was 110 bpm and BP was 100/60mmHG. All the following are true about type 1 respiratory failure except:

A. Decreased PaO2
B. Normal PaCO2
C. Decreased PaCO2
D. Normal A-a gradient

Explanation:

- **Type 1 Respiratory Failure**: Respiratory failure is defined as inadequate gas exchange due to malfunction of one or more components of the respiratory system. There are two main types of acute respiratory failure: hypoxemic and hypercarbic. Hypoxemic respiratory failure is defined by arterial O2 saturation.
- In type 1 respiratory failure A-a is increased because PaO2 is reduced.

Ans. D

132. A 60 year old man gives history of working in the mining industry for the past 20 years. He complaints of chronic cough and breathlessness. All the following are recognized features of asbestosis, except:

A. Restrictive pattern in PFT
B. Calcification of pleura
C. Risk of mesothelioma
D. Egg shell calcification

Explanation:

- In addition to exposures to asbestos that may occur during the production of asbestos products (from mining to manufacturing), common occupational asbestos exposures occur in shipbuilding and other construction trades (e.g., pipefitting, boilermaking) and in the manufacture of safety garments and friction materials (e.g., brake and clutch linings). Along with worker exposure in these areas, bystander exposure (e.g., spouses) can be responsible for some asbestos related lung diseases. A range of respiratory diseases has been associated with asbestos exposure. Pleural plaques indicate that asbestos exposure has occurred, but they are typically not symptomatic. Interstitial lung disease, often referred to as asbestosis, is pathologically and radiologically similar to idiopathic pulmonary fibrosis; it is typically accompanied by a restrictive ventilatory defect with reduced diffusing capacity of the lung for carbon monoxide (DLCO) on pulmonary function testing. Asbestosis, which is directly related to the intensity and duration of exposure, usually develops at least 10 years after exposure, and no specific therapy is available.

Ans. D

133. A patient presents with dry cough and exertional dyspnea. Cryo-biopsy reveals interstitial lung disease. What is the auscultatory finding typical for this disease?

A. Early inspiratory crackle
B. Mid inspiratory crackle
C. Expiratory rhonchi
D. Late expiratory crackles

Explanation:

- Early inspiratory crackles are seen in airway disorders such as chronic bronchitis.
- Mid inspiratory coarse crackles are heard in bronchiectasis.
- Late inspiratory fine crackles are heard in ILD.

Ans. D

134. A 50 year old female had a accidental fall from the first floor of a building. Post the incident she developed breathlessness. What is the diagnosis for this patient? Chest radiograph of the patient is given below:

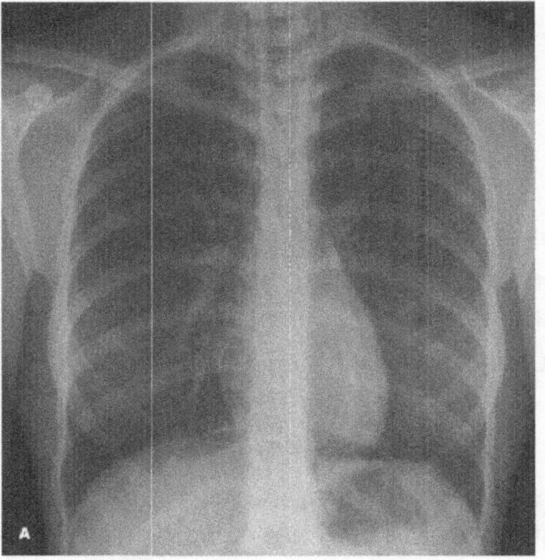

A. Pneumomediastinum | B. Hiatus hernia
C. COPD | D. Pulmonary embolism

Explanation:

- Chest X-ray shows continuous diaphragm sign indicating the presence of mediastinal gas outlining the superior surface of the diaphragm and separating it from the heart. This is seen in pneumomediastinum.
- Gas outlining the lateral margin of the descending aorta and extending laterally between the parietal pleura and medial left hemi diaphragm is known as V sign of Maclerio.

Ans. A

135. A 50 year old female presents to the OPD with chronic cough and breathlessness with frequent exacerbations. On examination she has clubbing and bilateral coarse crackles on auscultation. Her sputum shows classical triple layer seen in bronchiectasis. Investigation of choice for the diagnosis of bronchiectasis:

A. Chest X-ray | B. Non contrast CT chest
C. HRCT chest | D. Contrast CT chest

Explanation:

- The diagnosis of bronchiectasis is based on clinical presentation with consistent CXR findings, such as parallel "tram tracks," a "signet-ring sign" (a cross-sectional area of the airway with a diameter at least 1.5 times that of the adjacent vessel), lack of bronchial tapering, bronchial wall thickening, or cysts emanating from the bronchial wall.
- HRCT chest is the most sensitive investigation of choice for bronchiectasis.

Ans. C

136. A 30 year old anxiety disorder patients presents with complaints of breathlessness. On examination she was tachypneic, while auscultation revealed normal vesicular breath sounds. Her PFT and DLCO levels were normal. Alveolar hyperventilation causes?

A. Respiratory acidosis
B. Respiratory alkalosis
C. Metabolic acidosis
D. Metabolic alkalosis

Explanation:

- Hyperventilation is caused by ventilation in excess of requirements based on CO2 production, leading to a reduced PaCO2. Although anxiety can contribute to the initiation and progression of hyperventilation, hyperventilation is not always related to anxiety. Hyperventilation can precede systemic illnesses such as diabetic ketoacidosis.
- Hyperventilation is caused by ventilation in excess of requirements based on CO2 production, leading to a reduced PaCO2. Although anxiety can contribute to the initiation and progression of hyperventilation, hyperventilation is not always related to anxiety. Hyperventilation can precede systemic illnesses such as diabetic ketoacidosis.
- Treatment of chronic hyperventilation is problematic. Identification of initiating factors and excluding alternative diagnoses can be helpful.

Ans. B

137. Not true about ventilation is:

A. RBC becomes fully oxygen saturated by time cell has traveled just 1/3rd length of alveolar capillary
B. Oxygen uptake from lung diffusion limited
C. Oxygen & CO2 tensions in capillary blood leaving normal alveolus are essentially equal to those in alveolar gas
D. In High altitude or High performance atheletes exerting maximal effort is Oxygen uptake from normal lungs diffusion limited

Explanation:

- Red blood cell becomes fully oxygen saturated by the time the cell has traveled just one-third the length of the alveolar capillary.
- Thus, uptake of alveolar oxygen is ordinarily limited by the amount of blood transiting the alveolar capillaries rather than by the rapidity with which oxygen can diffuse across the membrane; consequently, oxygen uptake from the lung is said to be "perfusion limited" rather than diffusion limited.
- co2 also equilibrates rapidly across the alveolar membrane.
- Therefore, the oxygen and co2 tensions in capillary blood leaving a normal alveolus are essentially equal to those in alveolar gas.
- Only in rare circumstances (e.g., at high altitude or in high-performance athletes exerting maximal effort) is oxygen uptake from normal lungs diffusion limited.

- Diffusion limitation can also occur in interstitial lung disease if substantially thickened alveolar walls remain perfused.

Ans. B

138. Most common cause of chylothorax is:

A. Tumors in the mediastinum
B. Trauma
C. Infections
D. SLE

Explanation:

- A chylothorax occurs when the thoracic duct is disrupted and chyle accumulates in the pleural space.
- Most common cause of chylothorax is trauma (most frequently thoracic surgery), but it also may result from tumors in the mediastinum.
- Patients with chylothorax present with dyspnea, and a large pleural effusion is present on the chest radiograph.
- Thoracentesis reveals milky fluid, and biochemical analysis reveals a triglyceride level that exceeds 1.2 mmol/L (110 mg/dL). Patients with chylothorax and no obvious trauma should have a lymphangiogram and a mediastinal CT scan to assess the mediastinum for lymph nodes.
- Treatment of choice for most chylothoraxes is insertion of a chest tube plus the administration of octreotide.
- If these modalities fail, percutaneous transabdominal thoracic duct blockage effectively controls most chylothoraces.
- An alternative treatment is ligation of the thoracic duct.
- Patients with chylothoraxes should not undergo prolonged tube thoracostomy with chest tube drainage because this will lead to malnutrition and immunologic incompetence.

Ans. B

139. Hamman's sign is seen in:

A. Pneumomediastinum
B. Pneumotorax
C. Ascites
D. Pedal edema

Explanation:

Pneumomediastinum

- In this condition, there is gas in the interstices of the mediastinum.
- The three main causes are (1) alveolar rupture with dissection of air into the mediastinum; (2) perforation or rupture of the esophagus, trachea, or main bronchi; and (3) dissection of air from the neck or the abdomen into the mediastinum. Typically, there is severe substernal chest pain with or without radiation into the neck and arms.
- Physical examination usually reveals subcutaneous emphysema in suprasternal notch and *Hamman's sign*, which is a crunching or clicking noise synchronous with heartbeat and is best heard in the left lateral decubitus position.
- Diagnosis is confirmed with the chest radiograph. Usually no treatment is required, but mediastinal air will be absorbed faster if the patient inspires high concentrations of oxygen.
- If mediastinal structures are compressed, the compression can be relieved with needle aspiration.

Ans. A

140. Lung cancer more common in nonsmokers and woman is:

A. Small cell carcinoma
B. Adenocarcinoma
C. Squamous cell carcinoma
D. Large cell carcinoma

Explanation:

- In lifetime never smokers or former light smokers (<10 pack-year history), women, and younger adults (<60 years), adenocarcinoma tends to be the most common form of lung cancer.

Ans. B

141. Differential diagnosis for nodular infiltrates in chest in immunocompromised patients include all except:

A. Aspergillus
B. Nocardia
C. Radiation pneumonitis
D. Recurrent tumor

Explanation:

Table: Differential diagnosis of chest infiltrates in immunocompromised patients

Infiltrate	Cause of Pneumonia	
	Infectious	Noninfectious
Localized	Bacterial (including *Legionella*, mycobacteria)	Local hemorrhage or embolism, tumor
Nodular	Fungi (e.g., *Aspergillus or Mucor*), Nocardia	Recurrent tumor
Diffuse	Viruses (especially cytomegalovirus), *Chlamydia, Pneumocystis, Toxoplasma gondii,* mycobacteria	Congestive heart failure, radiation pneumonitis, drug-induced lung injury, lymphangitic spread of cancer

Ans. C

142. There is a potential hypoventilation with all modes except:

A. ACMV
B. IMV
C. PSV
D. NIV

Explanation:

Table: Characteristics of the most commonly used form of mechanical ventilation

Ventilatory Mode	Variables Set by User (Independent)	Variables Monitored by User (Dependent)	Trigger Cycle Limit	Advantages	Disadvantages
ACMV (assist-control ventilation)	Tidal volume Ventilator rate	Peak, mean and plateau airway pressures	Patient effort	Patient control	Potential hyperventilation
	FiO_2	VE	Timer	Guaranteed ventilation	Barotrauma and volume trauma
	PEEP level Pressure limit	ABG I/E ratio	Pressure limit		Every effective breath generates a ventilator volume

Contd.

Contd.

IMV (intermittent mandatory ventilation)	Tidal volume Mandatory ventilator rate FiO_2 PEEP level Pressure limit Spontaneous breaths between assisted breaths	Peak, mean and plateau airway pressures VE ABG I/E ratio	Patient effort Timer Pressure limit	Patient control Comfort from spontaneous breaths Guaranteed ventilation	Potential dysynchrony Potential hypoventilation
PSV (pressure-support ventilation)	Inspiratory pressure level FiO_2 PEEP level Pressure limit	Tidal volume Respiratory rate VE ABG	Pressure limit Inspiratory flow	Patient control Comfort Assures synchrony	No timer backup Potential hypoventilation
NIV (noninvasive ventilation)	Inspiratory and expiratory pressure level FiO_2	Tidal volume Respiratory rate VE ABG	Pressure limit Inspiratory flow	Patient control	Mask interface may cause discomfort and facial bruising Leaks are common Hypoventilation

Ans. A

143. All suggest alternative diagnosis other than IPF on CT chest except:

A. Extensive ground glass opacities
B. Micronodules
C. Mosaic attenuation
D. Posterior basal predominance

Explanation:

- Chest CT findings include subpleural reticulation with a posterior basal predominance usually including more advanced fibrotic features, such as honeycombing and traction bronchiectasis.
- Collectively these imaging findings are referred to as a UIP pattern.
- Presence of extensive ground glass opacities, bronchovascular changes, micronodules, mosaic attenuation, or an upper lung predominance should raise suspicion for an alternative diagnosis.

Ans. D

144. Pleural effusion secondary to pulmonary embolism all are true except:

A. Most common overlooked Differential diagnosis in undiagnosed pleural effusion
B. Dyspnea is most common symptom
C. Pleural effusion is almost always transudate
D. Diagnosis done by CT Chest

Explanation:

- Diagnosis most commonly overlooked in the differential diagnosis of patient with an undiagnosed pleural effusion is pulmonary embolism.
- Dyspnea is the most common symptom.
- Pleural fluid is almost always an exudate. The diagnosis is established by spiral CT scan or pulmonary arteriography.

- Treatment of a patient with a pleural effusion secondary to pulmonary embolism is the same as it is for any patient with pulmonary emboli.
- If the pleural effusion increases in size after anticoagulation, the patient probably has recurrent emboli or another complication, such as a hemothorax or a pleural infection.

Ans. C

145. Most sensitive test for an interstitial lung disease is:

A. Chest X-ray
B. CT scan chest
C. DLCO
D. ABG

Explanation:

- Lung volumes, mechanics, and diffusion are all useful in evaluating interstitial lung diseases such as sarcoidosis.
- **Diffusion of carbon monoxide (DLCO) is the most sensitive test for an interstitial lung disease.**
- Reduced lung volumes are a reflection of the restrictive lung disease seen in sarcoidosis. However, a third of the patients presenting with sarcoidosis still have lung volumes within the normal range, despite abnormal chest roentgenograms and dyspnea.

Ans. C

146. All come under loads due to reduced lung compliance except:

A. Alveolar edema
B. Atelectasis
C. Intrinsic positive end-expiratory pressure
D. Abdominal distention

Explanation:

- Overall load on the respiratory system can be sub classified into resistive loads (e.g., bronchospasm), loads due to reduced lung compliance (e.g., alveolar edema, atelectasis, intrinsic positive end-expiratory pressure [auto-PEEP]—see below), loads due to reduced chest wall compliance (e.g., pneumothorax, pleural effusion, abdominal distention), and loads due to increased minute ventilation requirements (e.g., pulmonary embolus with increased dead-space fraction, sepsis).

Ans. D

147. Intubation and mechanical ventilation is best needed for:

A. Type I respiratory failure
B. Type II respiratory failure
C. Type III respiratory failure
D. Type IV respiratory failure

Explanation:

TYPE IV RESPIRATORY FAILURE

- This form results from hypo-perfusion of respiratory muscles in patients in shock.
- Normally, respiratory muscles consume <5% of total cardiac output and oxygen delivery. Patients in shock often experience respiratory distress due to pulmonary edema (e.g., in cardiogenic shock), lactic acidosis, and anemia.
- In this setting, up to 40% of cardiac output may be distributed to the respiratory muscles.
- **Intubation and mechanical ventilation can allow redistribution of the cardiac output away from the respiratory muscles and back to vital organs while the shock is treated.**

Ans. D

148. All are true about Exercise-induced asthma (EIA) except:

A. Exercise-induced asthma (EIA) typically begins at the beginning of exercise, and recovers spontaneously within about 30 min

B. EIA is worse in cold, dry climates than in hot, humid conditions

C. It may be prevented by prior administration of β2-agonists and antileukotrienes

D. Best prevented by regular treatment with ICS

Explanation:

- Exercise is a common trigger of asthma, particularly in children.
- Mechanism is linked to hyperventilation, which results in increased osmolality in airway lining fluid and triggers mast cell mediator release, resulting in bronchoconstriction.
- Exercise-induced asthma (EIA) typically begins after exercise has ended, and recovers spontaneously within about 30 min.
- EIA is worse in cold, dry climates than in hot, humid conditions.
- It is, therefore, more common in sports such as cross-country running in cold weather, overland skiing, and ice hockey than in swimming.
- It may be prevented by prior administration of β2-agonists and antileukotrienes, but is best prevented by regular treatment with ICS, which reduce the population of surface mast cells required for this response.

Ans. A

149. Most common organisms responsible for ventilator-associated pneumonia include all except:

A. Pseudomonas aeruginosa

B. Streptococcus

C. Enteric gram-negative rods

D. Staphylococcus aureus

Explanation:

- Endotracheal intubation and MV have direct and indirect effects on lung and upper airways, the cardiovascular and the gastrointestinal system.
- Pulmonary complications include barotrauma, nosocomial pneumonia, oxygen toxicity, tracheal stenosis, and deconditioning of respiratory muscles.
- Barotrauma and volutrauma overdistend and disrupt lung tissue; may be clinically manifest by pneumomediastinum, interstitial and subcutaneous emphysema, or pneumothorax; and can result in the liberation of cytokines from overdistended tissues, further promoting tissue injury.
- Clinically significant pneumothorax requires tube thoracostomy. Intubated patients are at high risk for ventilator-associated pneumonia as a result of aspiration from the upper airways through small leaks around the endotracheal tube cuff; most common organisms responsible for this condition are *Pseudomonas aeruginosa*, enteric gram-negative rods, and *Staphylococcus aureus*.
- Given the high associated mortality rates, when suspected, early initiation of empirical antibiotics directed against likely pathogens is recommended.
- *Hypotension* resulting from elevated intrathoracic pressures with decreased venous return is almost always responsive to intravascular volume repletion.

Ans. B

150. Prerenal causes of AKI are all except:

A. Cisplatin

B. ACEI

C. ARB

D. Cyclosporine

Explanation:

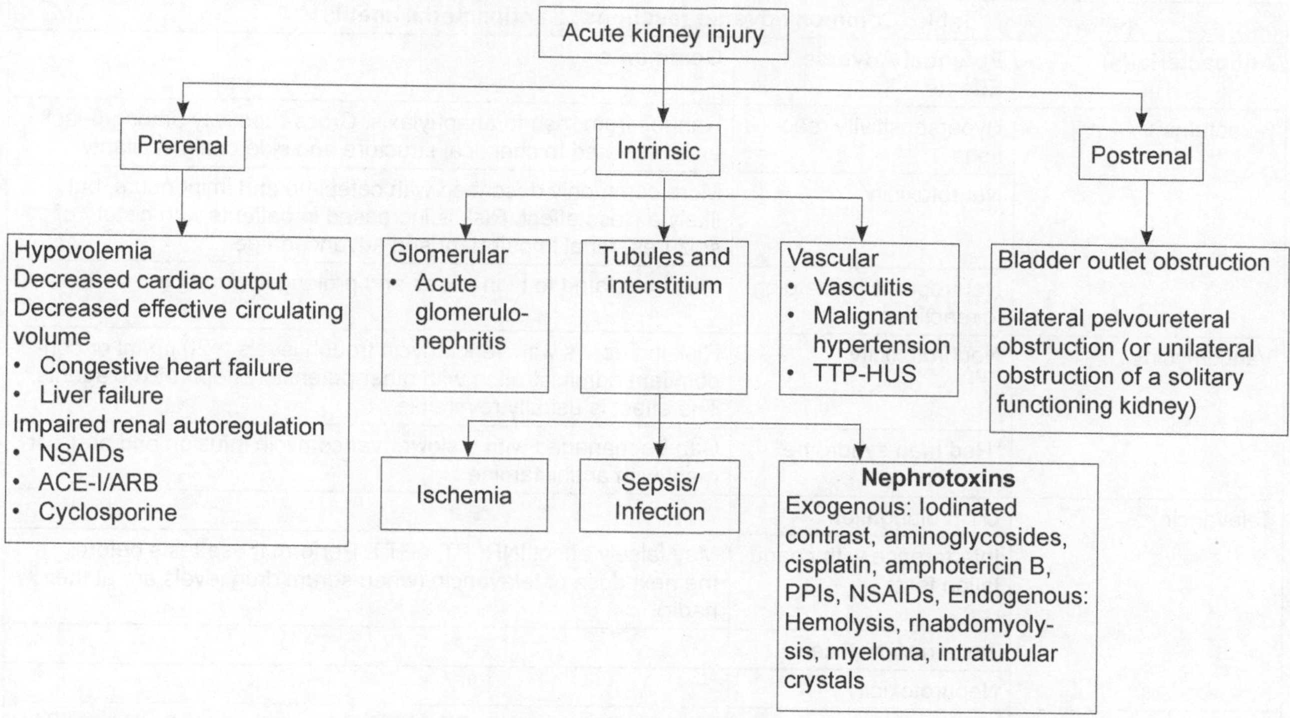

Ans. A

151. Most common cause of pleural effusion is:

A. Pneumonia
B. Chronic pancreatitis
C. Left ventricular failure
D. Malignant pleural effusion

Explanation:

- Most common cause of pleural effusion is left ventricular failure. Effusion occurs because increased amounts of fluid in lung interstitial spaces exit in part across visceral pleura; this overwhelms capacity of lymphatics in parietal pleura to remove fluid.
- Parapneumonic effusions are associated with bacterial pneumonia, lung abscess, or bronchiectasis and are probably the most common cause of exudative pleural effusion in United States.
- Empyema refers to a grossly purulent effusion.
- Malignant pleural effusions secondary to metastatic disease are the second most common type of exudative pleural effusion. The three tumors that cause ~75% of all malignant pleural effusions are lung carcinoma, breast carcinoma and lymphoma.

Ans. C

152. Orange discoloration of body fluids is seen with:

A. Vancomycin
B. Rifampin
C. Daptomycin
D. Fluoroquinolones

Explanation:

Table: Common adverse reactions to antibacterial agents		
Antibacterial(s)	**Potential Adverse Effects**	**Comments**
β-Lactams	Hypersensitivity reactions	Ranges from rash to anaphylaxis. Cross-reactivity among β-lactams is related to chemical structure and side chain similarity
	Neurotoxicity	More commonly described with cefepime and imipeneum, but likely a class effect. Risk is increased in patients with history of seizures, renal impairment and advanced age
	Neutropenia/hematologic reactions	May be related to high doses and prolonged duration
Vancomycin	Nephrotoxicity	Risk increases with vancomycin trough levels > 20 μg/ml or concomitant administration with other potentially nephrotoxic agents. The effect is usually reversible
	"Red man syndrome"	Can be managed with a slower vancomycin infusion and pretreatment with antihistamine
Telavancin	QT prolongation	
	Interference with coagulation tests	May falsely affect INR, PT, aPTT. Perform these tests before the next dose of telavancin (when serum drug levels are at their nadir)
	Taste disturbances	
	Nephrotoxicity	
Oritavancin	Interference with coagulation tests	May falsely affect INR, PT, aPTT, Perform these tests at least 24 hours after the dose is administered
	Gastrointestinal distress	
Dalbavancin	Gastrointestinal distress	
Deptomycin	Myopathy	Monitor CPK levels during therapy. Rhabdomyolysis has been reported but appears to be rare
	Eosinophilic pneumonia	
Aminoglycosides	Nephrotoxicity	Associated with prolonged use; usually reversible
	Ototoxicity	Can cause both vestibular and cochlear toxicity. Ototoxicity may be irreversible
Fluoroquinolones	QT_c prolongation	Moxifloxacin appears more likely than other quinolones to exert this effect. Risk of arrhythmia increases when these drugs are given concomitantly with other QT_c-prolonging agents
	Tendinitis	Risk is greater among the elderly and patients receiving steroids
	Dysglycemia	
	Exacerbation of myasthenia gravis	
Rifampin	Hepatotoxicity	Risk is greater when drug is given with other antituberculosis agents. When rifampin is given alone, LFT values may be transiently elevated without symptoms
	Orange discoloration of body fluids	
Tetracyclines and glycylcylines	Photosensitivity	
	Gastrointestinal distress	High incidence of diarrhea, nausea, vomiting
Macrolides	Gastrointestinal distress	Erythromycin is occasionally used as a therapeutic agent for some gastric motility disorders
	QT_c prolongation	Azithromycin use is associated with an increased risk of death from cardiovascular causes among patients at high baseline risk

Contd.

Contd.

Metronidazole	Peripheral neuropathy	Associated with prolonged use
Clindamycin	Diarrhea and pseudo-membranous colitis	
Linezolid, tedizolid	Myelosuppression	Associated with prolonged used
	Optic and peripheral neuropathy	Associated with prolonged use
	Lactic acidosis	
TMP-SMX	Hypersensitivity reactions	Allergy usually associated with sulphonamide moiety
	Nephrotoxicity	Associated with high doses
	Hematologic effects	Associated with prolonged use
Nitrofurantoin	Pneumonitis and other pulmonary reactions	Associated with prolonged use
	Peripheral neuropathy	Associated with accumulation of nitrofurantoin in renal failure. Avoid use in renal impairment
Fosfomycin	Gastrointestinal effects	
Polymyxins	Nephrotoxicity	Associated with high dose
	Neurotoxicity	Neuromuscular blockade and muscle weakness are well described and usually reversible
Quinupristin-dalfopristin	Arthralgias and mylgias	
Chloramphenicol	Bone marrow suppression	Aplastic anemia or hematopoietic toxicity

Ans. B

153. All are true regarding cystic fibrosis of the pancreas except:

A. Fat soluble vitamin insufficiency

B. Low levels of serum immunoreactive trypsinogen

C. Loss of pancreatic islet mass

D. Poor growth

Explanation:

- Complete name of the disease, *cystic fibrosis of the pancreas*, refers to profound tissue destruction of the exocrine pancreas, with fibrotic scarring and/or fatty replacement, cyst proliferation, loss of acinar tissue, and ablation of normal pancreatic architecture.
- As in the lung, tenacious exocrine secretions (sometimes termed *concretions*) obstruct pancreatic ducts and impair production and flow of digestive enzymes to the duodenum.
- Sequelae of exocrine pancreatic insufficiency include chronic malabsorption, poor growth, fat-soluble vitamin insufficiency, high levels of serum immunoreactive trypsinogen (a diagnostic test used in newborn screening), and loss of pancreatic islet cell mass. Cf-related diabetes mellitus is a manifestation in over 30% of adults with the disease and is likely multifactorial in nature (attributable to progressive destruction of endocrine pancreas, insulin resistance due to stress hormones, and additional factors).

Ans. B

154. Worst prognosis is associated with:

A. Idiopathic pulmonary fibrosis

B. Nonspecific interstitial pneumonia

C. Systemic sclerosis associated ILD

D. Respiratory bronchiolitis associated ILD

Explanation:

Table: Common interstitial lung disease findings

	IPF	Nonspecific Interstitial Pneumonia	Respiratory Bronchiolitis Associated ILD	Systemic Sclerosis Associated ILD	Sarcoidosis
Clinical symptoms	Gradual onset of SOB, dry cough. Unusual in younger adults	Subacute onset of SOB, dry cough. Frequently associated with other conditions	Can be asymptomatic, or have SOB and cough	Gradual onset of SOB, dry cough. Fatigue, tightening of skin, exaggerated cold response, reflux, and difficulty swallowing	Can be asymptomatic, or have SOB, and cough. Can also have fatigue, palpitations, eye, skin and joint findings
Physical examination findings	Frequent rales at lung bases, digital clubbing is common	Frequent rales. Clubbing is less common	Rales common. Clubbing is rare	Can have rales in isolation. Also skin thickening, joint swelling and telangiectasias	Can be normal, rales may be present. Can have skin findings, joint pain and enlarged lymph nodes
Exposures	Idiopathic but many exposed to smoke. Genetic findings may explain >1/3 of the risk of the disease	Can be idiopathic but should prompt consideration for associated conditions	Strong association with smoking	Mostly unknown, some debate about solvent and silicate exposures	Mostly unknown, although silicate dusts thought to play a role in some cases
HRCT findings	Bilateral subpleural reticular changes most prominent in lower, posterior lung zones. Traction bronchiectasis and honeycombing common. Classic UIP pattern is considered diagnostic	Peripheral subpleural ground glass and reticular pattern. Traction bronchiectasis is common but honeycombing is rare. HRCT not diagnostic	Diffuse patchy centrilobular ground glass nodules	Can have UIP or NSIP patterns, also dilated esophagus, occasional mediastinal calcifications, and pulmonary vascular enlargement	Can have mediastinal and hilar lymphadenopathy. Peribrochovascular reticular-nodular findings
Histopathology	UIP pattern including fibroblastic foci, temporal and spatial heterogeneity, honeycombing	Cellular or fibrotic pattern of NSIP. More uniform than a UIP pattern	Respiratory bronchiolitis with adjacent inflammatory and fibrosing changes. Pigment laden macrophages	Both UIP or NSIP patterns can occur	Non-caseating granulomas
Clinical course	50% 3-5 years mortality	18% 5-year mortality	25% 7-year mortality	20-30% 10-year mortality	Generally low but varies by state

Ans. A

155. Factors indicating requirement for thoracentesis are all except:

A. Pleural fluid pH <7.2

B. Loculated pleural effusion

C. Pleural fluid glucose >60 mg/dl

D. Gross pus in the pleural space

Explanation:

Factors indicating the likely need for a procedure more invasive than a thoracentesis (in increasing order of importance) include the following:

1. Loculated pleural fluid
2. Pleural fluid pH <7.20
3. Pleural fluid glucose <3.3 mmol/L (<60 mg/dL)
4. Positive Gram stain or culture of the pleural fluid
5. Presence of gross pus in the pleural space

Ans. C

156. Most widely used drug for induction of lung post transplantation is:

A. Alemtuzumab

B. Tacrolimus

C. Basiliximab

D. Adalimumab

Explanation:

- Interleukin-2 receptor antagonist basiliximab has been the most widely used drug (~50% of recipients), but the antilymphocyte globulins and alemtuzumab have been used, as well.
- Three-drug maintenance immunosuppressive regimen that includes a calcineurin inhibitor (cyclosporine or tacrolimus), a purine synthesis antagonist (azathioprine or a mycophenolic acid precursor), and prednisone is traditional; the triad of tacrolimus, mycophenolate, and prednisone is the most commonly prescribed regimen.
- Subsequently, other drugs such as sirolimus or everolimus may be substituted for various reasons.

Ans. C

157. A 30 year old man known case of bronchial asthma was on steroid, now stopped abruptly for 15 days, comes to the hospital with fatigability. His BP is 90/60mm Hg, his PR – 92/min, regular. Serum sodium – 130mEq/l, potassium – 5.5 mEq/l. Cortisol level is low. What is the diagnosis?

A. Primary adrenal failure

B. Normal adrenal function

C. Corticosteroid related adrenal suppression

D. SIADH

Explanation:

- It is due to the corticosteroid use for bronchial asthma. It leads to adrenal suppression thereby causing postural hypotension, hyponatremia low cortisol levels. The treatment is gradual tapering and stopping the corticosteroids.

Ans. C

158. Fluid management in ARDS include all except:

A. Low LA pressure improves outcomes

B. Aggressive fluid restriction is indicated

C. Hypotension is less if fluid restriction done

D. Low left atrial filling pressure minimizes pulmonary edema

Explanation:

- Increased pulmonary vascular permeability leading to interstitial and alveolar edema fluid rich in protein is a central feature of ARDS.
- In addition, impaired vascular integrity augments the normal increase in extravascular lung water that occurs with increasing left atrial pressure.
- Maintaining a low left atrial filling pressure minimizes pulmonary edema and prevents further decrements in arterial oxygenation and lung compliance; improves pulmonary mechanics; shortens ICU stay and duration of mechanical ventilation.
- Thus, aggressive attempts to reduce left atrial filling pressures with fluid restriction & diuretics should be an important aspect of ARDS management, limited only by hypotension & hypoperfusion of critical organs such as kidneys.

Ans. C

159. All are true about Assist control ventilation except:

A. Respiratory alkalemia
B. Non synchronous with inspiration
C. Dynamic hyperinflation
D. Barotrauma

Explanation:

- ACMV is the most widely used mode of ventilation. In this mode, an inspiratory cycle is initiated either by the patient's inspiratory effort or, if none is detected within a specified time window, by a timer signal within the ventilator.
- Every breath delivered, whether patient- or timer-triggered, consists of operator-specified tidal volume. Ventilatory rate is determined either by the patient or by the operator-specified backup rate, whichever is of higher frequency.
- ACMV is commonly used for initiation of MV because it ensures a backup minute ventilation in the absence of an intact respiratory drive and allows for synchronization of the ventilator cycle with the patient's inspiratory effort.
- Problems can arise when ACMV is used in patients with tachypnea due to nonrespiratory or nonmetabolic factors, such as anxiety, pain, and airway irritation. Respiratory alkalemia may develop and trigger myoclonus or seizures.
- Dynamic hyperinflation leading to increased intrathoracic pressures (so-called auto-PEEP) may occur if the patient's respiratory mechanics are such that inadequate time is available for complete exhalation between inspiratory cycles.
- Auto-PEEP can limit venous return, decrease cardiac output, and increase airway pressures, predisposing to barotrauma.

Ans. B

160. Cause of low pressure pulmonary edema is:

A. Heart failure
B. Intravascular volume overload
C. ARDS
D. Renal failure

Explanation:

- Pulmonary edema can be further categorized as occurring due to elevated pulmonary microvascular pressures, as seen in heart failure and intravascular volume overload or ARDS (low-pressure pulmonary edema)

Ans. C

161. Causes of type II respiratory failure include all except:

A. Gastric Aspiration
B. Brainstem injury
C. Severe hypothyroidism
D. Myopathy

Explanation:

- Type 2 respiratory failure is a consequence of alveolar hypoventilation and results from the inability to eliminate carbon dioxide effectively.
- Mechanisms are categorized by impaired central nervous system (CNS) drive to breathe, impaired strength with failure of neuromuscular function in the respiratory system, and increased load(s) on the respiratory system. Reasons for diminished CNS drive to breathe include drug overdose, brainstem injury, sleep-disordered breathing and severe hypothyroidism.
- Reduced strength can be due to impaired neuromuscular transmission (e.g., myasthenia gravis, Guillain-Barré syndrome, amyotrophic lateral sclerosis) or respiratory muscle weakness (e.g., myopathy, electrolyte derangements, fatigue).

Ans. A

162. All combination about HRCT findings are correct except:

A. Bilateral subpleural reticular changes most prominent in lower, posterior lung zones in IPF
B. Peripheral subpleural ground glass and reticular patterns. Traction bronchiectasis is common but honeycombing is rare in nonspecific interstitial pneumonia
C. Diffuse patchy centrilobular ground glass nodules in systemic sclerosis associated ILD
D. Can have mediastinal and hilar lymphadenopathy. Peribronchovascular reticular-nodular findings in sarcoidosis

Explanation:

Table: Common interstitial lung disease findings

	IPF	Nonspecific Interstitial Pneumonia	Respiratory Bronchiolitis Associated ILD	Systemic Sclerosis Associated ILD	Sarcoidosis
Clinical symptoms	Gradual onset of SOB, dry cough. Unusual in younger adults	Subacute onset of SOB, dry cough. Frequently associated with other conditions	Can be asymptomatic, or have SOB and cough	Gradual onset of SOB, dry cough. Fatigue, tightening of skin, exaggerated cold response, reflux, and difficulty swallowing	Can be asymptomatic, or have SOB, and cough. Can also have fatigue, palpitations, eye, skin and joint findings
Physical examination findings	Frequent rales at lung bases, digital clubbing is common	Frequent rales. Clubbing is less common	Rales is common. Clubbing is rare	Can have rales in isolation. Also skin thickening, joint swelling and telangiectasias	Can be normal, rales may be present. Can have skin findings, joint pain and enlarged lymph nodes
Exposures	Idiopathic but many exposed to smoke. Genetic findings may explain >1/3 of the risk of the disease	Can be idiopathic but should prompt consideration for associated conditions	Strong association with smoking	Mostly unknown, some debate about solvent and silicate exposures	Mostly unknown, although silicate dusts thought to play a role in some cases

Contd.

Contd.

HRCT findings	Bilateral subpleural reticular changes most prominent in lower, posterior lung zones. Traction bronchiectasis and honeycombing common. Classic UIP pattern is considered diagnostic	Peripheral subpleural ground glass and reticular patterns. Traction bronchiectasis is common but honeycombing is rare. HRCT not diagnostic	Diffuse patchy centrilobular ground glass nodules	Can have UIP or NSIP patterns, also dilated esophagus, occasional mediastinal calcifications, and pulmonary vascular enlargement	Can have mediastinal and hilar lymphadenopathy. Peribrochovascular reticular-nodular findings
Histopathology	UIP pattern including fibroblastic foci, temporal and spatial heterogeneity, honeycombing	Cellular or fibrotic pattern of NSIP. More uniform than a UIP pattern	Respiratory bronchiolitis with adjacent inflammatory and fibrosing changes. Pigment laden macrophages	Both UIP or NSIP patterns can occur	Non-caseating granulomas
Clinical course	50% 3-5 years mortality	18% 5-year mortality	25% 7-year mortality	20-30% 10-year mortality	Generally low but varies by state

Ans. C

163. Strongly associated with smoking is:

A. IPF

B. Nonspecific interstitial pneumonia

C. Systemic sclerosis associated ILD

D. Respiratory bronchiolitis associated ILD

Explanation:

Table: Common interstitial lung disease findings

	IPF	Nonspecific Interstitial Pneumonia	Respiratory Bronchiolitis Associated ILD	Systemic Sclerosis Associated ILD	Sarcoidosis
Clinical symptoms	Gradual onset of SOB, dry cough. Unusual in younger adults	Subacute onset of SOB, dry cough. Frequently associated with other conditions	Can be asymptomatic, or have SOB and cough	Gradual onset of SOB, dry cough. Fatigue, tightening of skin, exaggerated cold response, reflux, and difficulty swallowing	Can be asymptomatic, or have SOB, and cough. Can also have fatigue, palpitations, eye, skin and joint findings
Physical examination findings	Frequent rales at lung bases, digital clubbing is common	Frequent rales, Clubbing is less common	Rales is common. Clubbing is rare	Can have rales in isolation. Also skin thickening, joint swelling and telangiectasias	Can be normal, rales may be present. Can have skin findings, joint pain and enlarged lymph nodes

Contd.

Contd.

Exposures	Idiopathic but many exposed to smoke. Genetic findings may explain >1/3 of the risk of the disease	Can be idiopathic but should prompt consideration for associated conditions	Strong association with smoking	Mostly unknown, some debate about solvent and silicate exposures	Mostly unknown, although silicate dusts thought to play a role in some cases
HRCT findings	Bilateral subpleural reticular changes most prominent in lower, posterior lung zones. Traction bronchiectasis and honeycombing common. Classic UIP pattern is considered diagnostic	Peripheral subpleural ground glass and reticular patterns. Traction bronchiectasis is common but honeycombing is rare. HRCT not diagnostic	Diffuse patchy centrilobular ground glass nodules	Can have UIP or NSIP patterns, also dilated esophagus, occasional mediastinal calcifications, and pulmonary vascular enlargement	Can have mediastinal and hilar lymphadenopathy. Peribrochovascular reticular-nodular findings
Histopathology	UIP pattern including fibroblastic foci, temporal and spatial heterogeneity, honeycombing	Cellular or fibrotic pattern of NSIP. More uniform than a UIP pattern	Respiratory bronchiolitis with adjacent inflammatory and fibrosing changes. Pigment laden macrophages	Both UIP or NSIP patterns can occur	Non-caseating granulomas
Clinical course	50% 3-5 years mortality	18% 5-year mortality	25% 7-year mortality	20-30% 10-year mortality	Generally low but varies by state

Ans. D

164. Below have increased mortality after Lung volume reduction surgery except:

A. Patients with an FEV1 <20% of predicted and diffusely distributed emphysema on CT scan

B. Patients with an FEV1 <20% of predicted and diffusing capacity of lung for carbon monoxide (DLCO) <20% of predicted

C. Patients with upper lobe–predominant emphysema and a low post-rehabilitation exercise capacity

D. All above category of patients have increased mortality after procedure

Explanation:

- In carefully selected patients with emphysema, surgery to remove the most emphysematous portions of lung improves exercise, lung function, and survival.
- Anatomic distribution of emphysema and post-rehabilitation exercise capacity are important prognostic characteristics.
- Patients with upper lobe–predominant emphysema and a low post-rehabilitation exercise capacity are most likely to benefit from LVRS.
- Patients with an FEV1 <20% of predicted and either diffusely distributed emphysema on CT scan or diffusing capacity of lung for carbon monoxide (DLCO) <20% of predicted have increased mortality after the procedure, and thus are not candidates for LVRS.
- Methods of achieving lung volume reduction by using bronchoscopic techniques are under investigation.

Ans. C

165. Drug associated with ILD is:

A. Gefitinib
B. Avelumab
C. Everolimus
D. Busulfan

Explanation:

- Molecular targeted agents, imatinib, erlotinib, and gefitinib are potent inhibitors of tyrosine kinases. These drugs may cause interstitial lung disease (ILD).
- In the case of gefitinib, preexisting fibrosis, poor performance status, and prior thoracic irradiation are independent risk factors; this complication has a high fatality rate.

Ans. A

166. Wheezing is uncommon in most forms of ILD but can be present in below conditions except:

A. Sarcoidosis
B. HP
C. Eosinophilic GPA
D. IPF

Explanation:

- End-inspiratory fine crackles, or rales, noted at the lung bases are found in most patients with IPF and may be one of the earliest signs of disease.
- However, rales are nonspecific and can be found in many forms of ILD and other disorders.
- Wheezing is uncommon in most forms of ILD but can be present in some disorders, such as sarcoidosis, HP, and eosinophilic GPA.
- Signs of advanced disease include cyanosis, digital clubbing, and cor pulmonale.

Ans. D

167. All are common abnormalities of anterior mediastinum except:

A. Teratomatous neoplasm
B. Hernia through foramen of Morgagni
C. Lymphomas
D. Bronchogenic cysts

Explanation:

Table: The three compartments of the mediastinum

	Anterior Compartment	**Middle Compartment**	**Posterior Compartment**
Anatomical boundaries	Manubrium and sternum anteriorly, pericardium, aorta and brachiocephalic vessels posteriorly	Anterior mediastinum anteriorly, posterior mediastinum posteriorly	Pericardium and trachea anteriorly; vertebral column posteriorly
Contents	Thymus gland, anterior mediastinal lymph nodes, internal mammary arteries and veins	Pericardium, heart, ascending and transverse arch of aorta, superior and inferior vena cavae, brachiocephalic arteries and veins, phrenic nerves, trachea, and main bronchi and their contiguous lymph nodes, pulmonary arteries and veins	Descending thoracic aorta, esophagus, thoracic duct, azygos and hemiazygos veins, sympathetic chains, and the posterior group of mediastinal lymph nodes
Common abnormalities	Thymoma, lymphomas, teratomatous neoplasms, thyroid masses, parathyroid masses, mesenchymal tumors, giant lymph node hyperplasia, hernia through foramen of Morgagni	Metastatic lymph node enlargement, granulomatous lymph node enlargement, pleuropericardial cysts, bronchogenic cysts, masses of vascular origin	Neurogenic tumors, meningocele, meningomyelocele, gastroenteric cysts, esophageal diverticula, hernia through foramen of Bochdalek, extramedullary hematopoiesis

Ans. D

168. All are true about aspirin sensitive asthma except:

A. Asthma is triggered by COX inhibitors, but is persistent even in their absence

B. All nonselective COX inhibitors should be avoided, but selective COX2 inhibitors are safe to use when an anti-inflammatory analgesic is needed

C. Aspirin-sensitive asthma doesn't respond to usual therapy with ICS

D. Although antileukotrienes should be effective in these patients, they are no more effective than in allergic asthma

Explanation:

- Small proportion (1–5%) of asthmatics become worse with aspirin and other COX inhibitors, although this is much more commonly seen in severe cases and in those patients with frequent hospital admission.
- Aspirin-sensitive asthma is a well defined phenotype of asthma that is usually preceded by perennial rhinitis and nasal polyps in nonatopic patients with a late onset of disease.
- Aspirin, even in small doses, characteristically provokes rhinorrhea, conjunctival injection, facial flushing, and wheezing.
- There is a genetic predisposition to increased production of cysteinyl-leukotrienes with functional polymorphism of *cys*-leukotriene C4 synthase.
- Asthma is triggered by COX inhibitors, but is persistent even in their absence.
- All nonselective COX inhibitors should be avoided, but selective COX2 inhibitors are safe to use when an anti-inflammatory analgesic is needed.
- Aspirin-sensitive asthma responds to usual therapy with ICS.
- Although antileukotrienes should be effective in these patients, they are no more effective than in allergic asthma.
- Occasionally, aspirin desensitization is necessary, but this should only be undertaken in specialized centers.

Ans. C

169. FEV1/FVC diagnostic of obstruction is:

A. <50%

B. <70%

C. <90%

D. 100%

Explanation:

- Diminished-forced expiratory volume in 1 s (FEV1)/forced vital capacity (FVC) (often defined as <70%) is diagnostic of obstruction. In addition to measuring FEV1 and FVC, the clinician should examine the flow-volume loop (which is less effort-dependent).
- Plateau of the inspiratory and expiratory curves suggests large-airway obstruction in extrathoracic and intrathoracic locations, respectively.

Ans. B

170. Oxygen uptake from normal lungs diffusion limited is seen in:

A. ILD

B. Asthma

C. Emphysema

D. High altitude

Explanation:

- Oxygen and CO2 tensions in capillary blood leaving a normal alveolus are essentially equal to those in alveolar gas.

- Only in rare circumstances (e.g., at high altitude or in high-performance athletes exerting maximal effort) is oxygen uptake from normal lungs diffusion limited.
- Diffusion limitation can also occur in interstitial lung disease if substantially thickened alveolar walls remain perfused.

Ans. D

171. R_{aw} is expressed as cmH20/L/s is increased in:

A. Emphysema
B. Asthma
C. Pulmonary fibrosis
D. Moderate obesity

Explanation:

- During an episode of acute asthma, luminal narrowing due to smooth muscle constriction as well as inflammation and thickening within the small- and medium-sized bronchi raise frictional resistance and reduce airflow.
- "Scooping" of flow-volume loop is caused by reduction of airflow, especially at lower lung volumes.
- Often, airflow obstruction can be reversed by inhalation of β2-adrenergic agonists acutely or by treatment with inhaled steroids chronically. TLC usually remains normal (although elevated TLC is sometimes seen in long-standing asthma), but FRC may be dynamically elevated.
- RV is often increased due to exaggerated airway closure at low lung volumes, and this elevation of RV reduces FVC.
- Because central airways are narrowed, Raw is usually elevated.
- Mild arterial hypoxemia is often present due to perfusion of relatively under ventilated alveoli distal to obstructed airways (and is responsive to oxygen supplementation), but DICO is normal or mildly elevated.

Ans. B

172. All are features of proliferative phase of ARDS except:

A. Recover rapidly
B. Organization of alveolar exudates
C. Type 1 pneumocytes proliferate along basement membrane
D. Synthesize new pulmonary surfactant

Explanation:

- **Proliferative** phase of ARDS usually lasts from day 7 to day 21.
- Most patients recover rapidly and are liberated from mechanical ventilation during this phase.
- Despite this improvement, many patients still experience dyspnea, tachypnea, and hypoxemia.
- Some patients develop progressive lung injury and early changes of pulmonary fibrosis during the proliferative phase.
- Histologically, the first signs of resolution are often evident in this phase, with the initiation of lung repair, the organization of alveolar exudates, and a shift from neutrophil- to lymphocyte-predominant pulmonary infiltrates.
- As part of the reparative process, type II pneumocytes proliferate along alveolar basement membranes.
- These specialized epithelial cells synthesize new pulmonary surfactant and differentiate into type I pneumocytes

Ans. C

173. Not true about Chrug strauss syndrome is:

A. Extravascular granuloma formation
B. Disease can occur at any age with possible exception of infants
C. Mononeuritis multiplex is most common manifestation
D. Increased level of fibrinogen or alpha2 globulins can be found in 81% of patients

Explanation:

- Patients with eosinophilic granulomatosis with polyangiitis (Churg-Strauss) often exhibit nonspecific manifestations such as fever, malaise, anorexia, and weight loss, which are characteristic of a multisystem disease.
- Pulmonary findings in eosinophilic granulomatosis with polyangiitis (Churg-Strauss) clearly dominate the clinical picture with severe asthmatic attacks and the presence of pulmonary infiltrates.
- Mononeuritis multiplex is the second most common manifestation and occurs in up to 72% of patients.
- Allergic rhinitis and sinusitis develop in up to 61% of patients and are often observed early in the course of disease.
- Clinically recognizable heart disease occurs in ~14% of patients and is an important cause of mortality.
- Skin lesions occur in ~51% of patients and include purpura in addition to cutaneous and subcutaneous nodules.
- Renal disease in eosinophilic granulomatosis with polyangiitis (Churg-Strauss) is less common and generally less severe than that of granulomatosis with polyangiitis and microscopic polyangiitis.

Ans. C

174. A 50 year old male who is known case of COPD developed right sided pneumothorax following rupture of an apical bulla. An ICD was inserted on the right 5th intercostal space in the mid-axillary line. Since he had persistent air leak for more than 1 week, he was advised to under go VATS. Which among the following statements regarding VATS (Video assisted thoracic surgery) is false?

A. It is used to diagnose pleural lesions and peripheral pulmonary infiltrates and nodules.
B. It requires single lung ventilation during the procedure
C. It has largely replaced open biopsy which requires a thoracotomy
D. None of the above

Explanation:

- VATS, also known as thoracoscopy, is widely used for the diagnosis of pleural lesions as well as pesripheral parenchymal infiltrates and nodules. VATS, which requires that the patient tolerate single-lung ventilation during the procedure, involves passing a rigid scope with a camera through a trocar and into the pleural space; instruments can be inserted and manipulated through separate intercostal incisions. VATS has largely replaced "open biopsy", which requires a thoracotomy.

Ans. D

175. A 15 year old female was brought to the ER with acute onset breathlessness and wheeze. The wheeze is predominantly expiratory in nature. Wheezing is seen in all these conditions except:

A. Congestive heart failure
B. Upper airway obstruction by tumor
C. Churg -Strauss syndrome
D. COPD

Explanation:

- Differential diagnosis of asthma includes other disorders that can cause wheezing and dyspnea. Upper airway obstruction by tumor or laryngeal edema can mimic asthma, but stridor in the large airways is typically noted on physical examination.

- Localized wheezing in the chest may indicate an endobronchial tumor or foreign body. Congestive heart failure can cause wheezing but is typically accompanied by bibasilar crackles.
- Eosinophilic pneumonias and Churg-Strauss syndrome (eosinophilic granulomatosis with polyangiitis) may present with wheezing.
- Vocal cord dysfunction can mimic severe asthma and may require direct laryngoscopy to assess.
- When asthma involves chronic airflow obstruction, distinguishing it from chronic obstructive pulmonary disease (COPD) can be very difficult, and some pts have both asthma and COPD (asthma-COPD overlap syndrome).

Ans. B

176. A 18 year old male was advised to undergo PFT to assess the degree of airway obstruction. PFT showed obstructive airway disease with bronchodilator reversibility. Which among the following statements regarding asthma is false?

A. Bronchodilator reversibility is demonstrated by an increase in FEV1 by ≥200 mL or ≥12% from baseline FEV1 15 min after a short-acting β agonist

B. Peak expiratory flow rate (PEFR) can be used by the pt to track asthma control objectively at home

C. Exhaled nitric oxide levels can provide an assessment of eosinophilic airway inflammation

D. Diffusing capacity for carbon monoxide is usually normal

Explanation:

- Spirometry often shows airflow obstruction, with a reduction in forced expiratory volume in 1 s (FEV1) and FEV1 /forced vital capacity (FVC) ratio.
- However, spirometry may be normal, especially if asthma symptoms are adequately treated.
- Bronchodilator reversibility is demonstrated by an increase in FEV1 by ≥200 mL and ≥12% from baseline FEV1 15 min after a short-acting β agonist (often albuterol metered-dose inhaler two puffs or 180 μg).
- Many but not all asthmatics will demonstrate significant bronchodilator reversibility; optimal pharmacologic treatment may reduce bronchodilator reversibility.
- Airway hyperresponsiveness is characteristic of asthma; it can be assessed by exposure to direct bronchoconstrictors such as methacholine or histamine.
- Greater airway responsiveness is associated with increased asthmatic symptoms.
- Peak expiratory flow rate (PEFR) can be used by the patient to track asthma control objectively at home.
- Measurement of lung volumes is not typically performed, but increases in total lung capacity and residual volume may be observed. The diffusing capacity for carbon monoxide is usually normal.

Ans. A

177. A 40 year old with frequent exacerbations of bronchial asthma was advised to take omalizumab injections every month. She had poor symptom control while on treatment with beta 2 agonist, steroids and anti histamines. Mechanism of action of Omalizumab is:

A. Anti IL 5

B. Beta 2 adrenergic agonists

C. Anti IgE

D. Anti IgM

Explanation:

- Omalizumab is a blocking antibody that neutralizes IgE; with SC injection every 2–4 weeks, it appears to reduce acute asthma exacerbation frequency in severe asthmatics. However, it is expensive and considered only for highly selected pts with elevated total serum IgE levels and refractory asthma symptoms despite maximal inhaled bronchodilator and ICS therapy. Antibodies that block IL-5 (mepolizumab, reslizumab) or its receptor (benralizumab) markedly reduce blood and tissue eosinophils and reduce exacerbations in pts who have persistently increased sputum eosinophils despite maximal ICS therapy.

- Most widely used class of bronchodilators is β2 -adrenergic agonists, which relax airway smooth muscle by activating β2 -adrenergic receptors. Two types of inhaled β2 agonists are widely used in asthma treatment: short-acting β2 agonists (SABAs) and long-acting β2 agonists (LABAs). SABAs, which include albuterol, have rapid onset of action and last for up to 6 h. SABAs are effective rescue medications, but excessive use indicates inadequate asthma control. SABAs can prevent exercise-induced asthma if administered before exercise. LABAs, which include salmeterol and formoterol, have a slower onset of action but last for >12 h. LABAs have replaced regularly scheduled use of SABAs, but they do not control airway inflammation and should not be used without inhaled corticosteroid (ICS) therapy.
- Combinations of LABAs with ICS reduce asthma exacerbations and provide an excellent long-term treatment option for asthma severity of moderate persistent degree or greater.
- No role of any Anti IgM therapy in asthma.

Ans. C

178. A 60 year old chronic smoker was diagnosed as COPD since on clinical examination he had a barrel shaped chest, pursed lip breathing and tripod sign was positive. What are the 2 diseases included in COPD?

A. Chronic bronchitis and Asthma
B. Chronic bronchitis and Bronchiolitis
C. Chronic bronchitis and Bronchiectasis
D. Chronic bronchitis and Emphysema

Explanation:

- Chronic obstructive pulmonary disease (COPD) is a syndrome characterized by chronic airflow obstruction. COPD includes emphysema (lung parenchymal destruction), chronic bronchitis (chronic cough and phlegm production), and small airway disease (fibrosis and destruction of small airways) in varying combinations in different pts.
- Presence of airflow obstruction is determined by a reduced ratio of the forced expiratory volume in 1 s (FEV1) to the forced vital capacity (FVC).

Ans. D

179. A 70 year old was brought to the ER with acute exacerbation of COPD. His Saturation was 90%, pulse rate was 120 bpm and blood pressure was 90/60 mmhg. Which among the following is not a sign in COPD?

A. Barrel shaped chest
B. Poor diaphragmatic excursion
C. Expiratory wheezing
D. Digital clubbing

Explanation:

- Physical examination may be normal until COPD is fairly advanced.
- As disease progresses, signs of hyperinflation may become more prominent, including barrel chest and poor diaphragmatic excursion.
- Expiratory wheezing may be observed, but it does not predict the severity of obstruction or response to therapy.
- Digital clubbing raises the possibility of lung cancer, since it is not a sign of COPD.
- During COPD exacerbations, signs of respiratory distress may be prominent, including tachycardia, tachypnea, use of accessory muscles of respiration, and cyanosis.

Ans. D

180. HRCT of a 40 year old male showed pan acinar emphysema. His PFT was suggestive of obstructive airway disease while his FeNO levels were normal. Which among the following statements regarding Alpha 1 antitrypsin deficiency is true?

A. Alpha 1 anti trypsin protects the lower airways from damage caused by proteolytic enzymes such as elastase

B. Characteristic radiographic pattern is pan acinar emphysema with bullous changes more prominent at the base of lung

C. Investigation of choice is by measuring the serum levels of Alpha 1 antitrypsin

D. All of the above

Explanation:

- α1 Antitrypsin (α1 AT) testing, typically by measurement of the protein level in the bloodstream, is recommended to exclude severe α1 AT deficiency.
- Augmentation therapy (a weekly IV infusion) is available for individuals with severe α1 AT deficiency (e.g., PI Z) who have developed airflow obstruction and/or emphysema.

Ans. D

181. A 50 year old chronic smoker with 20 pack years, presents to the ER with signs of respiratory distress including tachycardia, tachypnoea and cyanosis. The FEV1/FEC ratio is reduced to <0.7. There is an increase in total lung capacity and reduction in DLCO. What is your diagnosis?

A. Bronchial asthma

B. Lung cancer

C. Pneumothorax

D. Emphysema

Explanation:

- During COPD exacerbations, signs of respiratory distress may be prominent, including tachycardia, tachypnea, use of accessory muscles of respiration, and cyanosis.
- Objective documentation of airflow obstruction is essential for diagnosing COPD. Standardized staging of COPD is based on post-bronchodilator spirometry. In COPD, the FEV1 /FVC ratio is reduced to <0.7.Increase in total lung capacity and residual volume, as well as reduced diffusion capacity for carbon monoxide (DLCO) are typically seen in emphysema.

Ans. D

182. An obstructive sleep apnea patient was advised auto CPAP since his AHI (Apnea Hypopnea Index) was 30. Contraindications for NIV(non-invasive ventilation) include all except:

A. PaCO2 >45mmHg

B. Cardiovascular instability

C. Unconscious patient

D. Craniofacial abnormalities or facial trauma

Explanation:

- NIV (non-invasive ventilation) includes methods such as CPAP and BPAP. It is a form of positive pressure ventilation delivered through a non-invasive interface (e.g. Nasal mask, face mask, nasal plug). The main indications include:
  1. Acute exacerbation of COPD
  2. Acute cardiogenic pulmonary edema
  3. Pneumocystis pneumonia
  4. Viral pneumonitis (MERS, COVID 19)
  5. Obstructive sleep apnea
- Numerous studies suggest that noninvasive mask ventilation (noninvasive ventilation [NIV]) can improve outcomes in acute COPD exacerbations with respiratory failure (PaCO2 >45 mmHg). Contraindications to NIV include cardiovascular instability, impaired mental status, inability to cooperate, copious secretions, craniofacial abnormalities or facial trauma, extreme obesity, or significant burns. Progressive hypercarbia, refractory hypoxemia, or alterations in mental status that compromise ability to comply with NIV therapy, hemodynamic instability, and respiratory arrest may necessitate endotracheal intubation for mechanical ventilation.

Ans. A

183. A 60 yr old man presents to the OPD with history of insidious onset of breathlessness which is aggravated on exertion. Chest radiograph shows bilateral lung parenchymal fibrosis and holly leaf sign. Patient has an occupational history of working in mining industry for the past 30 years. What is your diagnosis?

A. Silicosis
B. Asbestosis
C. Byssinosis
D. Berylliosis

Explanation:

- Asbestosis specifically refers to the pneumoconiosis caused by inhalation of asbestos fibres.
- Disease is characterised by slowly progressive, diffuse pulmonary fibrosis.
- Exposure to asbestos occurs during the mining and milling of fibres, in industrial applications of asbestos (EG. Ship building, work with cement). And in non occupational settings with airborne asbestos (e.g. demolition of asbestos containing buildings).
- Holly leaf sign refers to the typical chest radiograph appearance of calcified pleural plaque.

Ans. B

184. A 50 year old male with history of working in a stone quarry, presents to the OPD with history of chronic cough and breathlessness. Which of the following statements regarding this disease is false?

A. Melanoptysis is present
B. Egg shell calcification is seen in chest radiograph
C. Progressive massive fibrosis is seen in CT chest
D. These patients are at increased risk of tuberculosis, atypical mycobacterial infection and fungal infection

Explanation:

- Longer-term exposure to free silica can result in simple silicosis, with small rounded opacities in the upper lobes of the lungs.
- Calcification of hilar lymph nodes can give a characteristic "eggshell" appearance on radiographic studies.
- Progressive nodular fibrosis can result in masses >1 cm in diameter in complicated silicosis. When such masses become very large, the term progressive massive fibrosis is used to describe the condition.
- Due to impaired cell-mediated immunity, silicosis pts are at increased risk of tuberculosis, atypical mycobacterial infections, and fungal infections. Silica may also be a lung carcinogen.
- Melanoptysis is classically seen in coal workers pneumoconiosis.

Ans. A

185. A 55-year-old male with 30 pack years of smoking presents to the OPD with complaints of cough and breathlessness for more than three months. Chest radiograph shows bilateral hyper inflation and PFT shows obstructive airway disease. Which among the following statements is false?

A. Smoking cessation does not improve survival.
B. Intervention should include psycho social support and pharmacological treatment
C. Nicotine replacement therapy may increase the success rate
D. Varenicline is superior to psycho social support alone

Explanation:

- Diagnosis is COPD. Elimination of tobacco smoking has been convincingly shown to reduce decline in pulmonary function and to prolong survival in pts with COPD; complete smoking cessation is essential for all COPD pts. Although lung function does not typically improve substantially after smoking cessation, the rate of decline in FEV1 often reverts to that of non-smokers. Pharmacologic treatment to assist with smoking cessation is often beneficial. Use of nicotine replacement therapy (available as a transdermal patch, gum, lozenge, nasal spray, and oral inhaler) can increase rates of smoking cessation; oral bupropion also produces significant benefit and can be combined successfully with nicotine replacement. Varenicline, a partial agonist for nicotinic acetylcholine receptors, also can promote smoking cessation. All adult, non-pregnant smokers without specific contraindications should be offered pharmacologic treatment to assist with smoking cessation.

Ans. A

186. Caplan syndrome is associated with:

A. Seropositive rheumatoid arthritis
B. Seronegative rheumatoid arthritis
C. Seropositve SLE
D. Seronegative SLE

Explanation:

- Caplan syndrome first described in coal miners but subsequently in patients with silicosis, is the combination of pneumoconiotic nodules and seropositive rheumatoid arthritis.
- Silica is often present in anthracitic coal dust and its presence may contribute to risk of PMF.

Ans. A

187. All are true about COPD and α1AT except:

A. S allele, associated with slightly reduced α1AT levels
B. Z allele, associated with markedly reduced α1AT levels
C. Individuals with two Z alleles or one Z and one null allele are referred to as PiZ, which is the most common form of severe α1AT deficiency
D. Alpha-1 antitrypsin augmentation therapy is recommended for use in PiMZ subjects

Explanation:

- Risk of lung disease in heterozygous PiMZ individuals, who have intermediate serum levels of α1AT (~60% of PiMM levels), has been controversial.
- Several recent large studies have demonstrated that PiMZ subjects who smoke are likely at increased risk for the development of COPD.
- However, alpha-1 antitrypsin augmentation therapy is not recommended for use in PiMZ subjects.

Ans. D

188. All can be used in acute severe asthma except:

A. Slow infusion of aminophylline
B. IV magnesium sulphate
C. IV ceftrioxone
D. Halothane

Explanation:

- A high concentration of oxygen should be given by facemask to achieve oxygen saturation of >90%.
- Mainstay of treatment are high doses of SABA given either by nebulizer or via a MDI with a spacer.
- In severely ill patients with impending respiratory failure, IV β2-agonists may be given. A nebulized anticholinergic may be added if there is not a satisfactory response to β2-agonists alone, as there are additive effects.
- In patients who are refractory to inhaled therapies, a slow infusion of aminophylline may be effective, but it is important to monitor blood levels, especially if patients have already been treated with oral theophylline.
- Magnesium sulfate given intravenously or by nebulizer is effective when added to inhaled β2-agonists, and is relatively well tolerated but is not routinely recommended.
- Prophylactic intubation may be indicated for impending respiratory failure, when the PCO2 is normal or rises.
- For patients with respiratory failure, it is necessary to intubate and institute ventilation.
- These patients may benefit from a general anesthetic, such as halothane, if they have not responded to conventional bronchodilators.
- Sedatives should never be given as they may depress ventilation. Antibiotics should not be used routinely unless there are signs of pneumonia.

Ans. C

189. All are true about other organ involvement in cystic fibrosis except:

A. Multilobular cirrhosis in 4–15% of patients with CF is seen
B. Meconium ileus, presentation in 10–20% of new-borns with CF
C. Upto 58 % of males with CF are infertile
D. Radiographic evidence of sinusitis occurs in most CF patients

Explanation:

- As in CF lung and pancreas, thick and tenacious secretions compromise numerous other exocrine tissues.
- Obstruction of intrahepatic bile ducts and parenchymal fibrosis are commonly observed in pathologic specimens, with multilobular cirrhosis in 4–15% of patients with CF and significant hepatic insufficiency as a resulting manifestation among adults.
- Contents of the intestinal lumen are often difficult to excrete, leading to meconium ileus (a presentation in 10–20% of newborns with CF) or distal intestinal obstructive syndrome in older individuals.
- Men typically exhibit complete involution of the vas deferens and infertility (despite functioning spermatogenesis), and ~99% of males with CF are infertile.

Ans. C

190. Increased mortality prediction in ARDS is done by:

A. Severity as by Berlin definition
B. PEEP
C. Respiratory system compliance
D. Extent of alveolar infiltrates on chest radiography

Explanation:

- Increasing severity of ARDS, as defined by the consensus Berlin definition, predicts increased mortality.
- Surprisingly, there is little additional value in predicting ARDS mortality from other parameters of lung injury, including the level of PEEP (≥10 cm H2O), respiratory system compliance (≤40 mL/cm H2O), the extent of alveolar infiltrates on chest radiography, and the corrected expired volume per minute (≥10 L/min) (as a surrogate measure of dead space).

Ans. A

191. Round pneumonia is seen with:

A. Pneumococcal pneumonia in children
B. Pneumococcal pneumonia in adults
C. Staphylococcal pneumonia
D. Coxiella pneumonia

Explanation:

- In children, "round pneumonia", a distinctly spherical consolidation on chest radiography, is associated with a pneumococcal etiology.
- Round pneumonia is uncommon in adults.
- S. pneumoniae is not the only cause of such lesions; other causes, especially cancer, should be considered.

Ans. A

192. Silicosis increases the risk of all except:

A. TB
B. RA
C. Scleroderma
D. Sarcoidosis

Explanation:

- Because silica causes alveolar macrophage dysfunction, patients with silicosis are at greater risk of acquiring lung infections that involve these cells as a primary defense (*Mycobacterium tuberculosis*, atypical mycobacteria and fungi).
- Because of the increased risk of active tuberculosis, the recommended treatment of latent tuberculosis in these patients is longer.
- Silica has immunoadjuvant properties and another potential clinical complication of silicosis is autoimmune connective tissue disorders such as rheumatoid arthritis and scleroderma.
- In addition, there are sufficient epidemiologic data that the International Agency for Research on Cancer lists silica as a probable lung carcinogen.

Ans. D

193. Most common clinical presentation of bronchiectasis is:

A. Persistent productive cough with ongoing production of thick, tenacious sputum

B. Recurrent episodes of fever with productive sputum

C. Long standing exertion breathlessness and non productive cough

D. Frequent episodes of hemoptysis and breathlessness lasting for 2 to 3 weeks during each episode

Explanation:

- Most common clinical presentation is a persistent productive cough with ongoing production of thick, tenacious sputum.
- Physical findings often include crackles and wheezing on lung auscultation, and some patients with bronchiectasis exhibit clubbing of the digits. Mild to moderate airflow obstruction is often detected on pulmonary function tests, overlapping with that seen at presentation with other conditions, such as chronic obstructive pulmonary disease (copd).
- Acute exacerbations of bronchiectasis are usually characterized by changes in nature of sputum production, with increased volume and purulence.
- However, typical signs and symptoms of lung infection, such as fever and new infiltrates, may not be present.

Ans. A

194. Differential diagnosis for nodular infiltrates in chest in immunocompromised patients include all except:

A. Aspergillus

B. Nocardia

C. Radiation pneumonitis

D. Recurrent tumor

Explanation:

Table: Differential diagnosis of chest infiltrates in immunocompromised patients

Infiltrate	Cause of Pneumonia	
	Infectious	**Noninfectious**
Localized	Bacteria (including *Legionella,* mycobacteria)	Local hemorrhage or embolism, tumor
Nodular	Fungi (e.g., *Aspergillus or Mucor*), *Nocardia*	Recurrent tumor
Diffuse	Viruses (especially cytomegalovirus), *Chlamydia, Pneumocystis, Toxoplasma gondii,* mycobacteria	Congestive heart failure, radiation pneumonitis, drug-induced lung injury, lymphangitic spread of cancer

Ans. C

195. Scooping of flow volume loop is caused by:

A. Emphysema
B. Acute asthma
C. Myasthenia gravis
D. Pulmonary fibrosis

Explanation:

- During an episode of acute asthma, luminal narrowing due to smooth muscle constriction as well as inflammation and thickening within the small- and medium-sized bronchi raise frictional resistance and reduce airflow.
- "Scooping" of the flow-volume loop is caused by reduction of airflow, especially at lower lung volumes.
- Often, airflow obstruction can be reversed by inhalation of β2-adrenergic agonists acutely or by treatment with inhaled steroids chronically.
- TLC usually remains normal (although elevated TLC is sometimes seen in long-standing asthma), but FRC may be dynamically elevated.
- RV is often increased due to exaggerated airway closure at low lung volumes, and this elevation of RV reduces FVC.
- Because central airways are narrowed, Raw is usually elevated.
- Mild arterial hypoxemia is often present due to perfusion of relatively underventilated alveoli distal to obstructed airways (and is responsive to oxygen supplementation), but DlCO is normal or mildly elevated

Ans. B

196. Which of the following is not a goal for initial management of ARDS?

A. Tidal volume </=6ml/kg PBW
B. Plateau pressure </=30 cm H20
C. RR</=35bpm
D. FiO2 >/=0.6

Explanation:

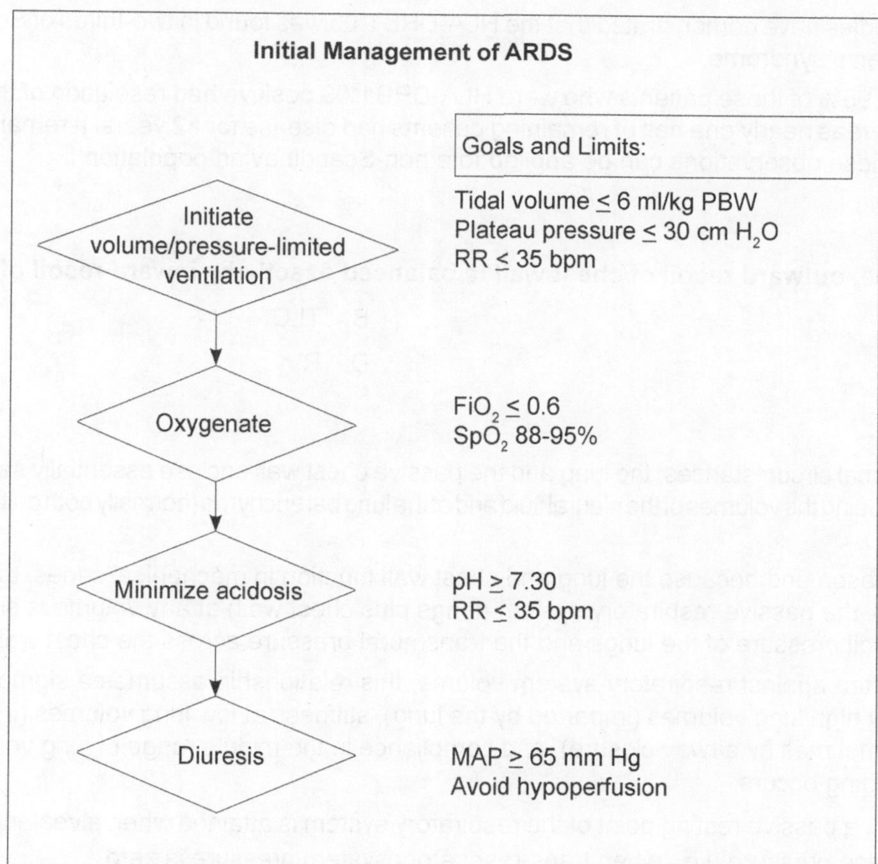

Ans. D

197. In which type pulmonary edema diuretic contraindicated?

A. High pressure pulmonary edema

B. Low pressure pulmonary edema

C. Re expansion pulmonary edema

D. High altitude pulmonary edema

Explanation:

- Re-expansion pulmonary edema can develop after removal of long-standing pleural space air or fluid.
- These patients may develop hypotension or oliguria with pulmonary edema resulting from rapid fluid shifts into the lung.
- Diuretics and preload reduction are contraindicated, and intravascular volume repletion often is needed while supporting oxygenation and gas exchange.

Ans. C

198. Not true regarding Löfgren's syndrome is:

A. Erythema nodosum & hilar adenopathy on chest X-ray

B. Associated with bad prognosis

C. HLA DRB1*01 was found in two thirds

D. More common in Scandinavian patients

Explanation:

- One form of the disease, *Löfgren's syndrome*, consists of erythema nodosum and hilar adenopathy on chest roentgenogram.
- In some cases, periarticular arthritis may be identified without erythema nodosum. Löfgren's syndrome is associated with a good prognosis, with >90% of patients experiencing disease resolution within 2 years.
- Recent studies have demonstrated that the HLA-DRB1*03 was found in two-thirds of Scandinavian patients with Löfgren's syndrome.
- More than 95% of those patients who were HLA-DRB1*03 positive had resolution of their disease within 2 years, whereas nearly one half of remaining patients had disease for >2 years. It remains to be determined whether these observations can be applied to a non-Scandinavian population.

Ans. B

199. At this volume, outward recoil of chest wall is balanced exactly by inward recoil of lung:

A. FRC

B. TLC

C. VC

D. RV

Explanation:

- Under normal circumstances, the lung and the passive chest wall enclose essentially same volume, the only difference being the volumes of the pleural fluid and of the lung parenchyma (normally both quite small in the absence of disease).
- For this reason and because the lung and chest wall function in mechanical series, the pressure required to displace the passive respiratory system (lungs plus chest wall) at any volume is simply the sum of the elastic recoil pressure of the lungs and the transmural pressure across the chest wall.
- When plotted against respiratory system volume, this relationship assumes a sigmoid shape, exhibiting stiffness at high lung volumes (imparted by the lung), stiffness at low lung volumes (imparted by the chest wall or sometimes by airway closure), and compliance in the middle range of lung volumes where normal tidal breathing occurs.
- In addition, a passive resting point of the respiratory system is attained when alveolar gas pressure equals body surface pressure (i.e., when trans-respiratory system pressure is zero).

- At this volume (called the *functional residual capacity* [FRC]), the outward recoil of the chest wall is balanced exactly by the inward recoil of the lung.
- As these recoils are transmitted through the pleural fluid, the lung is pulled both outward and inward simultaneously at FRC, and thus its pressure falls below atmospheric pressure (typically, −5 cmH2O).

Ans. A

200. Excursion between full and minimal lung inflation is called as:

A. VC
B. FRC
C. TLC
D. All of the above

Explanation:

- Excursion between full and minimal lung inflation is called *vital capacity* (VC; =and is readily seen to be the difference between volumes at two unrelated stiffness extremes—one determined by the lung (TLC) and the other by the chest wall or airways (RV). Thus, although VC is easy to measure (see below), it provides little information about the intrinsic properties of the respiratory system. As will become clear, it is much more useful for the clinician to consider TLC and RV individually.

Ans. A

201. Alveolar hypoventilation is indicated when pCO2 Exceeds ____mm Hg.

A. 30
B. 40
C. 50
D. 60

- If the Paco2 falls much below 40 mmHg, alveolar hyperventilation is present; if the Paco2 exceeds 40 mmHg, alveolar hypoventilation is present. Ventilatory failure is characterized by extreme alveolar hypoventilation.

Ans. B

202. Not true about topical pulmonary eosinophilia is:

A. Pronounced blood eosinophilia (>3000 eosinophils/μL)
B. PFT Suggestive of obstructive pattern in most of the cases
C. Total serum IgE levels (4-40 KIU/ml)
D. Antifilarial antibody levels are markedly elevated

Explanation:

- Main features include a history of residence in filaria-endemic regions, paroxysmal cough and wheezing (usually nocturnal and probably related to the nocturnal periodicity of microfilariae), weight loss, low-grade fever, lymphadenopathy, and pronounced blood eosinophilia (>3000 eosinophils/μL).
- Chest X-rays or CT scans may be normal, but generally show increased bronchovascular markings. Diffuse miliary lesions or mottled opacities may be present in the middle and lower lung fields.
- Tests of pulmonary function show restrictive abnormalities in most cases and obstructive defects in half. Characteristically, total serum IgE levels (4–40 KIU/mL) and antifilarial antibody levels are markedly elevated

Ans. B

203. A 70 year old patient with Pancoast tumor involving his upper lobe of lung invading brachial plexus is least likely to present with which of the following symptoms?

A. Sensory loss over medial forearm and hand
B. Weakness of intrinsic muscles of hand
C. Ipsilateral horners
D. Weakness of shoulder

Explanation:

- Pancoast tumor of the upper lobe of the lung may invade or compress the lower trunk
- Pancoast tumors typically present as an insidious onset of pain in the upper arm, sensory disturbance in the medial aspect of the forearm and hand, and weakness and atrophy of the intrinsic hand muscles along with an ipsilateral Horner's syndrome.
- Shoulder weakness occurs due to upper plexus involvement

Ans. D

204. Respiratory quotient for typical American diet is:

A. 0.65
B. 0.75
C. 0.85
D. 1

Explanation:

- As a consequence of oxygen uptake of alveolar gas into capillary blood, alveolar oxygen tension falls below that of inspired gas.
- Rate of oxygen uptake (determined by the body's metabolic oxygen consumption) is related to the average rate of metabolic CO2 production, and their ratio—the "respiratory quotient" (R = V.CO2/ V.O2)—depends largely on the fuel being metabolized.
- For a typical American diet, R is usually around 0.85.

Ans. C

205. A 60-year-old man undergoes pulmonary function testing as part of a routine health screening test. He had no pulmonary complaints. He is a non-smoker and had a prior history of working in ship building industry. His pulmonary function test results are as follows:

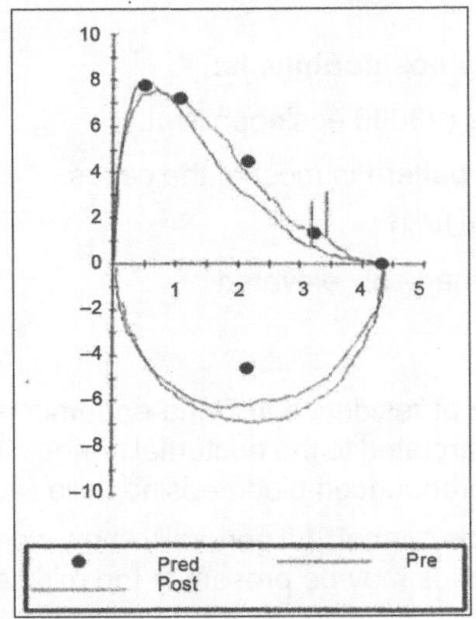

	Pre bronchodilator			Post bronchodilator
Test	Actual	Predicted	Predicted %	
FVC (L)	4.39	4.32	102%	-1
FEV1 (L)	3.20	3.37	95%	7
FEV1/FVC (%)	73	78		8

His spirometry graph. What's the interpretation?

A. Restrictive lung disease
B. Obstructive lung disease
C. Normal spirometry
D. Inadequate effort

Explanation:

- This case demonstrates an example of normal pulmonary function tests.
- FVC and the FEV1 are 102% and 95% of predicted, respectively, values well above the lower limit of normal. Based on this normal spirometry pattern, you would conclude that there is no evidence of air-flow obstruction.

Ans. C

206. A 75-year-old man presents with progressive dyspnea on exertion over the past one year. He reports a dry cough but no wheezes, sputum production, fevers or hemoptysis. He is a non-smoker and worked as a lawyer until retiring 3 years ago. His pulmonary function testing is as follows:

	Pre-Bronchodilator (BD)		
Test	**Actual**	**Predicted**	**% Predicted**
FVC (L)	1.57	4.46	35
FEV_1 (L)	1.28	3.39	38
FEV_1/FVC (%)	82	76	
FRC	1.73	3.80	45
RV (L)	1.12	2.59	43
TLC (L)	2.70	6.45	42
RV/TLC (%)	41	42	
DLCO corr	5.06	31.64	16

His flow-volume loop is as follows:

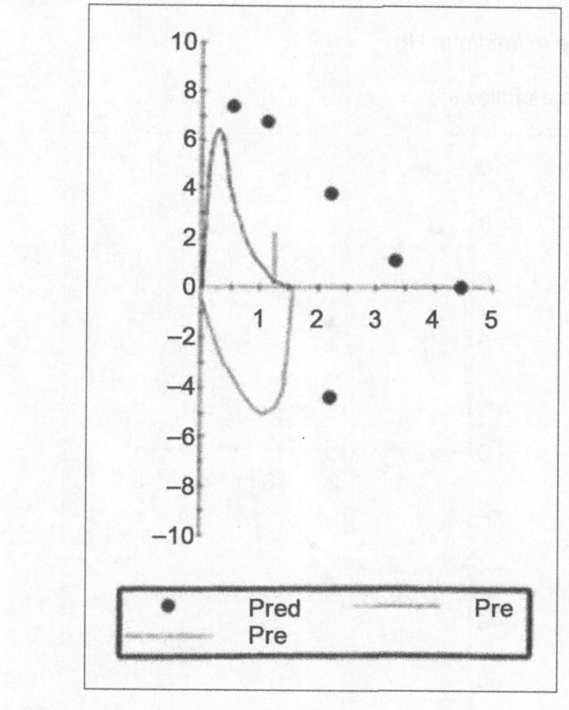

What's the diagnosis?

A. Restrictive lung disease

B. Obstructive lung disease

C. Normal spirometry

D. Inadequate effort

Explanation:

- This patient has a reduced FEV1 and FVC with a preserved FEV1/FVC ratio. The total lung capacity is reduced and the patient, therefore, has a restrictive defect.
- Flow-volume loop also has the characteristic appearance of a restrictive process – tall, narrow and a short expiratory phase.
- Based on the fact that his TLC is below 50% predicted, this would be classified as a "severe" restrictive defect. His DLCO is also markedly reduced indicating he has a reduced alveolar- capillary interface for gas exchange and suggesting that the cause of his restrictive process lies within the lung parenchyma.

Ans. A

207. A 64-year-old man presents to his primary care provider with complaints of increasing dyspnea on exertion. He has a 40 pack-year history of smoking and is retired following a career as a building contractor. His pulmonary function testing is as follows:

	Pre-Bronchodilator (BD)			Post-BD	
Test	**Actual**	**Predicted**	**% Predicted**	**Actual**	**% Change**
FVC (L)	1.89	4.58	41	3.69	96
FEV_1 (L)	0.89	3.60	25	1.89	112
FEV_1/FVC (%)	47	79			
RV (L)	5.72	2.31	248		
TLC (L)	7.51	6.41	117		
RV/TLC (%)	76	37			
DLCO corr	20.73	33.43	62		

The units for DLCO are ml/min/mm Hg

His flow volume loop is as follows:

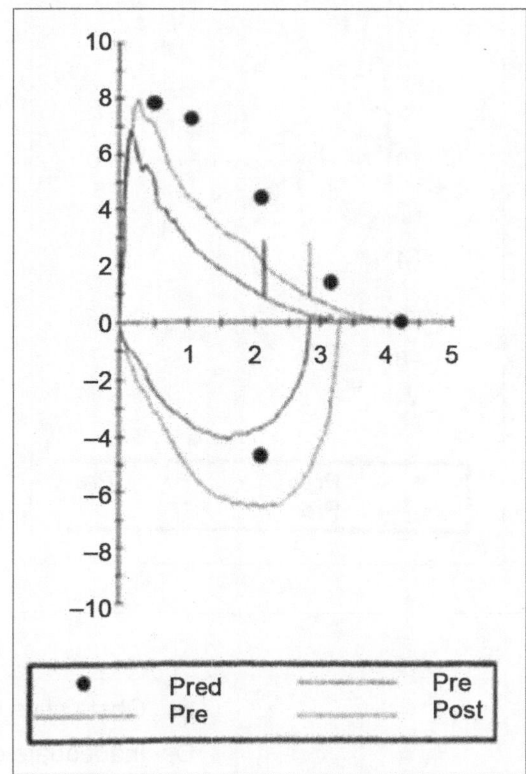

What is the interpretation?

A. Restrictive lung disease
B. Obstructive lung disease
C. Pulmonary embolism
D. All of the above

Explanation:

- This patient has markedly abnormal spirometry.
- FVC is only 41% predicted while the FEV1 is only 25% predicted, well below the lower limit of normal of 80% predicted. In addition, the FEV1/FVC ratio is markedly reduced.
- Combination of the low FEV1, FVC and reduced FEV1/FVC ratio is consistent with a diagnosis of airflow obstruction.
- With an FEV1 of 25% predicted, this would be classified as "severe" airflow obstruction.

Ans. B

208. A 25-year-old man presents to his physician with complaints of dyspnea and wheezing. He is a non-smoker. Two years ago, he was in a major motor vehicle accident and was hospitalized for 3 months. He had a tracheostomy placed because he remained on the ventilator for a total of 7 weeks. His tracheostomy was removed 2 months after his discharge from the hospital. His pulmonary tests are as follows:

	Pre-Bronchodilator (BD)		
Test	Actual	Predicted	% Predicted
FVC (L)	4.73	4.35	109
FEV_1 (L)	2.56	3.69	69
FEV_1/FVC (%)	54	85	

His flow volume loops is as follows:

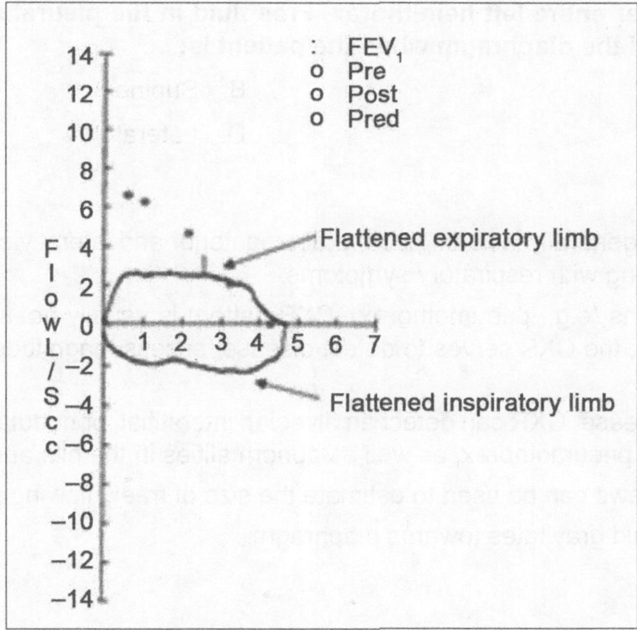

Interpretation this situation?

A. Fixed airway obstruction
B. Tracheal stenosis
C. Both A & B
D. Restrictive lung disease

Explanation:

- Noteworthy feature of his flow volume loop is that there is flattening of both the inspiratory and expiratory limbs.
- This pattern is seen in patients who have a fixed upper airway obstruction.
- In a patient with a prior history of tracheostomy, you would be very suspicious that this patient has developed tracheal stenosis, a known long-term complication of tracheostomy tubes.

Ans. C

209. Mr. Panda is 67-year-old male who was originally seen by the pulmonologist after a chest X-ray revealed a right upper-lobe lung mass. On further examination neck swelling noted in the morning, hoarseness of voice during the past week, purplish discoloration across his chest, thick vessels under his tongue, increased dyspnea on exertion. physical findings are as follows: blood pressure 124/64, respirations 20, pulse 72 regular, temperature 97.8°; diffuse edema in the neck; dilated, engorged blood vessels on the chest and under the tongue; and edema in the left arm and hand. What is the most probable clinical diagnosis?

A. Cervical adenopathy
B. Superior vena cava obstruction
C. Horner syndrome
D. Chylothorax

Explanation:

- Superior vena cava syndrome consists of various symptoms due to compression of the SVC.
- Early signs and symptoms include cough, dyspnea, hoarseness, chest pain, jugular vein distention, and edema of the hands, face, and/or neck.
- Because SVCS is a life-threatening emergency, early diagnosis and appropriate intervention are imperative.

Ans. B

210. A 25 year old male, with complaints of dull aching chest pain on left. On examination there is stony dull on percussion over entire left hemithorax. Free fluid in the pleural cavity is affected by gravity. Fluid gravitates toward the diaphragm when the patient is:

A. Erect
B. Supine
C. Right oblique
D. Lateral

Explanation:

- Chest X-ray (CXR), generally including both posteroanterior and lateral views, is often the first diagnostic study in pts presenting with respiratory symptoms.
- With some exceptions (e.g., pneumothorax), CXR pattern is usually not sufficiently specific to establish a diagnosis; instead, the CXR serves to detect disease, assess magnitude, and guide further diagnostic investigation.
- With diffuse lung disease, CXR can detect an alveolar, interstitial, or nodular pattern. CXR can also detect pleural effusion and pneumothorax, as well as abnormalities in the hila and mediastinum.
- Lateral decubitus views can be used to estimate the size of freely flowing pleural effusions.
- Erect chest X-ray fluid gravitates towards diaphragm.

Ans. A

211. A 40 year old female with complaints of productive cough, dyspnoea and fever for 1 week. Her X-ray picture is of right middle lobe consolidation. In this, major fissure forms the ____right middle lobe boundary.

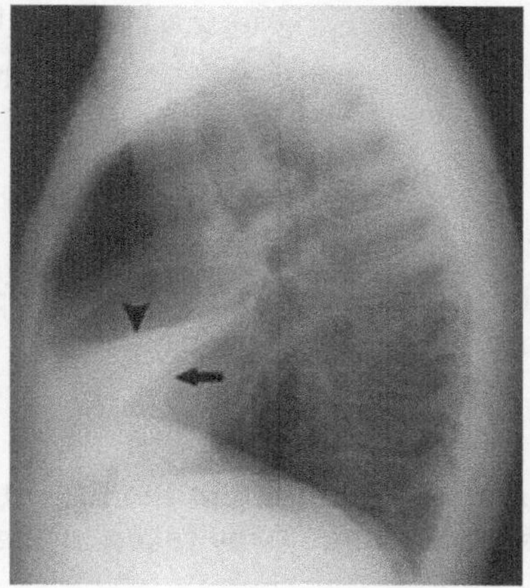

A. Superior
B. Posterior
C. Anterior
D. Inferior

Explanation:

- Superior margin of the right middle lobe is the minor fissure (arrowhead) and the posterior margin is the major fissure (arrow).

Ans. B

212. A 40 year old male presented to the OPD with complaints of chronic cough and breathlessness. Patient was advised to take chest X-ray for recurrent night time cough. Identify the structure on X-ray shown below.

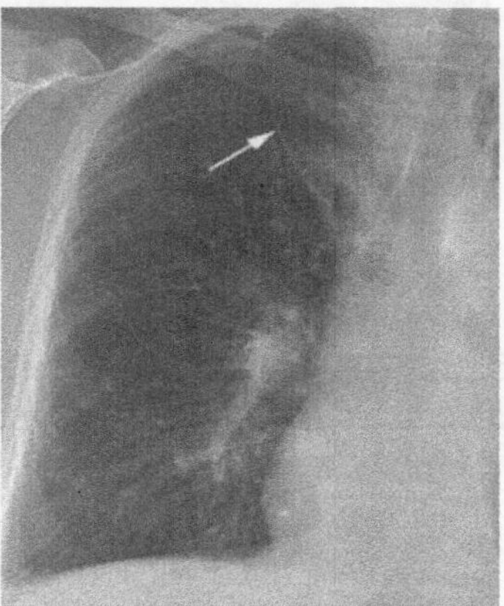

A. Visceral pleura
B. Parietal pleura
C. Azygos fissure
D. Minor fissure

Explanation:

- There are three accessory fissures seen occasionally in normal individuals. The azygos fissure is formed by an anomalous development of the azygos vein. The vein "migrates through" the medial right upper lobe, dragging visceral and parietal pleura with it. The azygos lobe is separated from the rest of the upper lobe by the azygos fissure.

Ans. C

213. A 40 year old male presented to the OPD with complaints of purulent cough for 2 weeks duration. Chest radiograph showed air bronchogram sign. Visualization of air in the intrapulmonary bronchi on a chest roentgenogram is called the air bronchogram sign. Presence of an air bronchogram indicates:

A. Normal lung
B. Interstitial thickening
C. Emphysema
D. Alveolar consolidation

Explanation:

- **Air bronchogram** refers to the phenomenon of **air**-filled bronchi (dark) being made visible by the opacification of surrounding alveoli (grey/white).
- It is almost always caused by a pathologic airspace/alveolar process, in which something other than **air** fills the alveoli. Its commonly seen in alveolar consolidation.

Ans. D

214. A 60 year old male, chronic smoker, admitted in the ER with complaints of shortness of breath. This is his third admission in this year. Chest X-ray taken at the time of admission is shown. What is the probable diagnosis?

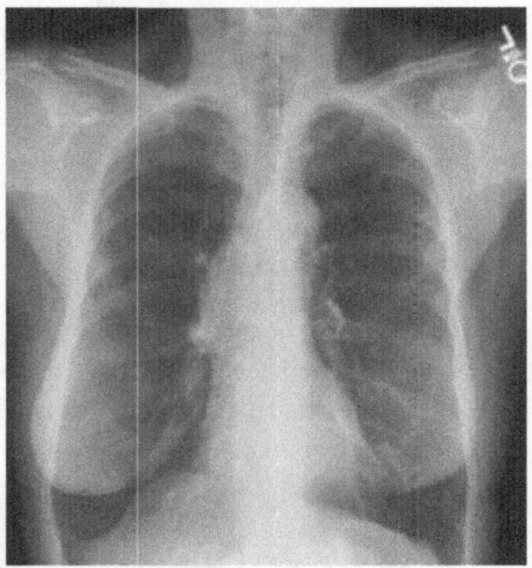

A. Pneumothorax
B. Pleural effusion
C. Emphysema
D. Idiopathic pulmonary fibrosis

Explanation:

- Classic radiographic appearance of hyperinflation is manifested by increased radiolucency of the lungs; low, flat diaphragms; exaggerated verticality of the heart; increased AP diameter of the chest; and widening of the retrosternal lucent space in emphysema.

Ans. C

215. A 60-year-male with viral pneumonia, has rapidly deteriorating symptoms. He was advised mechanical ventilation. What is the ventilator strategy followed in case of ARDS to prevent trauma to the lungs?

A. High PEEP
B. High tidal volume
C. Low tidal volume
D. Low PEEP

Explanation:

- Strategy of using VTs that avoid volutrauma is commonly referred to as low tidal volume ventilation (LTVV) or lung protective ventilation (LPV). in mechanical ventilation should be kept within a safe range to prevent volutrauma or VILI. The recommended size of VT is 6 ml/kg of IBW (not actual body weight). IBW is determined by knowing a patient's gender, weight, and height, and tables with formulas for calculating IBW are readily available.

Ans. C

216. A 70-year-old woman who has been sent from a nursing home with confusion and shortness of breath. Her history is notable for end-stage renal disease caused by hypertension and a recent stroke, which has resulted in left-sided hemiplegia. The emergency physician ordered a chest X-ray examination, which revealed a right lower lobe infiltrate and a right pleural effusion. On physical examination, the patient is somnolent. Her vital signs are temperature, 35° C; blood pressure, 85/50 mm Hg; and heart rate, 130 beats/min. What's the probable diagnosis?

A. Community acquired pneumonia
B. Health care associated pneumonia
C. Pulmonary thromboembolism
D. COPD

Explanation:

- Community-acquired pneumonia is defined as pneumonia that is acquired outside the hospital.
- Most commonly identified pathogens are Streptococcus pneumoniae, Haemophilus influenzae, atypical bacteria (i.e., Chlamydia pneumoniae, Mycoplasma pneumoniae, Legionella species) and viruses.
- Symptoms and signs are fever, cough, sputum production, pleuritic chest pain, dyspnea, tachypnea, and tachycardia.
- Diagnosis is based on clinical presentation and chest X-ray.
- Treatment is with empirically chosen antibiotics.
- Prognosis is excellent for relatively young or healthy patients, but many pneumonias, especially when caused by S. pneumoniae, Legionella, Staphylococcus aureus, or influenza virus, are serious or even fatal in older, sicker patients.

Ans. A

217. A 70 year old male chronic smoker with 100 pack years has come complaints of progressive breathlessness for 6 months. Which of the following is tobacco related lung disease?

A. Pulmonary Lanhergancell histiocytosis
B. RB ILD
C. DIP
D. All the above

Explanation:

- Although the association is rarer than with obstructive lung disease, first-hand tobacco smoke inhalation can lead to three types of ILD in susceptible individuals: RB-ILD, DIP, and PLCH.
- In RB-ILD, macro- phages accumulate in the respiratory bronchioles leading to bronchiolar remodeling and fibrosis of adjacent alveoli.
- In DIP, the increased macro- phages fill the alveoli, manifesting as restrictive impairment on pulmonary function testing and diffuse ground-glass attenuation on high-resolution CT imaging.

Ans. D

218. A 50 year old male gives history of working in mining and automobile industry for 15 years each. Which of the following occupational lung disease is more prone for developing tuberculosis?

A. Coal workers pneumoconiosis
B. Asbestosis
C. Silicosis
D. Farmers lung

Explanation:

- Important to recognize the association of silicosis with lung cancer and active tuberculosis.
- At increased risk for lung cancer, and the risk is increased when combined with exposure to tobacco smoke, diesel exhaust, or radon gas.
- Patients with silicosis develop active tuberculosis 2 to 30 times more frequently than co-workers without silicosis.

- This association is especially important in societies with a high incidence of human immunodeficiency virus infection, which markedly increases the risk for silicosis-associated active tuberculosis.

Ans. C

219. A 50 year old undergone diagnostic thoracentesis for right moderate effusion. The protein value of the pleural fluid is 2.0 g/dl. The following are the causes of transudative effusion except:

A. Congestive heart failure
B. Nephrotic syndrome
C. Malignancy
D. Cirrhosis

Explanation:

- Malignant disease is the most common cause of large unilateral pleural effusions among persons older than 60 years. Common cancers that form malignant pleural effusions include lung cancer and breast cancer, although any cancer can metastasize to the pleural surface. The effusions usually are lymphocyte predominant; malignant cells are found during cytologic examination of the pleural fluid.
- Some malignant pleural effusions, such as those from lymphoma, respond to therapy for the malignant disease.
- However, most patients with symptomatic malignant pleural effusions need primary therapy with pleurodesis.
- Pleurodesis occurs when the visceral and parietal pleural membranes are fused by talc, other chemicals, or surgery to obliterate the pleural space.

Ans. C

220. A 68-year-old man presents to the clinic with the concern of developing lung cancer in the future. He currently smokes one pack of cigarettes per day and has smoked for 45 years. He does not cough or feel shortness of breath. He has a history of high blood pressure and high cholesterol. He is otherwise in his regular state of health. Should this man have lung cancer screening? If yes, what is the screening?

A. No screening needed
B. Self assessment is enough
C. Low dose CT chest
D. Six minute walk test

Explanation:

- U.S. Preventive Services Task Force gave low-dose CT chest screening a grade B recommendation for high-risk individuals (age 55 to 80 and at least 30 pack-years of current smoking [pack years = the number of packs per day × years smoked], or at least 30 pack-years of former smoking and quit within 15 years).

Ans. C

221. A 30 year old male, following RTA received multiple blood transfusions and developed severe breathlessness and fall in saturation, criteria to diagnose ARDS is:

A. Fio2/PaO2 <= 300 mmHg
B. Absence of elevated left atrial pressure
C. Basal pulmonary infiltrates on Chest X-ray
D. Acute onset within 1 month of a clinical insult

Explanation:

- Key diagnostic criteria for ARDS include (1) diffuse bilateral pulmonary infiltrates on CXR; (2) PaO2 (arterial partial pressure of oxygen in mmHg)/FIO2 (inspired O2 fraction) ≤300 mmHg; (3) absence of elevated left atrial pressure; and (4) acute onset within 1 week of a clinical insult or new or worsening respiratory symptoms and treat/remove cause.

Ans. B

222. A 60 year old male was brought to the ER with complaints of sudden onset of breathlessness following a RTA. BLUE protocol was followed to assess the patient. Ultrasound chest can detect all of the following except:

A. Pneumothorax
B. Pleural effusion
C. Pulmonary edema
D. Pulmonary hypertension

Explanation:

- Diagnostic Ultrasound is not useful for assessing the pulmonary parenchyma or pulmonary vasculature, but it can detect and localize pleural abnormalities such as pleural effusion and pneumothorax.

Ans. D

223. A 52 year old male presented to the OPD with complaints of cough, breathlessness and right sided pleuritic chest pain. Chest X-ray shows Ellis curve on the right lung suggestive of right sided pleural effusion. Which among the following statements regarding chest X-ray is false?

A. Posteroanterior and lateral views are most often used to diagnose respiratory symptoms
B. Anteroposterior view is routinely taken in bed-ridden patients
C. Lateral decubitus view can be used to estimate the size of freely flowing pleural effusion
D. None of the above

Explanation:

- Chest X-ray (CXR), generally including both postero-anterior and lateral views, is often the first diagnostic study in patients presenting with respiratory symptoms.
- With diffuse lung disease, CXR can detect an alveolar, interstitial, or nodular pattern.
- CXR can also detect pleural effusion and pneumothorax, as well as abnormalities in the hila and mediastinum.
- Lateral decubitus views can be used to estimate the size of freely flowing pleural effusions.

Ans. D

224. A 50 year old male who is known case of COPD developed right sided pneumothorax following rupture of an apical bulla. An ICD was inserted on the right 5th intercostal space in the mid-axillary line. Since he had persistent air leak for more than 1 week, he was advised to undergo VATS. Which among the following statements regarding VATS (Video assisted thoracic surgery) is false?

A. It is used to diagnose pleural lesions and peripheral pulmonary infiltrates and nodules
B. It requires single lung ventilation during the procedure
C. It has largely replaced open biopsy which requires a thoracotomy
D. None of the above

Explanation:

- VATS, also known as thoracoscopy, is widely used for the diagnosis of pleural lesions as well as pesripheral parenchymal infiltrates and nodules. VATS, which requires that the patient tolerate single-lung ventilation during the procedure, involves passing a rigid scope with a camera through a trocar and into the pleural space; instruments can be inserted and manipulated through separate intercostal incisions. VATS has largely replaced "open biopsy", which requires a thoracotomy.

Ans. D

225. A 40 year old male was diagnosed with samter triad of aspirin sensitivity, nasal polyposis and asthma. Intrinsic asthma is associated with all except:

A. Atopic dermatitis
B. Allergic rhinitis
C. Allergic conjunctivitis
D. None of the above

Explanation:

- Majority of asthmatics have childhood-onset disease. Most asthmatics have atopy, and they often have atopic dermatitis (eczema) and/or allergic rhinitis. This phenotype is known as extrinsic asthma. A minority of asthmatic pts do not have atopy (negative skin prick tests to common allergens and normal serum total IgE levels). These individuals, occasionally referred to as intrinsic asthmatics, often have adult-onset disease.

Ans. D

226. A 50 year old male was advised bed rest for 1 month following an RTI. ECHO done after 1 month shows right ventricular hypokinesia with tricuspid regurgitation and hypotension. What is the diagnosis?

A. Pulmonary hypertension
B. Pulmonary embolism.
C. AV malformation
D. Infective endocarditis

Explanation:

- In PE, a normal chest X-ray (CXR) is common. Although not commonly observed, focal oligemia and peripheral wedge-shaped densities on CXR are well-established findings in PE.
- Chest CT with IV contrast has become primary diagnostic imaging test for PE.
- Ventilation-perfusion lung scanning is primarily used for subjects unable to tolerate IV contrast.
- Transthoracic echocardiography can identify right ventricular hypokinesis with moderate-to-large PE, but it is not typically useful for diagnosing the presence of a PE.
- Transesophageal echocardiography can be used to identify large central PE when IV contrast chest CT scans are not appropriate (e.g., renal failure or severe contrast allergy). With the advent of contrast chest CT scans for PE diagnosis, pulmonary angiography studies are rarely performed.

Ans. B

227. A 20-year-old brought to ER with acute exacerbations of Bronchial Asthma, she was treated with oxygen, IV Steroids and bronchodilators and discharged with inhaled corticosteroids and oral leukotrienes. Regarding Inhaled corticosteroids (ICS) true statements include:

A. Avoid using spacer devices as they prevent effective drug delivery
B. Avoid rinsing the mouth after using ICS to increase contact time and absorption of ICS
C. Avoid using LABAs without ICS
D. Combinations of low dose theophylline and ICS must be avoided as they increase risk of exacerbations

Explanation:

- ICS side effects include hoarseness and oral candidiasis; these effects may be minimized by use of a spacer device and by rinsing out mouth after taking ICS.
- LABAs have replaced regularly scheduled use of SABAs, but they do not control airway inflammation and should not be used without inhaled corticosteroid (ICS) therapy. Combinations of LABAs with ICS reduce asthma exacerbations and provide an excellent long-term treatment option for asthma severity of moderate persistent degree or greater.
- Low doses of theophylline may have additive effects with ICS at levels below the standard therapeutic range, and this can be a useful treatment option for severe asthma.

Ans. C

228. A 32 year female with known history of Bronchial asthma, now presented with tachypnea, wheezing, and chest tightness. Regarding acute asthma exacerbations all are true except:

A. Pulmonary function testing reveals a reduction in FEV1 and PEF
B. Asthma exacerbation treatment includes high doses of SABAs and systemic corticosteroids

C. Pco2 is usually increased due to hypoventilation

D. Normal or rising PCO_2 can signal impending respiratory failure

Explanation:

- Mainstays of asthma exacerbation treatment are high doses of SABAs and systemic corticosteroids. In case of acute asthma exacerbations pulmonary function testing reveals a reduction in FEV1 and PEF. Hypoxemia can result; PCO_2 is usually reduced due to hyperventilation. Normal or rising PCO_2 can signal impending respiratory failure.

Ans. C

229. A 30 year old female had an acute exacerbation of asthma during pregnancy. Last exacerbation occurred 10 years back. Regarding the radiographic findings of an asthma patient true is all except:

A. Chest X-ray will have multiple infiltrates

B. In acute exacerbations, pneumothorax may be identified

C. In BPA, eosinophillic pulmonary infiltrates may be observed

D. CT chest may show central bronchiectasis

Explanation:

- Chest X-ray is usually normal. In acute exacerbations, pneumothorax may be identified. In BPA, eosinophilic pulmonary infiltrates may be observed.
- Chest CT scan is not typically performed in routine asthma but may show central bronchiectasis in BPA.

Ans. A

230. A 18 year old male was advised to undergo PFT to assess the degree of airway obstruction. PFT showed obstructive airway disease with bronchodilator reversibility. Which among the following statements regarding asthma is false?

A. Bronchodilator reversibility is demonstrated by an increase in FEV1 by ≥100 mL or ≥12% from baseline FEV1 15 min after a short-acting β agonist

B. Peak expiratory flow rate (PEFR) can be used by patient to track asthma control objectively at home

C. Exhaled nitric oxide levels can provide an assessment of eosinophilic airway inflammation

D. Diffusing capacity for carbon monoxide is usually normal

Explanation:

- Spirometry often shows airflow obstruction, with a reduction in forced expiratory volume in 1s (FEV1) and FEV1/forced vital capacity (FVC) ratio.
- However, spirometry may be normal, especially if asthma symptoms are adequately treated.
- Bronchodilator reversibility is demonstrated by an increase in FEV1 by ≥200 mL and ≥12% from baseline FEV1 15 min after a short-acting β agonist (often albuterol metered-dose inhaler two puffs or 180 μg).
- Many but not all asthmatics will demonstrate significant bronchodilator reversibility; optimal pharmacologic treatment may reduce bronchodilator reversibility.
- Airway hyper-responsiveness is characteristic of asthma; it can be assessed by exposure to direct bronchoconstrictors such as methacholine or histamine.
- Greater airway responsiveness is associated with increased asthmatic symptoms. The peak expiratory flow rate (PEFR) can be used by the patient to track asthma control objectively at home.
- Measurement of lung volumes is not typically performed, but increases in total lung capacity and residual volume may be observed. The diffusing capacity for carbon monoxide is usually normal.

Ans. A

231. A 50 year old female was diagnosed with right upper lobe mass lesion. Which among the following is the non ionizing imaging modality that will aid in taking a biopsy from the mass?

A. Chest X-ray
B. CT scan
C. PET CT
D. Ultrasound

Explanation:

- Diagnostic ultrasound is a non ionizing imaging approach which is safe to perform on pregnant women and children. It can detect and localize pleural abnormalities and guide thoracocentesis of a pleural effusion.

Ans. D

232. A 50 year old female had a accidental fall from the first floor of a building. Post the incident she developed breathlessness. What is the diagnosis for this patient? Chest radiograph of the patient is given below:

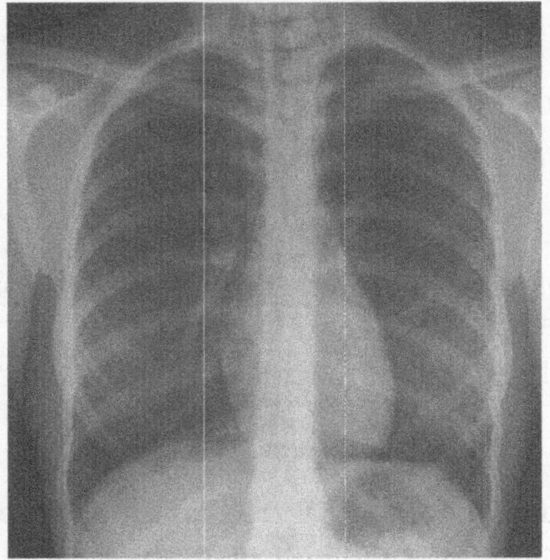

A. Pneumomediastinum
B. Hiatus hernia
C. COPD
D. Pulmonary embolism

Explanation:

- Chest X-ray shows continuous diaphragm sign indicating the presence of mediastinal gas outlining the superior surface of the diaphragm and separating it from the heart. This is seen in pneumomediastinum.
- Gas outlining the lateral margin of the descending aorta and extending laterally between the parietal pleura and medial left hemi diaphragm is known as V sign of Maclerio.

Ans. A

233. Most common cause of pleural effusion is:

A. Left ventricular failure
B. ARDS
C. Liver cirrhosis
D. Malignancy

Explanation:

- Most common cause of pleural effusion is left ventricular failure.
- Effusion occurs because the increased amounts of fluid in lung interstitial spaces exit in part across the visceral pleura; this overwhelms capacity of the lymphatics in the parietal pleura to remove fluid.
- In patients with heart failure, diagnostic thoracentesis should be performed if the effusions are not bilateral and comparable in size, if patient is febrile, or if the patient has pleuritic chest pain to verify that the patient has a transudative effusion.

Ans. A

CHAPTER 3

CARDIOLOGY

1. Patient was on ketoconazole for treatment of fungal infection after complaining heartburn, after checking ECG then, which came out normal. Doctor prescribes him a drug, he developed palpitation and light headedness, repeat ECG have shown following pattern, which drug the doctor have given?

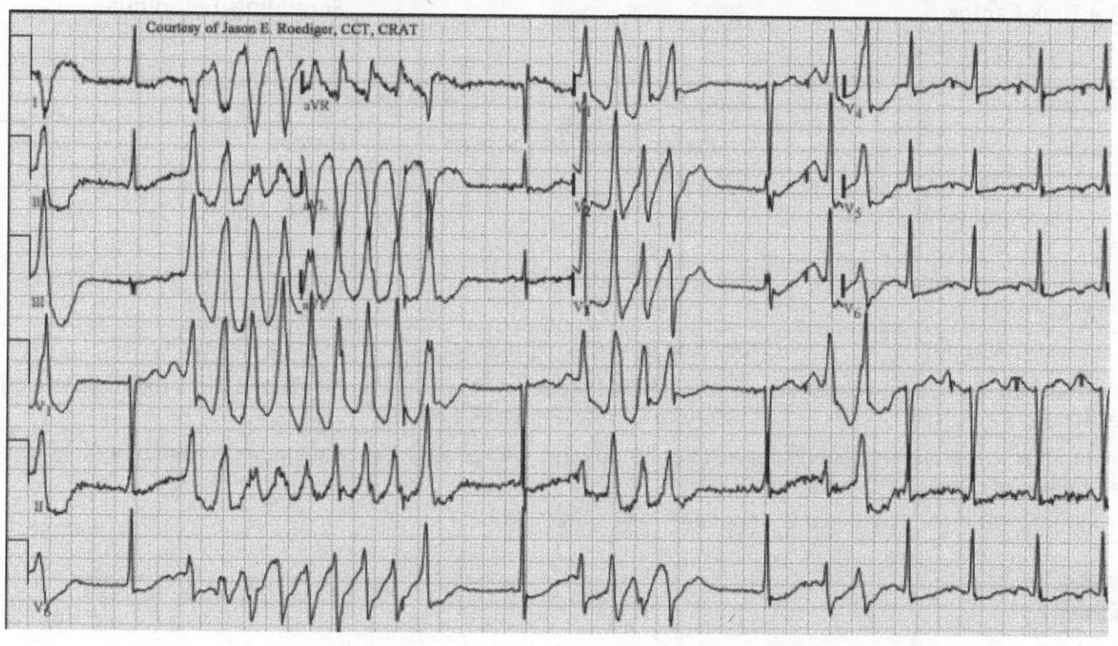

A. Omeprazole

B. Cisapride

C. Metoclopramide

D. Domperidone

Explanation:

- Patient on ketoconazole for treatment of fungal infection, after giving history of heartburn* and doctor have prescribed, prokinetic* cisapride, after checking normal ECG finding and anticipating Gastro-esophageal reflux disease*
- Patient develops "TORSADES – DE – POINTES* [Long QT interval* polymorphic ventricular tachycardia*]
- ECG showing polymorphous ventricular tachycardia figuring torsades de pointes, which runs the risks of sudden cardiac death*

Ans. B

2. All of the following are major risk factors for sudden cardiac death in Hypertrophic cardiomyopathy except:

A. Syncope

B. LV thickness >25mm

C. Abnormal BP response to exercise

D. Family H/O sudden cardiac death

Explanation:

Risk Factors for Sudden Death in Hypertrophic Cardiomyopathy (HCM):

- History of cardiac arrest or spontaneous sustained ventricular tachycardia
- Syncope
- Family history of sudden cardiac death
- Spontaneous nonsustained ventricular tachycardia
- LV thickness >30 mm (ECHO finding)
- Abnormal BP response to exercise

Table: Risk factors for sudden death in hypertrophic cardiomyopathy

Major Risk Factor		Screening Technique
History of cardiac arrest or spontaneous sustained ventricular tachycardia[a]		History
Syncope	Nonvagal, often with or after exertion	History
Family history of sudden cardiac death		Family history
Spontaneous nonsustained ventricular tachycardia[b]	>3 beats at rate > 120	Exercise or 24- to 48-h ambulatory recording
LV thickness >30 mm	Present in <10% of patients	Echocardiography
Abnormal blood pressure response to exercise	Systolic blood pressure fall or failure to increase at peak exercise	Maximal upright exercise testing

[a] Implantable cardioverter-defibrillator adviser for patients with prior arrest or sustained ventricular tachycardia regardless of other risk factors.

[b] Prognostic value most applicable to patients < 40 years old.

Ans. B

3. Pseudo P pulmonale seen in:

A. Hypokalaemia

B. Hyperkalaemia

C. Hypomagnesemia

D. Hypercalcaemia

Explanation:

P Pulmonale can be observed in patients with Hypokalemia- Transient & concomitant

Tall P waves are considered to be called as Pseudo P pulmonale

Notched (or bifid) p-wave known as "p mitrale", indicative of left atrial hypertrophy which may be caused by mitral stenosis. There may be tall peaked p-waves. This is called "p-pulmonale" and is indicative of right atrial hypertrophy often secondary to tricuspid stenosis or pulmonary hypertension. **A similar picture can be seen in hypokalemia (known as "pseudo p-pulmonale").**

ECG CHANGES	
HYPERKALAEMIA 1. Absent P-wave 2. Widening of QRS complex 3. Bizarre, intraventricular conduction disturbance 4. Tall, peaked T-waves 5. Disappearance of the ST segment	**HYPOKALAEMIA** 1. Disappearance of T-wave 2. Progressive increase in amplitude of U-wave 3. First and second degree AV block 4. ST segment depression
HYPOCALCAEMIA Prolonged QT interval (due to an increase in duration of ST segment). QT prolongation is inversely proportional to serum calcium level. T-waves are normal.	**HYPERCALCEMIA** Shortening of QT interval (due to shortening of ST segment). T-waves may also become flattened or inverted.

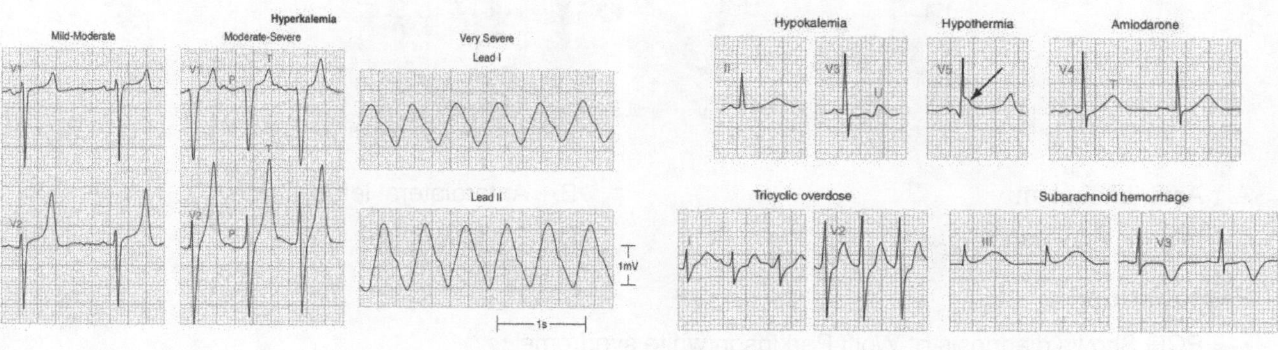

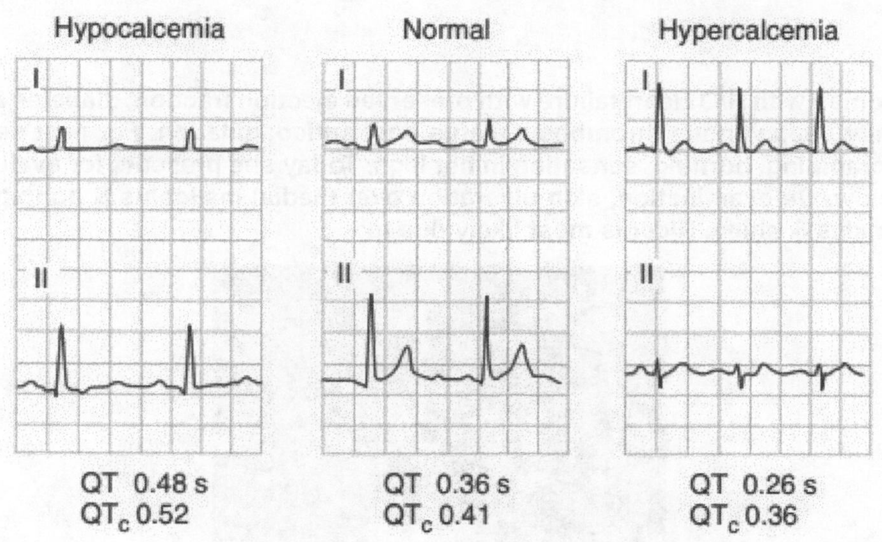

Ans. A

4. **A 22 yr old owner who presents to you for evaluation of palpitations. Her ECG picture is given. She likely has bypass accessory tract located at:**

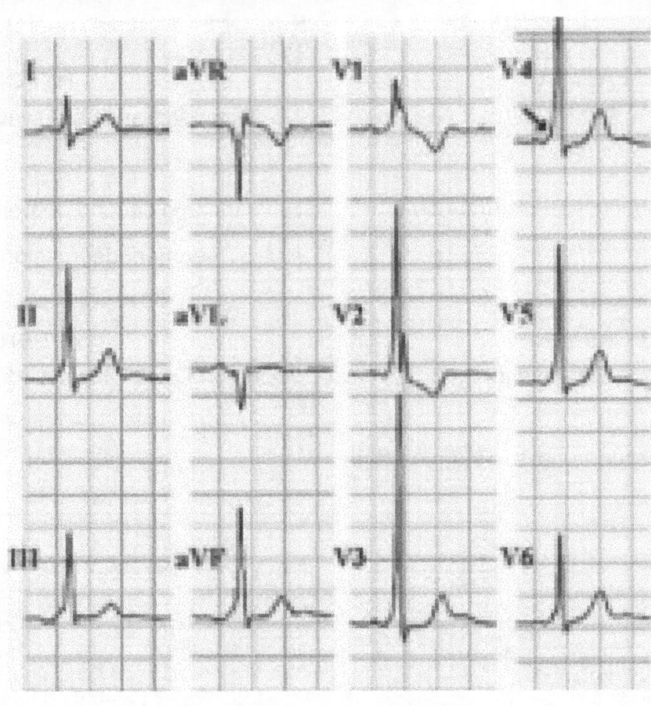

A. Anterior septum
B. Anterolateral left ventricle
C. Inferior left ventricle
D. Right ventricle

Explanation:

- ECG Shows diagnosis of Wolff Parkinson white syndrome
- Presence of left bundle appearing delta wave/QRS complex localizes this accessory tract to right ventricle

Ans. D

5. **A 77 yr old woman with H/O Heart failure with preserved ejection fraction, diabetes mellitus & prior left lower extremity deep venous thrombosis status post anticoagulation. For past several months, she complained cramping, burning sensation in her legs. Today she presents for evaluation of skin ulcer as shown below. On examination, skin ulceration over medial malleolus & nonpitting woody edema of bilateral ankles & shins. Ulcer is most likely due to:**

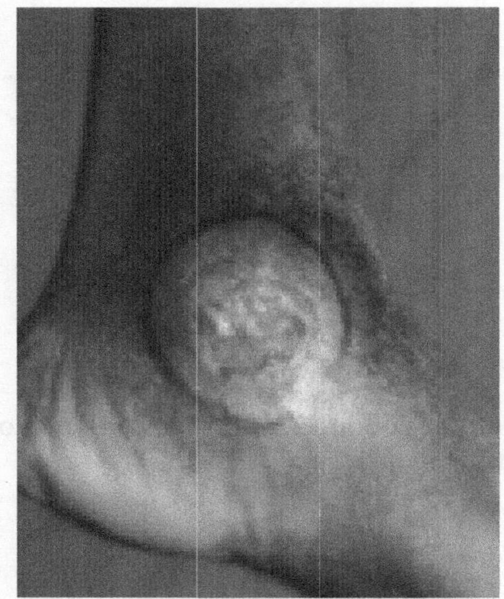

A. Arachnid envenomation
B. Chronic venous insufficiency
C. Diabetic foot ulcer
D. Bacillus anthracis infection

Explanation:

- Classic clinical picture of chronic venous insufficiency is active venous ulcer.
- Phlebectasia corona is fan shaped pattern of intradermal veins near ankle on foot

Ans. B

6. **A 32 yr old man presents with exertional pain in his both forearms & hands. He smokes one pack of cigarettes per day, but otherwise has no past medical history. He has palpable brachial pulse but very faint radial and ulnar pulses. Picture of hand is shown below. Angiography of upper extremity reveals smooth tapering segmental lesions in small distal arterial vessels. Which treatments has greatest chance of success?**

A. Cilostazol
B. Enoxaparin
C. Cessation of smoking
D. Prednisone

Explanation:

- Patient has Classic presentation of TAO
- Inflammatory vascular occlusive disorder involving small and medium size arteries and veins in distal upper and lower extremities.
- No specific treatment is present for this condition, except Cessation of smoking.

Ans. C

7. **A 32 yr old guitarist with no past medical H/O presents with chest pain after suffering from coryza, cough, fever & muscle aches for past week. He describes pain as constant & radiating to left shoulder & exacerbated by lying flat 7 during deep breaths. Examination reveals rasping extracardiac sound present in three components per heart beat. ECG is depicted in picture. Troponin I levels are undetectable on presentation & 6 hours later. BP, Heart rate & oxygenation are normal. Most appropriate next step is:**

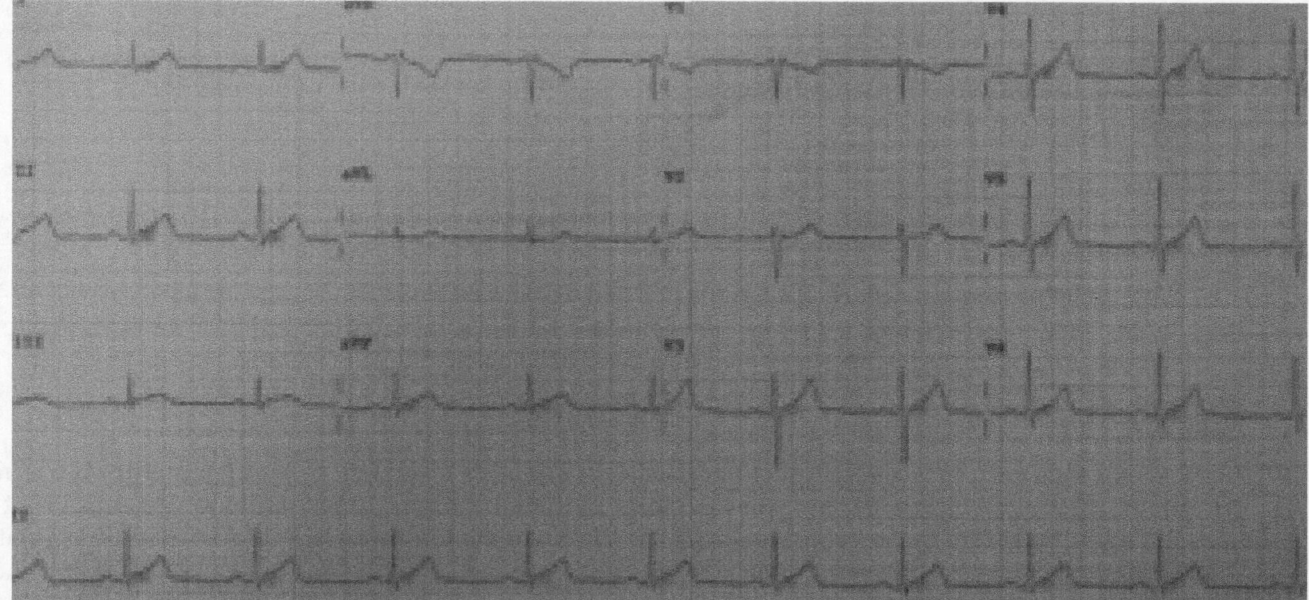

A. Aspirin 81mg daily, metoprolol 25mg twice daily & atorvastatin 80mg daily
B. Aspirin 1g every 8 hours with omeprazole 20mg daily

C. Heparin, aspirin, clopidogrel with immediate coronary angiography
D. Prednisone 40mg daily for 2 weeks followed by taper over ensuing 2 months

Explanation:

- ECG Shows diffuse ST Elevation with PR Depression & negative cardiac – Typically suggesting acute pericarditis
- No specific treatment is present for acute pericarditis
- Aspirin with Gastric protection is given in majority of conditions

Ans. B

8. Not associated with Orthopnea among following?

A. Abdominal Obesity
B. Abdominal Ascites
C. Diaphragmatic Weakness
D. Hepatopulmonary Syndrome

Explanation:

- Orthopnea-Dyspnea occurring in recumbent position & usually a feature of heart failure than exertional dyspnea.
- Relieved by sitting upright or sleeping with additional support
- Orthopnea can also occur with abdominal obesity, ascites & pulmonary disease patients Hepatopulmonary syndrome
- Leads to Orthodeoxia→ Hypoxia in upright position
- Leads to Platypnea→ Sensation of shortness of breath when upright

Ans. C

9. All the following are upregulated in heart failure with ejection fraction reduced except:

A. Angiotensin II
B. BNP
C. Calcium uptake in sarcoplasmic reticulum
D. Norepinephrine

Explanation:

- **Following are upregulated in failing heart-** Angiotensin II, Aldosterone, Arginine vasopressin along with norepinephrine
- Brain natriuretic peptide is also upregulated that aids in reducing systemic vascular resistance & natriuresis.
- In heart failure, transcriptional & post transcriptional changes in myocyte leads to calcium leakage through sarcoplasmic reticular membrane & therefore decreased calcium uptake in sarcoplasmic reticulum.

Ans. C

10. A 68 yr old man with H/O myocardial infarction & congestive heart failure that is comfortable at rest. However when walking to his car, he develops dyspnea, fatigue & palpitations. He must rest for several minutes before these symptoms resolve. Which of the following is New York Heart Association classification?

A. Class I
B. Class II
C. Class III
D. Class IV

Explanation:

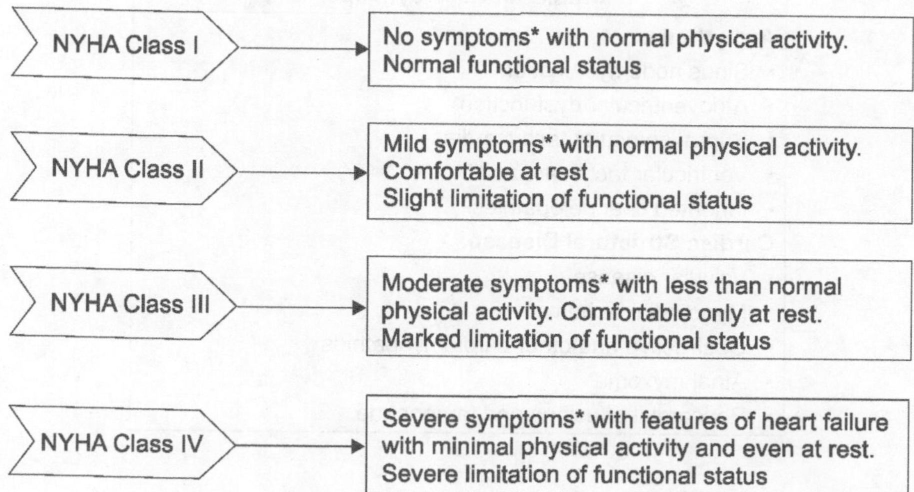

Ans. C

11. A 64-year-old woman with a history of poorly controlled diabetes, hypertension, and tobacco use is admitted 6 hours after acutely developing right hemiparesis, visual field deficit on the right, and expressive aphasia. Workup for stroke etiology reveals no evidence of atrial fibrillation, normal transthoracic echo, and a computed tomography angiogram that shows 80% stenosis of the left common carotid artery and 60% stenosis of the right common carotid artery. Which of the following is the next best step?

A. Treat the patient medically with an antiplatelet agent

B. Treat the patient medically with anticoagulation

C. Perform a left carotid endarterectomy (CEA)

D. Perform a right CEA

Explanation:

- Patient has a symptomatic left carotid artery stenosis. There is approximately a 9% ipsilateral stroke risk in the next 2 years with CEA versus a 26% risk if medically treated alone, based on the North American Symptomatic Carotid Endarterectomy Trial study. Given this information, the patient should undergo a left CEA, preferably within 2 weeks from symptom onset. Given that the right carotid is asymptomatic and <70% stenosed, there is no indication for a right CEA or CAS at this time.
- In the absence of atrial fibrillation or mechanical heart valve, there is no indication for medical management with anticoagulation.
- Carotid artery stenting is often used for patients who are poor operative candidates for CEA or in cases such as stenosis induced from radiation therapy.

Ans. C

12. Not a cause of cardiac syncope is:

A. Sinus node dysfunction

B. AV Node dysfunction

C. AV dysfunction

D. Supraventricular tachycardias

Explanation:

Table: Cardiac syncope
Arrhythmias
• Sinus node dysfunction
• Atrioventricular dysfunction
• Supraventricular tachycardias
• Ventricular tachycardias
• Inherited channelopathies
Cardiac Structural Disease
• Valvular disease
• Myocardial ischemia
• Obstructive and other cardiomyopathies
• Atrial myxoma
• Pericardial effusions and tamponade

Ans. B

13. Pain is often absent in which type of pericarditis?

A. Viral
B. Postirradiation
C. SLE
D. Syphilis

Explanation:

- Pain is often absent in slowly developing tuberculosis, postirradiation, neoplastic and uremic pericarditis.
- These conditions are slowly developing and there onset is subacute to chronic and most of the time present as subacute effusive constrictive pericarditis in which there is thickened pericardium and pericardial effusion and thus there is no inflamed pericardium, and no stretching of parietal and visceral pleura and hence no pericardial rub is heard.

Ans. B

14. Most common Haemophilus species to cause HACEK endocarditis:

A. H.parainfluenzae
B. H.influenzae type B
C. H.hemolyticus
D. Non-typable H.influenzae

Explanation:

- Haemophilus parainfluenzae is the most common Haemophilus species isolated from cases of HACEK endocarditis.
- Of patients with HACEK endocarditis due to Haemophilus species, 60% have been ill for <2 months before presentation, and 19–50% develop congestive heart failure.
- Mortality rates as high as 30–50% were reported in older series; however, more recent studies have documented mortality rates of <5%.
- H. parainfluenzae has been isolated from other infections, such as meningitis; brain, dental, pelvic, and liver abscess; pneumonia; urinary tract infection; and septicemia.

Ans. A

15. Following is ECG of a patient with Uncontrolled diabetes. What is the cause?

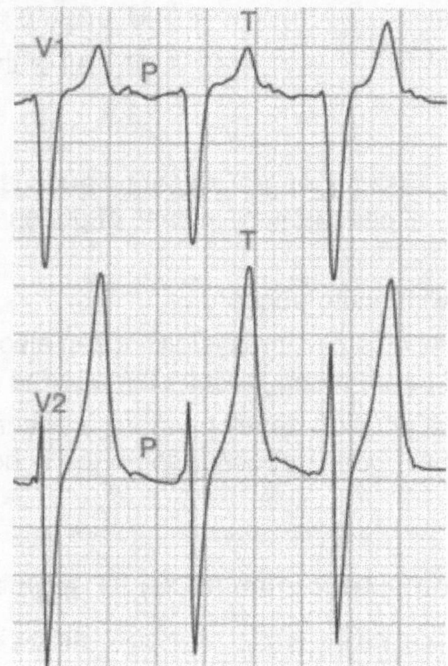

A. Hyperkalemia

B. Hypothermia

C. Hypernatremia

D. Hypercalcaemia

Explanation:

- Hyperkalemia produces a sequence of changes , usually beginning with narrowing and peaking (tenting) of the T waves.
- Further elevation of extracellular K+ leads to AV conduction disturbances, diminution in P-wave amplitude & widening of QRS interval.
- Severe hyperkalemia eventually causes cardiac arrest with a slow sinusoidal type of mechanism ("sine-wave" pattern) followed by asystole.

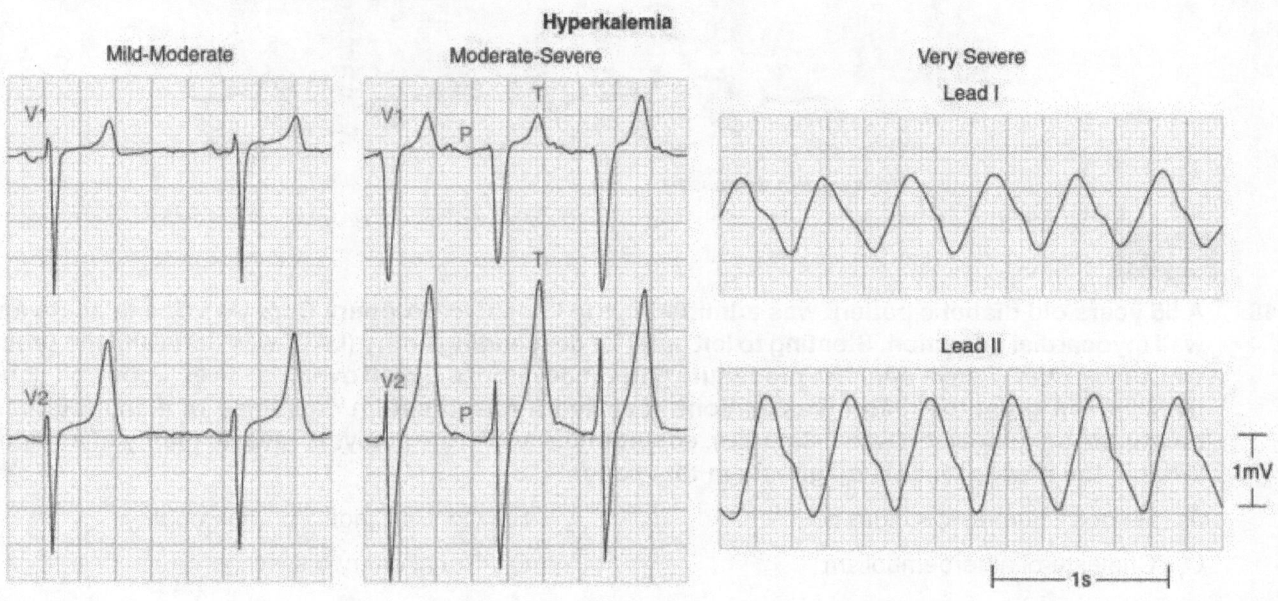

Ans. A

16. **Pericardial rub heard in which condition:**

A. Cardiac tamponade
B. Acute pericarditis
C. Pericardial effusion
D. All of the above

Explanation:

- Pericardial rub is an scratching, rasping, or grating sound audible due to scratching of two inflamed layers of pericardium (parietal & visceral pericardium) in case of pericarditis heard at end expiration with patient upright and leaning forward.
- It is heard in 85 % of patients with acute pericarditis.
- It is triphasic i.e. midsystolic, mid diastolic, presystolic. It can also be heard in acute myocardial infarction, Dressler's syndrome. It is best heard along the left sternal edge in third and fourth intercostal space.
- When tamponade or pericardial effusion develops there is accumulation of fluid in between parietal and visceral pericardium so scratching does not occur so no rub is heard.

Ans. B

17. **In case of acute pericarditis Electrocardiogram (ECG) ST segment elevation is seen in which stage?**

A. Stage 1
B. Stage 2
C. Stage 3
D. Stage 4

Explanation:

- ST segment elevation with concavity upwards is seen in stage 1 in two or three limb leads and v2-v6 and PR segment depression is also seen indicating atrial involvement.

  Whereas in case of myocardial infarction there is ST segment elevation with convexity upwards is seen and thus helps in differentiating it from acute pericarditis as both conditions are similar in presentation.

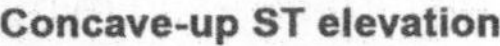

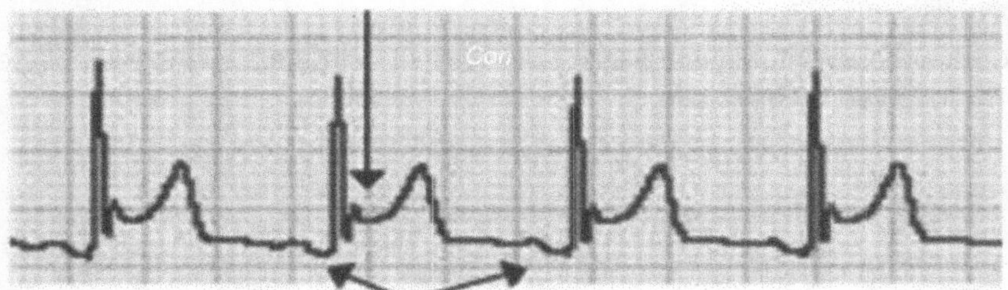

Ans. A

18. **A 55 years old diabetic patient was admitted in the Intensive Coronary Care Unit due to acute anterior wall myocardial infarction. Stenting to left anterior descending artery (LAD) was done and the procedure was uneventful. 2 days after the procedure patient developed a rash over his lower limbs and gangrene over his left great toe. Lab investigations revealed a raised serum creatinine of 4.5mg/dL (baseline creatinine on admission was 0.8mg/dL), eosinophilia and urine analysis reveals plenty of eosinophils. What is the most probable diagnosis in this patient?**

A. Hemolytic uraemic syndrome
B. Contrast induced nephropathy
C. Cholesterol atheroembolism
D. Renal artery dissection

Explanation:

- This is a classical scenario of ***atheroembolic renal disease*** which commonly presents after vascular procedures (coronary angiography, aortic instrumentation).

- This patient is presenting with acute kidney injury, livedo reticularis, eosinophilia and eosinophils in urine analysis.
- Emboli are cholesterol-rich and lodge in medium and small renal arteries, with a consequent eosinophil-rich inflammatory reaction. Patients with atheroembolic acute renal failure often have a normal urinalysis, but the urine may contain eosinophils and casts.
- Diagnosis can be confirmed by renal biopsy, but this procedure is often unnecessary when other stigmata of atheroemboli are present (livedo reticularis, distal peripheral infarcts, eosinophilia)

Ans. C

19. In the above ECG what is the diagnosis:

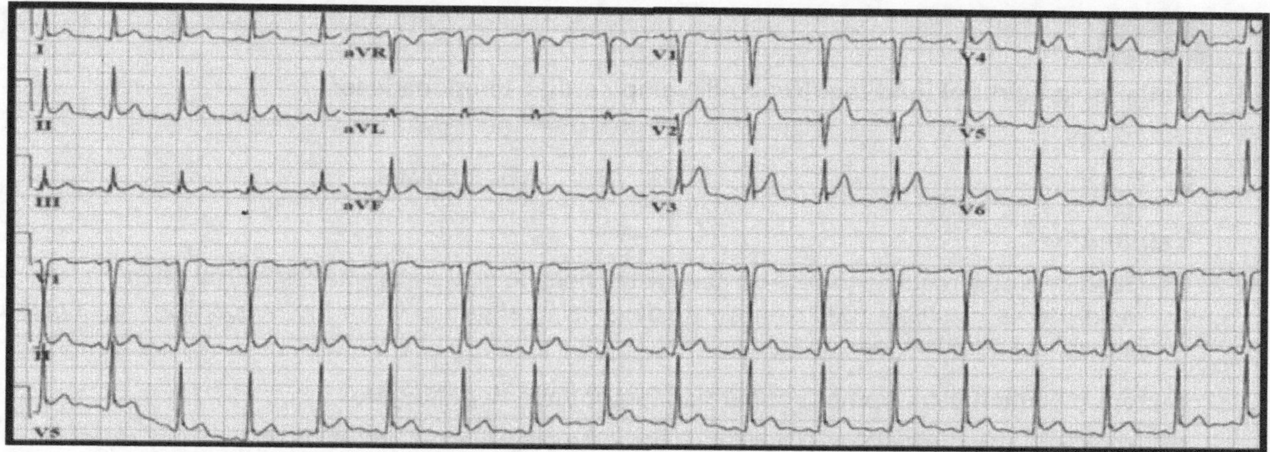

A. Acute myocardial infarction

B. Paroxysmal supraventricular tachycardia

C. Acute pericarditis

D. Brugada syndrome

Explanation:

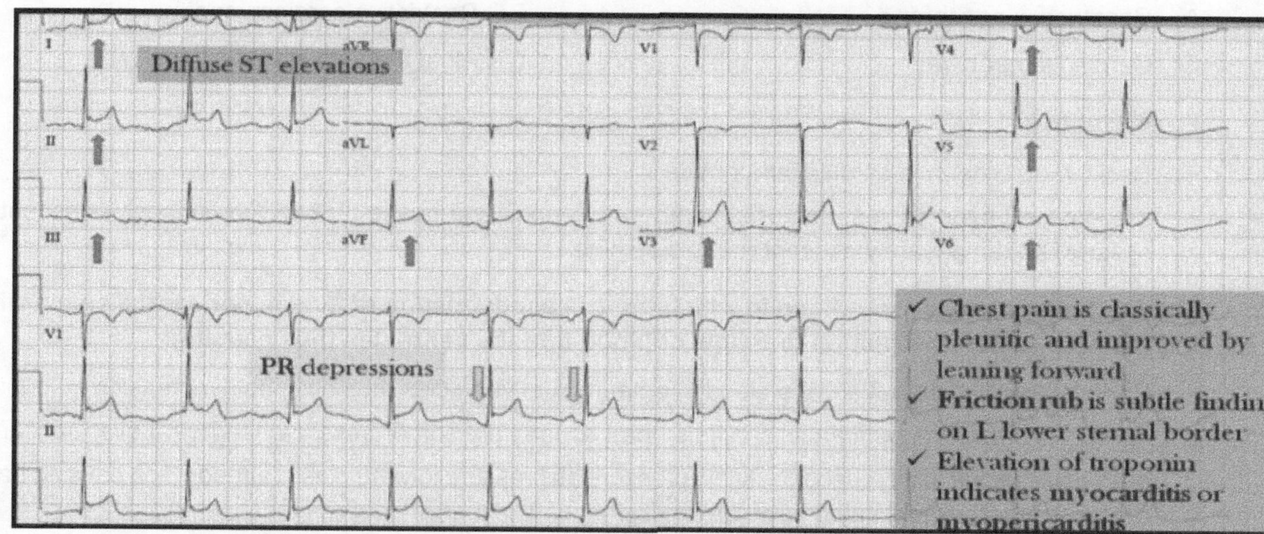

- As shown in above ECG there is ST segment elevation in lead 1, 2 , 3 and V2-V6 with concavity upwards. Also PR depression in V1. Finding are suggestive of acute pericarditis. In acute pericarditis there are 4 stages which can be seen in ECG.
- Stage 1- ST segment elevation with concavity upwards, involving two or three limb leads and V2-V6, with reciprocal depression only in aVR and sometimes V1. Also there is depression of PR segment below TP segment, reflecting atrial involvement.

- Stage 2-After several days ST segment return to normal.
- Stage 3-T wave is inverted.
- Stage 4-weeks or months after the onset of acute pericarditis ECG returns to normal.
- In myocardial infarction the ST segment elevation is there with convexity upwards whereas in case of acute pericarditis ST segment elevation is with concavity upwards. Also there is q waves present inn case of old MI.
- In case of paroxysmal supraventricular tachycardia, there is no ST elevation seen and rate is high.
- Brugada syndrome is heritable arrythmia syndrome characterised by AD inheritance, and sodium channelopathy. In this ECG is characteristically consist of coved – type of ST elevation followed by T wave inversion right sided precordial leads (n V1-V3) and with RBBB (right bundle branch block).

Ans. C

20. Minimum amount of fluid required to develop cardiac tamponade is:

A. 200 ml
B. 300 ml
C. 500 ml
D. 1000 ml

Explanation:

- Quantity of fluid required to develop cardiac tamponade may be as small as 200 ml when the fluid develops rapidly to as much as 2000ml in slowly developing effusions when the pericardium has opportunity to stretch and adapt increasing volume.

Factors on which development of cardiac tamponade depends are:

- Rapidly developing fluid can cause serious obstruction when fluid fills the space very rapidly.
- Amount of fluid which is filling the space.

Ans. A

21. Becks triad is seen in which condition?

A. Constrictive pericarditis
B. Restrictive cardiomyopathy
C. Cardiac tamponade
D. All of the above

Explanation:

- Becks triad is seen in cardiac tamponade.
- It comprised hypotension, soft or absent heart sounds and raised JVP with prominent x descent (early systolic) but an absent y descent (early diastolic).

Cardiac tamponade is a condition in which there is accumulation of fluid in pericardial space which is sufficient to cause obstruction to inflow of blood into the ventricles thus causing:

1. Reduced cardiac output as less blood in entering into ventricles thus causing hypotension
2. As fluid is present in pericardial sac thus heart sounds are soft or absent when heard over pericardium.
3. JVP is raised due to increased backflow pressure as pressure in ventricles is already high causing backflow of blood and thus right sided hear failure.

Ans. C

22. All are true regarding AV block except:

A. Atrioventricular block is probably the most common cause of arrhythmic cardiac syncope.
B. Complete AV block occurs primarily in elderly patients.

C. The patient is pale and, if standing, falls down, often with resultant injury.

D. Clinical features of complete AV block include a slow collapsing pulse and decrease of the jugular venous pressure

Explanation:

- Atrioventricular block is probably the most common cause of arrhythmic cardiac syncope. The term Stokes-Adams attack describes disturbances of consciousness occurring in association with a complete AV block.
- Complete AV block occurs primarily in elderly patients. The onset of a Stokes-Adams attack generally is sudden, although a number of visual, sensory, and perceptual premonitory symptoms may be experienced.
- During the syncopal attack, the pulse disappears and no heart sounds are audible. The patient is pale and, if standing, falls down, often with resultant injury.
- If the attack is sufficiently prolonged, respiration may become labored, and urinary incontinence and clonic muscle jerks may occur. Prolonged confusion and neurological signs of cerebral ischemia may be present.
- Regaining of consciousness generally is rapid. The clinical features of complete AV block include a slow-collapsing pulse and elevation of the jugular venous pressure, sometimes with cannon waves. The first heart sound is of variable intensity, and heart sounds related to atrial contractions may be audible.
- An ECG confirming the diagnosis demonstrates independence of atrial P waves and ventricular QRS complexes. During Stokes-Adams attacks, the ECG generally shows ventricular standstill, but ventricular fibrillation or tachycardia also may occur.

Ans. D

23. Most common supraventricular tachycardia is:

A. Sinus tachycardia
B. Atrial fibrillation
C. Atrial flutter
D. Paroxysmal supraventricular tachycardia

Explanation:

- Most common supraventricular tachycardia is sinus tachycardia in response to physiologic stress, such as exercise, but it can also be a manifestation acute illness.
- Defining feature: normal sinus mechanism precipitated by exertion, stress, concurrent illness.
- First step in diagnosis of supraventricular tachycardia is to consider possibility of sinus tachycardia.
- Therapy is then determined by the clinical findings.
- If the arrhythmia is ongoing and is not due to sinus tachycardia, initial assessment determines whether immediate therapy is needed.

Ans. A

24. Most common cause for high cardiac output hypotension:

A. Sepsis
B. Liver failure
C. Burns
D. Severe Pancreatitis

Explanation:

- Signs of increased cardiac output include a widened pulse pressure (particularly with a reduced diastolic pressure), warm extremities with bounding pulses, and rapid capillary refill.
- In hypotensive patients with clinical evidence of increased cardiac output, a search for causes of decreased SVR is appropriate.
- Most common cause of high-cardiac-output hypotension is sepsis.
- Other causes include liver failure, severe pancreatitis, burns, trauma, anaphylaxis, thyrotoxicosis, and peripheral arteriovenous shunts.

Ans. A

25. Paroxysmal supraventricular tachycardia can be terminated by:

A. Valsalva Maneuver
B. Carotid sinus massage
C. Adenosine
D. All of the above'

Explanation:

- Maneuvers that increase AV block, such as carotid sinus massage, Valsalva maneuver, or administration of AV nodal–blocking agents, such as adenosine, are useful to create AV block that will expose the p wave.
- Increasing vagal tone produces the AV block.
- AV nodal reentry tachycardia (AVNRT) is the most common form of paroxysmal supraventricular tachycardia (PSVT).
- Most forms of AVNRT utilize a slowly conducting AV nodal pathway (right inferior extension) that extends from the compact AV node near His bundle, inferiorly along the tricuspid valve annulus to the floor of coronary sinus.
- Reentry wavefront propagates up this slowly conducting pathway to the compact AV node and then exits from the fast pathway at the top of the AV node.
- Path back to the slow pathway probably involves the left atrial septum which has connections to the coronary sinus musculature.

Ans. D

26. A 19-year-old woman from Guatemala presents to your office for a routine screening physical examination. At age 4 years, she was diagnosed with acute rheumatic fever. She does not recall the specifics of her illness and remembers only that she was required to be on bed rest for 6 months. She has remained on penicillin V orally at a dose of 250 mg twice a day since that time. She asks if she can safely discontinue this medication. She has had only one other flare of her disease, at age 8, when she stopped taking penicillin at the time of her emigration to the United States. She is currently working as a day care provider. Her physical examination is notable for normal point of maximal impulse (PMI) with a grade III/VI holosystolic murmur that is heard best at the apex of the heart and radiates to the axilla. What do you advise the patient to do?

A. An echocardiogram should be performed to determine the extent of valvular damage before deciding if penicillin can be discontinued
B. Penicillin prophylaxis can be discontinued because she has had no flares in 5 years
C. She should change her dosing regimen to intramuscular benzathine penicillin every 8 weeks
D. She should continue on penicillin indefinitely as she had a previous recurrence, has presumed rheumatic heart disease, and is working in a field with high occupational exposure to group A Streptococcus

Explanation:

- Episodes of rheumatic fever are most common in first 5 yrs after initial diagnosis. Penicillin prophylaxis is recommended for at least this period.
- After the first 5 years, secondary prophylaxis is determined on an individual basis.
- Ongoing prophylaxis is currently recommended for patients who have had recurrent disease, have rheumatic heart disease, or work in occupations that have a high risk for re-exposure to group A streptococcal infection.
- Prophylactic regimens are penicillin V, PO 250 mg twice a day (bid); benzathine penicillin, 1.2 million units intramuscularly (IM) every 4 weeks; and sulfadiazine, 1 g PO daily. Polyvalent pneumococcal vaccine has no cross-reactivity with group A Streptococcus.

Ans. D

27. A 50 year old male was advised bed rest for 1 month following an RTI. ECHO done after 1 month shows right ventricular hypokinesia with tricuspid regurgitation and hypotension. What is the diagnosis?

A. Pulmonary hypertension
B. Pulmonary embolism.
C. AV malformation
D. Infective endocarditis

Explanation:

- In PE, a normal chest X-ray (CXR) is common. Although not commonly observed, focal oligemia and peripheral wedge-shaped densities on CXR are well-established findings in PE. Chest CT with IV contrast has become the primary diagnostic imaging test for PE. Ventilation-perfusion lung scanning is primarily used for subjects unable to tolerate IV contrast. Transthoracic echocardiography can identify right ventricular hypokinesis with moderate-to-large PE, but it is not typically useful for diagnosing the presence of a PE. Transesophageal echocardiography can be used to identify large central PE when IV contrast chest CT scans are not appropriate (e.g., renal failure or severe contrast allergy). With the advent of contrast chest CT scans for PE diagnosis, pulmonary angiography studies are rarely performed.

Ans. B

28. Electrical alternans is seen in which of the following condition?

A. Cardiac tamponade
B. Constrictive pericarditis
C. Restrictive cardiomyopathy
D. All of the above

Explanation:

- Electric alternans is seen in cardiac tamponade. Electrical alternans is seen in cases of pericardial effusion especially when it is associated with tamponade.
- In ECG there will be periodic beat to beat shift in the QRS axis, low voltage QRS complexes will be is seen.There will be alternating amplitude of QRS complexes will be present. This is seen due to mechanical swinging of the heart to and fro in the large pericardial fluid.

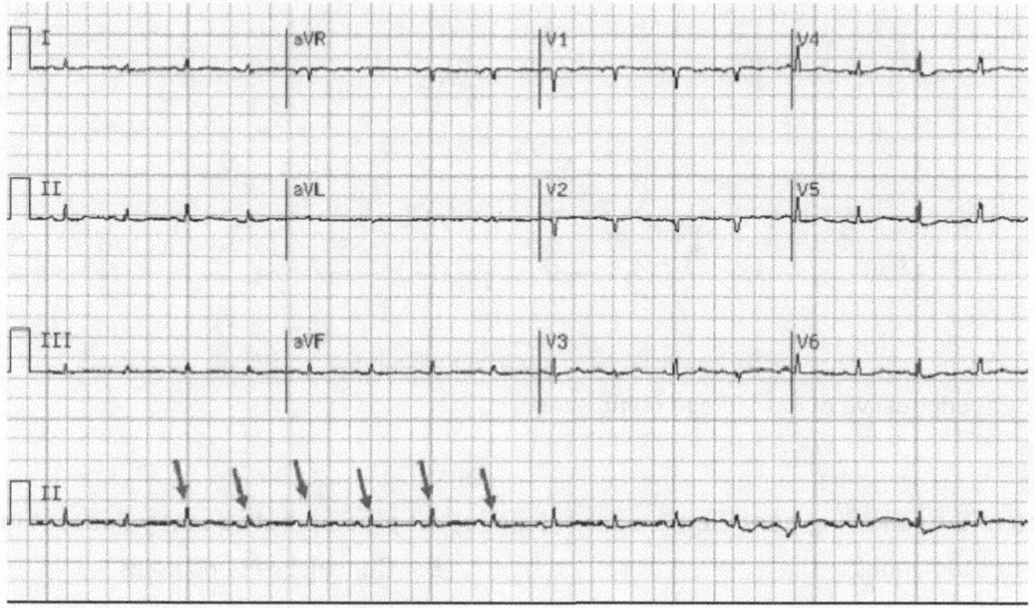

ECG shown above is case of cardiac tamponade.

In this ECG findings are:

1. Red and blue arrow indicating alternating amplitude of QRS complexes that is called as Electrical alternans.
2. Sinus tachycardia.
3. Low voltage complexes defined as:
   a. The amplitude of all the QRS complexes in the limb leads are < 5 mm or
   b. The amplitude of all the QRS complexes in the precordial leads (v1-v6) are <10 mm.

These above mentioned findings in ECG are seen in cases of large pericardial effusion and cardiac tamponade.

Ans. A

29. Low voltage complexes in ECG are seen in:

A. Cardiac tamponade
B. Pericardial effusion
C. Restrictive cardiomyopathy
D. All of the above

Explanation:

Low voltage complexes defined as

- The amplitude of all the QRS complexes in the limb leads are < 5 mm **or**
- The amplitude of all the QRS complexes in the precordial leads (v1-v6) are < 10 mm.

Common causes are cardiac tamponade, restrictive cardiomyopathy, pericardial effusion. Other causes like pleural effusion, constrictive pericarditis, emphysema, pneumothorax obesity.

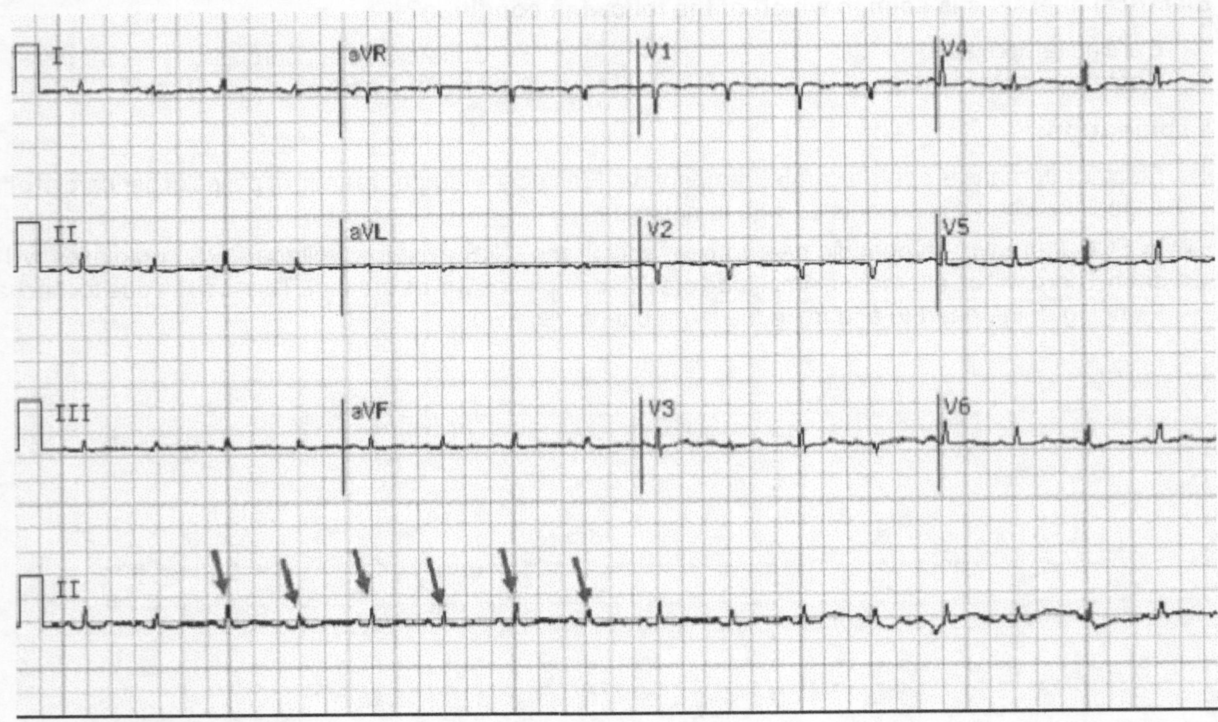

Above ECG suggestive of low voltage complexes.

Ans. D

30. In which of the following condition prominent x descent present but absent y descent in JVP?

A. Cardiac tamponade
B. Constrictive pericarditis
C. Restrictive cardiomyopathy
D. Right ventricular wall myocardial infarction

Explanation:

- In JVP the prominent x descent and absent y descent is seen in cardiac tamponade .Whereas in case of constrictive pericarditis there is both prominent x and y descent present.
- Filling pressure of the heart (myocardial transmural pressure) =
- Intracavitary pressure (ventricular) – pericardial pressure.
- In cardiac tamponade pericardial pressure is more than intracavitary pressure thus it reduced venous return to heart thus causing alteration in JVP. Normally venous return occurs in two phases: i.e. systolic and diastolic. In cardiac tamponade the pericardial pressure is elevated in both the phases except in the short brief period in systolic phase where pericardial pressure decreases and venous filling occurs causing prominent x descent, but pericardial pressure does not decreases in diastolic phase so no prominent y descent is present.

- In contrast to cardiac tamponade, in constrictive pericarditis pericardial pressure falls in both during the systolic phase and during initial one third of diastolic phase thus both x and y prominent descent are present

Table: Features that distinguish cardiac tamponade from constrictive pericarditis and similar clinical disorders

Characteristic	Tamponade	Constrictive Pericarditis	Restrictive Cardiomyopathy	RVMI	Effusive Constrictive Pericarditis
Clinical					
Pulsus paradoxus	+++	+	+	+	+++
Jugular veins					
• Prominent y descent	–	++	+	+	–
• Prominent x descent	+++	++	+++	+	+++
• Kussmaul's sign	–	+++	+	+++	++
Third heart sound	–	–	+	+	+
Pericardial knock	–	++	–	–	–
Electrocardiogram					
Low ECG voltage	++	++	+	–	+
Electrical alternans	++	–	–	–	–
Echocardiogram					
Thickened pericardium	–	+++	–	–	++
Pericardial calcification	–	++	–	–	–
Pericardial effusion	+++	–	–	–	++
RV size	Usually small	Usually normal	Usually normal	Enlarged	Usually normal
Exaggerated respiratory variation in flow velocity	+++	+++	–	+++	+
CT/MRI					
Thickened pericardium	–	+++	–		++
Equalization of diastolic pressures	+++	+++	–	++	++

Ans. A

31. In dilated cardiomyopathy Left ventricular diastolic dimension is:

A. > 60 mm

B. > 55 mm

C. > 50 mm

D. >65 mm

Explanation:

In DCMP the left ventricular diastolic dimension is greater or equal to 60 mm. Normally it is < 55mm.

Thus in DCMP there is systolic dysfunction as ventricles are dilated and not able to contract sufficiently.

Table: Presentation with symptomatic cardiomyopathy

	Dilated	Restrictive	Hypertrophic
Ejection fraction (normal > 55%)	Usually < 30% when symptoms severe	25-50%	> 60%
Left ventricular diastolic dimension (normal < 55 mm)	≥ 60 mm	<60 mm (may be decreased)	Often decreased
Left ventricular wall thickness	Normal or decreased	Normal or increased	Markedly increased
Atrial size	Increased, may also be primarily affected	Increased; may be massive	Increased; related to elevated filling pressures

Contd.

Valvular regurgitation	Related to annular dilation; mitral appears earlier during decompensation; tricuspid regurgitation with right ventricular dysfunction	Related to endocardial involvement; frequent mitral and tricuspid regurgitation, rarely severe	Related to valve-septum interaction; mitral regurgitation
Common first symptoms	Exertional intolerance	Exertional intolerance, fluid retention early, may have dominant right-sided symptoms	Exertional intolerance; may have chest pain
Congestive symptoms[a]	Left before right, except right prominent in young adults	Right often dominates	Left sided congestion at rest may develop late
Arrhythmias	Ventricular tachyarrhythmia; conduction block in Chagas' disease, and some families, Atrial fibrillation	Ventricular uncommon except in sarcoidosis, conduction block in sarcoidosis and amyloidosis, Atrial fibrillation	Ventricular tachyarrhythmias; atrial fibrillation

Ans. A

32. Which of the following infection causes dilated cardiomyopathy?

A. Borrelia burgdorferi

B. T.cruzi

C. Toxoplasma

D. All of the above

Explanation:

- All of the above mentioned infections causes DCMP. Other common causes are given in the box below.

Table: Major causes of dilated cardiomyopathy (with common examples)

Inflammatory Myocarditis

- **Infective**
  - Viral (coxsackie,[a] adenovirus,[a] HIV, hepatitis C)
  - Parasitic (*T. cruzi*–Chagas' disease, trypanosomiasis, toxoplasmosis)
  - Bacterial (diphtheria)
  - Spirochetal (*Borrelia burgdorferi*–Lyme disease)
  - Rickettsial (Q fever)
  - Fungal (with systemic infection)
- **Noninfective**
  - Granulomatous inflammatory disease
    - Sarcoidosis
    - Giant cell myocarditis
  - Eosinophilic myocarditis
  - Polymyositis, dermatomyositis
  - Collagen vascular disease
  - Checkpoint inhibitor chemotherapy
  - Transplant rejection

Toxic

- Alocohol
- **Catecholamines:** Amphetamines, cocaine
- Chemotherapeutic agents (anthracyclines, trastuzumab)
- Interferon
- Other therapeutic agents (hydroxychloroquine, chloroquine)
- Drugs of misuse (emetine, anabolic steroids)
- **Heavy metals:** Lead, mercury
- **Occupational exposure:** Hydrocarbons, arsenicals

Metabolic[a]
• **Nutritional deficiencies:** Thiamine, selenium, carnitine • **Electrolyte deficiencies:** Calcium, phosphate, magnesium • **Endocrinopathy** – Thyroid disease – Pheochromocytoma – Diabetes • Obesity • Hemochromatosis
Inherited Metabolic Pathway Defects[a] **Familial[a] (See Table 254-3)**
• Skeletal and cardiac myopathy • Dystrophin-related dystrophy (Duchenne's, Becker's) • Mitochondrial myopathies (e.g., Kearns-Sayre syndrome) • Arrhythmogenic ventricular cardiomyopathy • Hemochromatosis • Associated with other systemic diseases • Susceptibility to immune-mediated myocarditis
Overlap with Nondilated Cardiomyopathy
• "Minimally dilated cardiomyopathy" • Hemochromatosis[a] • Amyloidosis[a] • Hypertrophic cardiomyopathy[a] ("burned-out")
"Idiopathic"[a] **Miscellaneous (Shared Elements of Above Etiologies)**
• Peripartum cardiomyopathy • Left ventricular noncompaction[a] • Tachycardia-related cardiomyopathy – Supraventricular arrhythmias with uncontrolled rate – Very frequent nonsustained ventricular tachycardia or high premature ventricular complex burden

Ans. D

33. Chagas disease causes which of the following abnormalities?

A. SA node dysfunction
B. AV node dysfunction
C. Right bundle branch block
D. All of the above

Explanation:

- Features typical of Chagas disease are SA NODE and AV NODE dysfunction and RBBB. Atrial fibrillation and ventricular tachyarrhythmias also occur. Small ventricular aneurysms are also present at the apex.
- It is caused by T.CRUZI protozoan transmitted by the bite of reduviid bug, endemic in south and Central America.
- The acute phase of Chagas disease manifests as acute myocarditis or meningoencephalitis.
- Chronically it manifest in the cardiac and gastrointestinal systems.
- Most common infective cause of cardiomyopathy.
- Treatment given is antiparasitic with benznidazole and nifurtimox.

Ans. D

34. Peri partum cardiomyopathy develops during:

A. Within first 6 months
B. Within first 6 weeks
C. Within first 6 days
D. Within 1 year

Explanation:

- Peripartum cardiomyopathy develops during last trimester or with in first 6 months after pregnancy.
- It is reversible type of cardiomyopathy.
- High risk factors include increased maternal age, increased parity, twins pregnancy, malnutrition.
- Preclampsia.

Ans. A

35. Alcohol induced dilated cardiomyopathy occurs when alcohol consumed in amount:

A. 5 to 6 drinks daily for 5 – 10 years
B. 3 to 4 drinks daily for 5 – 10 years
C. 2 to 3 drinks daily for 5 – 10 years
D. None of the above

Explanation:

- Alcohol consumption sufficient to cause dilated cardiomyopathy is in an otherwise normal heart is 5 to 6 drinks (1 drink = 10 g of ethanol) daily to 5 to 10 years but frequent binge alcohol drinking (> 5 drinks in male and > 4 drinks in females within 2 hours) also causes.
- Alcohol is the most common toxin causing dilated cardiomyopathy. Toxicity is due to alcohol and its metabolite acetaldehyde.
- Atrial fibrillation occurs commonly both early in disease (holiday heart) and in advanced stages. Sudden death is seen. It is reversible if cessation of alcohol is done.
- Even with severe disease, marked improvement can occur within 3 to 6 months of abstinence.
- Other toxic compounds causing dilated cardiomyopathy are cocaine, amphetamines and related catecholaminergic stimulants.

Ans. A

36. Which of the following causes reversible dilated cardiomyopathy?

A. Alcohol induced
B. Peripartum
C. Beri beri heart disease
D. All of the above

Explanation:

Reversible dilated cardiomyopathy is seen in conditions like:

1. Alcohol induced
2. Nutritional deficiencies like selenium, thiamine, carnitine deficiency
3. Peripartum
4. Tachycardia induced like in hyperthyroidism, hyperdynamic circulatory states (anemia, fever)
5. Drug induced
6. Toxin induced like alcohol, cocaine, amphetamines, lead, mercury, arsenic.

In all above conditions when the causative agent is removed then cardiomyopathy is reversed & normal cardiac function is restored.

Ans. D

37. Systolic dysfunction is seen in which of the following condition?

A. Dilated cardiomyopathy
B. Restrictive cardiomyopathy
C. Hypertrophic cardiomyopathy
D. Infilterative cardiomyopathy

Explanation:

Table: Presentation with symptomatic cardiomyopathy

	Dilated	Restrictive	Hypertrophic
Ejection fraction (normal > 55%)	Usually < 30% when symptoms severe	25-50%	>60%
Left ventricular diastolic dimension (normal < 55 mm)	≥ 60 mm	< 60 mm (may be decreased)	Often decresed
Left ventricular wall thickness	Normal or decreased	Normal or increased	Markedly increased
Atrial size	Increased, may also be primarily affected	Increased; may be massive	Increased; related to elevated filling pressures
Valvular regurgitation	Related to annular dilation; mitral appears earlier during decompensation; tricuspid regurgitation with right ventricular dysfunction	Related to endocardial involvement; frequent mitral and tricuspid regurgitation, rarely severe	Related to valve-septum interaction; mitral regurgitation
Common first symptoms	Exertional intolerance	Exertional intolerance, fluid retention early, may have dominant right-sided symptoms	Exertional intolerance; may have chest pain
Congestive symptoms[a]	Left before right, except right prominent in young adults	Right often dominates	Left-sided congestion at rest may develop late
Arrhythmias	Ventricular tachyarrhythmia; conduction block in Chagas' disease and some families, Atrial fibrillation	Ventricular uncommon except in sarcoidosis, conduction block in sarcoidosis and amyloidosis, Atrial fibrillation	Ventricular tachyarrhythmias; atrial fibrillation

- In case of dilated cardiomyopathy systolic dysfunction is seen as there is reduced contractility of heart due to dilated left ventricular diastolic dimension causing impaired pumping.
- In cases of restrictive and Hypertrophic cardiomyopathy there is diastolic dysfunction.
- Infiltrative cardiomyopathy are among the causes of restrictive cardiomyopathy thus causing diastolic dysfunction.

Ans. A

38. Takotsubo Cardiomyopathy is also known as:

A. Apical ballooning syndrome
B. Stress induced cardiomyopathy
C. Both A and B
D. Arrythmogenic right ventricular dysplasia

Explanation:

- Takotsubo cardiomyopathy is also known as stress induced cardio myopathy or apical ballooning syndrome, which occurs typically in older women with sudden outburst of intense emotional or physical stress.

- Ventricles shows global ventricular dilation with basal contractions, forming shape of the narrow -necked jar (takotsubo) used in japan to trap octopuses.
- Presentation include pulmonary edema, hypotension, and chest pain with ECG suggestive of ST elevation and or deep T wave inversion.
- On performing angiography no obstruction is evident in coronary vessels.
- It is an reversible condition, all the changes reverse within days to weeks.
- It occurs due to release of catecholaminergic compounds present in body after physical stress or emotional stress causing contraction of coronary vessels.
- Managed by combined alpha plus beta blockers rather than selective beta blocker.

Ans. C

39. A 28 years old male patient came with history of angina on exertion since 5 days, dyspnea since 4 days in emergency. His BP and other vitals were normal. CXR was normal. ECG done suggestive of left ventricular hypertrophy so nitrate was given sublingually which did not relieved the pain instead aggravated it. He also gave history of recurrent chest pains on exertion. What is your probable diagnosis?

A. Unstable angina
B. Hypertrophic obstructive cardiomyopathy
C. Mitral valve prolapse
D. Aortic stenosis

Explanation:

- In above question the patient is young with past history of similar angina, dyspnea episodes along with angina not relieved with nitrates with ECG suggestive of LVH most likely HOCM.
- HOCM is seen in young adults and it is the leading cause of sudden death in young.
- Most commonly it is asymptomatic, clinical features include angina, dyspnea, palpitations.
- Family history of sudden death or similar complaints is often present.
- ECG s/o left ventricular hypertrophy changes
- 2 D ECHO is best test to diagnose HOCM suggestive of asymmetrical septal hypertrophy with systolic anterior movement of mitral valve
- Pain is not relieved by nitrates in HOCM.
- An harsh diamond shaped systolic murmur is heard in HOCM best heard in left sternal border.
- Murmur of HOCM decreases in intensity with maneuvers that increase venous return and thus increasing blood in left ventricle causing movement of muscular obstruction protruding into the outflow tract away from the opposite wall decreasing the obstruction and thus the murmur. So hand grip, squatting, supine position with legs elevated causes decrease in murmur as they all increase venous return to heart .
- Opposite will occur with manuevers like Valsalva, standing, exercise, amyl nitrite, as these causes reduced blood in left ventricle causing decrease in left ventricular size thus increases the outflow obstruction and intensity of murmur.
- HOCM is managed with beta blockers.
- In case of unstable angina pain is very severe and occurs at rest, lasting more than 10 minutes, follows crescendo pattern. ECG is usually normal, but may show ST depression, flat or inverted T waves. Nitrates reduces pain and do not aggravate pain.
- In case of mitral valve prolapse patients are most commonly asymptomatic and clinical features like palpitation, syncope, chest pain can occur. It is commonly seen in young females mid to late systolic clicks heard.
- In case of aortic stenosis, angina , dyspnea ,syncope are the cardinal symptoms. Nitrates do not aggravate pain in AS.

Ans. B

40. Heart failure with reduced ejection fraction is called when ejection fraction is:

A. < 30%
B. < 35%
C. < 40%
D. < 45%

Explanation:

Table: Etiologies of heart failure	
Depressed Ejection Fraction (<40%)	
Coronary artery disease • Myocardial infarction[a] • Myocardial ischemia[a] Chronic pressure overload • Hypertension[a] • Obstructive valvular disease[a] Chronic volume overload • Regurgitant valvular disease • Intracardiac (left-to-right) shunting • Extracardiac shunting Chronic lung disease • Cor pulmonale • Pulmonary vascular disorders	Nonischemic dilated cardiomyopathy • Familial/genetic disorders • Infiltrative disorders[a] Toxic/drug-induced damage • Metabolic disorder[a] • Viral Chagas' disease Disorders of rate and rhythm • Chronic bradyarrhythmias • Chronic tachyarrhythmias
Preserved Ejection Fraction (>40-50%)	
• Pathologic hypertrophy • Primary (hypertrophic cardiomyopathies) • Secondary (hypertension) Aging Endomyocardial disorders	Restrictive cardiomyopathy • Infiltrative disorders (amyloidosis, sarcoidosis) • Storage diseases (hemochromatosis) Fibrosis
High-Output States	
Metabolic disorders • Thyrotoxicosis • Nutritional disorders (beriberi)	Excessive blood flow requirements • Systemic arteriovenous shunting • Chronic anemia
[a]Indicates conditions that can also lead to heart failure with a preserved ejection fraction.	

- Heart failure is now classified as heart failure with reduced ejection fraction (< 40%) and heart failure with preserved ejection fraction (> 40%)

Ans. C

41. Sudden death is seen in which of the following condition?

A. HOCM
B. Dilated cardiomyopathy
C. Mitral valve relapse
D. All of the above

Explanation:

- Sudden death is seen in HOCM, dilated cardiomyopathy, mitral valve prolapse.
- Other condition like aortic stenosis, arrhythmogenic right ventricular cardiomyopathy /dysplasia.
- Family history of sudden death in often present in HOCM, dilated cardiomyopathy.

Ans. D

42. Anginal pain is not relieved with nitrates in which condition?

A. Aortic stenosis
B. Mitral regurgitation
C. Hypertrophic obstructive cardiomyopathy
D. Aortic regurgitation

Explanation:

- Nitrates causes reduction in pre load thus causing reduced venous return, so less blood will enter left ventricle causing decrease in left ventricular size that will cause more protrusion of obstruction into outflow tract thus increases the outflow obstruction and thus aggravates pain.
- Maneuvers that increase venous return and thus increasing blood in left ventricle causing movement of muscular obstruction protruding into the outflow tract away from the opposite wall decreasing the obstruction and thus the murmur. So hand grip, squatting, supine position with legs elevated causes decrease in murmur as they all increase venous return to heart.
- Opposite will occur with manuevers like Valsalva, standing, exercise, amyl nitrite. As these causes reduced blood in left ventricle causing decrease in left ventricular size thus increases the outflow obstruction and intensity of murmur.
- In all other options pain is relieved with nitrates.

Ans. C

43. All are true about Infective endocarditis due to P. aeruginosa except:

A. Disease is more indolent than Staphylococcus aureus endocarditis
B. Patients experience chest pain and hemoptysis more than seen by Staphylococcus aureus endocarditis
C. Infective endocarditis due to P. aeruginosa is a disease of IV drug users whose native valves are involved
D. Skin manifestations are rare in this disease, but ecthyma gangrenosum is seen

Explanation:

- Infective endocarditis due to *P. aeruginosa* is a disease of IV drug users whose native valves are involved.
- This organism has also been reported to cause prosthetic-valve endocarditis.
- Sites of prior native-valve injury due to the injection of foreign material such as talc or fibers probably serve as niduses for bacterial attachment to the heart valve.
- Manifestations of *P. aeruginosa* endocarditis resemble those of other forms of endocarditis in IV drug users except that the disease is more indolent than *Staphylococcus aureus* endocarditis.
- While most disease involves the right side of the heart, left-sided involvement is not rare and multivalvular disease is common.
- Fever is a common manifestation, as is pulmonary involvement (due to septic emboli to the lungs).
- Thus, patients may also experience chest pain and hemoptysis.
- Involvement of the left side of the heart may lead to signs of cardiac failure, systemic emboli, and local cardiac involvement with sinus of Valsalva abscesses and conduction defects.
- Skin manifestations are rare in this disease, and ecthyma gangrenosum is not seen.
- Diagnosis is based on positive blood cultures along with clinical signs of endocarditis.

Ans. D

44. For the management of patients post myocardial infarction, which is correct?

A. Pioglitazone should be started in patients post MI
B. Metformin should be stopped in all patients post MI
C. Metformin can be used in patients with congestive heart failure
D. Metformin should be stopped in patients who have an unstable congestive heart failure

Explanation:

- Unstable congestive heart failure increases the risk of hypoperfusion and acute kidney injury. These are the risk factors for the development of lactic acidosis in patients on metformin and should be avoided in these patients.

Ans. D

45. False about treatment of carotid atherosclerosis is:

A. Endarterectomy is most beneficial when performed within 4 weeks of symptom onset

B. Benefit is more pronounced in patients >75 years

C. Men appear to benefit more than women

D. An institutional perioperative morbidity and mortality rate of ≤6% generally should undergo carotid endarterectomy

Explanation:

- Recent meta-analysis of the NASCET and ECST trials demonstrated that endarterectomy is most beneficial when performed within 2 weeks of symptom onset.
- In addition, benefit is more pronounced in patients >75 years, and men appear to benefit more than women.

Ans. A

46. Postoperative low cardiac output syndrome is seen after:

A. Drainage of massive pleural effusion

B. Drainage of massive ascites

C. Drainage of pericardial effusion

D. Drainage of spinal fluid

Explanation:

- Thoracoscopic pericardial fenestration can be employed for benign causes; however, 60% of malignant pericardial effusions recur after this procedure.
- In a subset of patients, drainage of the pericardial effusion is paradoxically followed by worsening hemodynamic instability.
- This so-called "postoperative low cardiac output syndrome" occurs in up to 10% of patients undergoing surgical drainage and carries poor short-term survival.

Ans. C

47. A 50 year old female was diagnosed with right upper lobe mass lesion. Which among the following is the non ionizing imaging modality that will aid in taking a biopsy from the mass?

A. Chest X-ray

B. Computed tomography scan

C. PET CT

D. USG

Explanation:

- Diagnostic ultrasound is a non ionizing imaging approach which is safe to perform on pregnant women and children. It can detect and localize pleural abnormalities and guide thoracocentesis of a pleural effusion.

Ans. D

48. Which of the following do not cause heart failure with reduced ejection fraction?

A. Myocardial infarction

B. Cor pulmonale

C. Chagas disease

D. Restrictive cardiomyopathy

Explanation:

Table: Etiologies of heart failure	
Depressed Ejection Fraction (< 40%)	
Coronary artery disease • Myocardial infarction[a] • Myocardial ischemia[a] Chronic pressure overload • Hypertension[a] • Obstructive valvular disease[a] Chronic volume overload • Regurgitant valvular disease • Intracardiac (left-to-right) shunting • Extracardiac shunting Chronic lung disease • Cor pulmonale • Pulmonary vascular disorders	Nonischemic dilated cardiomyopathy • Familial/genetic disorders • Infiltrative disorders[a] Toxic/drug-induced damage • Metabolic disorder[a] • Viral Chagas' disease Disorders of rate and rhythm • Chronic bradyarrhythmias • Chronic tachyarrhythmias
Preserved Ejection Fraction (>40-50%)	
Pathologic hypertrophy • Primary (hypertrophic cardiomyopathies) • Secondary (hypertension) Aging Endomyocardial disorders	Restrictive cardiomyopathy • Infiltrative disorders (amyloidosis, sarcoidosis) • Storage diseases (hemochromatosis) Fibrosis
High-Output States	
Metabolic disorders • Thyrotoxicosis Nutritional disorders (beriberi)	Excessive blood flow requirements • Systemic arteriovenous shunting • Chronic anemia
[a]Indicates conditions that can also lead to heart failure with a preserved ejection fraction.	

- *MI, Chagas disease, Cor pulmonale all can cause reduced ejection.*
- Restrictive cardiomyopathy causes heart failure with preserved ejection fraction. It causes diastolic heart failure and systolic function of heart is well preserved.

Ans. D

49. Thrombolysis in myocardial infarction score (TIMI score) is used in assessment of risk of ischemic events or risk of mortality in case of:

A. ST elevated Myocardial infarction
B. Non ST segment elevated Myocardial infarction
C. Unstable angina
D. Both B and C

Explanation:

- TIMI score stands thrombolysis in myocardial infarction is used to predict early risk of death (30 days) and risk of ischemic events in case of NSTEMI/UA.

Includes following risk factors:

1. Age >/= 65 years
2. >/=3 CAD risk factors
3. Known CAD
4. Prior aspirin use
5. >/=2 anginal episodes in prior 24 hours
6. ST deviation >/=0.5mm of initial ECG
7. Increased cardiac biomarkers

Additional risk factors in TIMI score:

1. CHF
2. Hypertension
3. Age >/= 75 Years
4. Diabetes Mellitus
5. Prior Stroke
6. Prior Cabg
7. Peripheral Artery Disease
8. Egfr < 60 ml/min /1.732 m2
9. Current smoking

Ans. D

50. In HEART score, which of the following carry 2 points in ECG Changes?

A. ST segment elevation
B. Significant ST depression
C. Non specific abnormality
D. T wave inversion

Explanation:

Heart Score		
History	Highly suspicious	2
	Moderately suspicious	1
	Slightly suspicious	0
ECG	Significant ST-depression	2
	Non-specific abnormality	1
	Normal	0
Age	≥ 65 years	2
	45-< 65 years	1
	< 45 years	0
Risk factors	≥ Risk factors	2
	1-2 Risk factors	1
	None	0
Troponin (serial)	≥ 3 × 99th percentile	2
	1-< 3 × 99th percentile	1
	≤ 99th percentile	0
	Total	
Low-risk: 0-3 Not low risk: ≥4		

North America Chest Pain Rule	
High Risk Criteria	**Y/N**
Typical symptoms for ischemia	
ECG: Acute ischemic changes	
Age ≥ 50 years	
Known coronary artery disease	
Troponin (serial) ≥ 99th percentile	
Low-risk: All No **Not Low-risk:** Any Yes	

	Heart Score	North America Chest Pain Rule
Captured as Low-risk (%)	20.2	4.4
Sensitivity	99.1	100
Specificity	25.7	5.6

Ans. B

51. A patient presented with presyncopal attacks and palpitations and diagnosed as POTS (Postural Orthostatic Tachycardia syndrome). Which is false?

A. Increase in heart rate to >120/min or by 30 beats/min in standing position

B. Women are more affected

C. Associated with orthostatic fall of BP

D. Treated with propranolol and fludrocortisone

Explanation:

- POTS- Increase in heart rate to >120/min or by 30 beats/min in standing position without hypotension
- Associated with presyncopal symptoms
- Pathogenesis- sympathetic denervation distally in the legs with preserved cardiovascular function

Ans. C

52. A 50 year old male develops acute MI after contracting COVID 19 infection. He develops cardiogenic shock secondary to MI. Inotropic agents to be used in shock include all except:

A. Norepinephrine is first-line agent in distributive shock

B. Dobutamine as second choice in distributive/septic shock

C. Dobutamine can be used in cardiogenic shock

D. Norepinephrine can also be used in cardiogenic shock

Explanation:

Vasopressor and/or Inotropic Agents used in shock

- Norepinephrine is first-line agent in distributive shock
- Consider vasopressin as second choice in distributive/septic shock
- Consider dobutamine in cardiogenic shock (can combine with norepinephrine, if needed for BP support).

Ans. B

53. All the following are upregulated in heart failure with ejection fraction reduced except:

A. Angiotensin II

B. BNP

C. Calcium uptake in sarcoplasmic reticulum

D. Norepinephrine

Explanation:

- **Following are upregulated in failing heart–** Angiotensin II, Aldosterone, Arginine vasopressin along with norepinephrine.
- Brain natriuretic peptide is also upregulated that aids in reducing systemic vascular resistance & natriuresis.
- In heart failure, transcriptional & post transcriptional changes in myocyte leads to calcium leakage through sarcoplasmic reticular membrane & therefore decreased calcium uptake in sarcoplasmic reticulum.

Ans. C

CHAPTER 4

ENDOCRINOLOGY

1. True about autoimmune polyendocrine syndrome type 1 is:

A. Polygenic

B. Late onset

C. Equivalent sex distribution

D. No defined immunodeficiency

Explanation:

APS-1	APS-2
Early onset: Infancy	Later onset
Siblings often affected and at risk	Multigenerational
Equivalent sex distribution	Females > males affected
Monogenic: *AIRE* gene, chromosome 21, autosomal recessive	Polygenic: *HLA, MICA, PTNP22, CTLA4*
Not HLA associated for entire syndrome, some specific component risk	DR3/DR4 associated; other HLA class III gene associations noted
Autoantibodies to type 1 interferons and IL-17 and IL-22	No autoantibodies to cytokines
Autoantibodies to specific target organs	Autoantibodies to specific target organs
Asplenism	No defined immunodeficiency
Mucocutaneous candidiasis	Association with other nonendocrine immunologic disorders like myasthenia gravis and idiopathic thrombocytopenic purpura

Ans. C

2. Fasting plasma glucose levels above which OHA will not be efficacious is:

A. 5.6 mmol/L

B. 7 mmol/L

C. 9.8 mmol/L

D. 11.1 mmol/L

Explanation:

- FPG is near the normal range, oral diabetes agents (e.g., sulfonylureas, metformin) may be sufficient to reduce hyperglycemia.
- If the FPG is >11.1 mmol/L (200 mg/dL), oral agents are usually not efficacious, and insulin therapy is required.

Ans. D

3. **T4 is given in case of congenital hypothyroidism at a dose of:**

A. 1-5 µg/kg per day
B. 10-15 µg/kg per day
C. 15-20 µg/kg per day
D. 20- 30 µg/kg per day

Explanation:

- When diagnosis is confirmed, T4 is instituted at a dose of 10–15 µg/kg per day, and the dose is adjusted by close monitoring of TSH levels.
- T4 requirements are relatively great during the first year of life, and a high circulating T4 level is usually needed to normalize TSH.
- Early treatment with T4 results in normal IQ levels, but subtle neurodevelopmental abnormalities may occur in those with the most severe hypothyroidism at diagnosis or when treatment is delayed or suboptimal.
- If transient hypothyroidism is suspected, or the diagnosis is unclear, treatment can be stopped safely after the age of 3 years followed by further evaluation.

Ans. B

4. **Not true about silent thyroiditis is:**

A. Painless thyroiditis that occurs in patients underlying autoimmune thyroid disease
B. Occurs in upto 5% of women 3-6 months after pregnancy & is then termed as postpartum thyroiditis
C. TPO +ve more common in women with Type 1 Diabetes mellitus
D. Glucocorticoid is treatment of choice

Explanation:

- *Painless thyroiditis*, or "*silent*" *thyroiditis*, occurs in patients with underlying autoimmune thyroid disease and has a clinical course similar to that of subacute thyroiditis.
- Condition occurs in up to 5% of women 3–6 months after pregnancy and is then termed *postpartum thyroiditis*.
- Typically, patients have a brief phase of thyrotoxicosis lasting 2–4 weeks, followed by hypothyroidism for 4–12 weeks, and then resolution; often, however, only one phase is apparent.
- Condition is associated with the presence of TPO antibodies antepartum, and it is three times more common in women with type 1 diabetes mellitus.
- As in subacute thyroiditis, the uptake of 99mTc pertechnetate or radioactive iodine is initially suppressed. In addition to the painless goiter, silent thyroiditis can be distinguished from subacute thyroiditis by a normal ESR and the presence of TPO antibodies.
- Glucocorticoid treatment is not indicated for silent thyroiditis.
- Severe thyrotoxic symptoms can be managed with a brief course of propranolol, 20–40 mg three or four times daily.
- Thyroxine replacement may be needed for the hypothyroid phase but should be withdrawn after 6–9 months, as recovery is the rule.
- Annual follow-up thereafter is recommended, because a proportion of these individuals develop permanent hypothyroidism.
- Condition may recur in subsequent pregnancy

Ans. D

5. **A 62-year-old female with a history of poorly controlled diabetes presents with left leg weakness. This initially began with severe left hip pain. Over the course of several weeks, she had weakness in her left leg and loss of muscle mass in the left thigh. She has minimal numbness, but has noted significant weight loss. Her examination demonstrates weakness of left hip flexion, knee flexion, and knee extension, but normal foot plantar flexion and dorsiflexion. Left patellar and ankle reflexes were**

absent. There was no incontinence. Magnetic resonance imaging of her lumbar spine and lumbosacral plexus were normal. Laboratory work, including complete blood count, complete metabolic panel, sedimentation rate, and C-reactive protein (CRP) were normal. Which of the following is true of this condition?

A. Standard treatment involves 1 gram of intravenous methylprednisolone over 5 days

B. Standard treatment involves physical therapy

C. Sural nerve biopsy is necessary for the diagnosis

D. Genetic testing for SEPT9 gene should be performed

Explanation:

- This patient has diabetic radiculoplexopathy, formerly known as diabetic amyotrophy. This is a condition usually occurring in patients over the age of 50, usually during times of uncontrolled diabetes. Initially, it presents with severe hip, back, or leg pain for a few days and is followed by weight loss and muscle atrophy in the proximal leg that eventually stabilizes. Over the course of several months, most have improvement in their strength. This can be a similar presentation to a vasculitic neuropathy; but with normal sedimentation rate and CRP, vasculitis is unlikely. A sural biopsy would be normal because the pathological abnormality is in the lumbosacral plexus.
- In cases of vasculitis, findings are more widespread, so biopsies can be helpful. SEPT9 mutations are seen in hereditary neuralgic amyotrophy, which typically affects the upper extremities. Diabetic radiculoplexopathy is generally a single event and does not require long-term immunosuppression.

Ans. B

6. **HLA Associated with congenital adrenal hyperplasia is:**

A. B51

B. B47

C. DR2

D. B57

Explanation:

Behçet's disease	B51
Congenital adrenal hyperplasia	B47
Narcolepsy	DR2
Goodpasture's syndrome (anti-GBM)	DR2
Abacavir hypersensitivity	B57

Ans. B

7. **Total number of Aminoacids in amyloid polypeptide protein secreted by Pancreatic beta cells is:**

A. 21

B. 30

C. 37

D. 52

Explanation:

- **Pancreatic beta cells co-secrete islet amyloid polypeptide (IAPP) or amylin, a 37-amino-acid peptide, along with insulin.**
- Role of IAPP in normal physiology is incompletely defined, but it is major component of the amyloid fibrils found in the islets of patients with type 2 diabetes, and an analogue is sometimes used in treating type 1 and type 2 DM.
- Human insulin is produced by recombinant DNA technology; structural modifications at one or more amino acid residues modify insulin's physical and pharmacologic characteristics.

Ans. C

8. Type of MODY that responds to Sulfonylurea is:

A. MODY 1
B. MODY 3
C. MODY 4
D. MODY 5

Explanation:

- Individuals with an HNF-1mutation (MODY 3) have a progressive decline in glycemic control but may respond to sulfonylureas.

Ans. B

9. All are common endocrine abnormality in both autoimmune poly endocrine syndrome type 1 & 2 except:

A. Addison disease
B. Hypoparathyroidism
C. Grave's disease
D. Type 1 diabetes

Explanation:

Table: Disease associations with autoimmune polyendocrine syndromes

Autoimmune Polyendocrine Syndrome Type 1	Autoimmune Polyendocrine Syndrome Type 2	Other Autoimmune Polyendocrine Disorders
Endocrine	**Endocrine**	IPEX (immune dysfunction polyendocrinopathy X-linked)
• Addison's disease	Addison's disease	Thymic tumors
• Hypoparathyroidism	Type 1 diabetes	Anti-insulin receptor antibodies
• Hypogonadism	Graves' disease or autoimmune thyroiditis	POEMS syndrome
• Graves' disease or autoimmune thyroiditis • Type 1 diabetes	Hypogonadism	Insulin autoimmune syndrome (Hirata's syndrome) Adult combined pituitary hormone deficiency (CPHD) with anti-Pit 1 autoantibodies Kearns-Sayre syndrome DIDMOAD syndrome
Nonendocrine	**Nonendocrine**	Congenital rubella associated with thyroiditis and/or diabetes
Mucocutaneous candidiasis	Celiac disease, dermatitis herpetiformis	
Chronic active hepatitis	Pernicious anemia	
Pernicious anemia	Vitiligo	
Vitiligo	Alopecia	
Asplenism	Myasthenia gravis	
Ectodermal dysplasia	IgA deficiency	
Alopecia	Parkinson's disease	
Malabsorption syndromes IgA deficiency	Idiopathic thrombocytopenia	

Ans. B

10. Which of the following conditions need insulin for survival?

A. GDM

B. Type 2 DM

C. Cushing's syndrome

D. None of the above

Explanation:

Type of Diabetes	Normal glucose tolerance	Hyperglycemia			
		Pre-diabetes*	Diabetes Mellitus		
		Impaired fasting glucose of impaired glucose tolerance	Not insulin requiring	Insulin required for control	Insulin required for survival
Type 1	→	→	→	→	→
Type 2	←	←	← →	→	
Specific types	←	←	← →	→	
Gestational diabetes	←	←	← →	→	
Time (years)	→	→	→	→	→
FPG	<5.6 mmol/l (100 mg/dl)	5.6-6.9 mmol/l (100-125 mg/dl)		≥70 mmol/l (126 mg/dl)	
2-h PG	<7.8 mmol/l (140 mg/dl)	7.8-11.0 mmol/l (140-199 mg/dl)		≥11.1 mmol/l (200 mg/dl)	
HbA1C	<5.6%	5.7-6.4%		≥6.5%	

- Spectrum from normal glucose tolerance to diabetes in type 1 DM, type 2 DM, specific types of diabetes, and gestational DM is shown from left to right. In most types of DM, the individual traverses from normal glucose tolerance to impaired glucose tolerance to overt diabetes (these should be viewed not as abrupt categories but as a spectrum).
- Arrows indicate that changes in glucose tolerance may be bidirectional in some types of diabetes. For example, individuals with type 2 DM may return to the impaired glucose tolerance category with weight loss; in gestational DM, diabetes may revert to impaired glucose tolerance or even normal glucose tolerance after delivery.
- Fasting plasma glucose (FPG), the 2-h plasma glucose (PG) after a glucose challenge, and the hemoglobin A1c (HbA1c) for the different categories of glucose tolerance are shown at the lower part of the figure. These values do not apply to the diagnosis of gestational DM.

Ans. D

11. Most common presenting feature of adult hypopituitarism:

A. Hypogonadism

B. Growth retardation

C. Hypoglycemia

D. Mental retardation

Explanation:

- **Hypogonadism is most common presenting** feature of adult hypo-pituitarism even when other pituitary hormones are also deficient.
- It is often a harbinger of hypothalamic or pituitary lesions that impair GnRH production or delivery through the pituitary stalk.
- Hypogonadotropic hypogonadism is a common presenting feature of hyperprolactinemia.

Ans. A

12. Major portion of postprandial glucose is used by:

A. Adipocytes
B. Brain
C. Skeletal muscle
D. Liver

Explanation:

- Glucagon, secreted by pancreatic alpha cells normally only when blood glucose or insulin levels are low or during exercise, is increased in DM and stimulates glycogenolysis and gluconeogenesis by liver and to a small degree by the renal medulla.
- Postprandially, the glucose load elicits a rise in insulin and fall in glucagon, leading to a reversal of these processes.
- Insulin, an anabolic hormone, promotes the storage of carbohydrate and fat and protein synthesis.
- Major portion of postprandial glucose is used by skeletal muscle, an effect of insulin-stimulated glucose uptake.
- Other tissues, most notably the brain, use glucose in an insulin independent fashion.
- Factors secreted by skeletal myocytes, adipocytes (leptin, resistin, adiponectin, etc.), and bone also influence glucose homeostasis.

Ans. C

13. Which of the following is indicative of beta cell dysfunction?

A. C peptide
B. Proinsulin
C. Amylin
D. Preproinsulin

Explanation:

- Insulin, produced by the beta cells of the pancreatic islets, is initially synthesized as a single-chain 86-amino-acid precursor polypeptide, preproinsulin.
- Subsequent proteolytic processing removes the amino-terminal signal peptide, giving rise to proinsulin.
- Proinsulin is structurally related to insulin-like growth factors I and II, which bind weakly to the insulin receptor.
- Cleavage of an internal 31-residue fragment from proinsulin generates C-peptide with A (21 amino acids) and B (30 amino acids) chains of insulin being connected by disulfide bonds.
- Mature insulin molecule and C-peptide are stored together and co-secreted from secretory granules in the beta cells.
- Because C-peptide is cleared more slowly than insulin, it is a useful marker of insulin secretion and allows discrimination of endogenous and exogenous sources of insulin in the evaluation of hypoglycaemia.
- Elevated levels of serum proinsulin have been observed in both type 1 and 2 DM and are thought to be indicative of beta cell dysfunction.
- Pancreatic beta cells co-secrete islet amyloid polypeptide (IAPP) or amylin, a 37-amino-acid peptide, along with insulin.
- Role of IAPP in normal physiology is incompletely defined, but it is major component of amyloid fibrils found in islets of patients with type 2 DM, and an analogue is sometimes used in treating type 1 & type 2 DM.

Ans. B

14. ATP sensitive K channels in beta cells of Pancreas is important in the action of which drug:

A. Voglibose
B. Meglitinides
C. GLP-1 analogues
D. IV glucose

Explanation:

Glucose is the key regulator of insulin secretion by the pancreatic beta cell, although amino acids, ketones, various nutrients, gastrointestinal peptides, and neurotransmitters also influence insulin secretion. Glucose levels >3.9 mmol/L (70 mg/dL) stimulate insulin synthesis, primarily by enhancing protein translation and processing.

- Glucose stimulation of insulin secretion begins with its transport into the beta cell by a facilitative glucose transporter .Glucose phosphorylation by glucokinase is the rate-limiting step that controls glucose-regulated insulin secretion.
- Further metabolism of glucose-6phosphate via glycolysis generates ATP, which inhibits the activity of an ATP-sensitive K+ channel. This channel consists of two separate proteins: one is the binding site for certain oral hypoglycemics (e.g., sulfonylureas, meglitinides); other is an inwardly rectifying K+ channel protein (Kir6.2). Inhibition of this K+ channel induces beta cell membrane depolarization, which opens voltage-dependent calcium channels (leading to an influx of calcium) and stimulates insulin secretion. Insulin secretory profiles reveal a pulsatile pattern of hormone release, with small secretory bursts occurring about every 10 min, superimposed upon greater amplitude oscillations of about 80–150 min.

Ans. B

15. Assertion(A): Patient diagnosed with diabetes doesn't need insulin for 2 years.
Reason(R): The diabetes mellitus type 1 has reserve beta cells.

A. Both (A) and (R) are correct and (R) explains (A)
B. Both (A) and (R) are correct but (R) doesn't explain (A)
C. (R) is correct But (A) is false
D. (A) is correct But (R) is false

Explanation:

Events that trigger the transition from glucose intolerance to frank diabetes are often associated with increased insulin requirements, as might occur during infections or at puberty. After the initial clinical presentation of type 1 DM, a "honeymoon" phase may ensue during which time glycemic control is achieved with modest doses of insulin or, rarely, insulin is not needed.

- However, this fleeting phase of endogenous insulin production from residual beta cells disappears and the individual becomes insulin deficient.
- Many individuals with longstanding type 1 DM produce a small amount of insulin (as reflected by C-peptide production), and some individuals with 50 years of type 1 DM have insulin-positive cells in the pancreas at autopsy.

Ans. A

16. All the calcium absorption processes are stimulated directly by PTH or Vit D except:

A. Proximal tubule paracellular route
B. Loop of Henle paracellular route
C. Absorption by cTAL
D. Transcellular route in DCT

Explanation:

- Most filtered calcium (65%) is reabsorbed in the proximal tubules via a passive, paracellular route that is coupled to concomitant NaCl reabsorption and not specifically regulated.
- Cortical thick ascending limb of Henle's loop (cTAL) reabsorbs roughly another 20% of filtered calcium, also via a paracellular mechanism.
- Calcium reabsorption in the cTAL requires a tight-junctional protein called paracellin-1 and is inhibited by increased blood concentrations of calcium or magnesium, acting via CaSR, which is highly expressed on basolateral membranes in this nephron segment.
- Operation of the renal CaSR provides a mechanism, independent of those engaged directly by PTH or 1,25(OH)2D, by which serum ionized calcium can control renal calcium reabsorption.
- Finally, ~10% of filtered calcium is reabsorbed in the distal convoluted tubules (DCTs) by a transcellular mechanism.
- Calcium enters the luminal surface of the cell through specific apical calcium channels (TRPV5), whose number is regulated. It then moves across cell in association with a specific calcium-binding protein (calbindinD28k) that buffers cytosolic calcium concentrations from the large mass of transported calcium.

Ca2+-ATPases and Na+/Ca2+ exchangers actively extrude calcium across basolateral surface and thereby maintain transcellular calcium gradient.

- All these processes are stimulated directly or indirectly by PTH.

Ans. C

17. Target BP in Type 2 DM patient with dyslipidemia & microalbuminuria is:

A. 130/80 mmHg
B. 140/90 mmHg
C. 120/80 mmHg
D. 150/90 mmHg

Explanation:

- Blood pressure should be maintained at <140/90 mmHg in individuals with diabetes and possibly <130/80 in individuals at increased risk for CVD and CKD progression.

Ans. A

18. Protective HLA for Type 1 Diabetes mellitus is:

A. DQ8
B. DR3
C. DR4
D. DR2

Explanation:

- **HLA risk factor for Type 1 DM**
- In decreasing order of risk DQ8 > DR4 > DR3
- DR2 - Strong negative association, that is, genetic association with protection from diabetes. This is the only PROTECTIVE HLA known as of now.

Ans. D

19. Most common mutation that can cause Pancreatic agenesis is:

A. GATA 6
B. Kir 6.2
C. ABCC 8
D. ICA 512/IA-2

Explanation:

- Mutations in the transcription factor GATA6 are the most common cause of pancreatic agenesis. Homozygous glucokinase mutations cause a severe form of neonatal diabetes, while mutations in mitochondrial DNA are associated with diabetes and deafness.

Ans. A

20. Increased levels of Thyroxine in Graves disease is caused by:

A. Thyroid stimulating immunoglobulin
B. Thyrotropin binding inhibitory immunoglobulin
C. Thyroglobulin antibodies
D. Thyroid peroxidase antibodies

Explanation:

- Hyperthyroidism of Graves' disease is caused by thyroid- stimulating immunoglobulin (TSI) that are synthesized in the thyroid gland as well as in bone marrow and lymph nodes.
- Such antibodies can be detected by bioassays or by using the more widely available thyrotropin-binding inhibitory immunoglobulin (TBII) assays.
- Presence of TBII in a patient with thyrotoxicosis implies the existence of TSI, and these assays are useful in monitoring pregnant Graves patients in whom high levels of TSI can cross placenta and cause neonatal thyrotoxicosis.

- Other thyroid autoimmune responses, similar to those in autoimmune hypothyroidism (see above), occur concurrently in patients with Graves' disease. In particular, thyroid peroxidase (TPO) and thyroglobulin (Tg) antibodies occur in up to 80% of cases.
- Because the coexisting thyroiditis can also affect thyroid function, there is no direct correlation between the level of TSI and thyroid hormone levels in Graves' disease.

Ans. A

21. Hyperglycemia in acute pancreatitis is due to all except:

A. Insulin resistance
B. Decreased insulin release
C. Increased glucagon release
D. Increased glucocorticoid & catecholamine

Explanation:

- Hemoconcentration may be the harbinger of more severe disease (i.e., pancreatic necrosis), whereas azotemia is a significant risk factor for mortality.
- Hyperglycemia is common and is due to multiple factors, including decreased insulin release, increased glucagon release, and an increased output of adrenal glucocorticoids and catecholamines.
- Hypocalcemia occurs in ~25% of patients, and its pathogenesis is incompletely understood. Although earlier studies suggested that the response of the parathyroid gland to a decrease in serum calcium is impaired, subsequent observations have failed to confirm this phenomenon.

Ans. A

22. 40 year old male came to the hospital with complaints of swelling in the front of his neck. O/E no evidence of opthalmopathy or dermopathy. TFT showed TSH 0.05 (0.3-5.5 mIU/ml), FT4 1.9ng/dl (0.93-1.79 ng/dl). USG neck revealed 3 × 2.5 cm nodule in the lower pole of the left lobe of thyroid. What is the treatment?

A. Lobectomy
B. Near total thyroidectomy
C. Radioiodine ablation
D. Sorafinib

Explanation:

- This is a case of toxic adenoma. Thyrotoxicosis is usually mild and is generally detected when nodule>3cm. Radioiodine ablation is the treatment of choice.

23. Plasma prolactin levels are normal in:

A. Tonic clinic seizures
B. Complex partial seizures
C. Syncope
D. Pshycogenic seizures

Explanation:

- Plasma prolactin concentrations frequently are elevated after tonic clonic seizures, peaking in 15 to 20 minutes, and less frequently after complex partial seizures.
- Serum prolactin levels almost invariably are normal after psychogenic seizures, although such a finding does not exclude the diagnosis of true epileptic seizures
- Elevated prolactin levels, however, also may be present after syncope and with the use of drugs such as antidepressants, estrogens, bromocriptine, ergots, phenothiazines, and antiepileptic drugs.

Ans. D

24. All are true about thyroid C cells except:

A. Neural crest derivatives from the ultimobranchial body give rise to thyroid C cells

B. Thyroid C cells produce calcitonin a calcium lowering hormone

C. Their density is greatest in juncture of the upper one-third and lower two-thirds of the thyroid gland

D. C-cells are important because of their involvement in papillary thyroid cancer

Explanation:

- Neural crest derivatives from the ultimobranchial body give rise to thyroid medullary C cells that produce calcitonin, a calcium-lowering hormone. The C cells are interspersed throughout the thyroid gland, although their density is greatest in the juncture of the upper one-third and lower two-thirds of the gland. Calcitonin plays a minimal role in calcium homeostasis in humans but the C-cells are important because of their involvement in medullary thyroid cancer.

Ans. D

25. NIS is present in all except:

A. Salivary glands

B. Prostate

C. Placenta

D. Thyroid gland

Explanation:

- NIS is most highly expressed in the thyroid gland, but low levels are present in the salivary glands, lactating breast, and placenta. The iodide transport mechanism is highly regulated, allowing adaptation to variations in dietary supply. Low iodine levels increase the amount of NIS and stimulate uptake, whereas high iodine levels suppress NIS expression and uptake. The selective expression of NIS in the thyroid allows isotopic scanning, treatment of hyperthyroidism, and ablation of thyroid cancer with radioisotopes of iodine, without significant effects on other organs.
- Mutation of the *NIS* gene is a rare cause of congenital hypothyroidism, underscoring its importance in thyroid hormone synthesis. Another iodine transporter, pendrin, is located on the apical surface of thyroid cells and mediates iodine efflux into the lumen. Mutation of the *pendrin* gene causes *Pendred syndrome*, a disorder characterized by defective organification of iodine, goiter, and sensorineural deafness.

Ans. B

26. Regarding Carney complex all are true except:

A. Pituitary adenoma -50%

B. Atrial myxoma

C. Lentigines

D. Adrenal hyperplasia

Explanation:

- Carney complex is characterized by spotty skin pigmentation, myxomas, and endocrine tumors, including testicular, adrenal, and pituitary adenomas. Acromegaly occurs in ~20% of these patients.
- A subset of patients have mutations in the R1α regulatory subunit of protein kinase A (PRKAR1A).

Ans. A

27. A 36 year old woman is evaluated for a palpable thyroid nodule. USG shows a 2 × 2 cm hypoechoic nodule with coarse calcifications. USG does not show any evidence of nodal metastasis. FNAC is suggestive of medullary thyroid carcinoma. She has family history of MEN 2B and RET mutation in this patient is positive. Work up for pheochromocytoma us negative. What is the appropriate surgical plan?

A. Total thyroidectomy with bilateral central resection and an ipsilateral lateral neck dissection

B. Total thyroidectomy

C. Total thyroidectomy with central resection

D. Total thyroidectomy with ipsilateral lateral neck dissection

Explanation:

- Prophylactic thyroidectomy, with lifelong thyroxine replacement, has dramatically improved outcomes in patients with MEN 2 and MEN 3, such that ~90% of young patients with *RET* mutations who had a prophylactic thyroidectomy have no evidence of persistent or recurrent MTC at 7 years after surgery. In patients with clinically evident MTC, a total thyroidectomy with bilateral central resection is recommended, and an ipsilateral lateral neck dissection should be undertaken if the primary tumor is >1 cm in size or there is evidence of nodal metastasis in the central neck. Surgery is the only curative therapy for MTC.

Ans. A

28. A woman with history of genetically proven MEN 2B [Ex16 (918)] delivers a male child. When should the child be considered for RET mutational analysis and prophylactic thyroidectomy?

A. As Soon As Possible and <1 year
B. < 3 years
C. < 2 years
D. < 5 years

Explanation:

Table: Recommendations for tests and surgery in Men 2 and Men 3[a]

		Recommended Age (Years) for Test/Intervention				
RET Mutation, Exon (EX) Location and Codon involved	Risk[b]	*RET* Mutational Analysis	First Serum Calcitonin and Neck Ultrasound	Prophylactic Thyroidec-tomy	Screening for Pheochromo-cytoma	Screening for PHPT
Ex8 (533)[c]; Ex10 (609, 611, 618, 620)[c]; Ex11 (630, 631, 666)[c]; Ex13 (768, 790)[c]; Ex14 (804)[c]; Ex15 (891)[c]; Ex16 (912)[c]	+	<3-5	5	<5[d]	16[e]	16
Ex11 (634)[c]; Ex15 (883)[c]	++	<3	<3	<5[f]	11[c]	11
Ex15 (883)[g]; Ex16 (918)[g]	+++	ASAP and by <1	ASAP and by <0.5-1	ASAP and by <1	11[c]	____[h]

Ans. A

29. Disease accompanied by low T3 concentrations is:

A. Acute liver disease
B. Renal disease
C. Early stage of HIV infection
D. Acutely ill psychiatric patients

Explanation:

- Any severe illness can induce changes in thyroid hormone levels, but certain disorders exhibit a distinctive pattern of abnormalities.
- Acute liver disease is associated with an initial rise in total (but not unbound) T3 and T4 levels due to TBG release; these levels become subnormal with progression to liver failure.
- A transient increase in total and unbound T 4 levels, usually with a normal T3 level, is seen in 5–30% of acutely ill psychiatric patients.
- TSH values may be transiently low, normal, or high in these patients.
- In the early stage of HIV infection, T3 and T 4 levels rise, even if there is weight loss. T3 levels fall with progression to AIDS, but TSH usually remains normal.
- *Renal disease is often accompanied by low T3 concentrations, but with normal rather than increased rT3 levels, due to an unknown factor that increases uptake of rT3 into the liver.*

Ans. B

30. Least common among MEN 1 tumors is:

A. Gastrinoma
B. VIPoma
C. Insulinoma
D. Glucagonoma

Explanation:

Type (Chromosomal Location)	Tumors (Estimated Penetrance)	Gene And Most Frequently Mutated Codons
MEN 1 (11q13)	Parathyroid adenoma (90%)	*MEN1*
	Enteropancreatic tumor (30-70%)	83/84, 4-bp del (≈4%)
	• Gastrinoma (>50%)	119, 3-bp del (≈3%)
	• Insulinoma (10-30%)	209-211, 4-bp del (≈8%)
	• Nonfunctioning and PPoma (20-55%)	418, 3-bp del (≈4%)
	• Glucagonoma (<3%)	514-516, del or ins (≈7%)
	• VIPoma (M<1%)	Intron 4 ss (≈10%)
	Pituitary adenoma (15-50%)	
	• Prolactinoma (60%)	
	• Somatotrophinoma (25%)	
	• Corticotropinoma (<5%)	
	• Nonfunctioning (<5%)	
	Associated tumors	
	• Adrenal cortical tumor (20-70%)	
	• Pheochromocytoma (<1%)	
	• Bronchopulmonary NET (2%)	
	• Thymic NET (2%)	
	• Gastric NET (10%)	
	• Lipomas (>33%)	
	• Angiofibromas (85%)	
	• Collagenomas (70%)	
	• Meningiomas (8%)	

Ans. B

31. A 28 year old man with Klinefelter's syndrome is initiated on testosterone enanthate 150 mg once in 2 weeks. After 4 months, testosterone levels 1 week after injection is 200 ng/dl. What is the target testosterone range?

A. 200-400 ng/dl
B. 350-600 ng/dl
C. 150-450 ng/dl
D. 200-600 ng/dl

Explanation:

- In patients who are treated with testosterone enanthate or cypionate, testosterone levels should be 350–600 ng/dL 1 week after the injection. If testosterone levels are outside this range, adjustments should be made either in the dose or in the interval between injections. In men on transdermal patch, gel, or buccal testosterone therapy, testosterone levels should be in the mid- normal range (400–750 ng/dL) 4–12 h after application. If testosterone levels are outside this range, the dose should be adjusted. Multiple dose adjustments are often necessary to achieve testosterone levels in the desired therapeutic range.

Ans. B

32. A 20 year old man with hypergonodatropic hypogonadism is initiated on testosterone enanthate 150 mg every 2 weeks. After 3 months, the patient finds the fortnightly hospital visits cumbersome and wants to switch over to a longer acting preparation of testosterone. You decide to start him on testosterone undecanoate. What is the recommended dose of testosterone undecanoate?

A. Initial dose of 750 mg followed 2 weeks later by a second injection of 750 mg and then 750 mg every 10 weeks

B. Initial dose of 750 mg followed 2 weeks later by a second injection of 750 mg and then 750 mg every 12 weeks

C. Initial dose of 750 mg followed 8 weeks later by a second injection of 750 mg and then 750 mg every 10 weeks

D. Initial dose of 750 mg followed 4 weeks later by a second injection of 750 mg and then 750 mg every 10 weeks

Explanation:

- Testosterone esters are administered typically at doses of 75–100 mg intramuscularly every week, or 150–200 mg every 2 weeks. Testosterone undecanoate is administered at an initial dose of 750 mg followed 4 weeks later by a second injection of 750 mg and then 750 mg every 10 weeks.

Ans. D

33. A 32 year old man presents with primary infertility. On examination, he has typical features of klinefelters syndrome and Karyotyping reveals 47 XXY Karyotype. He is at increased risk of the following except:

A. Systemic Lupus Erythematosus
B. Osteoporosis
C. Diabetes Mellitus
D. Prostate cancer

Explanation:

- Men with Klinefelter syndrome are at increased risk of systemic lupus erythematosus, Sjögren's syndrome, breast cancer, diabetes mellitus, osteoporosis, non-Hodgkin's lymphoma, and some types of lung cancer, and reduced risk of prostate cancer. Periodic mammography for breast cancer surveillance is recommended for men with Klinefelter syndrome.

Ans. D

34. 18 year old male presented with complaints of failure to develop secondary sexual characters. O/E he was found to have tall stature with eunuchoid proportions and anosmia. What will be the likely diagnosis?

A. Klinefelter's syndrome
B. Kallman syndrome
C. Praderwilli syndrome
D. Bardet Biedel syndrome

Explanation:

- Kallman syndrome results from defective hypothalamic GnRH synthesis and is associated with anosmia or hyposmia and due to olfactory bulb agenesis. Males present with delayed puberty. Associated features are optic atrophy, color blindness, deafness, mirror movements. Most common genetic cause is X linked Kall gene mutation. Low LH, Low FSH, Low Testosterone are seen.

Ans. B

35. A 36 year old woman is seen in the infertility clinic and evaluated for ovarian reserve. Which of the following indicates an adequate ovarian reserve?

A. Day 3 FSH < 10 and AMH < 0.5 ng/ml
B. Day 3 FSH < 10 and AMH > 0.5 ng/ml
C. Day 3 FSH <10 and AMH > 1 ng/ml
D. Day 3 FSH < 10 and AMH < 1 ng/ml

Explanation:

- Measurement of FSH on day 3 of the cycle (an FSH level <10 IU/mL on cycle day 3 predicts adequate ovarian oocyte reserve) is the most cost-effective test. Other tests antral follicle count on ultrasound, and anti-müllerian hormone (AMH; <0.5 ng/ mL predicts reduced ovarian reserve although there is variability between labs). Importantly, tests of ovarian reserve help to predict the response to exogenous gonadotropins but do not predict ability to conceive.

Ans. B

36. 20 year old lady, 2 weeks post delivery came to the hospital with complaints of sudden onset visual loss with vomiting and abdominal pain. O/E hypoglycemia and hypotension was present. Hormonal profile revealed central hypothyroidism and central hypocortisolism. What is the diagnosis?

A. Empty sella
B. Lymphocytic hyophysitis
C. Pituitary apoplexy
D. Pituitary adenoma

Explanation:

- Pituitary apoplexy. Also known as Sheehan syndrome. Occur in pre-existing adenoma, postpartum period, sickle cell anemia or acute shock. It is an endocrine emergency, may present with shock, CNS hemorrhage, sudden visual loss and death. Hypopituitarism is common after apoplexy.

Ans. C

37. A 36 year old woman and her 40 year old husband consult you in the infertility clinic. They have been married for 9 months. What is the definition of infertility?

A. *Infertility* is the inability to conceive after 12 months of unprotected sexual intercourse or after 6 months in women ≥30
B. *Infertility* is the inability to conceive after 12 months of unprotected sexual intercourse or after 6 months in women ≥35
C. *Infertility* is the inability to conceive after 12 months of unprotected sexual intercourse or after 6 months in women ≥40
D. *Infertility* is the inability to conceive after 12 months of unprotected sexual intercourse or after 9 months in women ≥35

Explanation:

- *Infertility* is the inability to conceive after 12 months of unprotected sexual intercourse or after 6 months in women ≥35. This revised definition is based on data indicating that 50% of apparently normal couples will conceive within 3 months, 75–82% within 6 months, and 85–92% within 12 months, but recognizes the age-related decrease in fertility.

Ans. B

38. 45 year gentleman came to the hospital with complaints of headache and decrease in the temporal field of vision. MRI brain showed sellar mass. Hormonal profile showed Prolactin >500mcg/l. What is the initial treatment?

A. Trans-sphenoidal pituitary surgery
B. Radiotherapy
C. Pegvisomant
D. Cabergoline

Explanation:

- Diagnosis here is is prolatinoma. Oral dopamine agonists like cabergoline and bromocriptine are the main stay of treatment for the micro and maroprolatinomas. After starting treatment, normoprolactinemia occurs in 80% patients and mass effect including headache and visual disorders drastically improve.

Ans. D

39. A 40 year old woman came to the hospital with history of amenorrhea and galactorrhea. She is anxious to become pregnant and been trying to conceive for 9 months, without success. Her weight is 60KG, TSH 2.6mIU/L, FT4 1.5 ng/dl. BMI is 22, no acne or hirsutism. What is the diagnosis?

A. Pituitary microadenoma
B. Hypothyroidism
C. Hyperthyroidism
D. PCOS

Explanation:

- Symptoms are due to hyperprolcatinemia. Raised prolactin is due to microadenoma. She has amenorrhea, anovulation, can be reversed with Cabergoline, dopamine agonist.

Ans. A

40. 22 year old gentleman presented with complaints of increase in ring size and shoe size with coarsening of facial features. What is the investigation of choice?

A. Clonidine induced GH stimulation
B. Insulin induced hypoglycemia
C. Basal GH levels
D. OGTT

Explanation:

- Screening test for acromegaly are IGF 1 levels. Diagnosis is confirmed by OGTT. Acromegaly is diagnosed when failure to suppress GH <0.4mcg/l within 2 hours of oral Glucose load.

Ans. D

41. 40 year old gentleman with complaints of large hands and feet. IGF-1 levels were elevated. OGTT did not suppress growth hormone. Diagnosis of acromegaly was made. MRI revealed microadenoma. What is the treatment of choice?

A. Octreotide
B. Pegvisomant
C. Radiation
D. Trans-sphenoidal surgery

Explanation:

- Trans-sphenoidal surgical resection is the preferred primary treatment for both microadenoma and macroadenoma. Somatostatin analogues are used as an adjuvant for preoperative shrinkage of macroadenomas or patient who declines surgery or when the surgery fails.

Ans. D

42. A 52 year old woman, with history of established cardiovascular disease has attained menopause 6 months back. She enquires about Hormonal therapy. What is the effect of hormonal therapy on cardiovascular disease?

A. Estrogen has adverse effects on Coronary heart disease
B. Estrogen has beneficial effects on Coronary heart disease
C. Depends on the timing of estrogen therapy
D. Estrogen has no effect on Coronary heart disease

Explanation:

- A closer look at available data suggests that timing of initiation of HT may critically influence the association between such therapy and CHD. Estrogen may slow early stages of atherosclerosis but have adverse effects on advanced atherosclerotic lesions. It has been hypothesized that the prothrombotic and proinflammatory effects of estrogen manifest themselves predominantly among women with subclinical lesions who initiate

HT well after the menopausal transition, whereas women with less arterial damage who start HT early in menopause may derive cardiovascular benefit because they have not yet developed advanced lesions.

Ans. C

43. A 40 year old lady is brought to ER with head injury. CT brain does not show any trauma except enlargement of pituitary fossa. MRI brain revealed 1.5 cm pituitary adenoma. Neurological examination revealed bitemporal homonymous hemianopia. Which of the following anterior pituitary hormones has an inhibitory control by the hypothalamus?

A. ACTH
B. Prolactin
C. FSH
D. GH

Explanation:

- Pituitary hormones are secreted in a pulsatile manner after stimulation by hypothalamus releasing factors. Prolactin is the only anterior pituitary hormone whose secretion is inhibited by dopamine secreted by hypothalamus.

Ans. B

44. A 20 year old woman diagnosed with PCOS and significant hirsutism is started on combined oral contraceptive pills. She returns at 2 months and reports no improvement in hirsutism. What is the appropriate management?

A. Add on spironolactone to the current regimen
B. Add on flutamide to the current regimen
C. Continue the same oral contraceptive pills
D. Revisit the diagnosis of PCOS

Explanation:

- The effect of oral contraceptive pills on hair growth may not be evident for 6 months, and the maximum effect may require 9–12 months owing to the length of the hair growth cycle. Improvements in hirsutism are typically in the range of 20%, but there may be an arrest of further progression of hair growth.

Ans. C

45. A 20 year old woman presents with history of irregular menstrual cycles and increased terminal hair over the face, abdomen and chest. On examination, she has significant hirsutism.

Biochemical investigations are as follows:

FSH 5.4 IU/L

LH 3.3 IU/L

Testosterone 3.5 ng/dl

DHEAS 7600 μg/L

What is the most likely diagnosis?

A. Ovarian hyperthecosis
B. Polycystic ovarian syndrome
C. Adrenocortical carcinoma
D. Ovarian neoplasm

Explanation:

- A baseline plasma total testosterone level >12 nmol/L (>3.5 ng/mL) usually indicates a virilizing tumor, whereas a level >7 nmol/L (>2 ng/mL) is suggestive of tumor but may also be observed in women with hyperthecosis. A basal DHEAS level >18.5 μmol/L (>7000 μg/L) suggests an adrenal tumor.

Ans. A

46. 20 year lady came to the hospital with complaints of polyuria, polydipsia and nocturia. 24 hour urine volume was more than 40ml/kg and urine osmolality<300 mosm/l. AVP levels was undetectable. MRI brain showed pituitary bright spot. What is the likely diagnosis?

A. SIADH
B. Primary polydipsia
C. Nephrogenic DI
D. Pituitary DI

Explanation:

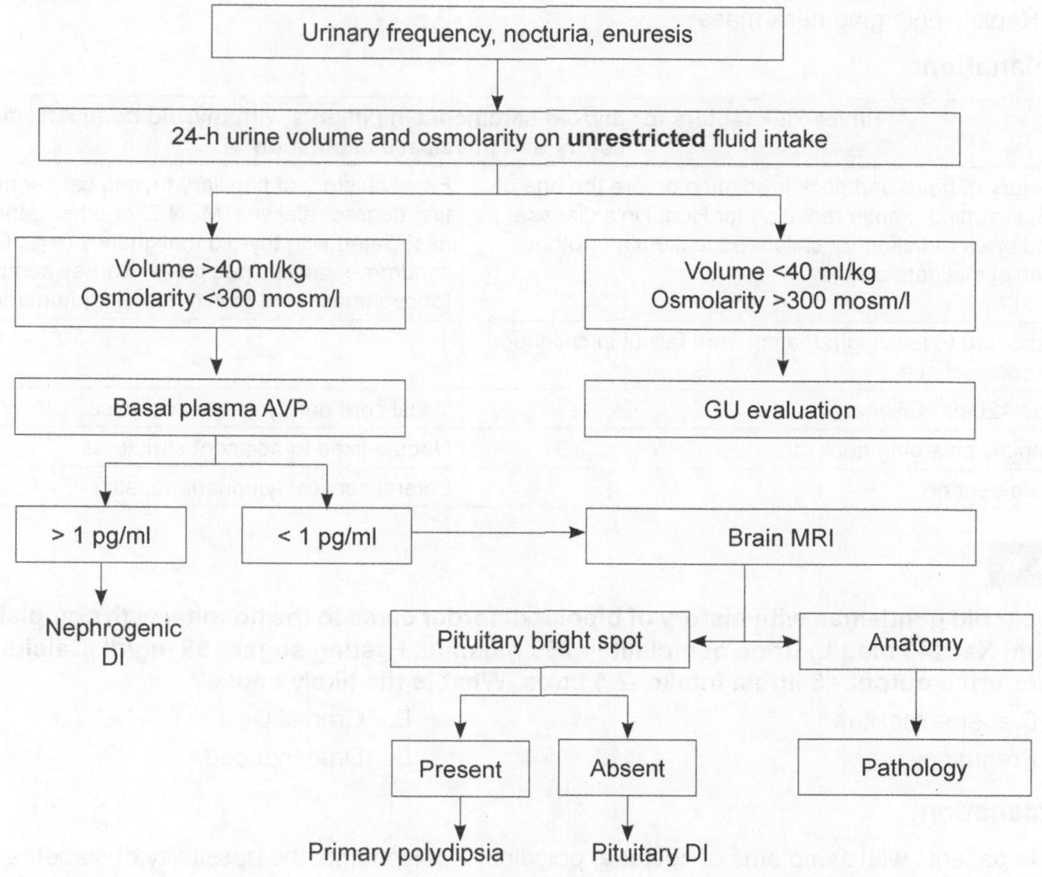

Ans. B

47. A 36 year old woman with a solitary nodule of thyroid is referred for evaluation. Ultrasound shows an isoechoic nodule of size 2x 1.8 cms. FNAC is done which is reported as Bethesda category IV. What is the risk of malignancy according to the FNAC result?

A. 15-30%
B. 5-10%
C. 10-20%
D. 60-70%

Table: Bethesda classification for thyroid cytology

Diagnostic category	Risk of malignancy
I. Nondiagnostic or unsatisfactory	1-5%
II. Benign	2-4%
III. Atypia or follicular lesion of unknown significance (AUS/FLUS)	5-15%
IV. Follicular neoplasm	15-30%
V. Suspicious for malignancy	60-75%
VI. Malignant	97-100%

Ans. A

48. A 22 year old woman is referred for evaluation of a solitary thyroid nodule. She has history of brain irradiation for childhood leukemia. Which one of the following is not a risk factor for thyroid cancer in patients with thyroid nodules?

A. History of head and neck irradiation before the age of 18, including, mantle radiation for Hodgkin's disease, and brain radiation for childhood leukemia or other cranial malignancies

B. Female gender

C. Age < 20 years or > 65 years

D. Rapidly enlarging neck mass

Explanation:

Table: Risk factors for thyroid carcinoma in patients with thyroid nodule from history and physical examination	
History of head and neck irradiation before the age of 18, including mantle radiation for Hodgkin's disease, and brain radiation for childhood leukemia or other cranial malignancies	Family history of papillary thyroid cancer in 2 or more first degree relatives, MEN 2, or other genetic syndromes associated with thyroid malignancy (e.g., Cowden's syndrome, familial polyposis, Carney complex, PTEN [phosphatase and tensin homolog] hamartoma tumor)
Exposure to ionizing radiation from fallout in childhood or adolescence	
Age <20 or >65 years	Vocal cord paralysis, hoarse voice
Rapidly enlarging neck mass	Nodule fixed to adjacent structures
Male gender	Lateral cervical lymphadenopathy

Ans. B

49. 35 year old gentleman with history of bipolar disorder came to the hospital with complaints of polyuria. Serum Na- 145 meq/L. Urine osmolality - 250 mosm/L. Fasting sugar - 99 mg/dl. Calcium -9.5 mg/dl. 24 hours urine output - 5 litres. Intake -2.5 litres. What is the likely cause?

A. Diabetes mellitus

B. Cranial DI

C. Pregnancy

D. Drug induced

Explanation:

- In patients with symptoms of nocturia, polydipsia, polyphagia, the possibility of diabetes insipidus should be suspected if urine osmolality <300 mosm/L and urine volume >50 ml/kg/day. In this patient, history of bipolar disorder gives clue that drug such as Lithium used in the treatment, is associated with nephrogenic diabetes insipidus.

Ans. D

50. A 31-year-old woman was referred to you for evaluation of a palpable left thyroid nodule. She had symptoms suggestive of thyrotoxicosis. Lab investigations showed raised T3, T4 with supressed TSH. Thyroid scintigraphy revealed a hyperfunctioning left-sided thyroid nodule, and ultrasonography revealed it to be 2.7 cm in greatest dimension, hyperechoic, and in the left lower lobe. What is the treatment of choice?

A. Radioiodine ablation

B. Antithyroid drugs

C. Lobectomy

D. Total Thyroidectomy

Explanation:

- Radioiodine ablation is usually the treatment of choice. Because normal thyroid function is suppressed, ^{131}I is concentrated in the hyperfunctioning nodule with minimal uptake and damage to nor- mal thyroid tissue. Relatively large radioiodine doses (e.g., 370–1110 MBq [10–29.9 mCi] ^{131}I) have been shown to correct thyrotoxicosis. in about 75% of patients within 3 months. Hypothyroidism occurs in <10% of those patients over the next 5 years. Surgical resection is also effective and is usually limited to lobectomy, thereby preserving thyroid function and minimizing risk of hypoparathyroidism or damage to the recurrent laryngeal nerves. Medical therapy using antithyroid drugs and beta blockers can normalize thyroid function but is not an optimal long-term treatment. Using ultrasound guidance, repeated percutaneous radiofrequency thermal ablation has been used successfully in some centers to ablate hyperfunctioning nodules, and this technique has also been used to reduce the size of nonfunctioning thyroid nodules.

Ans. A

51. Cortical sensation is mediated by which lobe:

A. Temporal
B. Frontal
C. Parietal
D. Occipital

Explanation:

- "Cortical" sensation is mediated by the parietal lobes and represents an integration of the primary sensory modalities; testing cortical sensation is only meaningful when primary sensation is intact.
- Double simultaneous stimulation is especially useful as a screening test for cortical function; with the patient's eyes closed, the examiner lightly touches one or both hands and asks the patient to identify the stimuli.
- With a parietal lobe lesion, the patient may be unable to identify stimulus on the contralateral side when both hands are touched.
- Other modalities relying on the parietal cortex include the discrimination of two closely placed stimuli as separate (two-point discrimination), identification of an object by touch and manipulation alone (stereognosis), and the identification of numbers or letters written on the skin surface (graphesthesia).

Ans. C

52. In MEN 2A, most common feature is:

A. Medullary thyroid cancer
B. Pheochromocytoma
C. Parathyroid carcinoma
D. Gastrinoma

Explanation:

Type (Chromosomal Location)	Tumors (Estimated Penetrance)	Gene And Most Frequently Mutated Codons
MEN 2 (10 cen-10q11.2) MEN 2A	MTC (90%) Pheochromocytoma (> 50%) Parathyroid adenoma (10-25%)	*RET* 634, e.g., Cys→Arg (~ 85%)
MTC only	MTC (100%)	*RET* 618, missense (>50%)
MEN 2B (also known as MEN 3)	MTC (>90%) Pheochromocytoma (>50%) Associated abnormalities (40-50%) • Mucosal neuromas • Marfanoid habitus • Medullated corneal nerve fibers • Megacolon	*RET* 918, Met→Thr (>95%)
MEN 4 (12q13)	Parathyroid adenoma[a] Pituitary adenoma[a] Reproductive organ tumors[a] (e.g., testicular cancer, neuroendocrine cervical carcinoma) ?Adrenal + renal tumors[a]	*CDKN1B;* no common mutations identified to date

Ans. A

53. 45 year old gentleman presented with loss of peripheral field of vision with holocranial headache. On examination, bitemporal hemianopia was present.

Hormonal profile

- **TSH 3.5 (0.3-5.5 mIU/ml)**
- **FT4 1.4 (0.93- 1.7 ng/dl)**
- **Prolactin 50ng/ml (4.04-15.2 ng/ml)**
- **IGF 1 70 (60-180ng/ml)**
- **Cortisol 7mcg/dl (6.27-18mcg/dl)**
- **MRI pituitary revealed pituitary macroadenoma.**

What is the diagnosis?

A. Non functioning pituitary adenoma
B. Prolactinoma
C. Acromegaly
D. Pitu tary apoplexy

Explanation:

- Prolactinoma is suspected only when prolactin levels more than 200mcg/dl. Non functioning pituitary adenoma secrete no pituitary hormones. They are usually macroadenomas at diagnosis. Most commonly present as visual disturbance due to optic chiasmal compression.

Ans. A

54. A 60 year old woman is diagnosed with severe, clinically active graves ophthalmopathy and is planned to be started on steroids. What is the dose of steroids recommended?

A. 250 mg IV methylprednisolone, once weekly for 12 weeks
B. 1 mg/kg of oral prednisolone
C. 500 mg IV methylprednisolone once a week for 6 weeks followed by oral steroids
D. 500 mg IV methylprednisolone once a week for 6 weeks followed by 250 mg IV methylprednisolone once a week for 6 weeks

Explanation:

- Severe ophthalmopathy, with optic nerve involvement or chemosis resulting in corneal damage, is an emergency requiring joint management with an ophthalmologist. Pulse therapy with IV methylprednisolone (e.g., 500 mg of methylprednisolone once weekly for 6 weeks, then 250 mg once weekly for 6 weeks) is preferable to oral glucocorticoids, which are used for moderately active disease.

Ans. D

55. A 45 year old patient presents with prognathism and interdental separation. Blood pressure is difficult to manage inspite of three anti hypertensive drugs. In addition, he was recently diagnosed to have impaired glucose tolerance. Which is the next investigation?

A. Basal GH measurement
B. Fasting glucose test with GH measurement
C. GTT including GH measurement
D. Serum prolactin

Explanation:

- The patient s symptoms are consistent with diagnosis of acromegaly. Diagnosis is made by measuring GH levels in response to glucose challenge.

Ans. C

56. 70 year old lady came to the hospital with complaints of diminished sensorium. O/E she had dry skin, hypothermia, anasarca and pericardial effusion. Thyroid profile showed TSH >150 mcg. What is the treatment of choice?

A. Oral Levothyroxine
B. Betablockers
C. Potassium iodide
D. IV levothyroxine with steroids

Explanation:

- Myxodema coma occurs in elderly patients, may present with reduced level of consciousness, seizures and hypothermia. Treatment of choice is IV levothyroxine since absorption is impaired for oral levothyroxine in myxedema. Parenteral hydrocortisone should be administered since there is impaired adrenal reserve in hypothyroidism.

Ans. D

57. 20 year lady known case of hypothyroidism on treatment G2P1L1 with gestational age 6 weeks, during her routine antenatal checkup had TSH of 3.5 mIU/ml (0.3-5.5 mIU/ml). What is the next step?

A. Her Thyroid function test is normal, no need of any further tests, continue the same dose of levothyroxine
B. To repeat TFT after 2 months
C. Increase levothyroxine dose
D. Stop levothyroxine as it is teratogenic

Explanation:

- TSH goal in pregnancy is less than 2.5 mIU/l. levothyroxine should be monitored every 4 weeks during the first half of pregnancy. Pregnant woman should be counseled to separate prenatal vitamins from levothyroxine.

Ans. C

58. 24 year old primigravida had hyperemesis gravidarum. Her gestational age was 20 weeks. Thyroid function test revealed TSH 0.01mIU/ml(0.3-5.5 mIU/ml). FT4- 2.03 (0.93-1.70 ng/dl). O/E goiter was present. What is the treatment of choice?

A. Propylthiouracil
B. Carbimazole
C. Levothyroxine
D. No treatment

Explanation:

- This is a case of Graves disease, treatment with antithyroid drugs such as propylthiouracil and carbimazole are indicated. They inhibit function of TPO. Due to heapatotoxicity of PTU, USFDA has limited its use to I trimester of pregnancy.

Ans. B

59. A 26 year old woman, case of graves disease, diagnosed 1.5 years back, euthyroid on 5 mg methimazole comes with 1.5 months of amenorrhea. Urine pregnancy test is positive. On examination, she has a grade 1 goitre. Her TFT Is normal. Her TSH receptor antibody is negative. What would you advise regarding methimazole?

A. Stop methimazole
B. Continue same dose of methimazole
C. Switch to propylthiouracil
D. Increase the dose of methimazole

Explanation:

- Antithyroid drugs should be used to manage Graves' disease in pregnancy. Because transplacental passage of these drugs may produce fetal hypothyroidism and goiter if the maternal dose is excessive, maternal antithyroid dose titration should target serum free or total T_4 levels at or just above the pregnancy reference range. If available, propylthiouracil should be used until 14–16 weeks' gestation because of the association of rare cases of methimazole/ carbimazole embryopathy, including *aplasia cutis* and other defects, such as choanal atresia and tracheoesophageal fistulae. Because of the potential for teratogenic effects, recent recommendations suggest discontinuation of antithyroid medication in a newly pregnant woman with Graves' disease, who is euthyroid on a low dose of methimazole (<5–10 mg/day) or PTU (<100–200 mg/day), after evaluating recent thyroid function tests, disease history, goiter size, duration of therapy, and TRAb measurement. Following cessation, careful monitoring of maternal thyroid function tests is essential.

Ans. A

60. Which is a cause of Primary Hyperthyroidism?

A. TSH Secreting pituitary adenoma
B. Struma ovary
C. Chorionic gonadotropin secreting tumors
D. Subacute thyroiditis

Explanation:

Table: Causes of thyrotoxicosis
Primary Hyperthyroidism
• Graves' disease • Toxic multinodular goiter • Toxic adenoma • Functioning thyroid carcinoma metastases • Activating mutation of the TSH receptor • Activating mutation of Gsα (McCune-Albright syndrome) • Struma ovarii **Drugs:** Iodine excess (Jod-Basedow phenomenon)
Thyrotoxicosis without Hyperthyroidism
• Subacute thyroiditis • Silent thyroiditis • Other causes of thyroid destruction: Amiodarone, radiation, infarction of adenoma • Ingestion of excess thyroid hormone (thyrotoxicosis factitia) or thyroid tissue
Secondary Hyperthyroidism
• TSH-secreting pituitary adenoma • Thyroid hormone resistance syndrome: Occasional patients may have features of thyrotoxicosis • Chorionic gonadotropin-secreting tumors[a] • Gestational thyrotoxicosis[a]

Ans. B

61. 19 year old lady came to the hospital with hyperemesis gravidarum during I trimester of pregnancy. O/E no goiter was present. TSH was 0.1 (0.3-5.5 mIU/ml). Total T4 16 mcg/dl (5.19-14.1 mcg/dl). What is the treatment?

A. Propylthiouracil
B. Carbimazole
C. Levothyroxine
D. No treatment

Explanation:

- During I trimester of pregnancy, rise in circulating HCG levels stimulate TSH receptor and there is a reciprocal fall of TSH levels. There is estrogen induced rise in TBG during I trimester, so total T4 and total T3 levels were 1.5 times higher throughout the pregnancy.

Ans. D

62. A 64 year old woman presents with history of anxiety, palpitations and weight loss. Her blood investigations showed raised T3,T4 values with supressed TSH. Technetium thyroid scintigraphy showed increased uptake in the thyroid gland. Her baseline differential white blood count is normal. She is started on carbimazole 30 mg/day. Agranulocytosis is a severe side effect of carbimazole. How often should she be monitored with blood counts for development of agranulocytosis?

A. 1 month after starting treatment and 3 monthly thereafter

B. 3 months after starting treatment and yearly thereafter

C. 2 weeks after starting treatment and monthly thereafter

D. Need not be monitored with regular blood counts

Explanation:

- The common minor side effects of antithyroid drugs are rash, urticaria, fever, and arthralgia (1–5% of patients). These may resolve spontaneously or after substituting an alternative antithyroid drug; rashes may respond to an antihistamine. Rare but major side effects include hepatitis (especially with propylthiouracil; avoid use in children) and cholestasis (methimazole and carbimazole); vasculitis; and, most important, agranulocytosis (<1%). It is essential that antithyroid drugs are stopped and not restarted if a patient develops major side effects. Written instructions should be provided regarding the symptoms of possible agranulocytosis (e.g., sore throat, fever, mouth ulcers) and the need to stop treatment pending an urgent complete blood count to confirm that agranulocytosis is not present. It is not useful to monitor blood counts prospectively, because the onset of agranulocytosis is idiosyncratic and abrupt.

Ans. D

63. 19 year nursing student came to the hospital with complaints of palpitations, weight loss and loose stools. O/E fine tremors were present with no goiter. TSH 0.05 (0.3-5.5 mIU/ml), FT4 1.8 ng/dl (0.93-1.70 ng/dl). Radio iodine uptake with Iodine123 showed low uptake. Circulating levels of thyroglobulin was detected to be low. What is the diagnosis?

A. Graves' disease

B. Thyroiditis

C. TSH secreting pituitary adenoma

D. Thyrotoxicosis factitia

Explanation:

- Causes of low radio iodine uptake are thyroiditis, thyrotoxicosis factitia, ectopic thyroid tissue, strauma ovary. Thyrotoxicosis can be differentiated from destructive thyroiditis by clinical features and low level of thyroiditis.

Ans. D

64. 60 year old male known diabetic, CAD was admitted in ICU for pneumonia. Thyroid function test in this patient was TSH 2.5 (0.3-5.5 mIU/ml), FT3 1.5pg/ml (2.2-4.4 pg/ml), FT4 1.5 (0.93-1.70 ng/dl). What is the treatment?

A. Tab Levothyroxine 100 mcg

B. Tab Levothyroxine 25 mcg

C. IV Levothyroxine

D. No treatment.

Explanation:

- This is a case of Sick Euthyroid Syndrome also called as nonthyroid illness where there is decrease in FT3, total T3, normal TSH.

Ans. D

65. Regarding Rhinocerebral mucormycosis all are true except:

A. High grade fever
B. Dull sinus pain
C. Diplopia
D. Proptosis

Explanation:

- Individuals with diabetes or immunocompromising conditions such as solid organ transplants or hematologic malignancies are at risk for invasive rhinocerebral mucormycosis.
- Patients present with low-grade fever, dull sinus pain, diplopia, decreased mental status, decreased ocular motion, chemosis, proptosis, dusky or necrotic nasal turbinates, and necrotic hard-palate lesions that respect the midline.
- Without rapid recognition and intervention, the process continues on an inexorable invasive course, with mortality rates of 50–85% or greater.
- Uncontrolled diabetes and increasing age are negative prognostic factors.

Ans. A

66. A 17 year old female presented with history of menstrual disturbances, palpitations, tremors and weight loss. On examination she has a grade 2 goitre. Her blood investigations showed raised T3,T4 values with supressed TSH. TSH receptor antibody was positive. Technetium thyroid scintigraphy showed increased uptake in the thyroid gland. She was diagnosed with graves disease and started on carbimazole 30 mg/day. The dose was titrated and continued for 18 months. At the end of 18 months, she was euthyroid on carbimazole 5 mg/day. TSH receptor antibody was positive. The predictors of relapse after stopping antithyroid drugs are the following except:

A. Young age
B. Female gender
C. Large goitre
D. Severe hyperthyroidism

Explanation:

- Maximum remission rates (up to 30–60% in some populations) are achieved by 12–18 months for the titration regimen and are higher in patients where TRAb levels are no longer detected, than in those with TRAb persistence. For unclear reasons, remission rates appear to vary in different geographic regions. Younger patients, males, smokers, and patients with a history of allergy, severe hyperthyroidism or large goiters are most likely to relapse when treatment stops, but outcomes are difficult to predict. All patients should be followed closely for relapse during the first year after treatment and at least annually thereafter.

Ans. B

67. 19 year old female comes to the hospital with complaints of swelling in the neck which is progressively enlarging in size. Thyroid function test are normal. USG neck shows 5 × 4 cm nodule in the lower pole of left lobe of thyroid with no lymph nodes. FNAC of the nodule reveals features suggestive of papillary carcinoma thyroid. What is the treatment of choice?

A. Lobectomy
B. Weight and watch
C. Iodine 131 ablation
D. Near total thyroidectomy

Explanation:

- Well differentiated thyroid cancer >1cm should be surgically excised. In tumours, more than 1 cm and less than 4 cm in the absence of metastasis either unilateral lobectomy or bilateral near total thyroidectomy can be done. However for tumours more than 4 cm, or in the presence of mets or extra thyroidal invasion, near total thyroidectomy needs to be done.

Ans. D

68. A 36 year old man with history of palpitations, weight loss and neck swelling is diagnosed with Graves' disease. He is started on nemercazole 20 mg/day. What is the optimum duration of treatment with antithyroid drugs?

A. Till patient achieves euthyroidism

B. Stopped once patient is biochemically hypothyroid

C. To be continued for 12-18 months with dose titration

D. To be stopped as soon as patient achieves euthyroidism and restarted if there is a relapse

Explanation:

- Maximum remission rates with antithyroid drugs (up to 30–60% in some populations) are achieved by 12–18 months for the titration regimen and are higher in patients where TRAb levels are no longer detected, than in those with TRAb persistence.

Ans. C

69. A 68 year old woman complaints of slowly enlarging mass in the anterior aspect of the neck associated with dysphagia. USG shows diffuse goiter. Biopsy reveals dense infiltration of the gland with fibrous material. Autoantibodies were negative. TSH 20IU/ml (0.3-5.5 IU/ml), FT4 0.4 (0.93-1.7ng/dl). What is the diagnosis?

A. Thyroid carcinoma

B. Reidel's thyroiditis

C. Hashimoto thyroiditis

D. Graves' disease

Explanation:

- Reidel's thyroiditis is a rare disorder, occurs in middle aged women, presents with painless goiter with compression of trachea, oesphagus, recurrent laryngeal nerve. Dense fibrosis disrupts the normal gland architecture. Surgical treatment is the choice. It is related to IgG4 disorders.

Ans. B

70. A 35 year old female complaints of constipation, cold intolerance, weight gain with irregular menses. Her PR is 58 bpm, dry skin with hungup reflex. TSH -1.5 MIU/ml(0.3-5.5 IU/ml), FT4 0.4ng/dl(0.93 – 1.7ng/dl). What is the next investigation?

A. FT3

B. USG thyroid

C. MRI pituitary

D. Anti TPO antibodies

Explanation:

- Secondary hypothyroidism is suspected when there is features of hypothyroidism but normal or low TSH. The diagnosis is confirmed by detecting free T4. The goal of the treatment is to maintain in the upper limit of reference interval because TSH cannot be used to maintain therapy.

Ans. C

71. A 28 year old woman is diagnosed with Graves' disease and started on carbimazole 30 mg/day. The dose of antithyroid drugs are titrated based on.

A. T4 levels 4-6 weeks after starting treatment

B. T4, TSH levels 4-6 weeks after starting treatment

C. T4 levels 10-12 weeks after starting treatment

D. T4, TSH levels 4-6 weeks after starting treatment

Explanation:

- Thyroid function tests and clinical manifestations are reviewed 4–6 weeks after starting treatment, and the dose is titrated based on unbound T_4 levels. Most patients do not achieve euthyroidism until 6–8 weeks after treatment is initiated. TSH levels often remain suppressed for several months and therefore do not provide a sensitive index of treatment response.

Ans. B

72. A 34 year old woman, case of graves' disease who presented with severe toxicosis about 3 months back is now euthyroid on carbimazole 40 mg/day. She is planned for radioiodine treatment. What is the best regimen of carbimazole in this case?

A. Continue carbimazole in the immediate pre and post radioiodine treatment period

B. Continue carbimazole till the day prior to radioiodine treatment and stop after treatment

C. Stop carbimazole 5-7 days prior to radioiodine treatment

D. Stop carbimazole 2-3 days prior to radioiodine treatment and restart 3-7 days after radioiodine treatment

Explanation:

- Carbimazole or methimazole must be stopped 2–3 days before radioiodine administration to achieve optimum iodine uptake, and can be restarted 3–7 days after radioiodine in those at risk of com- plications from worsening thyrotoxicosis. Propylthiouracil appears to have a prolonged radioprotective effect and should be stopped for a longer period before radioiodine is given, or a larger dose of radioiodine will be necessary.

Ans. D

73. A 32 year old lady presents to the hospital with flu-like illness and tenderness over her neck for the past 3 weeks. Her own medication is OCP only. O/E BP – 154/80 mm Hg, PR- 96/min, Fine tremor noted. There is tenderness over the anterior neck. TSH – 0.1 IU/L, FT4 2.04ng/dl. What is the diagnosis?

A. De Quervain's thyroiditis

B. Graves' disease

C. Hashimoto thyroiditis

D. Toxic multinodular goitre

Explanation:

- There is flu like symptoms, tenderness over the neck which point to the diagnosis. Antithyroid drugs are not used, beta blockers may be used in controlling the symptoms.

Ans. A

74. All are true statements except:

A. Cortisol values increase fivefold between midnight and dawn

B. Low testosterone and elevated LH levels suggest a primary gonadal problem

C. Free thyroxine and TSH are both low it is important to consider primary hypopituitarism

D. Elevated calcium and PTH levels suggest hyperparathyroidism

Explanation:

- Cortisol values increase fivefold between midnight and dawn; reproductive hormone levels vary dramatically during female menstrual cycle.
- Low testosterone and elevated LH levels suggest a primary gonadal problem, whereas a hypothalamic-pituitary disorder is likely if both LH and testosterone are low.
- Because TSH is a sensitive indicator of thyroid function, it is generally recommended as a first-line test for thyroid disorders. An elevated TSH level is almost always the result of primary hypothyroidism, whereas a low TSH is most often caused by thyrotoxicosis.

- These predictions can be confirmed by determining the free thyroxine level.
- In less common circumstance when free thyroxine and TSH are both low, it is important to consider secondary hypopituitarism caused by hypothalamic-pituitary disease.
- Elevated calcium and PTH levels suggest hyperparathyroidism, whereas PTH is suppressed in hypercalcemia caused by malignancy or granulomatous diseases. A suppressed ACTH in the setting of hyper-cortisolemia, or increased urine-free cortisol, is seen with hyper-functioning adrenal adenomas.

Ans. C

75. A 24 year married woman, diagnosed case of graves' disease, is treated with 10 mCi radioiodine. What should she be advised regarding conception?

A. She can safely conceive 3 months after radioiodine treatment

B. She can safely conceive 1 year after radioiodine treatment

C. She can safely conceive 6 months after radioiodine treatment

D. She can safely conceive 18 months after radioiodine treatment

Explanation:

- Pregnancy and breast-feeding are absolute contraindications to radioiodine treatment, but patients can conceive safely 6 months after treatment.

Ans. C

76. All below receptor mutations cause disease by functioning in an analogous dominant negative manner except:

A. Vitamin D receptors

B. Thyroid hormone receptor β

C. Thyroid hormone receptor α

D. PPARγ

Explanation:

- Mutations in the genes encoding TRα and PPARγ can also cause disease by functioning in an analogous dominant negative manner.

Ans. A

77. A 31 year old man is referred to the hospital because of recently discovered hypertension that is labile and difficult to control. Which of the following features is most likely to suggest a genetic syndrome is the cause for his hypertension?

A. Serum potassium level of 3.9

B. Serum calcium level of 9

C. Family history of medullary thyroid cancer

D. Family history of Papillary thyroid neoplasia

Explanation:

- Among endocrine causes of hypertension, only pheochromocytoma has a strong genetic heritability (Autosomal dominant). MEN 2 is strongly associated with a family history medullary thyroid cancer.

Ans. C

78. A 54 year old male is seen in the obesity clinic. He is worked up for metabolic syndrome. Which of the following do not constitute the NCEP ATP III 2001 criteria for metabolic syndrome?

A. Central obesity: waist circumference >102 cm (M), >88 cm (F)

B. Hypertriglyceridemia: triglyceride level ≥150 mg/dL or specific medication

C. Low HDL cholesterol: <50 mg/dL and <40 mg/dL for men and women, respectively, or specific medication

D. Hypertension: blood pressure ≥130 mmHg systolic or ≥85 mm Hg diastolic or specific medication

Explanation:

Table: NCEP: ATPIII 2001
Three or more of the following:
• *Central obesity:* Waist circumference >102 cm (M), >88 cm (F)
• *Hypertriglyceridemia:* Triglyceride level ≥150 mg/dl or specific medication
• *Low HDL[c] cholesterol:* <40 mg/dl and <50 mg/dl for men and women, respectively, or specific medication
• *Hypertension:* Blood pressure ≥130 mm Hg systolic or ≥85 mm Hg diastolic or specific medication
• Fasting plasma glucose level ≥100 mg/dl or specific medication or previously diagnosed type 2 diabetes

Ans. C

79. A 30 year old woman has come to the hospital with recurrent headaches, anxiety, sweating, palpitations. Her 24 hour urinary metanephrines are elevated. CT showed mass in the right adrenal medulla, BP-146/94 mm Hg. What is the treatment?

A. Urgent beta blockade, then unilateral adrenalectomy

B. Urgent alpha blockade, then beta blockade,unilateral adrenalectomy

C. Urgent beta blockade, then alpha blockade, unilateral adrenalectomy

D. Urgent adrenalectomy

Explanation:

- The patient has pheochromocytoma of the right adrenal medulla. It is characterized by headache, palpitations, hyperhidrosis. Preoperatively blood pressure is controlled with alpha adrenergic blockers.
- Beta blockers can be added later. Preoperatively BP should be < 160/90 mmHg consistently.

Ans. B

80. A 19 year old woman with poorly controlled type 1 diabetes presents with a temperature, dehydration and altered consciousness. Her initial biochemistry profile shows sodium 130 mEq/l, potassium 4.5 mEq/l, bicarbonate 14 mEq/l, pH of 7.02. What is the most immediate treatment?

A. IV bicarbonate

B. IV fluids

C. IV Insulin

D. IV potassium

Explanation:

- The patient has DKA. It is associated with mortality in patients with type 1 diabetes mellitus. Having poorly controlled diabetes mellitus is a risk factor for developing DKA. Immediate management is replacement with IV fluids aggressively followed by insulin therapy.

Ans. C

81. A 56 year old Indian man is seen in the obesity clinic. His BMI is 34 kg/m². He is worked up for metabolic syndrome. What is the waist circumference cut off used for South Asians in the Harmonizing definition of metabolic syndrome?

A. Men ≥ 102 cms, Women ≥ 88 cms

B. Men ≥ 90 cms, Women ≥ 80 cms

C. Men ≥ 100 cms, Women ≥ 88 cms

D. Men ≥ 102 cms, Women ≥ 90 cms

Explanation:

Table: Harmonizing definition[b]		
Three of the following: Waist circumference (cm)		
Men	**Women**	**Ethnicity**
≥94	≥80	Europid, sub-Saharan African, Eastern and Middle Eastern
≥90	≥80	South Asian, Chinese and ethnic South and Central American
≥85	≥90	Japanese
• Fasting triglyceride level >150 mg/dl or specific medication • HDL cholesterol level <40 mg/dl and <50 mg/dl for men and women, respectively, or specific medication • Blood pressure >130 mm systolic >85 mm diastolic or previous diagnosis or specific medication • Fasting plasma glucose level ≥100 mg/dl (alternative indication: drug treatment of elevated glucose levels)		

Ans. B

82. An obese, 56 year old patient with dyslipidemia, well controlled DM and hypertension has been on a low cholesterol diet for the last 6 months. LDL was 201g/dl, HDL was 39mg/dl, HbA1c 6.4. His latest LDL was 190g/dl and his triglycerides in the normal range. What is the next therapeutic step in his cholesterol management?

A. Add pioglitazone
B. Add gemfibrosil
C. Add metformin
D. Add statins

Explanation:

- For the primary prevention of CVD, statins should be offered to people with type II diabetes and who have a 10% or greater 10 year risk of developing CVD.

Ans. D

83. A 2 year old male child is brought with complaints of recurrent fasting hypoglycaemia. On examination he has hepatomegaly and proximal myopathy. A post prandial sample reveals high lactate levels. What is the likely diagnosis?

A. GSD Type 0
B. GSD Type VI
C. GSD Type III
D. GSD Type IV

Explanation:

- Although rare, disorders of glycogenolysis can result in fasting hypoglycemia. These disorders include glycogen storage disease (GSD) of types 0, I, III, and IV and Fanconi-Bickel syndrome. Patients with GSD types I and III characteristically have high blood lactate levels before and after meals, respectively. Both groups have hypertriglyceridemia, but ketones are high in GSD type III.

Ans. C

84. An obese patient with type II DM is seen in OP clinic. Despite following diet control measures, blood glucose not controlled. There is a strong family history of cardiovascular disease and the patient is anxious to modify the risk. His recent Hba1c is 6.7, BMI is 30, BP -110/80 mmHg. What is the first line of treatment?

A. Pioglitazone
B. GLP1 analogue
C. Long acting insulin
D. Metformin

Explanation:

- Metformin is used as a treatment in type 2 DM in obese patient when diet and exercise have failed to control glycemic levels. It reduces hepatic glucose output and has its predominant effects on fasting plasma glucose.

Ans. D

85. A 62 year old man with no known comorbidities is observing fasting during a religious tradition. At what glycemic threshold does glucagon increase as a defense against hypoglycaemia?

A. 80-85 mg/dl
B. 60-65 mg/dl
C. 65-70 mg/dl
D. 70-80 mg/dl

Explanation:

Table: Physiologic responses to decreasing plasma glucose concentrations

Response	Glycemic Threshold, mmol/l (mg/dl)	Physiologic ↓ Effects	Role in Prevention or Correction of Hypoglycemia (Glucose Counter Regulation)
↓ Insulin	4.4-4.7 (80-85)	↑ R_a (↓R_d), increased lipolysis; ↑ FFA ↑ Glycerol	Primary glucose regulatory factor/first defense against hypoglycemia
↑ Glucagon	3.6-3.9 (65-70)	↑ R_a	Primary glucose counterregulatory factor/ second defense against hypoglycemia
↑ Epinephrine	3.6-3.9 (65-70)	↑ R_a ↓ R_c increased lipolysis; ↑ FFA and Glycerol	Third defense against hypoglycemia, critical when glucagon is deficient
↑ Cortisol and growth hormone	3.6-3.9 (65-70)	↑ R_a ↓ R_c	Involved in defense against prolonged hypoglycemia; not critical
Symptoms	2.8-3.1 (50-55)	Recognition of hypoglycemia	Prompt behavioral defense against hypoglycemia (food ingestion)
↓ Cognition	<2.8 (<50)	–	Compromises behavioral defense against hypoglycemia

Ans. C

86. A 60 year old man with type 2 DM has been managed with metformin 500 mg twice daily and also has history of hypertension for which he is treated with ramipril 5mg BD. His BMI is 37, HBa1c 8.4. Which of the following is a contraindication to GLP1 analogue treatment?

A. Increased BMI
B. H/O gastroparesis
C. H/O hypoglycemia
D. Retinopathy

Explanation:

- GLP1 analogues can delay gastric emptying and can therefore exacerbate the symptoms of gastroparesis and are contraindicated in patients with history of gastroparesis.

Ans. B

87. A 62 year old man with no known comorbidities is observing fasting during a religious tradition. Which of the following hormones is not involved in the defense against acute hypoglycaemia?

A. Reduced Insulin levels
B. Increased Glucagon levels
C. Increased Epinephrine levels
D. Increased Cortisol levels

Explanation:

- As plasma glucose levels decline just below the physiologic range, glucose counterregulatory (plasma glucose–raising) hormones are released (Table 399-2; Fig. 399-1). Among these, pancreatic -cell glucagon, and adrenomedullary epinephrine play a primary role. Glucagon stimulates hepatic glycogenolysis and gluconeogenesis. Adrenomedullary epinephrine also stimulates hepatic glycogenolysis and gluconeogenesis (and renal gluconeogenesis), but limits peripheral uptake of glucose and stimulates lipolysis with production of glycerol and fatty acids. Epinephrine becomes critical when glucagon is deficient. When hypoglycemia is prolonged beyond ~4 h, cortisol and growth hormone also support glucose production and restrict glucose utilization to a limited amount (~20% compared to epinephrine). Thus cortisol and growth hormone play no role in defense against acute hypoglycemia.

Ans. D

88. A 20 year old woman is admitted to ER after a collapse. She is found to be hypoglycemic. She was collapsed at work and this has happened at least three times in the past 2 months. Blood glucose levels are 45mg/dl, blood insulin levels are high and serum c peptide levels are normal. Her father is obese and diagnosed with type 2 DM, taking insulin regularly. What is the diagnosis?

A. Glucagonoma
B. Metformin abuse
C. Insulinoma
D. Insulin abuse

Explanation:

- The marked elevation in insulin levels in the presence of a normal C peptide suggest that illicit use of insulin is the most likely diagnosis. Potential access to exogenous insulin as her father has a long standing diagnosis of type 2 DM and is likely to be taking insulin therapy makes the diagnosis most likely.

Ans. D

89. A 29 year old female comes to the hospital with recurrent episodes of sweating, palpitations, dizziness Detailed history revealed these episodes can occur at any time of the day but she has noticed them particularly at night. Her mother is a known case of type 1 diabetes mellitus. She was admitted for a 48 hour fasting glucose monitoring 12 hours after admission her glucose is noted to be 50mg/dl and elevated insulin levels. Which of the following investigation should be performed to confirm the diagnosis?

A. Glucose tolerance test
B. C – peptide levels
C. Insulin like growth factor 1 levels
D. Proinsulin

Explanation:

- The diagnosis is Insulinoma. It is the most common neuroendocrine tumour found in pancreatic islet cells. 90% are benign, while 10% are malignant. It is a feature of MEN type 1. Diagnosis is made by fasting glucose, C peptide, insulin and proinsulin levels. 72 hour fasting test is the diagnostic test .In self-administered insulin, C peptide levels are low. In Insulinoma, C peptide levels are normal while in sulphonyl urea abuse, elevated insulin levels are seen.

Ans. B

90. A 62 year old man with history of Type 2 Diabetes Mellitus since 5 years has an anterior wall MI. He undergoes percutaneous transluminal coronary angioplasty. 3 months later at review, he is referred to you in view of his uncontrolled glycemic status. He is on metformin 1 gm/day and glimiperide 2 mg/day His investigations are as follows:

HbA1c 10%

FBS 190 mg/dl

PPBS 260 mg/dl

Urea 24 mg/dl

Creatinine 0.73 mg/dl

What would be the best regimen in this scenario?

A. Metformin + Basal bolus insulin regimen
B. Metformin + Vildagliptin
C. Increase the dose of metformin and glimiperide
D. Metformin + Empagliflozin

Explanation:

- Based on recent demonstrations of a beneficial cardiovascular effect in certain individuals with type 2 DM and CVD, or at high-risk of CVD, empagliflozin, canagliflozin, and liraglutide should now be considered in these populations.

Ans. D

91. A 47 year old woman with type 2 DM has come to the hospital for review. She was diagnosed with type 2 diabetes mellitus after having an MI. She has history of gastroparesis but asymptomatic now. Current drugs are metformin 1g BD, simvastatin 40mg and asprin 75mg. His BMI is 33 kg/m2, gained 7kg in weight, BP 130/80 mm Hg. What is the additional drug for her?

A. Pioglitazone
B. Gliclazide
C. GLP1 analogue
D. Empagliflozin

Explanation:

- This is SGLT2 inhibitor. SGLT2 inhibitors act by increasing renal excretion of glucose and sodium. This leads to reduction in Hba1c, modest effects on weight and positive effects on blood pressure. Empagliflozin and Canagliflozin reduces cardiovascular events and all cause cardiovascular mortality in patients with type 2 DM and cardiovascular disease.

Ans. D

92. A 36 year old man is recently diagnosed with Type 2 Diabetes Mellitus and started on metformin. His HBA1c at diagnosis is 9%. How much HBA1c reduction is expected with metformin?

A. 0.5- 0.8%
B. 0.5-1.5%
C. 2-3%
D. 1-2%

Explanation:

Table: Agents used for treatment of type 1 or type 2 diabetes

	Mechanism of Action	Examples[a]	HBA_{1C} Reduction (%)[b]	Agent-Specific Advantages	Agent-Specific Disadvantages	Contra-indications
Oral						
Biguanides[C+]	↓ Hepatic glucose production	Metformin	1-2	Weight neutral, do not cause hypoglycemia, inexpensive, extensive experience, ↓CV events	Diarrhea, nausea, lactic acidosis, vitamin B_{12} deficiency	Renal insufficiency (see text for GFR < 45 ml/min), CHF, radiographic contrast studies, hospitalized patients, acidosis

Contd.

α-Glucosidase inhibitors[c++]	↓ GI glucose absorption	Acarbose, miglitol, voglibose	0.5-0.8	Reduce postprandial glycemia	GI flatulence, liver function tests	Renal/liver disease
Dipeptidyl peptidase IV inhibitors[c+++]	Prolong endogenous GLP-1 action; ↑Insulin ↓glucagon	Alogliptin, linagliptin, saxagliptin, sitagliptin, vildagliptin	0.5-0.8	Well tolerated, do not cause hypoglycemia	Angioedema/ urticarial and immune-mediated dermatologic effects	Reduced dose with renal disease
Insulin secretagogues: Sulfonylureas[c+]	↑ Insulin secretion	Glibomuride, gliclazide, glimepiride, glipizide, gliquidone, glyburide, glyclopyramide	1-2	Short onset of action, lower postprandial glucose, inexpensive	Hypoglycemia, weight gain	Renal/liver disease
Insulin secretagogues: Non-sulfonylureas[c+++]	↑ Insulin secretion	Mitiglinide nateglinide, repaglinide	0.5-1.0	Short onset of action, lower postprandial glucose	Hypoglycemia	Renal/liver disease
Sodium-glucose cotransporter 2 inhibitors[+++]	↑ Renal glucose excretion	Canagliflozin, dapagliflozin, empagliflozin, ertugliflozin	0.5-1.0	Do not cause hypoglycemia, ↓ weight and BP; see text for CVD effect	Urinary and genital infections, polyuria, dehydration, exacerbate tendency to hyperkalemia and DKA; see text	Moderate renal insufficiency, insulin-deficient DM
Thiazolidinediones[c+++]	↓ Insulin resistance, ↑ glucose utilization	Pioglitazone, rosiglitazone	0.5-1.4	Lower insulin requirements	Peripheral edema, CHF, weight gain, fractures, macular edema	CHF, liver disease
Parenteral						
Amylin agonists[c++++]	Slow gastric emptying, ↓glucagon	Pramlintide	0.25-0.5	Reduce postprandial glycemia, weight loss	Injection, nausea, ↑risk of hypoglycemia with insulin	Agents that also slow GI motility
GLP-1 receptor agonists[c+++]	↑Insulin, ↓glucagon, slow gastric emptying, satiety	Albiglutide, dulaglutide, exenatide, iraglutide, hxisenatide, semaglutide	0.5-1.0	Weight loss, do not cause hypoglycemia; see text for CVD effect	Injection, nausea, ↑ risk of hypoglycemia with insulin secretagogues	Renal disease, agents that also slow GI motility: medullary carcinoma of thyroid, pancreatic disease
Insulin[c++++]	↑Glucose utilization, ↓hepatic glucose production, and other anabolic actions	See text and Table 397-4	Not limited	Known safety profile	Injection, weight gain, hypoglycemia	
Medical nutrition therapy and physical activity[c+]	↓Insulin resistance, ↑Insulin secretion	Low-calorie, low-fat diet, exercise	1-3	Other health benefits	Complication difficult, long-term success low	

Ans. D

93. A 62 year old man undergoes a routine evaluation for complaints of generalised fatigue. His Fasting plasma glucose is 230 mg/dl and 240 mg/dl on 2 occasions. What is the best management in this case?

A. Metformin only

B. Combination therapy with 2 oral antidiabetic agents

C. Insulin

D. Insulin + oral antidiabetic agents

Explanation:

- Patients with mild hyperglycemia (FPG <7.0–11.0 mmol/L [126–199 mg/dL]) often respond well to a single, oral glucose-lowering agent, while those with moderate hyperglycemia (FPG 11.1–13.9 mmol/L [200–250 mg/dL]) will usually require more than one oral agent or insulin. Patients with more severe hyperglycemia (FPG >13.9 mmol/L [250 mg/dL]) may respond partially but are unlikely to achieve normoglycemia with oral therapy. Insulin can be used as initial therapy in individuals with severe hyperglycemia (FPG <13.9–16.7 mmol/L [250–300 mg/dL]) or in those who are symptom- atic from the hyperglycemia. This approach is based on the rationale that more rapid glycemic control will reduce "glucose toxicity" to the islet cells, improve endogenous insulin secretion, and possibly allow oral glucose-lowering agents to be more effective. If this occurs, the insulin may be discontinued.

Ans. B

94. A 50 year old gentleman is diagnosed with type 2 diabetes mellitus after being treated for lower limb cellulitis. She has a past history of bronchial asthma for which she takes salbutamol inhaler. BMI is 32 and creatinine is normal. Which is the initial intervention for controlling blood sugar?

A. Empagliflozin

B. Gliclazide

C. Metformin

D. Sitagliptin

Explanation:

- Metformin is the initial intervention to control blood sugar levels. It has got a positive effects on lipids and vascular inflammation which may account for positive effect on cardiovascular outcomes.

Ans. C

95. All are true about resistance to thyroid hormone (RTH) disorder except:

A. Autosomal dominant disorder

B. Elevated thyroid hormone levels

C. Inappropriately normal or elevated TSH

D. Signs and symptoms typical of hypothyroidism

Explanation:

- Resistance to thyroid hormone (RTH) is an autosomal dominant disorder characterized by elevated thyroid hormone levels and inappropriately normal or elevated TSH.
- Individuals with RTH do not, in general, exhibit signs and symptoms that are typical of hypothyroidism because hormone resistance is partial and is compensated by increased levels of thyroid hormone.
- Clinical features of RTH can include goiter, attention deficit disorder, mild reduction in IQ, delayed skeletal maturation, tachycardia, and impaired metabolic responses to thyroid hormone.
- Classical forms of RTH are caused by mutations in the TRβ gene.
- These mutations, located in restricted regions of the ligand-binding domain, cause loss of receptor function.
- However, because the mutant receptors retain the capacity to dimerize with RXRs, bind to DNA, and recruit co-repressor proteins, they function as antagonists of remaining normal TRβ and TRα receptors.
- This property, referred to as "dominant negative" activity, explains the autosomal dominant mode of transmission.
- Diagnosis is suspected when unbound thyroid hormone levels are increased without suppression of TSH.

- Similar hormonal abnormalities are found in other affected family members, although TRβ mutation arises de novo in about 20% of patients.
- DNA sequence analysis of TRβ gene provides a definitive diagnosis.
- RTH must be distinguished from other causes of euthyroid hyperthyroxinemia (e.g., FDH) and inappropriate secretion of TSH by TSH-secreting pituitary adenomas

Ans. D

96. A 20 year old man presents to the hospital complaints of tiredness, polyuria, thirst and recurrent thrush infections. He has a family history of type 2 diabetes with early onset in the second decades, O/E he looks slim, BMI of 22, no evidence of acanthosis nigricans. Islet cell, glutamic acid decarboxylase (GAD), insulin antibodies are all negative. Urine and blood ketone measurement are negative, but urinary dipstick shows 3+glucosuria.

A. Type 1 diabetes
B. Type 2 diabetes
C. MODY
D. Addison's disease

Explanation:

- MODY has an age of onset between 10 and 30 years, can be managed in many patients with the use of sulphonylureas alone. The strong family history of early onset diabetes without a history of insulin resistance or elevated BMI is also suggestive of MODY, as is the marked glucosuria.

Ans. C

97. Most common genetic alteration in papillary thyroid carcinoma is:

A. BRAF V600E
B. NRAS
C. RET
D. TRK1

Explanation:

- BRAF V600E mutations appear to be the most common genetic alteration in PTC.
- These mutations activate the kinase, which stimulates the mitogen activated protein kinase (MAPK) cascade.
- RAS mutations, which also stimulate MAPK cascade, are found in about 20–30% of thyroid neoplasms (NRAS > HRAS > KRAS), including both PTC follicular variant & FTC.
- Of note, simultaneous RET, BRAF, and RAS mutations rarely occur in the same tumor, suggesting that activation of the MAPK cascade is critical for tumor development, independent of the step that initiates the cascade.

Ans. A

98. A 17 year old male, diagnosed case of Type 1 Diabetes Mellitus since 2 years is poorly controlled on a split mix regimen. He is changed over to a basal bolus regimen with short acting insulin analogs and insulin glargine. When should he be advised to inject the short acting insulin analog?

A. Less than 10 minutes before meal
B. 30 minutes before meal
C. 20 minutes before meal
D. After meal

Explanation:

- Short-acting insulin analogues should be injected just before (<10 min) and regular insulin 30–45 min prior to a meal.

Ans. A

99. A well controlled 58 year old type 2 DM He has background diabetic retinopathy and currently takes metformin 500mg thrice daily, gliclazide twice daily and empagliflozin along with ramipril 10mg and aspirin 75mg. He complaints of weight gain and recurrent hypoglycemia. What is the causative drug?

A. Metformin
B. Gliclazide
C. Empagliflozin
D. Ramipril

Explanation:

- Insulin secretagogues like sulphonyl ureas are associated with hypoglycemia. Drugs like sulphonyl ureas and pioglitazone causes weight gain.

Ans. B

100. A 45 year old man, obese (BMI 35) has symptoms of nocturia and lethargy, fasting blood glucose of 150mg/dl. He has carried a 6 week trial of lifestyle modification including diet and regular evening walks. He has history of hypertension which is managed with ramipril 10mg daily. What is the initial treatment?

A. Pioglitazone
B. Sitagliptin
C. Gliclazide
D. Metformin

Explanation:

- Metformin is the initial treatment of choice for type 2 DM. It is a biguanide, one of the primary action of metformin is reduction of hepatic glucose output, it does not cause weight gain or hypoglycemia

Ans. D

101. A 58 year old man is newly diagnosed with Type 2 diabetes and started on metformin. What are the treatment targets recommended in Type 2 Diabetes Mellitus?

A. Fasting plasma glucose 80-130 mg/dl, Postprandial plama glucose <180 mg/dl, HBA1C < 6.5%

B. Fasting plasma glucose <100 mg/dl, Postprandial plama glucose <180 mg/dl, HBA1C < 7%

C. Fasting plasma glucose 80-130 mg/dl, Postprandial plama glucose <180 mg/dl, HBA1C < 7%

D. Fasting plasma glucose < 100 mg/dl, Postprandial plama glucose <200 mg/dl, HBA1C < 6.5%

Explanation:

Table: Treatment goals for adults with diabetes[a]

Index	Goal
Glycemic control[b]	
• HbA_{1c}	<7.0%[c]
• Preprandial capillary plasma glucose	4.4-7.2 mmol/l (80-130 mg/dl)
• Postprandial capillary plasma glucose[d]	<10.0 mmol/l (<180 mg/dl)
Blood pressure	<140/90 mm Hg[e]

Ans. C

102. A 57 year old man with type 2 diabetes mellitus presents to the clinic with HbA1c 8.4. His BP was 150/80 mm Hg. PR- 90/min, BMI 36. He is taking metformin 1g BD. He works as a bus driver . He was prescribed the drug which slows gastric emptying. What is the drug prescribed?

A. Empagliflozin
B. GLP agonist
C. Insulin
D. Pioglitazone

Explanation:

- GLP1 agonist act by slowing the gastric emptying, increasing insulin and decreasing glucagon levels.

Ans. B

103. A 59 year old man came to the hospital for review. He had type 2 DM for 10 years, treated with metformin, sitagliptin and gliclazide. His Hba1c is 12%. For the past 1 week, he had feelings of severe pain and paresthesia in the both feet and weight loss of 3 kgs. Which is the correct statement?

A. Insulin is the main treatment

B. The condition is common in type 1 diabetes

C. Weight loss is unlikely to be related to the diagnosis

D. Recovery from this condition will occur over 1 year

Explanation:

- Good glycemic control through the adjustment of diabetes medication is of prime importance in diabetic neuropathy. The patient is already on 3 drugs, poor glycemic control, insulin is the next treatment.

Ans. A

104. A 46 year old man undergoes a routine health check. His Fasting plasma glucose is 116 mg/dl, 2 hour plasma glucose value after a OGTT is 180 mg/dl. What is best advised in this scenario?

A. Start Metformin

B. Lifestyle modification only

C. Start on insulin

D. Repeat testing after 1 year

Explanation:

- Pharmacologic therapy for individuals with prediabetes is currently controversial because its cost-effectiveness and safety profile are not known. The ADA suggests that metformin be considered in individuals with both IFG and IGT who are at very high risk for progression to diabetes (age <60 years, BMI ≥35 kg/m^2, and women with a history of GDM).

Ans. B

105. A 50 year old woman on treatment for myasthenia gravis presents with intermittent postprandial hypoglycaemia. Critical sample at the time of hypoglycaemia reveals inappropriately raised insulin at RBS of 40 mg/dl. What is the most probable diagnosis?

A. Type A insulin Resistance

B. Type B insulin Resistance

C. Insulinoma

D. Reactive hypoglycemia

Explanation:

- Two distinct syndromes of severe insulin resistance have been described in adults: (1) type A, which affects young women and is characterized by severe hyperinsulinemia, obesity, and features of hyperandrogenism; and (2) type B, which affects middle-aged women and is characterized by severe hyperinsulinemia, features of hyperandrogenism, and autoimmune disorders. Individuals with the type A insulin resistance syndrome have an undefined defect in the insulin-signaling pathway; individuals with the type B insulin resistance syndrome have autoantibodies directed at the insulin receptor. These receptor autoantibodies may block insulin binding or may stimulate the insulin receptor, leading to intermittent hypoglycemia.

Ans. B

106. A 61 year old gentleman recovering from inferior MI in the cardiology ward, is found to have HbA1c 7.5. What is the correct statement among the following?

A. Metformin should be stopped if eGFR falls below 80ml/min

B. Metformin is contraindicated if angiography is planned

C. Metformin can be given even when cardiac angiogram is planned

D. No contraindication for metformin

Explanation:

- Metformin causes contrast nephropathy if administered before angiography. So it has to be stopped if angiogram is planned. Metformin should not be used if GFR<45ml/min, acidosis, unstable CHF, liver disease.

Ans. B

107. A 15 year old boy, diagnosed case of Type 1 Diabetes Mellitus since 3 months presents with recurrent hypoglycemia on a basal bolus insulin. What is the cause of recurrent hypoglycemias in Type 1 Diabetes Mellitus?

A. Autoimmune destruction of alpha cells

B. Altered pattern of hormone secretion from alpha cells

C. Iatrogenic hypoglycemia

D. None of the above

Explanation:

- Although other islet cell types (alpha cells [glucagon-producing], delta cells [somatostatin-producing], or PP cells [pancreatic polypeptide-producing]) are functionally and embry ologically similar to beta cells, they are spared from the autoimmune destruction. However, altered patterns of hormone secretion from these other cell types in type 1 DM likely contributes to metabolic instability. Alpha cell dysfunction as reflected by fasting hyperglucagonemia, hyperglucagonemia in the post-prandial state, and an impaired glu- cagon response to hypoglycemia. Pathologically, the pancreatic islets have modest infiltration of lymphocytes (a process termed *insulitis*). After beta cells are destroyed, it is thought that the inflammatory process abates and the islets become atrophic.

Ans. B

108. A 56 year old gentleman comes for review. He has type 2 DM for 5 years, currently on tab metformin 500 BD. His BMI is 34, BP -150/80 mm Hg. HbA1c- 8.4%. What is the next step in the management?

A. Basal insulin

B. Pioglitazone

C. Empagliflozin

D. Gliclazide.

Explanation:

- The patient is obese with worsening glycemic control, hence it requires treatment intensification without hazard of further weight gain. Empagliflozin, an SGLT2 inhibitor increases glucose excretion in urine. Other drugs causes weight gain.

Ans. C

109. A 65 year old diabetic is being admitted in comatose state. Examination revealed BP of 90/60 mm HG, PR -82/min and regular. Serum Na – 152 mEql/L, K – 5.5 mEql/L, Glucose 700 mg/dl, pH -7.35, bicarbonate -25 mmol/L. What is the diagnosis?

A. DKA

B. Drug overdose

C. Hyperosmolar hyperglycaemic coma

D. Acute stroke

Explanation:

- The bicarbonate and blood pH would be normal in hyperosmolar hyperglycaemic coma unlike DKA where it would be low. Rehydration with IV fluids is the intervention of choice.

Ans. C

110. A 62 year old man undergoes a routine health check up. He has no symptoms of note. His fasting plasma glucose is 110 mg/dl and 2 hour plasma glucose after an OGTT is 139 mg/dl. What is the diagnosis?

A. Impaired fasting glucose
B. Impaired glucose tolerance
C. Type 2 Diabetes Mellitus
D. Normal glucose tolerance

Explanation:

Type of Diabetes	Normal glucose tolerance	Hyperglycemia			
		Pre-diabetes*	Diabetes Mellitus		
		Impaired fasting glucose of impaired glucose tolerance	Not insulin requiring	Insulin required for control	Insulin required for survival
Type 1					
Type 2					
Specific types					
Gestational diabetes					
Time (years)					
FPG	<5.6 mmol/l (100 mg/dl)	5.6-6.9 mmol/l (100-125 mg/dl)		≥70 mmol/l (126 mg/dl)	
2-h PG	<7.8 mmol/l (140 mg/dl)	7.8-11.0 mmol/l (140-199 mg/dl)		≥11.1 mmol/l (200 mg/dl)	
HbA1C	<5.6%	5.7-6.4%		≥6.5%	

Ans. A

111. A 48 year old lady known case of DM and CKD had a DEXA scan done which showed osteoporosis. A drug was prescribed whose mechanism is antibody to RANK ligand. What is the drug prescribed?

A. Zolendronate
B. Denososumab
C. Abaloparatide
D. Romosozumab

Explanation:

- Denososumab is a monoclonal antibody to RANK ligand, FDA approved drug for osteoporosis.

Ans. B

112. A 26 year old woman is diagnosed with gestational diabetes in her 24th week of pregnancy and started on insulin. Insulin was withdrawn soon after delivery and 3 months post delivery, her fasting plasma glucose and 2 hour plasma glucose value during an OGTT were normal.

When should she be screened for development of Type 2 Diabetes/ prediabetes?

A. At next pregnancy
B. Lifelong screening every 3 years
C. Lifelong screening every year
D. Lifelong screening every 5 years

Explanation:

- Most women with GDM revert to normal glucose tolerance postpartum but have a sub- stantial risk (35–60%) of developing DM in the next 10–20 years. Currently, the ADA recommends that women with a history of GDM undergo lifelong screening for the development of diabetes or prediabetes at least every 3 years.

Ans. B

113. A 22 year old man with diabetes mellitus comes to the hospital for review. His BMI is 32, he was found to have MODY. Which of the following features in his history would lead to diagnosis of MODY?

A. BMI 32
B. Response to Gliclazide
C. Frequent admissions with DKA
D. Family history of diabetes mellitus

Explanation:

- A strong family history of diabetes is seen with MODY. MODY 3 is most common which is due to HNF1 alpha mutation. They respond to sulphonylureas and do not have recurrent DKA.

Ans. D

114. A 32 year old woman is seen in the obesity clinic. Her BMI is 32 kg/m2 and she is started on orlistat at a dose of 120 mg TID. What is the expected weight loss after 1 year?

A. 4-5%
B. 9-10%
C. 14-15%
D. 18-20%

Explanation:

- Multiple randomized, double-blind, placebo-controlled studies have shown that, after 1 year, orlistat produces a weight loss of ~9–10%, whereas placebo recipients have a 4–6% weight loss.

Ans. B

115. A 55 year old driver comes to the hospital for review. He had type 2 DM for the past 4 years, his blood glucose is poorly controlled on tab metformin 1 g BD and Gliclazide 80mg BD, a recent Hba1c was 8.7%. His BP is 150/80 mm Hg, PR- 80/min. He is reluctant to put on weight. Which is the appropriate intervention with respect to glycemic control?

A. Sitagliptin
B. Liraglutide
C. Basal insulin
D. Pioglitazone

Explanation:

- Liraglutide is associated with both improved glycemic control and weight loss. While Liraglutide use can cause hypoglycaemia when used with sulphonyl urea, dose of sulphonyl urea should be down titrated by 50%.

Ans. B

116. A 56 year old gentleman with history of uncontrolled T2DM, Systemic HTN, dyslipidemia, Osteoarthritis and severe obstructive sleep apnea is seen in the clinic. On examination his BMI is 41 kg/m2 and his BP is uncontrolled (170/90 mm Hg) on multiple antihypertensives. He enquires about bariatric surgery for weight loss:

Which group of patients should be considered for bariatric surgery?

A. BMI ≥ 40kg/m2 with multiple comorbidities
B. BMI ≥ 30kg/m2 with multiple comorbidities
C. BMI ≥ 35 kg/m2 with multiple comorbidities
D. BMI ≥ 35 kg/m2

Explanation:

- Bariatric surgery is indicated in patients with BMI ≥ 40 Kg/m2 or BMI ≥ 35 Kg/m2 with multiple comorbidities

Table: A guide to opting for treatment for obesity					
Treatment	BMI Category (kg/m²)				
	25-26.9	27-29.9	30-34.9	35-39.9	≥40
Diet, exercise, behavioral therapy	With comorbidities	With comorbidities	+	+	+
Pharmacotherapy	–	With comorbidities	+	+	+
Surgery	–	–	–	With comorbidities	+

Source: From the National Heart, Lung and Blood Institute, North American Association for the Study of Obesity (2000)

Ans. C

117. A 55 year old gentleman with obesity and type 2 DM comes for review. He is on tab metformin 1g BD, Ramipril 10mg and amlodipine 10mg OD. PR- 70/min, BMI is 36. HbA1c – 8.4%. He is started on sitagliptin? What is the mode of action of sitagliptin?

A. DPP IV inhibitor
B. GLP1 agonist
C. SGLT 2 inhibitor
D. Sulphonylurea

Explanation:

- DPP IV inhibitors inhibit breakdown of naturally occurring peptides including GLP1 , a gut peptide produced along with Gastric inhibitory peptide in the incretin response. The incretin response occurs in response to a meal and results in increased insulin release, feeling of satiety and slowed gastric emptying. DPP IV inhibitors result in reduction of HBA1C of between 0.6 and 0.9%.

Ans. A

118. A 9 month old female presented with hyponatremia and hypoglycemia following a three day history of fever. Her weight was above the 97th percentile for age. General physical examination revealed dark hair and dark roots. There was no hyperpigmentation of nipples or palmer creases. The remainder of her physical examination was normal.

This condition is caused by genetic mutation in:

A. MC4R
B. POMC
C. AgRP
D. LepR

Explanation:

- Mutations in the gene encoding proopiomelanocortin (POMC) cause severe obesity through failure to synthesize α-MSH and β- MSH, key neuropeptides that inhibit appetite in the hypothalamus. The absence of POMC also causes secondary adrenal insufficiency due to absence of adrenocorticotropic hormone (ACTH), as well as pale skin and red hair due to absence of α -MSH.

Ans. B

119. A 1 year old male child is brought with history of recurrent fractures. X-Ray forearm shows generalised osteopenia of the radius and ulna with intermembranous ossification. This condition is caused by genetic mutation in:

A. COL1A1
B. COL1A2
C. CRTAP
D. IFITM5

Explanation:

- The diagnosis in this case is Osteogenesis imperfect type 5. The characteristic features of OI Type 5 are calcification of the interosseous membranes in forearm and legs and/or hypertrophic callus. Variable bone deformity, normal sclerae and dentition. This is caused by mutation in the gene IFITM5

Table: Classification of osteogenesis imperfecta (OI)

Phenotype	Type	Typical Features	Inheritance	Gene/Protein Defect	Protein Defect
Non-deforming form	OI type 1	Mild to moderate bone fragility, normal or near normal stature, in most, blue sclerae, normal dentition in most hearing loss in ~50%.	AD	***COL1A1*** ***COL1A2***	Collagen I haploinsufficiency
Perinatally lethal form	OI type 2	Extreme bone fragility, short stature, long bone bowing	AD AR	***COL1A1*** ***COL1A2*** *CRTAP* *LEPRE1/P3H1* *PPIB/CYPB*	Collagen I structural mutations Collagen post-translational modification and folding machinery
Progressively deforming OI	OI type 3	Moderate to severe bone deformity, blue sclerae at birth, hearing loss and abnormal dentition common	AD AR	***COL1A1*** ***COL1A2*** *CRTAP* *LEPRE1/P3H1* *PPIB/CYPB* *FKBP10/FKBP65* *PLOD2/LH2* *SERPINH1/HSP47* *CREB3L1/OASIS* *SEC24D* *BMP1* *WNT1* *SERPINF1/PEDF* *TMEM38B/TRIC-B* *SP7/OSX*	Collagen I structural mutations Collagen post-translational modification and folding machinery Protein folding/ endoplasmic reticulum stress sensor COPII vesicle component collagen secretion Proteolytic removal of procollagen N-propeptide Wnt cell signaling pathway Signaling and collagen binding protein, important for mineralization Endoplasmic reticulum cation channel. Calcium homoestasis/collagen synthesis Transcription factor, bone formation

Common Variable OI with normal sclerae	OI type 4	Mild to moderate, bone fragility, normal sclerae, variable dentition, hearing loss in <10%.	AD AR	**COL1A1** **COL1A2** WNT1 CRTAP FKBP10/FKBP65 PPIB/CYPB SERPINF1/PEDF SPARC SP7/OSX	Collagen I structural mutations Wnt cell signaling pathway Collagen post-translational modification and folding machinery Signaling and collagen binding protein, important for mineralization Collagen binding/ extracellular matrix assembly Transcription factor, bone formation
OI with calcification of the interosseous membranes	OI type 5	Calcification of the interosseous membranes in forearm and legs and/or hypertrophic callus. Variable bone deformity, normal sclerae and dentition	AD	IFITM5	Transcription factor, bone formation
Bruck syndrome type 1	BRKS1	Contractures with pterygia, fractures in infancy or early childhood, postnatal short stature, severe limb deformity, and progressive scoliosis	AR	FKBP10/FKBP65	Collagen folding machinery
Bruck syndrome type 2	BRKS2	As for Bruck syndrome type 1	AR	PLOD2/LH2	Collagen post-translational modification of lysine

Note: Predominant OI gene mutations (>90%) are in **COL1A1** and **COL1A2** (in bold typeface).
Abbreviations: AD, autosomal dominant; AR, autosomal recessive.

Ans. D

120. A 70 year old lady with type 2 DM comes for review. She is on mixed insulin twice daily, anxious about weight gain. Other comorbids include ischemic heart disease and renal impairment. Her BMI is 33, eGFR 27m/min. Which is the suitable agent to add?

A. Gliclazide
B. Linagliptin
C. Metformin
D. Pioglitazone

Explanation:

- Linagliptin is used in renal impairment patients even without dose adjustment. It is excreted in faeces. It can cause modest weight loss also.

Ans. C

121. A 40 year old lady who works on a permanent night shift comes to the hospital for review. She is a known case of type 2 diabetes mellitus, on metformin 1g BD and Gliclazide 160mg BD. She suffers from frequent hypoglycaemia, weight gain and BMI is 32. Her BP is 150/90 mm Hg, Pulse is 78/min, regular. What is the next step with response to diabetes therapy?

A. Change gliclazide to pioglitazone
B. Change gliclazide to sitagliptin
C. Reduce gliclazide
D. Reduce metformin

Explanation:

- The patient has frequent episodes of hypoglycaemia and has weight gain. The most suitable option is to substitute sulphonylurea with DPPIV inhibitor which is weight neutral and does not result in hypoglycaemia.

Ans. B

122. A 25 year old man presents to diabetes clinic for review. He had recurrent balanitis and was found to have glycosuria. Family history revealed his father, one aunt, one uncle have had type 2 DM for more than 20 years. They had good glycemic control without complications. His BP 120/80 mm Hg and Pulse 80/min, regular. BMI is 20, HbA1c -5.9%, fasting plasma glucose – 140mg/dl. What is the diagnosis?

A. MODY 2
B. MODY 3
C. MODY 5
D. Type 1 diabetes

Explanation:

- MODY 2 is caused by mutations in glucokinase which acts as a glucose sensor for the beta cells. It increases the fasting plasma glucose. Microvascular complications are rare.

Ans. A

123. A 48 year old woman presents with low backache and hearing loss. X-Ray skull is shown in the picture. This condition is caused by mutations in the following genes except:

A. TCIRG1
B. TNFRSF11B
C. SQSTM1
D. CSF1

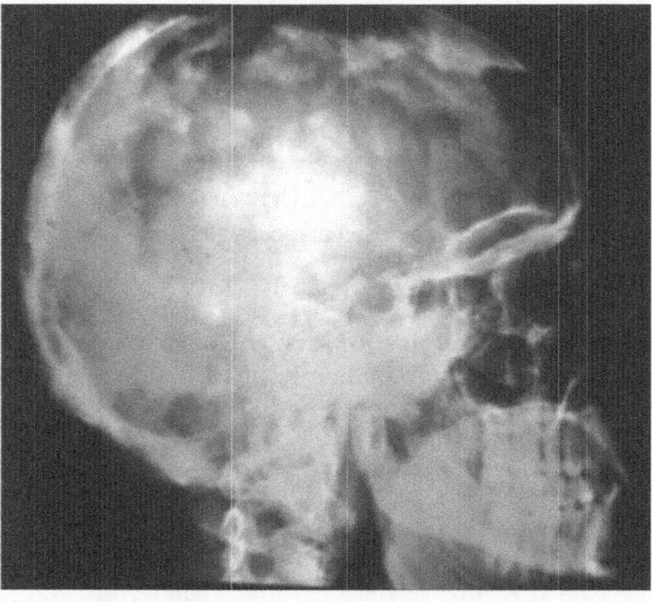

Explanation:

- The etiology of Paget's disease of bone remains unknown, but evidence supports both genetic and viral etiologies. A positive family history is found in 15–25% of patients and, when present, raises the prevalence of the disease seven- to tenfold among first-degree relatives.

- A clear genetic basis has been established for several rare familial bone disorders that clinically and radiographically resemble Paget's disease but have more severe presentation and earlier onset. A homozygous deletion of the *TNFRSF11B* gene, which encodes oste- oprotegrin causes *juvenile Paget's disease*, also known as *familial idiopathic hyperphosphatasia*, a disorder characterized by uncontrolled osteoclastic differentiation and resorption. Familial patterns of disease in several large kindred are consistent with an autosomal dominant pattern of inheritance with variable penetrance. *Familial expansile osteolysis, expansile skeletal hyperphosphatasia, and early-onset Paget's dis- ease* are associated with mutations in *TNFRSF11A* gene, which encodes RANK (receptor activator of nuclear factor-B), a member of the tumor necrosis factor superfamily critical for osteoclast differentiation. Finally, mutations in the gene for valosin containing protein cause a rare syndrome with autosomal dominant inheritance and variable penetrance known as *inclusion body myopathy with Paget's disease and frontotemporal dementia* (*IBMPFD*). The role of genetic factors is less clear in the more common form of late-onset Paget's disease. The most common mutations identified in familial and sporadic cases of Paget's disease have been in the *SQSTM1* gene (sequestasome-1 or p62 protein) in the C-terminal ubiquitin-binding domain. The other candidate genes include: CSF1 (1p13), which encodes macrophage colony stimulating factor (M-CSF), a cytokine that is required for osteoclast differentiation; RIN3 (14q32), which encodes a guanine exchange factor called Rab and Ras interactor 3; OPTN (10p13), which is involved in regulating NFB, TNFRSF11A (18q21) which encodes Receptor Activator of Nuclear Factor-B (RANK), a receptor that is essential for osteoclast differentiation; and TM7SF4, which encodes Dendritic Cell-Specific Transmembrane Protein (DC-STAMP), a molecule that is essential for fusion of osteoclast.
- *TCIRG1* gene mutation is found in about one-half of the patients with malignant infantile osteopetrosis. (Page 2963)

Ans. A

124. A 65 year old gentleman, long standing type 2 DM. His BMI is 28. Hba1c -8%, eGFR -29ml/min. He has a past history of ischemic heart disease and is on regular treatment for the same. He was prescribed long acting peakless insulin analog. What is the insulin prescribed?

A. Insulin glargine
B. NPH
C. Insulin Lispro
D. Insulin Aspart

Explanation:

- Short acting insulin analogs are aspart, lispro and glulysine. NPH is intermediate acting insulin, long acting insulin analogs are degludec, glargine, detemir. These long acting analogs are peakless and have decreased number of hypoglycemic episodes.

Ans. A

125. A 56 year old lady on evaluation for hypercalcemia is diagnosed with primary hyperparathyroidism. Preoperatively, Calcium is 13.5 mg/dl and PTH is 80 pg/ml. Her preoperative ^{99m}Tc sestamibi scan shows a right superior parathyroid adenoma. She is posted for surgery. Intra op PTH after parathyroid excision is 14 pg/ml. What level of intraoperative PTH post parathyroid excision suggests successful surgery?

A. Intraoperative sampling of PTH before and at 5-minute intervals after removal of a suspected adenoma to confirm a rapid fall (>50%) to normal levels of PTH

B. Intraoperative sampling of PTH before and at 5-minute intervals after removal of a suspected adenoma to confirm a rapid fall (>60%) to normal levels of PTH

C. Intraoperative sampling of PTH before and at 5-minute intervals after removal of a suspected adenoma to confirm a rapid fall (>75%) to normal levels of PTH

D. Intraoperative sampling of PTH before and at 5-minute intervals after removal of a suspected adenoma to confirm a rapid fall (>90%) to normal levels of PTH

Explanation:

- Preoperative ^{99m}Tc sestamibi scans with single- photon emission CT (SPECT) are used to predict the location of an abnormal gland and intraoperative sampling of PTH before and at 5-minute intervals after removal of a suspected adenoma to con- firm a rapid fall (>50%) to normal levels of PTH. In several centers, a combination of preoperative sestamibi imaging, cervical block anesthesia, minimal surgical incision, and intraoperative PTH measurements has allowed successful outpatient surgical management with a clear-cut cost benefit compared to general anesthesia and more extensive neck surgery.

Ans. A

126. A 50 year old gentleman during medical checkup is found to have fasting plasma glucose of 130 mg/dl. He has polyuria, polydipsia. He is obese with BMI of 31. The test is repeated couple of days later random blood sugar is found to be 210mg/dl. What is the diagnosis?

A. Normal
B. Diabetes mellitus
C. Impaired glucose tolerance
D. Obesity

Explanation:

- This patient has a fasting plasma glucose of 130mg/dl, random plasma glucose of 210mg/dl with symptoms. Both these values satisfy the clinical criteria for diagnosis of type 2 diabetes mellitus.

Ans. B

127. A 50 year old patient with long standing type 2 DM is found to have urinary albumin excretion of 300mg/l. His diabetes is well controlled with metformin and is normotensive with BP 122/80 mm Hg, PR_ 68/ min, regular. BMI is 32. Her Hba1c is 7.4%. which of the following drug is used to prevent progression of nephropathy?

A. Diltiazem
B. Gliclazide
C. Lisinopril
D. Nifedipine

Explanation:

- ACE Inhibitors are used to treat normotensive patients to retard the progression of nephropathy. Even in type 1 diabetes mellitus, ACE inhibitors offer some benefit in nephropathy.

Ans. C

128. A 45 Year old male presents with hypocalcemia post total thyroidectomy. He has been on long term proton pump inhibitors for Acid peptic disease. It is decided to start him on calcium supplements and activated Vitamin D. Which is the calcium preparation of choice?

A. Calcium Carbonate
B. Calcium Citrate
C. Calcium Acetate
D. Calcium phosphate

Explanation:

- Optimal rates of calcium absorption require gastric acid. This is especially true for weakly dissociable calcium supplements such as calcium carbonate. In fact, large boluses of calcium carbonate are poorly absorbed because of their neutralizing effect on gastric acid. In achlorhydric subjects and for those taking drugs that inhibit gastric acid secretion, supplements should be taken with meals to optimize their absorption. Use of calcium citrate may be preferable in these circumstances.

Ans. B

129. A 44 year old man with obesity, impaired fasting glucose and hypertension with a blood pressure of 150/92 mm Hg. BMI is 35. Which of the following drugs must be avoided?

A. Losartan
B. Lisinopril
C. Hydrochlorothiazide
D. Bisoprolol

Explanation:

- Drug and chemical induced diabetes. Thiazides negatively impact on progression to diabetes in patients with obesity/ impaired glucose tolerance. So hydrochlorothiazides should be avoided.

Ans. C

130. Hormonal production particularly sensitive to neuronal damage by lesions that affect the pituitary stalk or hypothalamus is:

A. Oxytocin
B. GH
C. TSH
D. FSH

Explanation:

- Posterior pituitary is supplied by the inferior hypophyseal arteries. In contrast to the anterior pituitary, the posterior lobe is directly innervated by hypothalamic neurons (supraoptico hypophyseal and tubero hypophyseal nerve tracts) via the pituitary stalk.
- Thus, posterior pituitary production of vasopressin (antidiuretic hormone [ADH]) and oxytocin is particularly sensitive to neuronal damage by lesions that affect the pituitary stalk or hypothalamus.

Ans. A

131. A 56 year old female presents with resistant hypertension, typical paroxysms suggestive of pheochromocytoma and an adrenal mass of 10 × 6 cm. Malignant pheochromocytoma is suspected. Criteria for making a diagnosis of malignant pheochromocytoma is:

A. Cellular atypia, presence of mitoses
B. Invasion of blood vessels or adjacent tissues
C. Lymph node or distant metastases
D. All of the above

Explanation:

- About 5–10% of pheochromocytomas and paragangliomas are malignant. The diagnosis of malignant pheochromocytoma is problematic. The typical histologic criteria of cellular atypia, presence of mitoses, and invasion of vessels or adjacent tissues are insufficient for the diagnosis of malignancy in pheochromocytoma. Thus, the term *malignant pheochromocytoma* is restricted to tumors with lymph node or distant metastases, the latter most commonly found by nuclear medicine imaging in lungs, bone, or liver locations suggesting a vascular pathway of spread.

Ans. C

132. A 50 year old man with history of type 2 DM had an anterior MI 4 years ago, on aspirin 150mg once daily and insulin twice daily. BMI is 34, BP -150/90 mm Hg, HbA1c- 6.9%. Which of the following drug is not FDA approved for obesity?

A. Orlistat
B. Lorcaserin
C. Liraglutide
D. Vitamin E

Explanation:

- FDA approved drugs for obesity are Lorcaserin, liraglutide, Phentermine/topiramate, naltrexone/bupropion, orlistat.

Ans. D

133. Pattern of hormone loss in cranial irradiation is:

A. GH deficiency is most common

B. gonadotropin deficiency is most common

C. ACTH deficiency deficiency is most common

D. ACTH followed by GH deficiency is most common

Explanation:

- Cranial irradiation may result in long-term hypothalamic and pituitary dysfunction, especially in children and adolescents, as they are more susceptible to damage after whole-brain or head and neck therapeutic irradiation.
- Development of hormonal abnormalities correlates strongly with irradiation dosage and the time interval after completion of radiotherapy.
- Up to two-thirds of patients ultimately develop hormone insufficiency after a median dose of 50 Gy (5000 rad) directed at the skull base.
- Development of hypopituitarism occurs over 5–15 years and usually reflects hypothalamic damage rather than primary destruction of pituitary cells.

Ans. A

134. A 50 year old man with long standing type 2 DM has come to the hospital with ulcer over the left foot great toe. O/E there is loss of sensation over the ulcer, his foot appears warm and there is some toe clawing. What is the etiology of his ulcer?

A. Trauma

B. Neuropathic ulcer

C. Arterial ulcer

D. Vasculitis

Explanation:

- The combination of painless ulcer in a pressure area with poorly controlled diabetes mellitus and neuropathy is suggestive of neuropathic ulcer. The lifetime risk of a person with diabetes developing a foot ulcer may be high as 25%. 50 percent of older patients with type 2 diabetes have one or more risk factors for foot ulceration.

Ans. B

135. A 65 year old gentleman presents to ER with deteriorating right eye vision over the past 24 hours. He has a long standing type 2 DM, hypertension, dyslipidemia. O/E he counts fingers in the right eye, 6/12 in the left eye. BP -150/90 mm Hg, PR -92/min, regular. Fundoscopy reveals retinal microaneurysms, blot hemorrhage and cottonwool spots. Optic disc appears normal. Which is the most common cause?

A. Non-proliferative diabetic retinopathy

B. Branch retinal vein occlusion

C. Branch retinal artery occlusion

D. Proliferative diabetic retinopathy

Explanation:

- Diabetic retinopathy is classified as non-proliferative and proliferative diabetic retinopathy. Non-proliferative diabetic retinopathy is characterized by retinal microaneurysms, blot hemorrhage and cotton wool spots. Neovascularisation is the hallmark of proliferative diabetic retinopathy.

Ans. A

136. Autoantibodies to Ro/SS-A and La/SS-B antigens in Sjögren's syndrome are associated with all except:

A. Usually present prior to diagnosis

B. Longer disease duration

C. More intense lymphocytic infiltration of major salivary glands

D. Extraglandular (systemic) manifestations

Explanation:

- Sera from patients with Sjögren's syndrome often contain autoantibodies to non-organ-specific antigens such as immunoglobulins (rheumatoid factors) and extractable nuclear and cytoplasmic antigens (Ro/ SS-A, La/SS-B). Ro/SS-A autoantigen consists of two polypeptides (52 and 60 kDa, respectively) in conjunction with cytoplasmic RNAs, whereas the 48-kDa La/SS-B protein is bound to RNA III polymerase transcripts.
- Autoantibodies to Ro/SS-A and La/SS-B antigens are usually present prior to diagnosis and are associated with earlier disease onset, longer disease duration, salivary gland enlargement, extraglandular (systemic) manifestations, and more intense lymphocytic infiltration of minor salivary glands.

Ans. C

137. A 40 year old male presents with uncontrolled HTN, headache, profuse sweating, palpitations and tachycardia. Pheochromocytoma is suspected and Plasma metanephrines is done which is 1.2 times the upper limit of normal. What is the next step in conformation of diagnosis?

A. CT adrenals

B. MIBG scan

C. MRI adrenals

D. Clonidine suppression test

Explanation:

- Catecholamines and metanephrines can be measured by different methods, including high-performance liquid chromatography, enzyme-linked immunosorbent assay, and liquid chromatography/ mass spectrometry. When pheochromocytoma is suspected on clinical grounds (i.e., when values are three times the upper limit of normal), this diagnosis is highly likely regardless of the assay used. However, as summarized in the sensitivity and specificity of available biochemical tests vary greatly, and these differences are important in assessing patients with borderline elevations of different compounds. Urinary tests for metanephrines (total or fractionated) and catecholamines are widely available and are used commonly for initial evaluation. Among these tests, those for the fractionated metanephrines and catecholamines are the most sensitive. Plasma tests are more convenient and include measurements of catecholamines and metanephrines. Measurements of plasma metanephrine are the most sensitive and are less susceptible to false-positive elevations from stress, including venipuncture. Although the incidence of false-positive test results has been reduced by the introduction of newer assays, physiologic stress responses and medications that increase catecholamine levels still can confound testing. Because the tumors are relatively rare, borderline elevations are likely to represent false-positive results. In this circumstance, it is important to exclude dietary or drug-related factors (withdrawal of levodopa or use of sympathomimetics, diuretics, tricyclic anti-depressants, alpha and beta blockers) that might cause false-positive results and then to repeat testing or perform a clonidine suppression test (i.e., the measurement of plasma normetanephrine 3 h after oral administration of 300 μg of clonidine). Other pharmacologic tests, such as the phentolamine test and the glucagon provocation test, are of relatively low sensitivity and are not recommended.

Ans. D

138. A 50 year old man is admitted with complaints of persistent vomiting, chronic fatigue, weight loss, hyperpigmentation and anorexia. A clinical diagnosis of primary adrenal insufficiency is made and a cosyntropin test is planned. What is the cortisol cut off after cosyntropin testing to establish adrenal insufficiency?

A. Cortisol values of < 3 μg/dl sampled 30-60 min after ACTH stimulation

B. Cortisol values of < 10-12 μg/dl sampled 30-60 min after ACTH stimulation

C. Cortisol values of < 16-18 μg/dl sampled 30-60 min after ACTH stimulation

D. Cortisol values of < 12-14 μg/dl sampled 30-60 min after ACTH stimulation

Explanation:

- The diagnosis of adrenal insufficiency is established by the short cosyntropin test, a safe and reliable tool with excellent predictive diagnostic value. The cut-off for adrenal failure is usually defined at cortisol levels of <450–500 nmol/L (16–18 μg/dL) sampled 30–60 min after ACTH stimulation.

Ans. C

139. A 65 year old gentleman has come for review. He is a known case of type 2 diabetes mellitus, taking metformin 2.5g/day since diagnosis. BMI is 30. His Hba1c is 8.4%. Other comorbids are systemic hypertension and dyslipidemia. What is the best choice for hyperglycemia and obesity in addition to metformin?

A. Insulin degludec

B. Gilbenclamide

C. Dapagliflozin

D. Acarbose

Explanation:

- The man has suboptimally controlled diabetes mellitus and obese. Dapagliflozin, an SGLT2 inhibitor will improve glycemic control in addition to promoting weight loss, lowering blood pressure and improving lipid profile. SGLT2 is a protein which facilitates glucose reabsorption in the kidney. SGLT2 inhibitors block the reabsorption of glucose in the kidney, increase glucose excretion and lower blood glucose levels.

Ans. C

140. A 56 year old postmenopausal woman undergoes CT abdomen for complaints of vague abdominal pain. An adrenal mass of 5 × 6 cm is incidentally detected and referred for evaluation. She is non hypertensive, non diabetic. The Investigations of choice would be

A. Plasma metanephrines, Midnight plasma cortisol and ACTH, DHEAS

B. Plasma metanephrines, Plasma aldosterone and renin, Midnight cortisol and ACTH, DHEAS

C. DHEAS, Midnight plasma cortisol and ACTH, Plasma aldosterone and renin

D. DHEAS and only

Explanation:

- Plasma metanephrines, midnight cortisol and ACTH should be done in all adrenal incidentalomas > 1 cm. DHEAS is done is adrenal masses > 4 cm.

- Plasma aldosterone and plasma renin is done in patients with hypertension and/or hypokalemia.

Algorithm for the Management of the Patient with an Incidentally Discovered Adrenal Mass

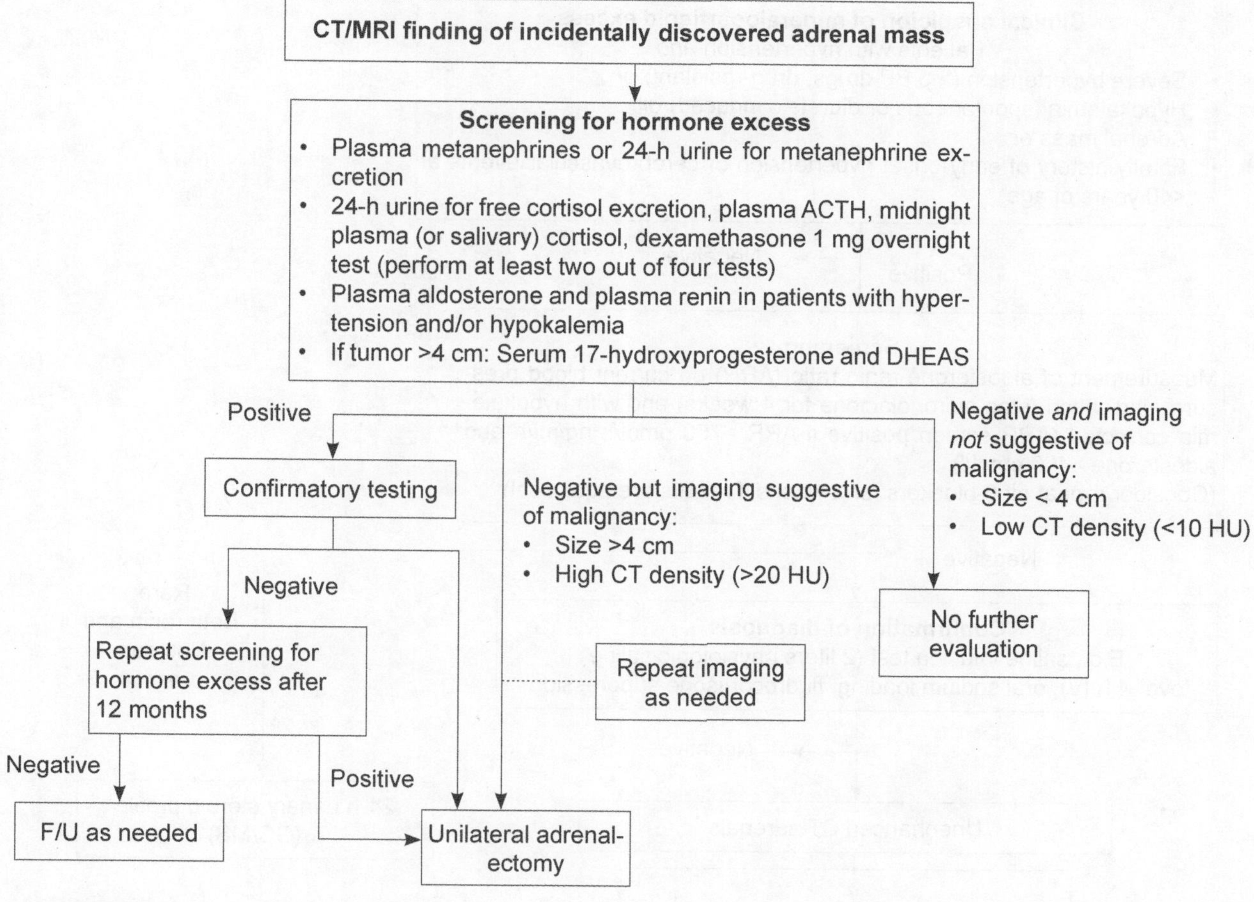

Ans. A

141. 26 year old male with history of resistant hypertension and hypokalemia is evaluated for primary hyperaldosteronism. Screening Plasma Aldosterone renin ratio is 1200 pmol/L: ng/mL/h. This is confirmed with a saline infusion test (post administration of 2L physiologic saline over a 4 hour period, aldosterone was 200 pmol/L). CT adrenals show a unilateral adrenal mass of 2 x 1.6 cms. Next course of action?

A. Adrenal venous sampling

B. Unilateral adrenalectomy

C. Treatment with mineralocorticoid receptor antagonists

D. Oral sodium loading test

Explanation:

- Patients with age < 40 years with confirmed primary hyperalsosteronism and unilateral adrenal mass on CT can be directly referred for unilateral adrenalectomy.

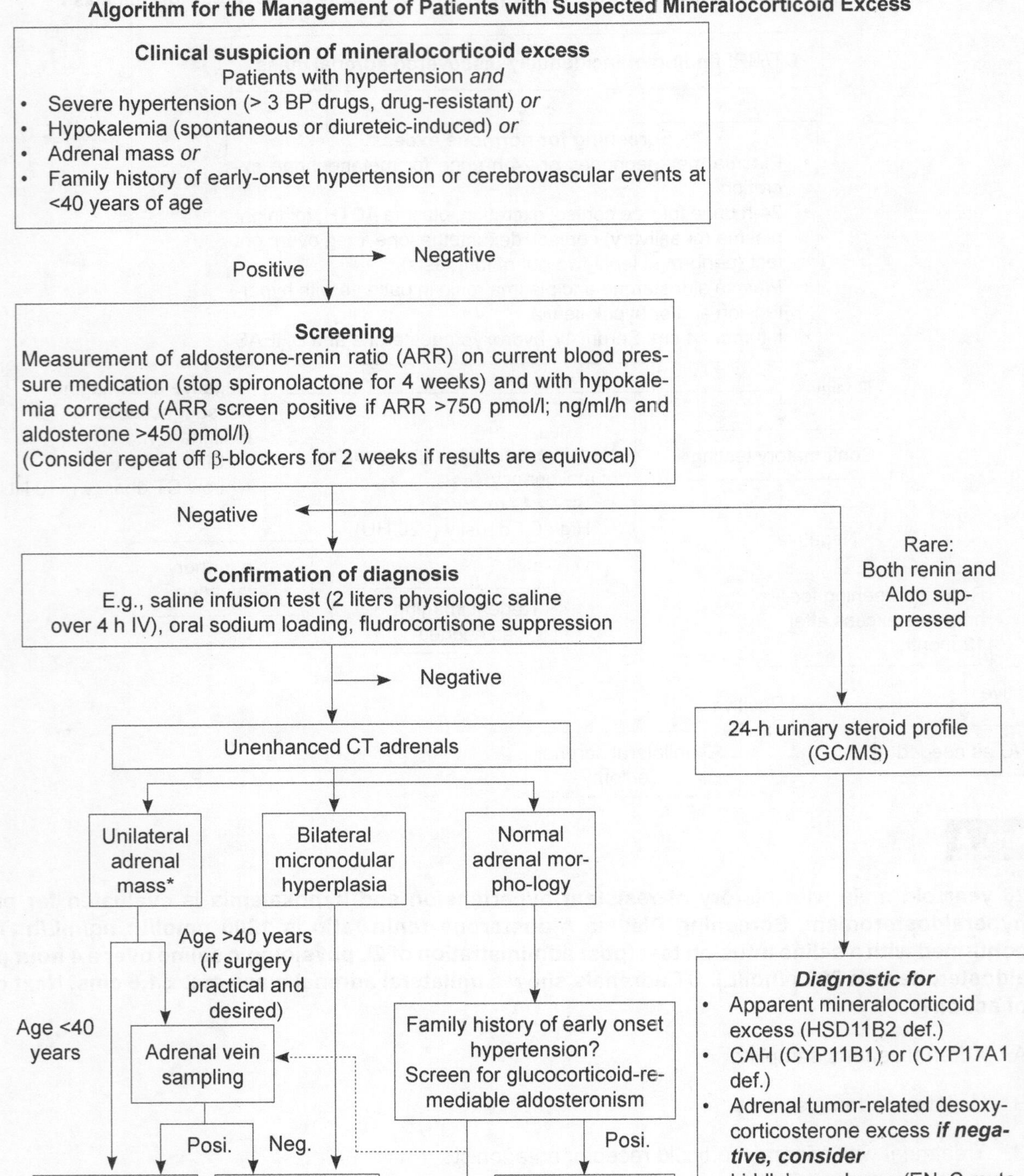

Ans. B

142. A 20 year old woman is referred to the hospital with abnormal fasting blood glucose levels. She has history of recurrent thrush, poorly responsive to 2 courses of fluconazole. Family history reveals her brother and her mother has diabetes. BMI is 22. Anti GAD and anti IA2 are negative. Which is the initial treatment?

A. Metformin
B. Gliclazide
C. Insulin
D. Pioglitazone

Explanation:

- The woman has a strong family history of diabetes mellitus with absence of ketones and negative antibodies. So the diagnosis is MODY. MODY3 is sensitive to treatment with sulphonyureas, gliclazide is the initial treatment.

Ans. B

143. 46 year old female, presents with features of weight gain, pinkish striae over the abdomen, amenorrhea and hirsutism. She has no history of exogenous steroid intake. Cushing's Syndrome is suspected. What is the screening test of choice and what is the cut off for making a diagnosis?

A. 8 am Cortisol > 140 nmol/L
B. 11 pm cortisol > 140 nmol/L
C. Midnight salivary cortisol > 5 nmol/L
D. 24 hour urinary free cortisol excretion increased 2 times above normal

Explanation:

The tests used for screening for Cushings syndrome are:

- 24-h urinary free cortisol excretion increased above normal (3x)
- Dexamethasone overnight test (Plasma cortisol >50 nmol/L at 8–9 am after 1 mg dexamethasone at 11 pm)
- Midnight plasma cortisol >130 nmol/L (or midnight salivary cortisol >5 nmol/L)

If further confirmation needed/desired:

- Low dose DEX test (Plasma cortisol >50 nmol/L after 0.5 mg dexamethasone q6h for 2 days).

Ans. C

144. A 30 year old lady known type 1 diabetes mellitus came to the hospital with weight loss and palpitations. O/E fine tremors of hand, staring look, diffuse goiter was present. BP 80/60 mm Hg. Lab investigations reveal hyperkalemia. Diagnosis of Addison's with Graves' disease was made. What is the likely diagnosis?

A. POEMS
B. APS 4
C. APS 2
D. MEN 4

Explanation:

- APS 2 more common than APS 1 in females. It is characterized by Addison's disease, Graves' disease and primary hypogonadism.

Ans. C

145. A 55 year old man with type 2 DM presents with diabetic retinopathy. His Hba1c is 9.2%, treated with metformin, liraglutide, basal insulin, but has history of non compliance to medication. BP is 160/90 mm Hg. Which of the following factors would worsen his diabetic retinopathy in the short term?

A. Rapid improvement in blood pressure control
B. Long term improvement in blood glucose control
C. Rapid improvement in blood glucose levels
D. Hypertriglyceridemia

Explanation:

- The intensive glycemic and blood pressure control will prevent diabetic retinopathy. Paradoxically during first 6-12 months of glycemic control, retinopathy may transiently worsen. Patients with type 2DM should have eye examination at the time of diagnosis, patients with type 1 DM should have eye examination within 5 years after onset of diabetes.

Ans. B

146. 5 year old boy presented with recurrent seizures. O/E hyperpigmentation was present with oral candidiasis. BP is 80/60 mm Hg. Lab investigations revealed hyperkalemia with hypocalcemia and hyperphosphatemia. What might be the likely diagnosis?

A. Addison's disease

B. MEN 4

C. MEN1

D. APS1

Explanation:

- Autoimmune polyglandular syndrome type 1 – major components are oral candidiasis, Addison's disease and hypoparathyroidism.

Ans. D

147. A 25 year old man with a new diagnosis of kallman syndrome is in the endocrine clinic. He has a mutation in the Kal1 gene. He has low FSH,LH and testosterone. Other pituitary hormones are normal. He is not keen on having children.

A. Oral testosterone

B. Regular injections of human chorionic gonadotropin

C. Regular injections of gonadotropins

D. Testosterone injectable.

Explanation:

- If fertility is not required, there is no need to stimulate spermatogenesis with GnRH, only testosterone replacement is required. Testosterone is available for oral use, but frequent dose is required. If he requires fertility in the future, then pulsed therapy with GnRH analogues can be given.

Ans. D

148. A 55 year old woman known case of type 2 DM comes to the hospital for review. She is on metformin 2g. Past history of note is an inferior MI 5 years back. BMI is 40, BP -150/90 mm Hg., her HBA1c – 8%. What is the appropriate treatment?

A. Behavioural therapy

B. Physical activity

C. Liraglutide

D. Bariatric surgery

Explanation:

- Bariatric surgery can be considered for patients with BMI>40 or BMI>35 with serious medical conditions. The types of Bariatric surgery are Roux-en-Y bypass and sleeve gastrectomy.

Ans. D

149. A 27 year old gentleman comes to the hospital. He is concerned as he has small testes and has a low libido and impotent. He also complains of having breasts despite being slim. He does not shave often. What is the most likely diagnosis?

A. Fragile X syndrome

B. Turner syndrome

C. Klinefelter syndrome

D. Androgen insensitivity syndrome

Explanation:

- The diagnosis is Klinefelters syndrome. Karyotype is XXY. In Fragile X syndrome, testes is large and mental retardation is seen. Turners syndrome is a female having male features. Its karyoptype is XO.

Ans. C

150. A 40 year old male presents with a decreased libido. His bloods reveal a low FSH, LH and testosterone level. His TSH – 3mIU/l. His prolactin level was 40 mcg/L. Which of the following is the most likely diagnosis?

A. Hypogonadotrophic hypogonadism
B. Hypergonadotrophic hypogonadism
C. Prolactinoma
D. Hypothyroidism

Explanation:

- The patient has hypogonadotrophic hypogonadism. In this condition, both FSH and LH are low. In hypergonadotrophic hypogonadism, FSH and LH are high but testosterone is low. In prolactinoma, serum prolactin>200mcg/L.

Ans. A

151. An obese (BMI - 30) 50 year old woman presents with myocardial infarction. Her mother has type 2 DM. Her cholesterol is 250 g/dl. Which of the following drugs acts by inhibiting cholesterol absorption?

A. Atorvastatin
B. Cholestyramine
C. Ezetimibe
D. Evolocumab

Explanation:

- Ezetimibe acts by inhibiting cholesterol absorption. Atorvastatin is an HMG CoA reductase inhibitor, Cholestyramine is a bile acid sequestrant, Evolocumab is a PCSK9 inhibitor.

Ans. C

152. A 40 year old woman post 4 months of her second child come to the hospital for review. She had gestational diabetes, wants to know how to reduce her future risk of type 2 diabetes. BMI is 29. Which is the appropriate intervention to reduce progression to type 2 DM?

A. Acarbose
B. Diet and exercise
C. Liraglutide
D. Orlistat

Explanation:

- Diet and exercise are associated with reduction in progression to type 2 diabetes mellitus.

Ans. B

153. A 66 year old gentleman known case of type 2 diabetes mellitus complaints of abdominal pain, weight loss, 6 episodes of malodorous stools in a day. He has previous history of biliary colic. O/E he is found to be anaemic. What is the most likely diagnosis?

A. Somatostatinoma
B. Glucagonoma
C. Insulinoma
D. VIPoma

Explanation:

- The clinical presentation of somatostatinoma is weight loss, steatorrhea, hypochlorhydria, diabetes mellitus. Site of the lesion is pancreas and duodenum. When present in the duodenum, obstructive features are seen.

Somatostatin levels are raised. In glucaogonoma, necrolytic migratory erythema is present. Insulinoma leads to hypoglycaemia.

Ans. A

154. An 20 year old girl presents with amenorrhoea for the last 8 months. She is asymptomatic otherwise. She exercises excessively and appears underweight with a BMI of 16. What is the most likely diagnosis?

A. Functional hypogonadism
B. Turner syndrome
C. Primary ovarian failure
D. Hypogonadotrophic hypogonadism.

Explanation:

- The patient has low BMI, amenorrhea and excessive exercise, so the diagnosis is functional hypogonadism due to Anorexia nervosa.

Ans. A

155. An 20 year old female comes to the hospital with symptoms of hypothyroidism. She has a short stature, webbed neck and has not yet commenced menstruation. Karyotyping reveals 45 X0. What is the most likely diagnosis?

A. Turner syndrome
B. Klinefelter syndrome
C. Noonan syndrome
D. Hypothyroidism

Explanation:

- Diagnosis is Turner syndrome and 45 XO karyotyping is diagnostic. There is hypothyroidism, genitourinary, cardiovascular abnormalities and gonadal failure. Noonan syndrome present similarly but the karyotyping is not 45XO.

Ans. A

156. A 23 year old patient admitted with diabetic ketoacidosis. GCS is 12 and her airway is not compromised, she has a respiratory rate of 30/min. BP – 100/60 mm Hg, PR- 80/min, RR- 28/min. Her main complaint is epigastric tenderness, commenced on oxygen therapy. Blood glucose is 360mg/dl. What is the next step in management?

A. Fluid and electrolyte replacement
B. IV insulin
C. Intubation
D. NG tube insertion

Explanation:

- The main cause of death in patients with DKA is due to hypovolemia and electrolyte disturbances. Early fluid and electrolyte replacement is necessary to prevent this complication. All patients with ketoacidosis will have potassium depletion. Insulin drives potassium to the intracellular space, increasing the risk of hypokalemia, even in oliguric patients. Potassium should be given with fluid from the second bag and stopped if oliguria is confirmed.

Ans. A

157. Familial nephrogenic SIAD (NSIAD) is common among:

A. Young boys
B. Young girls
C. Elderly male
D. Elderly female

Explanation:

- In some of them, all young boys, the inappropriate antidiuresis has been traced to a constitutively activating mutation of the V2 receptor gene.

- This unusual variant may be referred to as familial nephrogenic SIAD (NSIAD) to distinguish it from other possible causes of the syndrome.
- Inappropriate antidiuresis in these patients appears to be permanent, although hyponatremia is variable owing presumably to individual differences in fluid intake.

Ans. A

158. A 43 year old female is suffering from oligomenorrhoea. She complains of weight gain, cold intolerance, constipation on and off along with hair and nail changes. Investigations reveal low potassium and glucose. Hormonal profile shows serum FSH, LH and oestrogen levels are low. What is the cause of her amenorrhoea?

A. Hypothyroidism
B. Primary ovarian failure
C. Hypogonadotropic hypogonadism
D. Addison's disease

Explanation:

- The diagnosis is hypogonadotropic hypogonadism. There are symptoms of growth hormone, gonadotropin, adrenal and thyroid hormone deficiencies. Serum FSH , LH and estrogen levels are low thereby indicating hypothalamic cause of amenorrhea.

Ans. C

159. All are causes of hypokalemic hypertension except:

A. Type I syndrome of apparent mineralocorticoid excess
B. Type II syndrome of apparent mineralocorticoid excess
C. Liddle's syndrome
D. Congenital adrenal hyperplasia (CAH)

Explanation:

- Cortisol acts as a potent mineralocorticoid if it escapes efficient inactivation to cortisone by 11β-HSD2 in the kidney.
- This can be caused by inactivating mutations in *HSD11B2* gene resulting in syndrome of apparent mineralocorticoid excess (SAME) that characteristically manifests with severe hypokalemic hypertension in childhood. However, milder mutations may cause normokalemic hypertension manifesting in adulthood (type II SAME).
- Inhibition of 11β-HSD2 by excess licorice ingestion also results in hypokalemic hypertension, as does overwhelming of 11β-HSD2 conversion capacity by cortisol excess in Cushing's syndrome.
- DOC also binds and activates the MR and can cause hypertension if its circulating concentrations are increased. This can arise through autonomous DOC secretion by an ACC, but also when DOC accumulates as a consequence of an adrenal enzymatic block, as seen in congenital adrenal hyperplasia (CAH) due to CYP11B1 (11β-hydroxylase) or CYP17A1 (17α-hydroxylase) deficiency.

Ans. D

160. A 22 year old female presents with irregular periods, overweight and acne. She admits that she has to regularly bleach her upper lip hair and has a line of hair from her umbilicus to her pubic hair which she is embarrassed about. Her blood investigations reveal an elevated LH:FSH ratio and high testosterone and sex hormone binding globulin is low. Her fasting glucose is 120 mg/dl. What treatment can be advised?

A. Clomiphene
B. Meformin
C. Progesterone only pill
D. Orlistat

Explanation:

- The diagnosis is PCOS. The manifestations include acne, hirsutism, irregular menses and virilisation. It is associated with elevated LH, normal FSH, elevated LH:FSH ratio, normal or elevated testosterone and low sex hormone binding globulin. Insulin resistance may cause impaired fasting glucose. Metformin is used in this case as it will reduce androgen levels , thus improves hirsutism and acne and also improves insulin resistance.

Ans. B

161. A 55 year old gentleman is found to have a cholesterol of 250 mg/dl. Family history revealed that his mother and grandmother had hypercholesterolemia. He is thought to have familial hypercholesterolaemia. Which of the following features is highly suggestive of this?

A. Elevated HDL
B. Elevated LDL
C. Pancreatitis
D. Elevated triglycerides

Explanation:

- Familial hypercholesterolemia is an autosomal dominant condition. This is due to mutation of LDL receptors on chromosome 1 and mutations of apo B 100. Diagnosis is made by LDL>190 mg/dl in the absence of secondary etiology and hypercholesterolemia.

Ans. B

162. A 6 year old girl was brought to the hospital with complaints of breast development with 1 episode of bleeding per vagina. O/E she had tall stature with hyperpigmented macules on her trunk suggestive of Café au lait spots. What is the likely diagnosis?

A. Idiopathic
B. CNS infections
C. Hypothalamic hamartoma
D. McCune Albright syndrome

Explanation:

- Precocious puberty is defined as puberty in girls less than 8 years of age. Mc Cune Albright syndrome is a triad of café au lait spots, precocious puberty and fibrous dysplasia.

Ans. D

163. A 30 year old lady has 5 months of amenorrhea, weight gain, depression and constipation. She has noticed changes in her skin and hair. What is the cause of amenorrhea?

A. Elevated proalctin
B. Low estradiol
C. Elevated LH
D. Elevated FSH

Explanation:

- The symptoms seen in the patient are most likely due to hypothyroidism. Due to low T4, elevated TRH occurs which raises prolactin levels causing amenorrhea.

Ans. A

164. A 4 year old is brought to the hospital. His parents reveal that he is very small for his age. He has only just begun to walk and is not keen to, complains of pain while walking. O/E there is frontal bossing of the skull and bowing of the legs. Investigations reveal a slightly low calcium, low phosphate and high alkaline phosphatase, increased urinary phosphate. What is the diagnosis?

A. X-linked recessive hypophosphatemic rickets
B. X-linked dominant hypophosphatemic rickets
C. Osteomalacia
D. Vitamin D resistant rickets.

Explanation:

- X-linked dominant hypophosphatemic rickets. The child shows features of rickets and growth retardation due to low serum phosphate, high urinary phosphate suggestive of X-linked hypophosphatemic rickets. It occurs due to mutation in PHEX leading to abnormal phosphate handling. It is treated with phosphate supplementation and 1,25 hydroxylated vitamin D.

Ans. B

165. A 22 year old woman comes to the hospital with rapidly enlarging thyroid nodule. Histology suggest it is medullary thyroid carcinoma. Her BP is 156/90 mm Hg. What is the cause of hypertension?

A. Coarctation of aorta
B. Liddle's syndrome
C. Pheochromocytoma
D. Renal artery stenosis

Explanation:

- The medullary thyroid carcinoma leads to possibility of MEN2A and is associated with hyperparathyroidism, medullary thyroid carcinoma and pheochromocytoma.

Ans. C

166. 18 year old boy comes to the hospital worrying that his growth has stopped. Which hormone is responsible for epiphyseal fusion and cessation of growth?

A. GH
B. Testosterone
C. Oestrogen
D. Thyroxine

Explanation:

- The growth spurt at puberty is due to secretion of androgens in the male and estrogens in the female. Estrogens terminate growth by causing the epiphysis in the long bones to fuse. Oestrogens are responsible for skeletal maturation, epiphyseal fusion and cessation of growth in males and females.

Ans. C

167. A 65 year old woman presented with 6kg weight loss, polyuria and depressed mood for 2 months. Her serum Calcium levels were high, phosphate levels normal and PTH low. Her renal function is normal. What is the cause of raised calcium?

A. Hypercalcemia of malignancy
B. Vitamin D deficiency
C. Hyperthyroidism
D. Secondary hyperparathyroidism

Explanation:

- The high calcium, normal phosphate and suppressed PTH levels indicate malignancy. A detailed clinical history and examination will lead to the diagnosis. The causes of hypercalcemia can be classified according to elevated PTH or low PTH levels. Primary hyperparathyroidism and malignancy are the most common causes and account for 90% patients with hypercalcemia.

Ans. A

168. A 35 year old lady was diagnosed as an insulinoma. Her mother had a perforated duodenal ulcer at a young age. Her maternal aunt has a pituitary tumour. Which other features would be found in the hereditary syndrome?

A. Hirschprung s disease
B. Pheochromocytoma
C. Parathyroid hyperplasia
D. Medullary CA of thyroid

Explanation:

- Primary hyperparathyroidism is the most common feature of MEN1 with 90% penetrance by age 65 who have a mutation in Menin gene.

Ans. C

169. A 68 year old male has been suffering from a productive cough and shortness of breath. He is brought to ER as drowsy and confused state. Investigations reveal sodium of 112 mmol/L, normal renal function, with a plasma osmolality of 250 mOsmol/kg and urine osmolality of 450 mOsm/kg and urinary sodium of 45 mmol/L. What is the most likely cause of the hyponatraemia?

A. SIADH
B. Addison's disease
C. Hypothyroidism
D. Fluid overload

Explanation:

- The patient is diagnosed to have pneumonia. It can lead to SIADH. In SIADH, urine osmolality is elevated, serum osmolality is decreased, urine spot sodium is increased.

Ans. A

170. A 48 year old woman complaints of swelling in the neck, prominent on swallowing. O/E, there is a thyroid nodule at the neck. Family history revealed medullary thyroid carcinoma. Which other endocrine problem the patient requires screening is she has mutation in RET proto-oncogene?

A. Hypoparathyroidism
B. Pituitary adenoma
C. Pheochromocytoma
D. Type 2 Diabetes mellitus.

Explanation:

- MEN 2A is associated with thyroid anomaly, parathyroid disease and pheochromocytoma. So it should be screened with the family history of medullary thyroid neoplasm.

Ans. C

171. A 55 year old man presents with history of palpitations, sweating, flushing, headache. PR-120/min, BP-190/100 mm Hg. Urinary catecholamines are elevated over 24hour period. CT abdomen showed bilateral adrenal masses suggestive of pheochromocytoma. Syndromes associated with pheochromocytoma are all except:

A. VHL
B. NF-1
C. MEN2B
D. MEN 1

Explanation:

- Familial syndromes associated with pheochromocytoma are MEN 2A, MEN 2B, VHL, NF1 and mutation encoding several enzymes like SDH.

Ans. D

172. A 28 year old woman with non classical congenital adrenal hyperplasia due to11 beta hydroxylase has come to the hospital with oligomenorrhea and hirsutism. She is anxious to know which hormone is responsible for excess coarse hair growth?

A. Dehydroepiandrosterone
B. GnRH
C. Oestrogen
D. Cortisol

Explanation:

- Non classical CAH caused by the deficiency in the enzyme 11 beta hydroxylase results in the accumulation of sex steroids mainly DHEA. The symptoms are due to reduced production of cortisol and either over or under production of mineralocorticoids and androgens, depending on the enzyme deficiency.

Ans. A

173. While testing for ZES, PPI should be stopped atleast:

A. 7 days before testing
B. 5 days before testing
C. 10 days before testing
D. 3 days before testing

Explanation:

- Although a fasting gastrin >10 times normal is highly suggestive of ZES, two-thirds of patients will have fasting gastrin levels that overlap with levels found in the more common disorders outlined above, especially if a PPI is being taken by the patient.
- Effect of the PPI on gastrin levels and acid secretion will linger several days after stopping the PPI; therefore, it should be stopped for a minimum of 7 days before testing.
- During this period, the patient should be placed on a histamine H2 antagonist, such as famotidine, twice to three times per day.
- Although this type of agent has a short-term effect on gastrin and acid secretion, it needs to be stopped 24 h before repeating fasting gastrin levels.
- Patient may take antacids for the final day, stopping them ~12 h before testing is performed. Heightened awareness of complications related to gastric acid hypersecretion during the period of PPI cessation is critical.

Ans. A

174. A 30 year old woman presented with history of vomiting and abdominal pain for 3 days. She has a history of anorexia nervosa with diuretic abuse. Her PR – 90/min, BP – 106/74 mm Hg. Her weight is 55 kg. Serum sodium is 132 mEq/L, potassium is 5.6 mEq/L. What is the cause of hyperkalemia?

A. Bartter syndrome
B. Conn's syndrome
C. Diuretic abuse
D. Addison's disease

Explanation:

- The patient has hyperkalemia, hyponatremia typical of Addison's disease. There is no hypertension as relevant from findings. Conn's syndrome lead to hypertension. Diuretic abuse leads to hypokalemia and hyponatremia.

Ans. D

175. A 4 year old boy was brought by his mother to the hospital with complaints of development of pubic hair. O/E pubic hair was present with increase in penile length. His 17 hydroxyprogesterone level was elevated. There was no history of vomiting, abdominal pain or giddiness. What is the diagnosis?

A. 17 alpha hydroxylase deficiency
B. 21 alpha hydroxylase deficiency
C. 3betaHSD deficiency
D. 11 betahydroxylase deficiency

Explanation:

- 21 alpha hydroxylase deficiency is the most common cause of adrenal hyperplasia. 17 hydroxy progesterone levels are elevated. This is a case of simple virilising CAH.

Ans. B

176. A 45 year old man presents to the hospital with headache. His BP – 164/90 mm Hg. He has no history of drug intake, no comorbids. Fundoscopy reveals AV nicking. BMI is normal. Serum Na is 143 mEq/l, potassium is 2.5 mEq/l. Urea, creatinine and glucose levels are normal. What is the cause of his hypertension?

A. Cushing's disease
B. Primary hyperaldosteronism
C. Pheochromocytoma
D. Renal artery stenosis.

Explanation:

- It is the most common cause of secondary hypertension. The patient is hypokalemic, does not appear cushingoid or acromegalic on examination. Conn syndrome occurs in 5-15% of patients with secondary hypertension. Pheochromocytoma is not usually associated with hypokalemia and the patient does not describe any episodic features.

Ans. B

177. A 45 year old woman was brought to ER in an unconscious state. After recovery, she is found to have BP 90/60 mm Hg, hyponatremia (Na -128 mEq/l), hyperkalemia (K- 6.5mEq/l), amenorrhea for 4 years. What is the urgent treatment?

A. IV cefuroxime
B. IV hydrocortisone
C. IV phenytoin
D. IV thiamine

Explanation:

- The diagnosis is Addison's disease. She has hyponatremia, hyperkalemia, hypotension suggesting Addison's crisis. IV hydrocortisone is the life saving drug and must be given immediately. The causes of hypoadrenalism includes primary or secondary. Spontaneous hypoadrenalism is due to autoimmune destruction of the adrenal gland. Other causes include TB, HIV, hemorrhage into the adrenal glands.

Ans. B

178. Wolfram's syndrome includes all except:

A. DI
B. DM
C. Pancreatic tumor
D. Optic atrophy

Explanation:

- Third form is caused by mutations of the *WFS 1* gene responsible for Wolfram's syndrome (DI, diabetes mellitus, optic atrophy, and neural deafness [DIDMOAD]).

Ans. C

179. A type 1 DM patient is referred from CHC to your hospital. His 24 hour urine protein is 1.2 gm. His BP is 150/80 mm Hg. His HbAIC is 7.2%. Which of the following antihypertensives would you like to start in this patient?

A. HCTZ
B. Hydralazine
C. Enalapril
D. Clonidine

Explanation:

- Vast majority of patients with diabetic nephropathy require three or more antihypertensive drugs including ACE inhibitors or angiotensin receptor blockers (ARB) to achieve this goal.
- Drugs that inhibit the renin-angiotensin system, independent of their effects on systemic blood pressure, have been shown in numerous large clinical trials to slow the progression of diabetic nephropathy at early (microalbuminuria) and late (proteinuria with reduced glomerular filtration) stages.

- Since angiotensin II increases efferent arteriolar resistance and, hence, glomerular capillary pressure, one key mechanism for the efficacy of inhibitors of the renin angiotensin system is reducing glomerular hypertension.

Ans. C

180. A 48 year old man presents to ER with BP 90/60 mm Hg, skin pigmentation and Hashimoto thyroiditis. History of easy fatigability and abdominal pain persistent for many months. What is seen in the investigation?

A. Serum Glucose level of 350 g/dl

B. Serum Sodium level of 118 mEq/L

C. Serum potassium level of 2.3 mEq/L

D. Flat T waves on ECG

Explanation:

- The clinical picture of abdominal pain, low BP, hyperpigmentation, history of autoimmune disease is suggestive of Addison's disease. The biochemical features include hyponatremia, hyperkalemia, hypotension and hypoglycaemia.

Ans. B

181. A 62 year old gentleman recently been diagnosed with lung cell cancer presents with weight gain (mainly around the face and trunk), easy bruising, striae and dark skin. O/E he has a moon face, buffalo hump. His BP is 150/82 mm Hg. Blood investigations reveal hypokalaemia. What is the most likely diagnosis?

A. Exogenous steroids

B. Ectopic ACTH secretion

C. Addison's disease

D. Cushing' syndrome

Explanation:

- The diagnosis is Ectopic ACTH secretion. The patient has features of excess steroid secretion. Small cell lung cancer acts as an ectopic source of ACTH. It is differentiated from excess steroids by the presence of hyperpigmentation as ACTH has a melanocyte stimulating effect.

Ans. B

182. A 22 year old woman presents with nausea, dehydration and vomiting along with amenorrhea for few months. She has history of over the counter steroid drug abuse. She has cushingoid facies and postural hypotension. What is the cause of amenorrhea?

A. PCOS

B. Turner syndrome

C. Cushing's syndrome

D. Prolactinoma

Explanation:

- Excess steroids needs to suppression of gonadotropins with subsequent hypogonadism and amenorrhea.

Ans. C

183. A 30 year old woman complaints of weight gain, history of proximal myopathy. O/E she is obese with purple striae. BP is 150/100 mm Hg. Investigations reveal RBS 300 mg/dl. What is the investigation of choice for diagnosis?

A. FBS, PPBS

B. HBA1c

C. Cosyntropin test

D. Low dose dexamethasone suppression test.

Explanation:

- Diagnosis here is Cushing syndrome. For confirmation of diagnosis, 0.5mg of dexamethasone is given 6th hourly for 2 days. If plasma cortisol > 50nmol/l, diagnosis is made.

Ans. D

184. 18 year old male presented with delayed puberty with absent secondary sexual characteristics and micropenis. On evaluation patient was found to have colour blindness, anosmia and synkinesis.

Genetic mutation associated with it:

A. Anosmin 1/KAL 1
B. FGFR1
C. CHD7
D. All of the above

Explanation:

Kallmann syndrome

- X-linked KAL gene, mutations of which impair embryonic migration of GnRH neurons from the hypothalamic olfactory placode to the hypothalamus.
- **Other:** Autosomal recessive (i.e., GPR54, KISS1)
- Dominant (i.e., FGFR1) modes of transmission have been described
- **Other genes:** GNRH1, PROK2, PROKR2, CHD7, PCSK1, FGF8, NELF, WDR11, TAC3, TACR3, and SEMA3E.

Ans. D

185. A 39 year old female presented with history galactorrhea . On evaluation patient had history of over the counter medication for minor aliments. Drug causing hyperprolactemia is:

A. Verapamil
B. Cimetidine
C. α-Methyldopa
D. All of the above

Explanation:

Drug-induced hypersecretion

- Dopamine receptor blockers
  - Atypical antipsychotics: Risperidone
  - Phenothiazines: Chlorpromazine, perphenazine
  - Butyrophenones: Haloperidol
  - Thioxanthenes
  - Metoclopramide
- Dopamine synthesis inhibitors
  - α-Methyldopa
- Catecholamine depletors
  - Reserpine
- Opiates
- H_2 antagonists
  - Cimetidine, ranitidine
- Imipramines
  - Amitriptyline, amoxapine
- Serotonin reuptake inhibitors
  - Fluoxetine
- Calcium channel blockers
  - Verapamil
  - Estrogens
  - Thyrotropin-releasing hormone

Ans. D

186. A 45 year old male presented with history of headache, vomiting, blurring of vision, on perimetry: found to have b/l temporal hemianopia. MRI brain was ordered which showed a pituitary adenoma of 12*12 mm. PRL was 350 mcg/l Which is the best mode of treatment for this patient ?

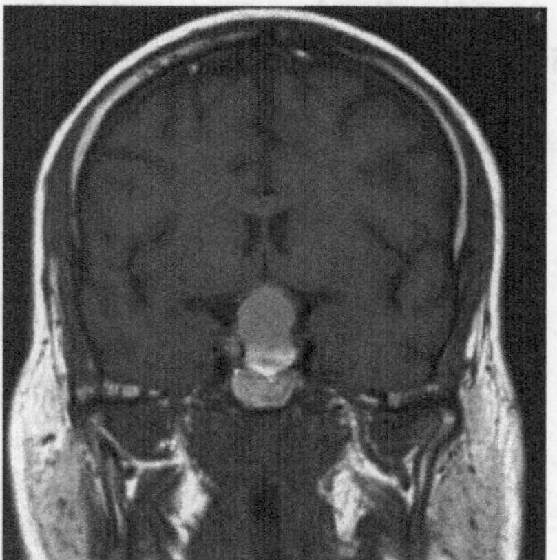

A. Medical treatment
B. Surgical management
C. Radiotherapy
D. No treatment necessary

Explanation:

- Oral dopamine agonists (cabergoline and bromocriptine) are the mainstay of therapy for patients with micro- or macroprolactinomas.

Ans. A

187. A 20 year old patient presented with history of 6 month amenorrhoea and hirsutism for which patient is undergoing treatment for the same in local hospital. She was referred to tertiary centre for further management. On evaluation she was found to have hypertension and virilisation with clitoromegaly. On evaluation she was found to have high DHEAS levels of 2500. On imaging showed large 10* 12cm large adrenal mass s/o ACC with hepatic and lung metastasis. Chemotherapy regimen used in ACC includes:

A. Mitatone
B. Cisplatin + doxorubicin
C. Etoposide
D. All of the above

Explanation:

- The established first-line chemotherapy regimen in ACC is the combination of cisplatin, etoposide, and doxorubicin plus continuing mitotane.

Ans. D

188. 68 year old female presented with excessive weight gain since 6 month. On probing she also has history of easy bruisability and difficulty climbing stairs. Newly diagnosed diabetes on OHA . On examination moon facies +, striae+ abdominal obesity +. Diagnosis of Cushing syndrome was made. Drug approved for treatment of hyperglycemia associated with Cushing's syndrome is:

A. Aminoglutethimide
B. Cyproheptadine
C. Etomidate
D. Mifepristone

Explanation:

- *Mifepristone* (300–1200 mg/d), a glucocorticoid receptor antagonist, blocks peripheral cortisol action and is approved to treat hyperglycemia in Cushing's disease

Ans. D

189. **62 year old known diabetic presents with history of polyuria and polydipsia of around 5-6 litres. Some local doctor had advised to take him more water in order to prevent urinary tract infection. Since then he is consuming 5 litres of water per day. On evaluation he was found to have serum sodium of 122, serum osmolarity 278, urine osmolarity of 64 and urine Na+ : 18. And his MRI imaging done. What is the probable diagnosis this patient is suffering?**

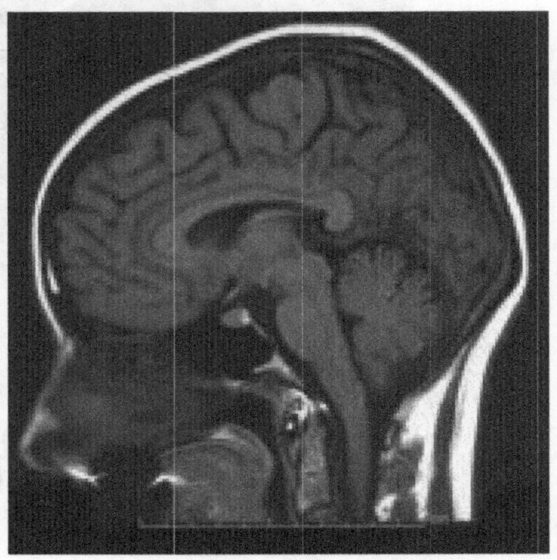

A. Diabetes mellitus
B. Nephrogenic DI
C. Central DI
D. Primary polydipsia

Explanation:

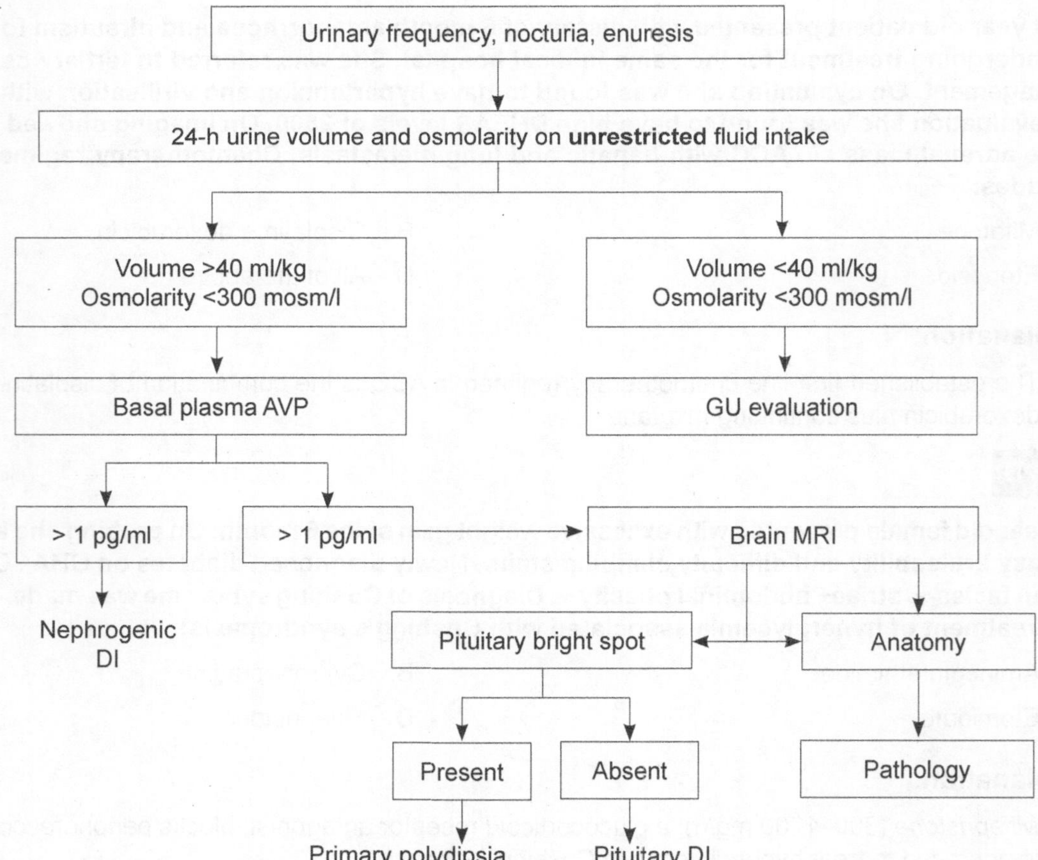

Ans. D

190. 22 year old patient presented with headache, blurring of vision mainly on the temporal side, nausea. On evaluation she was found to have pituitary macroadenoma. On biochemical investigation low 8 am cortisol, normal IGF1 and thyroid profile was noted and diagnosis of non functional pituitary adenoma was made. in the treatment of non functional pituitary adenoma, which of the following reduces FSH levels but do not have effect adenoma size?

A. Dopamine agonists
B. Octreotide
C. Nal-Glu-GnRH
D. None of the above

Explanation:

- The selective GnRH antagonist Nal-Glu GnRH suppresses FSH hypersecretion but has no effect on adenoma size.

Ans. C

191. All can cause primary adrenal insufficiency except:

A. Amyloidosis
B. TB
C. SLE
D. HIV

Explanation:

Primary adrenal insufficiency

1. **Autoimmune:** Addison's disease, polyglandular endocrinopathy
2. **Infectious:** HIV, cytomegalovirus, tuberculosis, disseminated fungal infection
3. **Infiltrative:** Amyloidosis, malignancy, metastatic cancer
4. **Drug-associated:** Heparin, low-molecular-weight heparin
5. **Hereditary:** Adrenal hypoplasia congenita, congenital lipoid adrenal hyperplasia, aldosterone synthase deficiency
6. Adrenal hemorrhage or infarction, including in antiphospholipid syndrome

Ans. C

192. 65 year old male presented with history of urosepsis and acute kidney injury on CKD with eGFR of 30ml/min. incidentally found to have corrected calcium level of 13.1 and Po4 of 2.21 and PTH of 31. Endocrinologists was consulted in view of acute hypercalcemia management. Which drug can be used in this patient to manage hypercalcemia?

A. Zoledronate
B. Denosumab
C. Pamidronate
D. Gallium nitrate

Explanation:

Table: Therapies for severe hypercalcemia				
Treatment	**Onset of Action**	**Duration of Action**	**Advantages**	**Disadvantages**
Most Useful Therapies				
Hydration with normal saline	Hours	During infusion	Rehydration invariably needed	Volume overload
Forced diuresis; normal saline plus loop diuretic	Hours	During treatment	Rapid action	Volume overload, cardiac decompensation, intensive monitoring, electrolyte disturbance, inconvenience

Contd.

Contd.

Pamidronate	1-2 days	10-14 days to weeks	High potency; intermediate onset of action	Fever in 20%, hypophosphatemia, hypocalcemia, hypomagnesemia, rarely jaw necrosis, atypical femoral fracture
Zolendronate	1-2 days	>3 weeks	Same as for pamidronate (lasts longer)	Same as pamidronate above
Denosumab	1-2 days	>3 weeks	Strongest antiresorptive	Occasional severe hypocalcemia, rarely jaw necrosis, skin infections, atypical femoral fracture
Special Use Therapies				
Calcitonin	Hours	1-2 days	Rapid onset of action; useful as adjunct in severe hypercalcemia	Rapid tachyphylaxis
Phosphate Oral	24 hours	During use	Chronic management (with hypophosphatemia); low toxicity if P < 4 mg/dl	Limited use except as adjuvant or chronic therapy
Glucocorticoids	Days	Days, weeks	Oral therapy, antitumor agent	Active only in certain malignancies, vitamin D excess and sarcoidosis; glucocorticoid side effects
Dialysis	Hours	During use and 24-48 hours afterward	Useful in renal failure; onset of effect in hours; can immediately reverse life-threatening hypercalcemia	Complex procedure, reserved for extreme or special circumstances

- **Denosumab is safe in renal failure**

Ans. B

193. Patient presented with polyuria polydipsia from last 6 month. On evaluation he was diagnosed with central diabetes insipidus which is due to deficient production ADH. At high concentration ADH action includes:

A. Smooth muscle contraction of blood vessels and GI tract

B. Glycogenolysis in liver

C. Potentiates ACTH release by CRH

D. All of the above

Explanation:

- At high concentrations, AVP also causes contraction of smooth muscle in blood vessels in the skin and gastrointestinal tract, induces glycogenolysis in the liver, and potentiates adrenocorticotropic hormone (ACTH) release by corticotropin-releasing factor.

Ans. D

194. 14 year old presented with history of polyuria, polydipsia and was diagnosed with young onset diabetes mellitus. On evaluation patient also had syndromic facies, optic atrophy, SN deafness, clinodactyly h/o consanguineous marriage in the family+. Younger sister also had similar history. MRI shows absent posterior pituitary bright spot s/o Diabetes insipidus. Gene involved in the above syndrome is:

A. WFS1
B. PROK2
C. FGF8
D. NECIDIN

Explanation:

- Mutations of the WFS 1 gene responsible for Wolfram's syndrome (DI, diabetes mellitus, optic atrophy, and neural deafness [DIDMOAD]). An X-linked recessive form linked to a region on Xq28

Ans. A

195. 56 year old male presented with polyuria, polydipsia, weight loss and diagnosed with uncontrolled glycemia. On evaluation he was found to have hyponatremia (s Na+ : 121) and RBS: 467. How much is the glucose corrected sodium in this patient?

A. 121
B. 131
C. 151
D. 149

Explanation:

- Formula used is : corrected Na+: $SNa + \frac{(S.\ glucose - 90)}{36}$

Ans. B

196. 76 year old patient admitted with history of headache, generalised weakness and on evaluation he was found to have hyponatremia. Lab investigation: serum sodium : 129 serum osmolarity: 260mosm/kg, urine sodium > 40meq/L, urine osmolarity 200 mosm/kg. The criteria used to diagnose SIADH is:

A. Schwartz and bartter criteria
B. Ferriman gallwey
C. IADPSG
D. HAPO

Explanation:

Criteria for SIADH

- Bartter and Schwartz (1967)
  - Hyponatraemia
  - Clinically euvolaemic
  - No diuretic use
  - Serum osmolality <275mOsm/mg
  - Urine osmolality >100 mOsm/kg
  - Urine sodium >40 mmol/l
  - Normal thyroid, adrenal and renal function

Ans. A

197. 7 day male child was evaluated in view of poor feeding, progressive indirect hyperbilurubenemia and found to have TSH of 67 with low Ft4. So diagnosis hypothyroidism was made. On evaluation the child was diagnosed to have athyreosis. Thyroid hormone synthesis normally begins at what time of

gestation?

A. About 6 weeks
B. About 11 weeks
C. About 28 weeks
D. About 16 weeks

Explanation:

- Thyroid hormone synthesis normally begins at about 11 weeks' gestation.

Ans. B

198. A newborn child was diagnosed with iodine deficiency hypothyroidism. Concomitant of which element contributes to neurologic manifestation of cretinism?

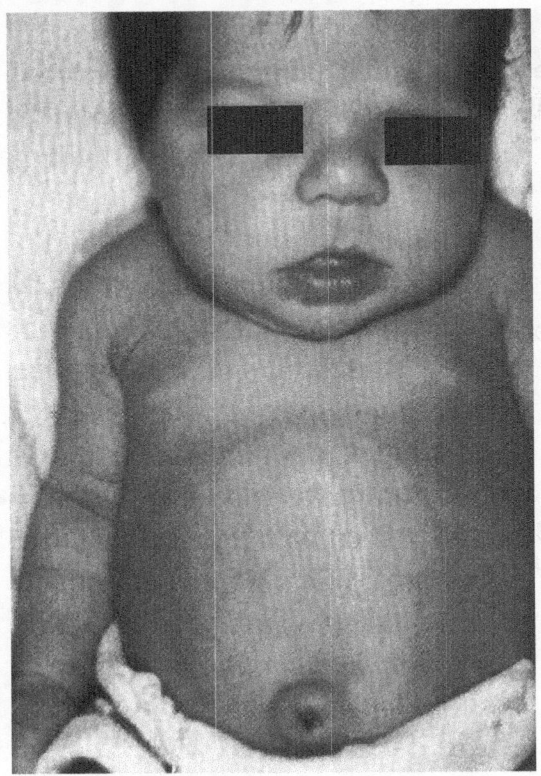

A. Manganese
B. Cobalt
C. Selenium
D. Copper

Explanation:

- Concomitant selenium deficiency may also contribute to the neurologic manifestations of cretinism.

Ans. C

199. Infant was diagnosed to have hypothyroidism and goitre. Diagnosis of pendred syndrome was made. Which of the following is false about pendred syndrome?

A. Due to deficiency of iodine transporter pendrin
B. Mutation in PENDRIN gene
C. Characterised by goitre and sensorineural deafness
D. None of the above

Explanation:

- Mutation of the pendrin gene causes Pendred syndrome, a disorder characterized by defective organification of iodine, goiter, and sensorineural deafness.

Ans. D

200. 25 year pregnant women with clinically euthyroid status . To maintain the euthyroid status recommended average daily intake of iodine in pregnant women is:

A. 100 mcg/day
B. 150 mcg/day
C. 220 mcg/day
D. 250 mcg/day

Explanation:

- The RDA is 220 µg iodine per day for pregnant women and 290 µg iodine per day for breastfeeding women.

Ans. C

201. 34 year old female presented with history of weight loss, increased appetite, palpitations, tremors. lab investigations s/o hyperthyroidism.

Extremely sensitive assays can detect TSH levels upto:

A. ≤ 0.004 mIU/L
B. < 0.04 mIU/L
C. < 0.4 mIU/L
D. < 0.0004 mIU/L

Explanation:

- Extremely sensitive assays can detect TSH levels ≤0.004 mIU/L,

Ans. A

202. 11 week primigravidae presented with recurrent episodes of vomiting. She was diagnosed to have gestational thyrotoxicosis. All are expected changes of TFT seen in normal pregnancy except:

A. Transient increase in hCG
B. The estrogen-induced decrease in TBG
C. Increased thyroid hormone metabolism by the placenta
D. Increase urinary iodide excretion

Explanation:

Five factors alter thyroid function in pregnancy:

1. Tthe transient increase in hCG during the first trimester, which weakly stimulates the TSH-R;
2. The estrogen-induced rise in TBG during the first trimester, which is sustained during pregnancy;
3. Alterations in the immune system, leading to the onset, exacerbation, or amelioration of an underlying autoimmune thyroid disease;
4. Increased thyroid hormone metabolism by the placenta;
5. Increased urinary iodide excretion, which can cause impaired thyroid hormone production in areas of marginal iodine sufficiency

Ans. B

203. Somatostatin inhibits:

A. POMC
B. PRL
C. TSH
D. FSH

Explanation:

Table: Anterior pituitary hormone expression and regulation					
Cell	**Corticotrope**	**Somatotrope**	**Lactotrope**	**Thyrotrope**	**Gonadotrope**
Tissue-specific transcription factor	T-Pit	Prop-1, Pit-1	Prop-1, Pit-1	Prop-1, Pit-1, TEF	SF-1, DAX-1
Fetal appearance	6 weeks	8 weeks	12 weels	12 weeks	12 weeks
Hormone	POMC	GH	PRL	TSH	FSH, LH
Protein	Polypeptide	Polypeptide	Polypeptide	Glycoprotein α, β subunits	Glycoprotein α, β subunits
Amino acids	266 (ACTH 1-39)	191	198	211	210, 204
Stimulators	CRH, AVP, gp-130 cytokines	GHRH, ghrelin	Estrogen, TRH, VIP	TRH	GnRH, activins, estrogen
Inhibitors	Glucocorticoids	Somatostatin, IGF-I	Dopamine	T_3, T_4, dopamine, somatostatin, glucacorticoids	Sex steroids, inhibin
Target gland	Adrenal	Liver, bone, other tissues	Breast, other tissues	Thyroid	Ovary, testis
Trophic effect	Steroid production	IGF-I, production, growth induction, insulin antagonism	Milk production	T_4 synthesis and secretion	Sex steroid production, follicle growth, germ cell maturation
Normal range	ACTH, 4-22 pg/l	<0.5 mg/l[a]	M < 15 µg/l F < 20 µg/l	0.1-5 mU/l	M, 5-20 IU/l; F (basal), 5-20 IU/l

Ans. C

204. Exogenous erythropoietic-stimulating agents maybe associated with an increased risk of all except:

A. Stroke
B. Arrhythmias
C. An increase in thromboembolic events
D. Faster progression of renal decline

Explanation:

- Use of exogenous erythropoiesis-stimulating agents can increase blood pressure and the requirement for antihypertensive drugs.
- Chronic ECFV overload is also a contributor to hypertension, and improvement in blood pressure can often be seen with the use of dietary sodium restriction, diuretics, and fluid removal with dialysis.
- Nevertheless, because of activation of the RAS and other disturbances in the balance of vasoconstrictors and vasodilators, some patients remain hypertensive despite careful attention to ECFV status.

Ans. B

205. Clinically euthyroid adult incidentally diagnosed with altered TFT. That is increased total T4 but free T4 was found to be normal. A diagnosis of euthyroid hyperthyroxinemia was made. All are acquired cause for euthyroid hyperthyroxinemia except:

A. Islet tumors
B. Oestrogen excess
C. Androgen excess
D. Cirrhosis

Explanation:

Table: Conditions associated with euthyroid hyperthyroxinemia			
Disorder	**Cause**	**Transmission**	**Characteristics**
Familial dysalbumi-nemic hyperthyroxinemia (FDH)	Albumin mutations, usually R218H	AD	Increased T_4 Normal unbound T_4 Rarely increased T_3
TBG			
• Familial excess	Increased TBG production	XL	Increased total T_4, T_3 Normal unbound T_4, T_3
• Acquired excess	Medications (estrogen), pregnancy, cirrhosis, hepatitis	Acquired	Increased total T_4, T_3 Normal unbound T_4, T_3
Transthyretin[a]			
• Excess	Islet tumors	Acquired	Usually normal T_4, T_3
• Mutations	Increased affinity for T_4 or T_3	AD	Increased total T_4, T_3 Normal unbound T_4, T_3
Medications: Propra-nolol, ipodate, iopanoic acid, amiodarone	Decreased $T_4 \rightarrow T_3$ conversion	Acquired	Increased T_4 Decreased T_3 Normal or increased TSH
Resistance to thyroid hormone (RTH)	Thyroid hormone receptor β mutations	AD	Increased unbound T_4, T_3 Normal or increased TSH Some patients clinically thyrotoxic

Ans. C

206. A patient who is a case of cutaneous T cell lymphoma received bexarotene treatment. He was found to have altered TFT. What is expected change in TFT in patient who is on bexarotene?

A. High TSH, low T4
B. Low TSH , low T4
C. High TSH, high T4
D. Low TSH , high T4

Explanation:

Table: Causes of hypothyroidism
Primary
• **Autoimmune hypothyroidism:** Hashimoto's thyroiditis, atrophic thyroiditis
• **Iatrogenic:** ^{131}I treatment, subtotal or total thyroidectomy, external irradiation of neck for lymphoma or cancer
• **Drugs:** Iodine excess (including iodine-containing contrast media and amiodarone), lithium, antithyroid drugs, *p*-aminosalicylic acid, interferon α and other cytokines, aminoglutethimide, tyrosine kinase inhibitors (e.g., sunitinib)
• **Congenital hypothyroidism:** Absent or ectopic thyroid gland, dyshormonogenesis, TSH-R mutation
• Iodine deficiency
• **Infiltrative disorders:** Amyloidosis, sarcoidosis, hemochromatosis, scleroderma, cystinosis, Riedel's thyroiditis
• Overexpression of type 3 deiodinase in infantile hemangioma and other tumors

Transient
• Silent thyroiditis, including postpartum thyroiditis • Subacute thyroiditis • Withdrawal of supraphysiologic thyroxine treatment in individuals with an intact thyroid • After ^{131}I treatment or subtotal thyroidectomy for Graves' disease
Secondary
• **Hypopituitarism:** Tumors, pituitary surgery or irradiation, infiltrative disorders, Sheehan's syndrome, trauma, genetic forms of combined pituitary hormone deficiencies • Isolated TSH deficiency or inactivity • **Bexarotene** treatment • **Hypothalamic disease:** Tumors, trauma, infiltrative disorders, idiopathic

Ans. B

207. Newborn child was diagnosed with congenital hypothyroidism secondary to thyroid agenesis. On examination infant was found to have choreoathetoid movements. Gene associated with this:

A. TTF1
B. TTF2
C. PAX8
D. NKX2-5

Explanation:

Table: Genetic causes of congenital hypothyroidism

Defective gene protein	Inheritance	Consequences
PROP-1	Autosomal recessive	Combined pituitary hormone deficiencies with preservation of adrenocorticotropic hormone
PIT-1	Autosomal recessive Autosomal dominant	Combined deficiencies of growth hormone, prolactin, thyroid-stimulating hormone (TSH)
TSHβ	Autosomal recessive	TSH deficiency
TTF-1 (TITF-1)	Autosomal dominant	**Variable thyroid hypoplasia, choreoathetosis, pulmonary problems**
TTF-2 (FOXE-1)	Autosomal recessive	Thyroid agenesis, choanal atresia, spiky hair
PAX-8	Autosomal dominant	Thyroid dysgenesis, kidney abnormalities
NKX2-1	Autosomal dominant	Thyroid dysgenesis, brain, lung abnormalities
NKX2-5	Autosomal dominant	Thyroid dysgenesis, heart abnormalities

Ans. A

208. 10 day child born to untreated hypothyroidism mother presented with history of decreased feeding, reduced activity, prolonged and severe jaundice and was diagnosed with hypothyroidism. The dose of thyroxine required to treat congenital hypothyroidism is:

A. 1.6 mcg/kg/day
B. 15 mcg/kg/day
C. 25 mcg/kg/day
D. 50 mcg/kg/day

Explanation:

- When the diagnosis of congenital hypothyroidism is confirmed, T4 is instituted at a dose of 10–15 μg/kg per day, and the dose is adjusted by close monitoring of TSH levels.

Ans. B

209. 56 year old female diagnosed with hypothyroidism. Has undergone PET scan for some other purpose. What are areas which are expected to show lower regional activity among patient with hypothyroidism?

A. Amygdala
B. Hippocampus
C. Perigenual anterior cingulated cortex
D. All of the above

Explanation:

- Experimentally, positron emission tomography (PET) scans examining glucose metabolism in hypothyroid subjects show lower regional activity in the amygdala, hippocampus, and perigenual anterior cingulated cortex, among other regions, and this activity corrects after thyroxine replacement.

Ans. D

210. 24 year old primigravidae presented with thyrotoxicosis. After evaluation a diagnosis of gestational thyrotoxicosis was made.

Gestational thyrotoxicosis is ---------

A. Primary hyperthyroidism
B. Secondary hyperthyroidism
C. Thyrotoxicosis without hyperthyroidism
D. Iatrogenic thyrotoxicosis

Explanation:

Table: Causes of thyrotoxicosis
Primary Hyperthyroidism
• Graves' disease • Toxic multinodular goiter • Toxic adenoma • Functioning thyroid carcinoma metastases • Activating mutation of the TSH receptor • Activating mutation of $G_{s\alpha}$ (McCune-Albright syndrome) • Struma ovarii • **Drugs:** Iodine excess (Jod-Basedow phenomenon)
Thyrotoxicosis Without Hyperthyroidism
• Subacute thyroiditis • Silent thyroiditis • Other causes of thyroid destruction: Amiodarone, radiation, infarction of adenoma • Ingestion of excess thyroid hormone (thyrotoxicosis factitia) or thyroid tissue
Secondary Hyperthyroidism
• TSH-secreting pituitary adenoma • **Thyroid hormone resistance syndrome:** Occasional patients may have features of thyrotoxicosis • Chorionic gonadotropin-secreting tumors • **Gestational thyrotoxicosis**

Ans. B

211. 26 year old female presented with history of weight loss, diarrhea, palpitation, irregular cycles, insomnia. On evaluation found to have diffuse goitre and TFT s/o hyperthyroidism. TSHrAb was found to be positive. Diagnosis of Graves disease was made condition associated with graves diseases are:

A. Post partum
B. IRIS after HAART
C. Patient on almetuzumab
D. All of the following

Explanation:

- Smoking is a minor risk factor for Graves' disease and a major risk factor for the development of ophthalmopathy.
- Sudden increases in iodine intake may precipitate Graves' disease,
- There is a threefold increase in the occurrence of Graves' disease in the postpartum period.
- Graves' disease may occur during the immune reconstitution phase after highly active antiretroviral therapy (HAART)
- Alemtuzumab treatment.

Ans. D

212. Young female known case of graves disease on irregular treatment presented with lesion on shin which is a noninflamed, indurated plaque with a deep pink or purple color and an "orange skin" appearance. Possibility of thyroid dermopathy was considered. Incidence of thyroid dermopathy in graves disease is:

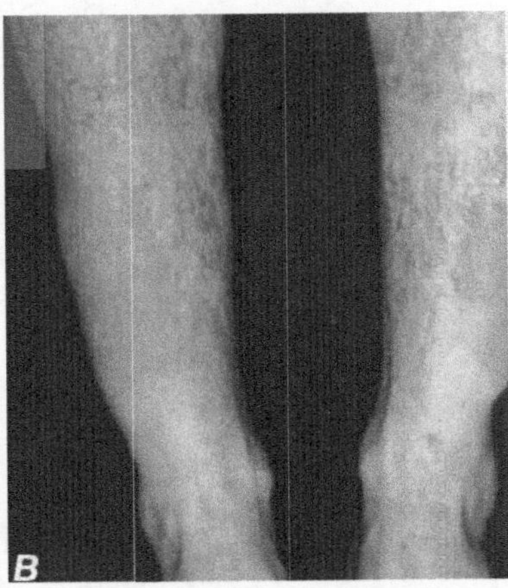

A. 21%
B. 5%
C. 10%
D. 15%

Explanation:

- Thyroid dermopathy occurs in <5% of patients with Graves' disease almost always in the presence of moderate or severe ophthalmopathy.
- frequent over the anterior and lateral aspects of the lower leg (hence the term pretibial myxedema)
- Skin changes can occur at other sites, particularly after trauma. The typical lesion is a noninflamed, indurated plaque with a deep pink or purple color and an "orange skin" appearance

Ans. B

213. Somatostatin inhibition is done by:

A. H1 receptors
B. H2 receptors
C. H3 receptors
D. H4 receptors

Explanation:

- Histamine also stimulates gastric acid secretion indirectly by activating the histamine H3 receptor on D-cells, which inhibits somatostatin release

Ans. C

214. 61 year old presented with new onset atrial fibrillation. On evaluation for AF, TFT was ordered which s/o primary hyperthyroidism. Patient was planned to start on warfarin. The required dose of warfarin in patient with hyperthyroidism is:

A. Decreased
B. Increased
C. Same as euthyroid patients
D. Based on Liver function

Explanation:

- Decreased warfarin doses are required when patients are thyrotoxic.
- If digoxin is used, increased doses are often needed in the thyrotoxic state.

Ans. A

215. 39 year old female presented with history excessive weight gain, irregular Cycles, constipation. on evaluation showed high TSH low T4. Diagnosis of primary hypothyroidism was made. Hypothyroidism screening should be done in women of what age?

A. 25 years
B. 30 years
C. 35 years
D. 45 years

Explanation:

Hypothyroidism	5-10%, women	TSH; confirm with free T_4
	0.5-2%, men	Screen women after age 35 and every 5 years thereafter

Ans. C

216. 71 year old postmenopausal women sustained femur fracture on trivial trauma. She was diagnosed to have osteoporotic fracture. Patient was managed surgically for the femur fracture.
Screening for osteoporosis should being at what age?

A. 55 years
B. 60 years
C. 65 years
D. 50 years

Explanation:

- Bone mineral density measurements in women >65 years or in postmenopausal women or men at risk.

Ans. C

217. 18 year old young male presented to OPD with history of not attaining pubertal changes when compared to his peer groups. On examination tall stature, long leg, b/l gynecomastia, small firm testis.
What Is the Investigation of choice to confirm the diagnosis?

A. LH, FSH levels
B. MRI sella
C. USG scrotum
D. Karyotyping

Explanation:

- Above clinical features suggestive of Klinefelter's syndrome.
- IOC is karyotyping .

Ans. D

218. OHA that causes weight gain is:

A. Metformin
B. Pramlintide
C. Lixisenatide
D. Glibornuride

Explanation:

	Mechanism of Action	Examples[a]	HBA_{sc} Reduction (*)[b]	Agent-Specific Advantages	Agent-Specific Disadvantages	Contra-indications
Oral						
Biguanides__	↓ Hepatic glucose production	Metformin	1-2	Weight neutral, do not cause hypoglycemia, inexpensive, extensive experience, ↓ CV events	Diarrhea, nausea, lectic acidosis, vitamin B_{12} deficiency	Renal insufficiency (see text for GFR <45 ml/min), CHF, radiographic contrast studies, hospitalized patients, acidosis
α-Glucosidase inhibitors***	↓ GI glucose absorption	Acarbose, miglitol, voglibose	0.5-0.8	Reduce postprandial glycemia	GI flatulence, liver function tests	Renal/liver disease
Dipeptidyl peptidase IV inhibitors***	Prolong endogenous GLP-1 action; ↑ Insulin, ↓ glucagon	Alogliptin, lingaliptin, saxagliptin, sitagliptin, villagliptin	0.5-0.8	Well tolerated, do not cause hypoglycemia	Angioedema/ urticarial and immune-mediated dermatologic effects	Reduce dose with renal disease
Insulin secretagogues: Sulfonylureas**	↑ Insulin secretion	Glibomuride, gliclazide, glimepride, glipizide, gliquidone, glyburide, glyclopyramide	1-2	Short onset of action, lower postprandial glucose, inexpensive	Hypoglycemia, weight gain	Renal/liver disease
Insulin secretagogues: Nonsulfonylureas***	↑Insulin secretion	Mitiglinide nateglinide, repaglinide	0.5-1.0	Short onset of action, lower postprandial glucose	Hypoglycemia	Renal/liver disease
Sodium-glucose cotransporter 2 inhibitors***	↑ Renal glucose excretion	Canagliflozin, dapagliflazin, empagliflazin, ertugliflazin	0.5-1.0	Do not cause hypoglycemia, ↓ weight and BP: see text for CVD effect	Urinary and genital infections, polyuria, dehydration, exacerbate tendency to hyperkalemia and DKA; see text	Moderate renal insufficiency, insulin-deficient DM
Thiazolidine-diones***	↓Insulin resistance, ↑glucose utilization	Pioglitazone, rosiglitazone	0.5-1.4	Lower insulin requirements	Peripheral edema, CHF, weight gain, fractures, macular edema	CHF, liver disease
Parenteral						
Amylin agonists***	Slow gastric emptying, ↓ glucagon	Pramlintide	0.25-0.5	Reduce postprandial glycemia, weight loss	Injection, nausea ↑ risk of hypoglycemia with insulin	Agents that also slow GI motility

GLP-1 receptor agonists***	↑ Insulin, ↓ glucagon, slow gastric emptying, satiety	Albiglutide, dulaglutide, exenatide, liraglutide, lixisenatide, semaglutide	0.5-1.0	Weight loss, do not cause hypoglycemia; see text for CVD effect	Injection, nausea, ↑ risk of hypoglycemia with insulin secretagogues	Renal disease, agents that also slow GI motility; medullary carcinoma of thyroid, pancreatic disease
Insulin***	↑ Glucose utilization ↓ hepatic glucose production, and other anabolic actions		Not limited	Known safety profile	Injection, weight gain, hypoglycemia	
Medical nutrition therapy and physical activity**	↓ Insulin resistance, ↑ Insulin secretion	Low-calorie, low-fat diet, exercise	1-3	Other health benefits	Compliance difficult, long-term success low	

Ans. D

219. 35 year old female presented with history of recurrent attacks of palpitation, headache and profuse sweating. h/o recurrent hospital visits + diagnosed to have anxiety attacks. Incidentally on evaluation found to have hypercalcemia with hypophosphatemia. On examination tachycardia +, goiter + , cervical lymphadenopathy + history of similar complaints in the family +.

Gene associated with the above syndrome is:

A. CDKN1B
B. RET
C. PRKAR1A
D. KLLN

Explanation:

Type (Chromosomal location)	Tumors (Estimated penetrance)	Gene and most frequently mutated codons
MEN2A (10 cen-10q11.2)	**MTC (90%) Pheochromocytoma (>50%) Parathyroid adenoma (10-25%)**	**RET 634, e.g., Cys→Arg (~85%)**

Ans. B

220. 8 year old male boy presented with history of polyuria polydipsia. After thorough evaluation other cause for polyuria, that is type 1 diabetes, rental tubular acidosis, central diabetes insipidus was ruled out. Probable diagnosis of nephrogenic DI was made. Mode of inheritance of nephrogenic DI due to v2 receptor mutation is:

A. Autosomal dominant
B. Autosomal recessive
C. Co dominant
D. X-linked recessive

Explanation:

- Nephrogenic DI due to V2 receptor mutation has X-linked recessive inheritance.

Ans. D

221. 14 year old child presented to orthopedics OPD with h/o lower limb deformity. On evaluation child was found to have inflamed costochondritis, inward movement of ICS on inspiration, pot belly, genu valgum. The hormone deficient in the above condition acts on which receptor?

A. GPCR
B. Tyrosine kinase
C. Serine threonine kinase
D. Nuclear receptor

Explanation:

- Above clinical picture s/o rickets
- Steroids, thyroid hormones, vitamin D, and retinoids are lipid-soluble and interact with intracellular nuclear receptors

Ans. D

222. 25 year old female presented with history of primary hypothyroidism was prescribed to take tab thyronorm 50mcg . But she missed one dose, treating physician advises her to take two doses together the next day. The half life of T4 is?

A. 50 mins
B. 4 days
C. 0.7 day
D. 7 days

Explanation:

Table: Characteristics of circulating T_4 and T_3

Hormone Property	T_4	T_3
Serum concentrations		
• Total hormone	8 µg/dl	0.14 µg/dl
• Fraction of total hormone in the unbound form	0.02%	0.3%
• Unbound (free) hormone	$21\times 10^{-12} M$	$6\times 10^{-12} M$
Serum half-life	**7 d**	2 d
Fraction directly from the thyroid	100%	20%
Production rate, including peripheral conversion	90 µg/d	32 µg/d
Intracellular hormone fraction	~20%	~70%
Relative metabolic potency	0.3	1
Receptor binding	$10^{-10} M$	$10^{-11} M$

Ans. D

223. 39 year old male presented with history of headache, holocranial from last 3 months. Associated with vomiting and blurring of vision. History of sustaining recurrent injuries while walking. On evaluation CT showed macroadenoma of pituitary with perimetry showing bitemporal hemianopia.

Which of the following is present in pituitary stalk?

A. Tuberohypophyseal nerve tract
B. Medial Hypophyseal nerve tract
C. Opticohypopyseal nerve tract
D. Cerebrohypopyhseal nerve tract

Explanation:

- The posterior lobe is directly innervated by hypothalamic neurons (supraopticohypophyseal and tuberohypophyseal nerve tracts) via the pituitary stalk.

Ans. A

224. Not true about effects if glucocorticoids on glucose hemostasis is:

A. Dose related
B. Usually reversible
C. Mostly pronounced in preprandial period
D. Impairs insulin secretion

Explanation:

- Glucocorticoids increase insulin resistance, decrease glucose utilization, increase hepatic glucose production, and impair insulin secretion.
- These changes lead to a worsening of glycemic control in individuals with DM and may precipitate hyperglycemia in other individuals.
- If new-onset hyperglycemia remains during chronic treatment with supraphysiologic doses of glucocorticoid (>5 mg of prednisone or equivalent), the DM may be called "steroid-induced diabetes."
- Effects of glucocorticoids on glucose homeostasis are dose-related, usually reversible, and most pronounced in the postprandial period.
- If FPG is near the normal range, oral diabetes agents (e.g., sulfonylureas, metformin) may be sufficient to reduce hyperglycemia.
- If the FPG is >11.1 mmol/L (200 mg/dL), oral agents are usually not efficacious, and insulin therapy is required. Short-acting insulin may be sufficient alone or together with long-acting insulin in order to control postprandial glucose excursions.

Ans. C

225. 43 year old male presented with history of headache, holocranial from last 8 months. Associated with vomiting and blurring of vision. On evaluation MRI showed microadenoma of pituitary which is T1 hypointense T2 hyperintense. The order of tropic hormone failure associated with pituitary compression by pituitary adenoma is:

A. ACTH>LH>GH>FSH>TSH
B. LH>GH>FSH>TSH>ACTH
C. TSH>ACTH>GH>FSH>LH
D. GH>FSH>LH>TSH>ACTH

Explanation:

- A Trophic hormone failure associated with pituitary compression or destruction usually occurs sequentially: growth hormone > folliclestimulating hormone > Luteinizing hormone > thyroid-stimulating hormone > adrenocorticotropic hormone.

Ans. D

226. 35 year old female presented with history irregular cycles, excessive weight gain, reduced appetite, constipation. Probable diagnosis of hypothyroidism was made. TFT was as follows TSH : 0.22, f T4: 0.6, f T3: 1.9. Diagnosis of central hypothyroidism was made.

Pit 1 mutation can cause deficiency of:

A. GH
B. Prolactin
C. TSH
D. All of the above

Explanation:

- Pit-1 mutations cause combined GH, prolactin (PRL), and TSH deficiencies.

Ans. D

227. 27 year old non pregnant female presented with history of galactorrhea and secondary amenorrhea. She denies of any drug intake. On evaluation her prolactin was found to be 210 mcg/dl.

Breast suckling increases prolactin levels that last for about:

A. 30-45 mins

B. 5-10 mins

C. 45-60 mins

D. 10-30 mins

Explanation:

- If breastfeeding is initiated, basal PRL levels remain elevated; suckling stimulates transient reflex increases in PRL levels that last for about 30–45 min.

Ans. A

228. 45 year old patient presented with weight gain from last 6 months. He was recently diagnosed with diabetes and hypertension and was on treatment. He also complaints of difficulty climbing stairs. On examination: abdominal obesity +, abdominal striae >1cm purple, depressing noted in thigh and abdomen. Paper like thin skin noted. Clinical diagnosis of Cushing syndrome was made. And it was noted that 11PM cortisol was found to be high. To confirm ONDST was ordered which confirmed Cushing syndrome. Mean basal ACTH was ordered. ACTH was found to be high. So diagnosis of ACTH dependent hypercortisolism was made. Which somatostatin receptor subtype preferentially suppress ACTH secretion?

A. SSTR2

B. SSTR3

C. SSTR4

D. SSTR5

Explanation:

- Pasireotide (600 or 900 µg/d subcutaneously), a somatostatin analogue with high affinity for SST5 > SST2 receptors, may control hypercortisolemia in a subset of patients with ACTH-secreting pituitary tumors

Ans. D

229. Patient presented with acromegalic features .on biochemical analysis found to have high IGF 1 levels to confirm diagnosis OGTT was ordered and found to have non suppressible GH levels . MRI shows pituitary macroadenoma. one of the drug used to control symptoms of acromegaly is pegvisomant. Pegvisomant best described as:

A. GH receptor antagonist

B. GH receptor protein

C. GHRH analogue

D. GHRH antagonist

Explanation:

- Pegvisomant antagonizes endogenous GH action by blocking peripheral GH binding to its receptor.

Ans. A

230. Half life of T4 is:

A. 2 days

B. 4 days

C. 7 days

D. 14 days

Explanation:

Table: Characteristics of circulating T_4 and T_3		
Hormone Property	T_4	T_3
• Serum concentrations • Total hormone • Fraction of total hormone in the unbound form • Unbound (free) hormone	 8 μg/dl 0.02% $21 \times 10^{-12} M$	 0.14 μg/dl 0.3% $6 \times 10^{-12} M$
Serum half-life	7 d	2 d
Fraction directly from the thyroid	100%	20%
Production rate, including peripheral conversion	90 μg/d	32 μg/d
Intracellular hormone fraction	~20%	~70%
Relative metabolic potency	0.3	1
Receptor binding	$10^{-10} M$	$10^{-11} M$

Ans. C

231. Patient presented with easy fatiguability and generalized tiredness. On evaluation found to have low BP, euvolemic hyponatremia. Found to have cortisol deficiency. Tissue specific transcription factor associated with corticotrope is:

A. T pit

B. Prop 1

C. Pit 1

D. All of the following

Explanation:

Table: Anterior pituitary hormone expression and regulation					
Cell	**Corticotrope**	**Somatotrope**	**Lactotrope**	**Thyrotrope**	**Gonadotrope**
Tissue-specific transcription factor	T-Pit	Prop-1, Pit-1	Prop-1, Pit-1	Prop-1, Pit-1, TEF	SF-1, DAX-1
Fetal appearance	6 weeks	8 weeks	12 weeks	12 weeks	12 weeks
Hormone	POMC	GH	PRL	TSH	FSH, LH
Protein	Polypeptide	Polypeptide	Polypeptide	Glycoprotein α, β subunits	Glycoprotein α, β subunits
Amino acids	266 (ACTH 1-39)	191	198	211	210, 204
Stimulators	CRH, AVP, gp-130 cytokines	GHRH, ghrelin	Estrogen, TRH, VIP	TRH	GnRH, activins, estrogen
Inhibitors	Glucocorticoids	Somatostatin, IGF-1	Dopamine	T_3, T_4, dopamine, somatostatin, glucocorticoids	Sex steroids, inhibin
Target gland	Adrenal	Liver, bone, other tissues	Breast, other tissues	Thyroid	Ovary, testis
Trophic effect	Steroid production	IGF-I production, growth induction, insulin antagonism	Milk production	T4 synthesis and secretion	Sex steroid production, follicle growth, germ cell maturation
Normal range	ACTH, 4-22 pg/l	<0.5 μg/l[a]	M <15 μg/l; F < 20 μg/l	0.1–5 mU/l	M, 5–20 IU/l; F (basal), 5–20 IU/l

[a] Hormone secretion integrated over 24 hours.

Ans. A

232. Glucose is transported by which glucose transporter in pancreatic islet cells?

A. GLUT 1
B. GLUT 3
C. GLUT 4
D. GLUT 5

Explanation:

- Glucose and other nutrients regulate insulin secretion by the pancreatic beta cell.
- Glucose is transported by a glucose transporter (GLUT1 and/or GLUT2 in humans, GLUT2 in rodents); subsequent glucose metabolism by the beta cell alters ion channel activity, leading to insulin secretion.
- SUR receptor is the binding site for some drugs that act as insulin secretagogues.

Ans. A

233. 7 year old child was referred to endocrinology department with history of not gaining height and increase weight. He was told to have hormone problem. Hormones promoting growth include all except:

A. GH
B. IGF1
C. IGF2
D. Cytokines

Explanation:

- Skeletal maturation and somatic growth is promoted by hormone stimuli like GH, IGF 1, sex steroids, thyroid hormones, paracrine growth factors, cytokines.

Ans. C

234. 16 year old child presented to pediatrics department with history of not attaining secondary sexual characteristics. On evaluation he was found to have truncal obesity, depressed nasal bridge, high arched palate and syndactyly. History similar complaints+ in the family. History of consanguineous marriage + a diagnosis of carpenter's syndrome was made. Carpenter's syndrome is associated with:

A. Primary hypogonadism
B. Secondary hypogonadism
C. Any of the above
D. None of the above

Explanation:

Table: A comparison of syndromes of obesity—Hypogonadism and mental retardation

Features	Syndrome				
	Prader-Willi	**Laurence-Moon-Biedl**	**Ahlstrom's**	**Cohen's**	**Carpenter's**
Inheritance	Sporadic; two-thirds have defect	Autosomal recessive	Autosomal recessive	Probably autosomal recessive	Autosomal recessive
Stature	Short	Normal; infrequently short	Normal; infrequently short	Short or tall	Normal
Obesity	Generalized Moderate to severe Onset 1-3 years	Generalized Early onset, 1-2 years	Truncal Early onset, 2-5 years	Truncal Mid-childhood, age 5	Truncal, gluteal
Craniofacies	Narrow bifrontal diameter Almond-shaped eyes Strabismus V-shaped mouth High-arched palate	Not distinctive	Not distinctive	High nasal bridge Arched palate Open mouth Short philtrum	Acrocephaly Flat nasal bridge High-arched palate

Contd.

Contd.

Limbs	Small hands and feet Hypotonia	Polydactyly	No abnormalities	Hypotonia Narrow hands and feet	Polydactyly Syndactyly Genu valgum
Reproductive status	1° Hypogonadism	1° Hypogonadism	Hypogonadism in males but not in females	Normal gonadal function or hypogonadotropic hypogonadism	2° Hypogonadism
Other features	Enamel hypoplasia Hyperphagia Temper tantrums Nasal speech			Dysplastic ears Delayed puberty	
Mental re-tar-dation	Mild to moderate		Normal intelligence	Mild	Slight

Ans. B

235. Which cranial nerve most commonly affected in diabetic neuropathy?

A. 3rd nerve
B. 7th nerve
C. 5th nerve
D. 6th nerve

Explanation:

- Mononeuropathy (dysfunction of isolated cranial or peripheral nerves) is less common than polyneuropathy in DM and presents with pain and motor weakness in the distribution of a single nerve.
- Mononeuropathies can occur at entrapment sites such as carpal tunnel or be non-compressive.
- Involvement of the third cranial nerve is most common and is heralded by diplopia.

Ans. A

236. 19 year old child presented to adolescent clinic with history of gaining weight. On probing he gives history of excessive junk food intake and minimal physical activity. MCC gene associated with obesity:

A. Ob
B. db
C. FTO
D. Trkb

Explanation:

Replicated loci linked to obesity have been identified, but together they account for <3% of interindividual **variation in BMI. The most replicated of these involves a region which includes several genes including FTO, which is of unknown function, but like many of the other recently described candidates, is expressed in the brain.**

Ans. C

237. 41 year male was referred to surgeon in view of morbid obesity with uncontrolled glycemia and dyslipidemia. Bariatric surgery is indicated when BMI is more than:

A. $30kg/m^2$
B. $35kg/m^2$
C. $40kg/m^2$
D. $45kg/m^2$

Explanation:

Table: A guide to opting for treatment for obesity					
Treatment	BMI Category (kg/m^2)				
	25-26.9	27-29.9	30-34.9	35-39.9	≥ 40
Diet, exercise, behavioral therapy	With comorbidities	With comorbidities	+	+	+
Pharmacotherapy	–	With comorbidities	+	+	+
Surgery	–	–	–	With comorbidities	+

Ans. C

238. 55 year old male who is a obese (BMI of 31) with metabolic syndrome. Endocrinologist advised life style modification with oral anti obesity medication. Which anti obesity drug was used in EQUIP trial?

A. PHEN/TPM
B. Lorcaserin
C. Liraglutide
D. Naltrexone

Explanation:

Table: Clinical trials for antiobesity medications									
	PHEN/TPM		Lorcaserin		Naltrexone SR/Bupropion SR			Liraglutide	
	Equip	Con-quer	Bloom	Blos-som	Cor-I	Cor-II	Cor-Bmod	Scale	Scale Mainte-nance
No. of participants (ITT-LOCF)	1230	2487	3182	4008	1742	1496	793	3731	422
BMI (kg/m^2)	≥ 35	27-45	27-45	30-45	30-45	30-45	30-45	>27	≥27
Age (y)	18-70	18-70	18-65	18-65	18-65	18-65	18-65	≥18	>18
Comorbid conditions (cardiovascular and metabolic)	≥1	≥2	≥1	≥1	≥1	≥1	≥1	≥1	≥1
Mean weight loss (%) with treatment vs placebo	10.9 vs 1.6	7.8 vs 1.2	5.8 vs 2.2	4.8 vs 2.8	6.1 vs 1.3	6.5 vs 1.9	9.3 vs 5.1	8.0 vs 2.6	6.2 vs 0.2
Placebo-sub-trac-ted weight loss (%)	9.3	6.6	3.6	3.0	4.8	4.6	4.2	5.4	6.0
Categorical change in 5% weight loss with treatment vs placebo	66.7 vs 17.3	62 vs 21	47.5 vs 20.3	47.2 vs 25	48 vs 16	50.5 vs 17.1	66.4 vs 42.5	63.2 vs 27.1	81.4 vs 48.9
Study completion rate, treatment vs placebo (%)	66.4 vs 52.9	69 vs 57	55.4 vs 45.1	57.2 vs 52	50	54	57.9 vs 58.4	71.9 vs 64.4	75 vs 69.5

Ans. A

239. 42 year old male with BMI of 42 was referred to bariatric surgeon from endocrinologist for bariatric surgery . Surgeon explains different surgery options available to him. Identify the procedure shown in the picture:

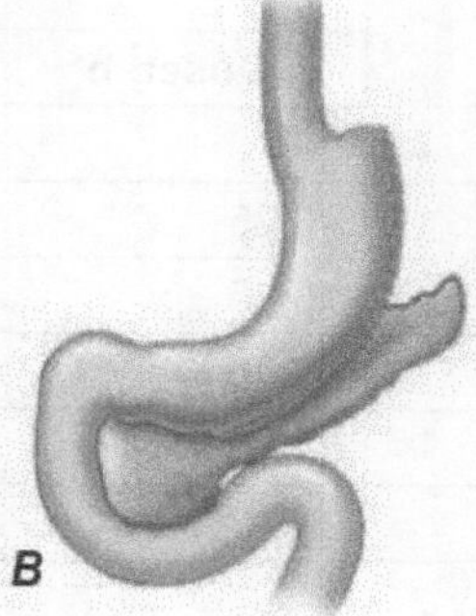

A. Laparoscopic sleeve gastrectomy
B. The Roux-en-Y gastric bypass
C. Biliopancreatic diversion with duodenal switch
D. Biliopancreatic diversion

Explanation:

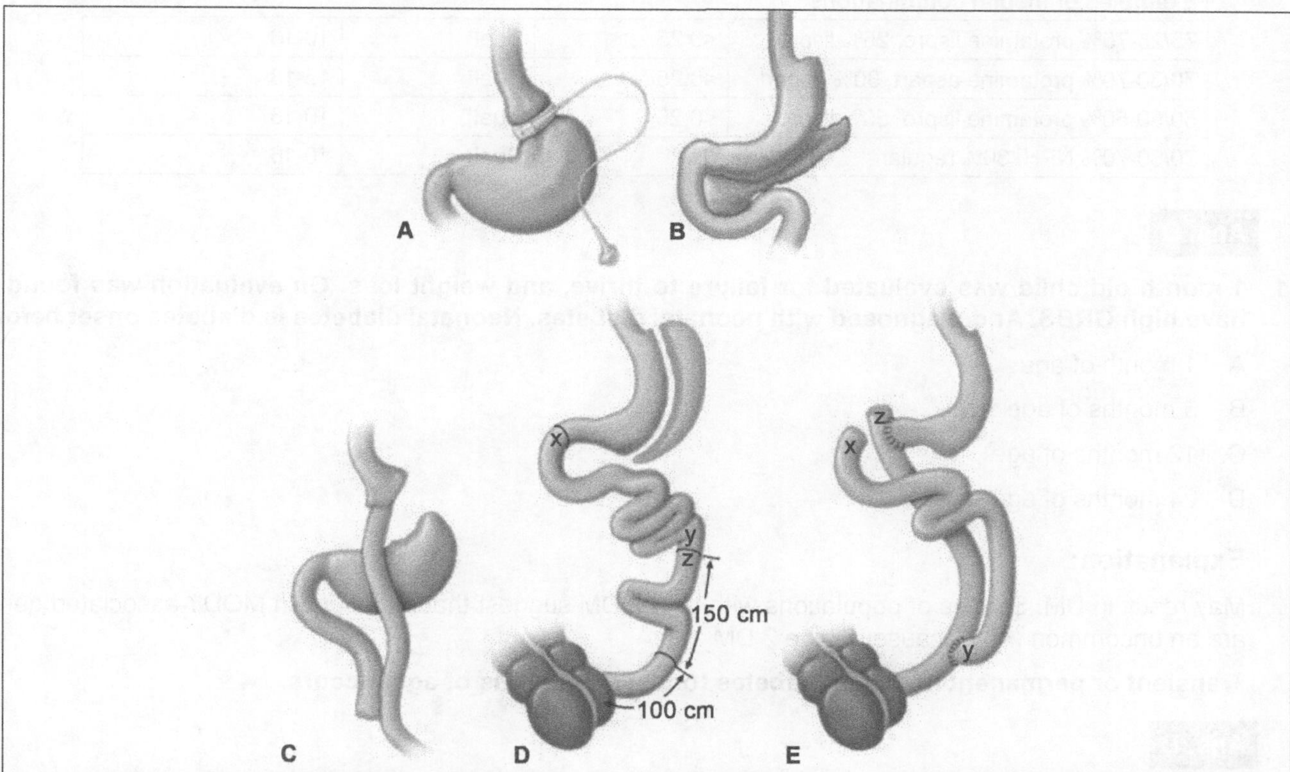

Figure: Bariatric surgical procedures. Examples of operative interventions used for surgical manipulation of the gastrointestinal tract. **A.** Laparoscopic adjustable gastric banding. **B.** Laparoscopic sleeve gastrectomy. **C.** The Roux-en-Y gastric bypass. **D.** Biliopancreatic diversion with duodenal switch. **E.** Biliopancreatic diversion

Ans. A

240. 51 year old male patient diagnosed with diabetes and found to non complaint to insulin. So physician prescribes him long acting insulin degludec. Effect of degludec lasts for:

A. 4 hours
B. 12 hours
C. 36 hours
D. 42 hours

Explanation:

Table: Properties of insulin preparations[a]			
Preparation	Time of Action		
	Onset, h	Peak, h	Effective Duration, h
Short-acting[b]			
Aspart	<0.25	0.5-1.5	2-4
Glulisine	<0.25	0.5-1.5	2-4
Lispro[†]	<0.25	0.5-1.5	2-4
Regular[g]	0.5-1.0	2-3	3-6
Inhaled human insulin	0.5-1.0	2-3	3
Long-acting[g]			
Degludec	**1-9**	____[c]	**42[d]**
Detemir	1-4	____[c]	12-24[d]
Glargine[f]	2-4	____[c]	20-24
NPH	2-4	4-10	10-16
Examples of Insulin combinations[e]			
75/25-75% protamine lispro, 25% lispro	<0.25	Dual[†]	10-16
70/30-70% protamine aspart, 30% aspart	<0.25	Dual[†]	15-18
50/50-50% protamine lispro, 50% lispro	<0.25	Dual[†]	10-16
70/30-70% NPH, 30% regular	0.5-1	Dual[†]	10-16

Ans. D

241. 1 month old child was evaluated for failure to thrive, and weight loss. On evaluation was found to have high GRBS. And diagnosed with neonatal diabetes. Neonatal diabetes is diabetes onset before:

A. 1 month of age

B. 6 months of age

C. 12 months of age

D. 24 months of age

Explanation:

May result in DM. Studies of populations with type 2 DM suggest that mutations in MODY-associated genes are an uncommon (<5%) cause of type 2 DM.

Transient or permanent neonatal diabetes (onset < 6 months of age) occurs.

Ans. B

242. 42 year old female patient diagnosed with type 2 diabetes mellitus. And she was prescribed T. Vildagliptin. Her query was how much this drug will reduce her HbA1C levels?

A. 0.5- 0.8

B. 0.5-1.0

C. 0.5-1.4

D. 1-2

Explanation:

	Mechanism of action	Examples	HBA_{1c} reduction (%)	Agent-specific advantages	Agent-specific disadvantages	Contraindications
Dipeptidyl peptidase IV inhibitors[c+++]	Prolong endogenous GLP-1 action; ↑ Insulin, ↓ glucagon	Alogliptin, linagliptin, saxagliptin, sitagliptin, vildagliptin	**0.5-0.8**	Well tolerated, do not cause hypoglycemia	Angioedema/ urticarial and immune-mediated dermatologic effects	Reduced dose with renal disease
Insulin secretagogues: Sulfonylureas[c+]	↑ Insulin secretion	Glibornuride, gliclazide, glimepiride, glipizide, gliquidone, glyburide, glyclopyramide	1-2	Short onset of action, lower postprandial glucose, inexpensive	Hypoglycemia, weight gain	Renal/liver disease
Insulin secretagogues: Nonsulfonyl-ureas[c+++]	↑ Insulin secretion	Mitiglinide nateglinide, repaglinide	0.5-1.0	Short onset of action, lower postprandial glucose	Hypoglycemia	Renal/liver disease
Sodium-glucose cotransporter 2 inhibitors[+++]	↑ Renal glucose excretion	Canagliflozin, dapagliflozin, empagliflozin, ertugliflozin	0.5-1.0	Do not cause hypoglycemia, ↓ weight and BP; see text for CVD effect	Urinary and genital infections, polyuria, dehydration, exacerbate tendency to hyperkalemia and DKA; see text	Moderate renal insufficiency, insulin-deficient DM

Ans. A

243. 40 year old male patient presented to OPD for routine health checkup. General practitioner askes for couple of tests. On among them is FBS .What does fasting mean in FBS?

A. No food intake for last 6 hours
B. No calorie intake for last 6hours
C. No food intake for last 8 hours
D. No calorie intake for last 8 hours

Explanation:

- Fasting state means : No calorie intake for last 8 hours

Ans. C

244. A 24 year old female presented with cyclical pattern of hematuria during menstrual cycle. True about episodic hematuria is:

A. Due to hormonal disturbances
B. Due to Trauma
C. Due to Invasion of urinary tract by endothelial implants
D. Due to OCP

Explanation:

As few as 3–5 red blood cells in the spun sediment from first-voided morning urine is suspicious. The diagnosis of glomerular injury can be delayed because patients will not realize they have *microscopic hematuria*, and only rarely with the exception of IgA nephropathy and sickle cell disease is *gross hematuria* present. When working up microscopic hematuria, perhaps accompanied by minimal proteinuria (<500 mg/24 h), it is important to exclude anatomic lesions, such as malignancy of the urinary tract, particularly in older men. Microscopic hematuria may also appear with the onset of benign prostatic hypertrophy, interstitial nephritis, papillary necrosis, hypercalciuria, renal stones, cystic kidney diseases, or renal vascular injury. However, when red blood cell casts or dysmorphic red blood cells are found in the sediment, glomerulonephritis is likely. A mean of 8–10 mg/24 h of albumin appears in the urine in the absence of kidney disease. In early nephropathy, such as in diabetic nephropathy, proteinuria increases to 30–300 mg/24 h and is called microalbuminuria and represents the presence of renal disease. Greater than 300 mg/24 h of albuminuria represents frank proteinuria and more advanced renal disease.

Ans. C

245. 16 year old female presented with recurrent vomiting. With history of polyuria, polydipsia, weight loss. GRBS was 600mg/dl, had ketosis and acidosis. She was found to have low C peptide, low insulin levels with ant GAD 65 antibody +. Diagnosed with type 1 DM.

Highest incidence type 1 DM is seen in:

A. China B. India

C. Scandinavia D. Africa

Explanation:

There is considerable geographic variation in the incidence of both type 1 and type 2 DM. Currently, Scandinavia has the highest incidence of type 1 DM; the lowest incidence is in the Pacific Rim where it is twenty- to thirty-fold lower. Northern Europe and the United States have an intermediate rate.

Ans. C

246. 55 year old male presented with excessive tiredness , sweating and palpitation and in emergency GRBS was done which showed 45mg/dl. He was recently prescribed antibiotics for his URTI. Drug causing hypoglycemia is:

A. Nicotinic acid B. ACEI

C. Pentamidine D. Diazoxide

Explanation:

Table: Etiologic classification of diabetes mellitus
I. Type 1 diabetes (immune-mediated beta cell destruction, usually leading to absolute insulin deficiency)
II. Type 2 diabetes (may range from predominantly insulin resistance with relative insulin deficiency to a predominantly insulin secretory defect with insulin resistance)
III. Specific types of diabetes
A. Genetic defects of beta cell development or function characterized by mutations in:
1. Hepatocyte nuclear transcription factor (HNF) 4α (MODY 1)
2. Glucokinase (MODY 2)
3. HNF-1α (MODY 3)
4. Insulin promoter factor-1, HNF-1β, Neuro D1, and others leading to other forms of MODY
5. Insulin, subunits of ATP-sensitive potassium channel leading to permanent neonatal diabetes
6. Mitochondrial DNA
7. Other pancreatic islet regulators/proteins such as *KLF11, PAX4, BLK, GATA4, GATA6, SLC2A2* (GLUT2), *RFX6, GLIS3*
B. Transient neonatal diabetes
C. Diseases of the exocrine pancreas–pancreatitis, pancreatectomy, neoplasia, cystic fibrosis, hemochromatosis, fibrocalculous pancreatopathy, mutations in carboxyl ester lipase
D. Genetic defects in insulin action, including type A insulin resistance, Leprechaunism, Rabson-Mendenhall syndrome, Lipodystrophy syndromes
E. Endocrinopathies–acromegaly, Cushing's syndrome, glucagonoma, pheochromocytoma, hyperthyroidism, somatostatinoma, aldosteronoma

Contd.

F. Drug- or chemical-induced–glucocorticoids, vacor (a rodenticide), pentamidine, **nicotinic acid**, diazoxide, β-**adrenergic agonists**, thiazides, calcineurin and mTOR inhibitors, **hydantoins**, asparaginase, α-interferon, protease inhibitors, antipsychotics (atypicals and others), epinephrine

G. Infections–congenital rubella, cytomegalovirus, coxsackievirus

H. Uncommon forms of immune-mediated diabetes–"stiff-person" syndrome, anti-insulin receptor antibodies

I. Other genetic syndromes sometimes associated with diabetes–Wolfram's syndrome, Down's syndrome, Klinefelter's syndrome, Turner's syndrome, Friedreich's ataxia, Huntington's chorea, Laurence-Moon-Biedl syndrome, myotonic dystrophy, porphyria, Prader-Willi syndrome

IV. Gestational diabetes mellitus (GDM)

Many other drugs have been associated with hypoglycemia. These include commonly used drugs such as angiotensin-converting enzyme inhibitors and angiotensin receptor antagonists, β-adrenergic receptor antagonists, quinolone antibiotics, indomethacin, quinine and sulfonamides.

Ans. B

247. 49 year old perimenopausal women presented with history of back pain. On evaluation DEXA scan suggestive of osteoporosis. The treating physician decided to rule out secondary cause for osteoporosis. All are the cause for secondary osteoporosis except:

A. Acromegaly
B. Adrenal insufficiency
C. Hypothyroidism
D. Diabetes mellitus

Explanation:

Table: Diseases associated with an increased risk of generalized osteoporosis in adults

Hypogonadal states	**Hematologic disorders/malignancy**
Turner's syndrome	Multiple myeloma
Klinefelter's syndrome	Lymphoma and leukemia
Anorexia nervosa	Malignancy-associated parathyroid hormone (PTHrP) production
Hypothalamic amenorrhea	Mastocytosis
Hyperprolactinemia	Hemophilia
Other primary or secondary hypogonadal states	Thalassemia
Endocrine disorders	**Selected inherited disorders**
Cushing's syndrome	Osteogenesis imperfecta
Hyperparathyroidism	Marfan's syndrome
Thyrotoxicosis	Hemochromatosis
Diabetes mellitus (both type 1 and 2)	Hypophosphatasia
Acromegaly	Glycogen storage diseases
Adrenal insufficiency	Homocystinuria
Nutritional and gastrointestinal disorders	Ehlers-Danlos syndrome
Malnutrition	Porphyria
Parenteral nutrition	Menkes' syndrome
Malabsorption syndromes	Epidermolysis bullosa
Gastrectomy	**Other disorders**
Severe liver disease, especially biliary cirrhosis	Immobilization
Pernicious anemia	Chronic obstructive pulmonary disease
Rheumatologic disorders	Pregnancy and lactation
Rheumatoid arthritis	Scoliosis
Ankylosing spondylitis	Multiple sclerosis
	Sarcoidosis
	Amyloidosis

Ans. C

248. 10 year old male child presented to OPD with history of recurrent attacks of sweating, tiredness and all these attacks are preceded by exercise. At the time of attacks child was found to have low GRBS (40mg/dl). Which subsided on consuming oral glucose. Mutation associated with exercise induced hypoglycemia is:

A. Monocarboxylate transporter 1
B. Glucokinase.
C. Defects in the carnitine cycle
D. Inherited fructose intolerance

Explanation:

Exercise-induced hypoglycemia, by definition, follows exercise. It results in hyperinsulinemia caused by increased activity of monocarboxylase transporter 1 and β cells.

Ans. A

249. 2 year old male child was brought to pediatrician with history of absent testis in the scrotum. On evaluation it was noted that bilateral testis was found in inguinal canal. Cryptorchidism is associated with:

A. INSL3 mutation
B. LGR8 mutation
C. Both of the above
D. None of the above

Explanation:

Of age. Androgens regulated predominantly the inguinoscrotal descent of the testes through degeneration of the cranio-suspensory ligament and a shortening of the gubernaculums, respectively. **Mutations in INSL3 and leucine-rich repeat family of G-protein-coupled receptor 8 (LGR8), which regulated transabdominal portion of testicular descent, have been found in some patients with cryptorchidism.**

Cryptorchidism is associated with increased risk of malignancy

Ans. C

250. 21 year old presented with history of excessive hair growth over face from last 6 month. Dermatologist prescribes finasteride. Finasteride is:

A. SRD5A1 Inhibitor
B. SRD5A2 Inhibitor
C. Both a+b
D. SRD5A3 inhibitor

Explanation:

In treating hirsutism, but concerns about the induction of hepatocellular dysfunction preclude its use. Finasteride is a competitive inhibitor of 5α-reductase type 2. Beneficial effects on hirsutism have been reported, but the predominance of 5α-reductase type 1 in the PSU appears to account for its limited efficacy.

Ans. B

251. 58 year old male patient presented with history of severe paraesthesia since 2 months. He is a known case of type 2 diabetes mellitus since 5 years on OHA. FDA approved drug for diabetic neuropathy are a/e:

A. Pregabalin
B. Gabapentin
C. Duloxitine
D. Tapentadol

Explanation:

Symptomatic treatment being available; evidence of the effectiveness of improved glycemic control in painful diabetic neuropathy is lacking. Two agents, duloxetine and pregabalin, have been approved by

the U.S. Food and Drug Administration (FDA) for pain associated with diabetic neuropathy. Tapentadol, a centrally acting opioid, is also FDA-approved, but has only modest efficacy and poses addiction risk, making it and other opioids less desirable

Ans. B

252. Till 6 weeks of intrauterine life gonads are bipotential. Later on they develop into either testos/ ovary. In the developing ovary, primordial germ cells (PGCs) proliferate and enter meiosis, whereas they proliferate and then undergo mitotic arrest in the developing testis. Which of the following prevents primordial germ cells in males from entering meiosis during embryological development?

A. CYP26B1
B. CYP26A1
C. CYP25B1
D. CYP25A1

Explanation:

Whereas they proliferate and then undergo mitotic arrest in the developing testis. PGC entry into meiosis is initiated by retinoic acid. The developing testis produces high levels of CYP26B1, an enzyme that degrades retinoic acid, preventing PGC entry into meiosis. Approximately 7 million germ cells are present in the fetal ovary in the second trimester, and 1 million remain at birth.

Ans. A

253. A child was referred to endocrinologist with ambiguous genitalia. Karyotyping was 46 XY. Child was found to have craniosynostosis and mid face hypoplasia, bowing of femur, radioulnar synostosis. A diagnosis of antler bixler syndrome was made. Antler bixler anomaly is associated with:

A. SOX9 mutation
B. POR deficiency
C. WNT4 mutation
D. SOX2 mutation

Explanation:

Gene	Inheritance	Gonad	Uterus	External genitalia	Associated features
CYB5A	AR	Testis	–	Ambiguous	Apparent isolated 17,20-lyase deficiency; methemoglobinemia
POR	**AR**	**Testis**	–	**Ambiguous or male**	**Mixed features of 21-hydroxylase deficiency and 17 α-hydroxylase/17,20-lyase deficiency, sometimes associated with Antley-Bixler craniosynostosis**
HSD17B3	AR	Testis	–	Female or ambiguous	Partial androgenisation at puberty,↑ androstenedione-to-testosterone ratio

Antle Bixler anomaly:

- POR deficiency
- Craniosynostosis
- Radio-ulnar synostosis
- Bowing of femur
- Mid-facial hypoplasia

Ans. B

254. A couple married for 5 years visited infertility clinic with h/o primary infertility. On evaluation the sperm count of male partner was found to be 5 million/ml. As per WHO classification he was diagnosed with severe male infertility. TOC for severe male factor infertility:

A. IUI

B. ICSI

C. Any of the above

D. None of the above

Explanation:

It may require IVF with or without intracytoplasmic sperm injection (ICSI). For men with a severe defect (sperm count of <10 × 10^6/ml, 10% motility), IVF with ICSI or donor sperm should be used. If ICSI is performed because of azoospermia due to congenital bilateral absence of the vas deferens, genetic testing for *CFTR* gene mutations and counseling should be provided because of the risk of cystic fibrosis.

Ans. B

255. A neonate was brought with h/o failure to thrive. On evaluation the child was noticed to have corneal clouding, hepatomegaly, with h/o seizures. Suspected to have mucopolysaccharidosis. All mucopolysaccharidosis are AR except:

A. Hunter's syndrome

B. Hurler's syndrome

C. Morquio disease

D. Scheie's disease

Explanation:

Advantages over HSCT alone

Hunter disease (MPS II) is an X-linked disorder due to deficiency in iduronate sulfate sulfatase and has manifestations similar to those of MPS I, including neurologic degeneration. There is no corneal clouding or other eye disease.

Hunter's syndrome:

- It is MPS type II
- XLR
- No corneal clouding
- Defect=L. iduronate sulphatase
- Increased heparen and dermatan sulphate

Ans. A

256. A 34-year-old woman has new onset hypertension. On evaluation her BP: 170/100 mm Hg. CT-Abdomen was done to r/o secondary hypertension; However it revealed adrenal adenoma. On further evaluation, her plasma aldosterone level was 55 ng/dl and PRA of 0.1 ng/ml/hour. 24-hr urinary cortisol, Serum DHEAS, plasma metanephrines was done and was found to be normal.

Steroid hormones are usually bound to specific transport proteins. Cortisol binding globulin (CBG) binds to:

A. Cortisol only

B. Cortisol and aldosterone

C. Cortisol, aldosterone, testosterone

D. Cortisol, aldosterone, testosterone, progesterone.

Explanation:

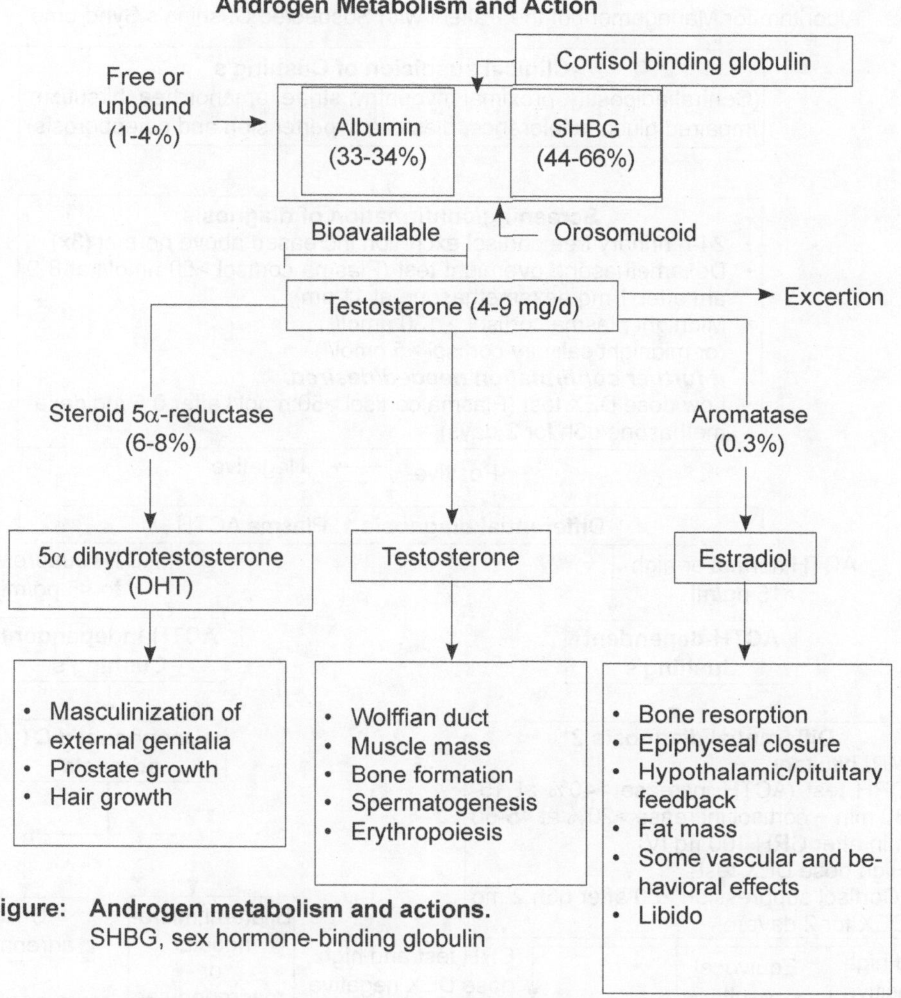

Figure: Androgen metabolism and actions. SHBG, sex hormone-binding globulin

Table: Circulating high-affinity protein carriers of steroid hormones

Protein Carrier	**Primary Ligand(s)**
Corticosteroid-binding globulin (CBG)	**Glucocorticoids, mineralocorticoids**
Sex hormone-binding globulin	Dihydrotestosterone, testosterone, estradiol
Thyroxine-binding globulin (TBG)	Thyroxine (T_4), triiodothyronine (T_3)
Vitamin A-binding protein(s)	Vitamin A (retinol)
Vitamin D-binding protein	25(OH) vitamin D_2, 25(OH) vitamin D_3, l,25(OH) vitamin D_2, 1,25 vitamin D_3

Ans. D

257. A 45-year-old female comes with history of excessive weight gain, increased bruisability, excessive facial hair and acne since 1 yr. Presently comes to casualty with h/o fall in bathroom and sustained vertebral fracture. O/e patient has cushingoid features. Patient denies taking any 'over the counter' medication. To support this, her 8 am serum cortisol was found to be high. Further investigation confirms Cushing syndrome by performing ONDST and 24hr urine cortisol. Plasma ACTH was 25 pg/ml. HDDST and CRH test were positive. Select the correct statement.

A. Get CT chest and abdomen to look for occult primary

B. ACTH receptor on adrenal gland is MC4R

C. POMC has 141AA

D. gp-130 stimulates ACTH secretion

Explanation:

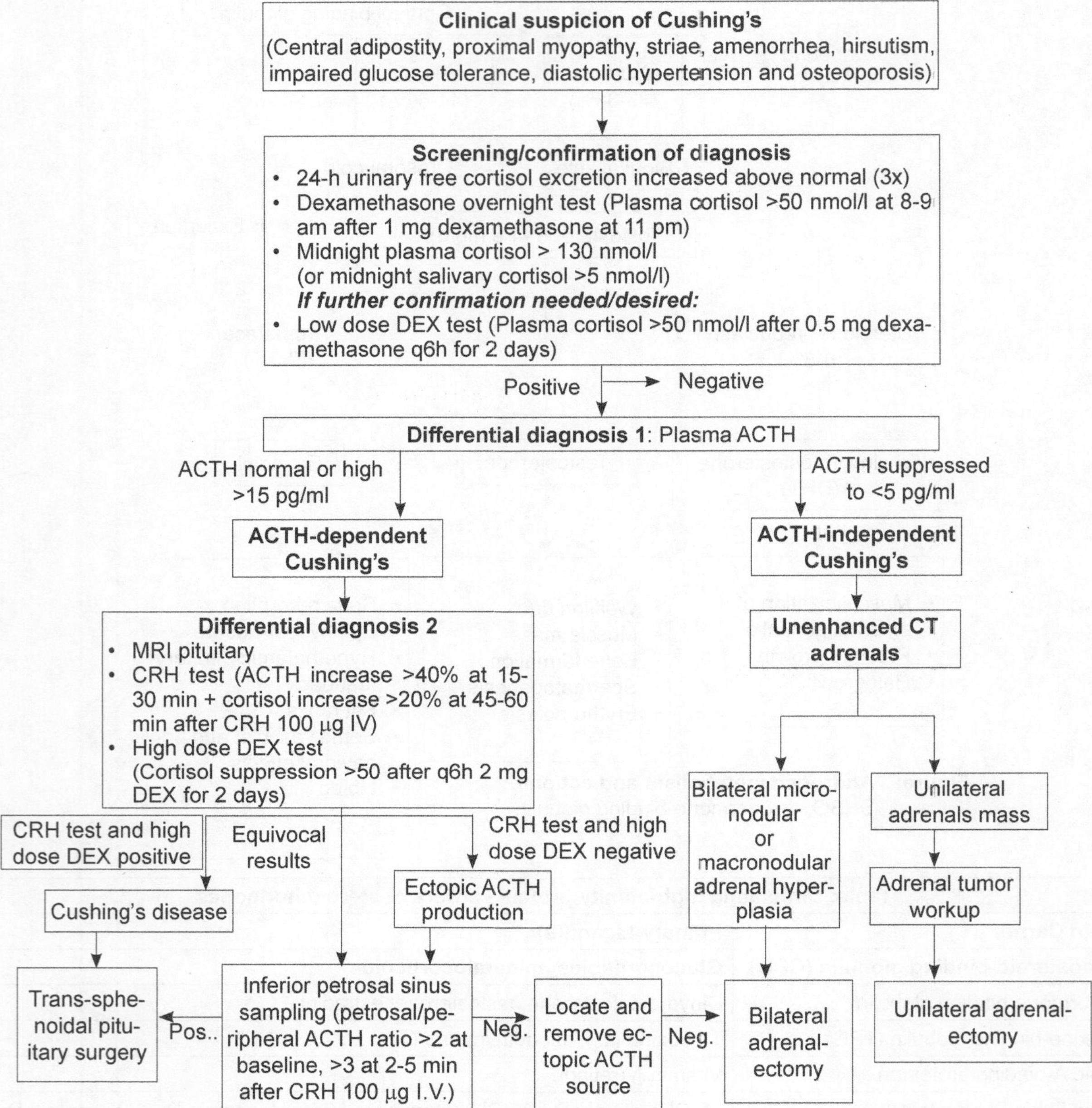

Table: Tissue distribution of melanocortin receptor (MCR) types	
MC Receptor Types	**Tissue**
MCR1	Skin, hair follicles
MCR2	**Adrenal cortex**
MCR3	Hypothalamus, limbic system
MCR4	Hypothalamus, various brain areas,[a] intestines
MCR5	Exocrine glands, skeletal muscle, adrenal cortex
[a]Cortex, thalamus, brainstem and spinal cord	

Next investigation here should be MRI pituitary since HDDST and CRH test is positive.

Table: Anterior pituitary hormone expression and regulation					
Cell	**Corticotrope**	**Somatotrope**	**Lactotrope**	**Thyrotrope**	**Gonadotrope**
Tissue-specific transcription factor	T-Pit	Prop-1, Pit-1	Prop-1, Pit-1	Prop-1, Pit-1, TEF	SF-1, DAX-1
Fetal appearance	6 weeks	8 weeks	12 weeks	12 weeks	12 weeks
Hormone	POMC	GH	PRL	TSH	FSH, LH
Protein	Polypeptide	Polypeptide	Polypeptide	Glycoprotein α, β subunits	Glycoprotein α, β subunits
Amino acids	**266** (ACTH 1-39)	191	198	211	210, 204
Stimulators	CRH, AVP, **gp-130** cytokines	GHRH, ghrelin	Estrogen, TRH, VIP	TRH	GnRH, activins, estrogen
Inhibitors	Glucocorticoids	Somatostatin, IGF-1	Dopamine	T_3, T_4, dopamine, somatostatin, glucocorticoids	Sex steroids, inhibin
Target gland	Adrenal	Liver, bone, other tissues	Breast, other tissues	Thyroid	Ovary, testis
Trophic effect	Steroid production	IGF-I production, growth induction, insulin antagonism	Milk production	T4 synthesis and secretion	Sex steroid production, follicle growth, germ cell maturation
Normal range	ACTH, 4-22 pg/l	<0.5 μg/l[a]	M <15 μg/l; F <20 μg/l	0.1-5 mU/l	M, 5-20 IU/l; F (basal), 5-20 IU/l

[a]Hormone secretion integrated over 24 hours.

Ans. D

258. A 25 year old male presented with h/o headache, vomiting, blurring of vision, and was diagnosed to have pituitary adenoma. On routine evaluation hypercalcemia and hypophosphatemia were noted. PTH was ordered which was 185 pg/ml and confirmed primary hyperparathyroidism. Sestamibi scan suggested left parathyroid adenoma. With above details, possibility of MEN-1 syndrome was considered. What is the incidence of lesion seen in the above picture in MEN-1 syndrome?

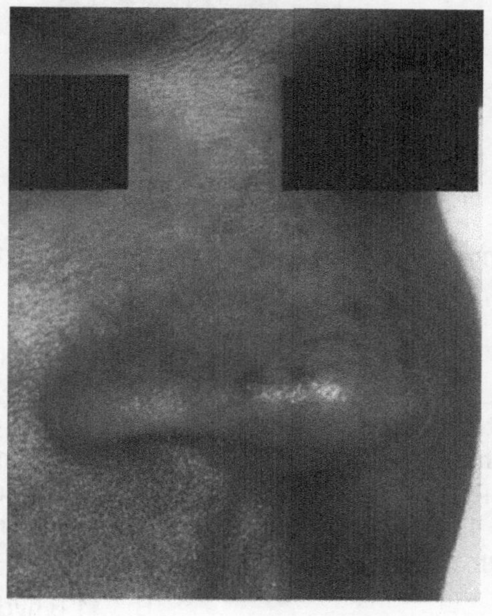

A. 58%
B. 74%
C. 25%
D. 85%

Explanation:

Table: MEN syndromes and their characteristic tumors and associated genetic abnormalities		
Type (Chromosome Location)	**Tumors (Estimated Penetrance)**	**Gene; Most Frequently Mutated Codons**
MEN1 (11q13)	• Parathyroid adenoma (90%) • Enteropancreatic tumor (30-70%) – Gastrinoma (40%) – Insulinoma (10%) – Nonfunctioning (20-55%) – Glucagonoma (<1%) – VIPoma (<1%) • Pituitary adenoma (30-40%) – Prolactinoma (20%) – Somatotropinoma (10%) – Corticotropinoma (<5%) – Nonfunctioning (<5%) • Associated tumors – Adrenal cortical tumor (20-40%) – Pheochromocytoma (<1%) – Bronchopulmonary NET (2%) – Thymic NET (2%) – Gastric NET (10%) – Lipomas (30%) – **Angiofibromas (85%)** – Collagenomas (70%) – Meningiomas (8%)	*MEN1* 83/.84, 4-bp del (≈4%) 119, 3-bp del (≈3%) 209-211, 4-bp del (≈8%) 418, 3-bp del (≈4%) 514-516, del or ins (≈7%) Intron 4 ss (≈10%)

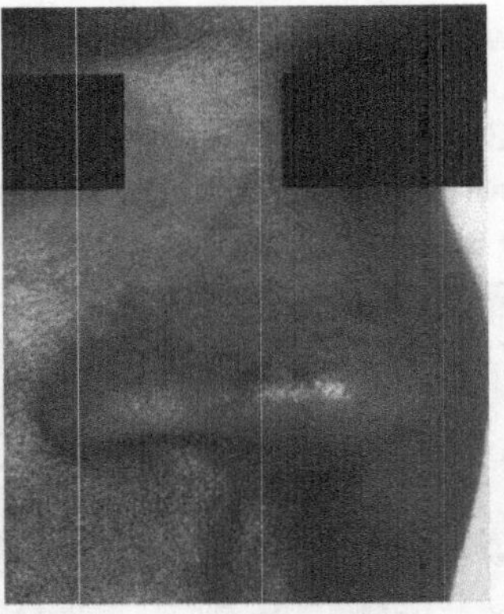

. Fig: Multiple angiofibromas in patient with multiple endocrine neoplasia type 1

Ans. D

259. A 6-year-old boy presented to paediatric endocrinologist with h/o axillary & pubic hair, increase in size of penis and testis. On GPE his BP was 140/100 mm Hg in both hands, rest of the CVS examination was found to be normal. On further evaluation his Bone Age was found to be 12 yrs. Laboratory evaluation revealed elevated levels of 17-OHP, testosterone and pubertal response to GnRH stimulation test. Which of the following enzyme is most likely to be deficient?

A. 21 α hydroxylase

B. 11 β hydroxylase

C. 3 β hydroxysteroid dehydrogenase

D. 17 α hydroxylase

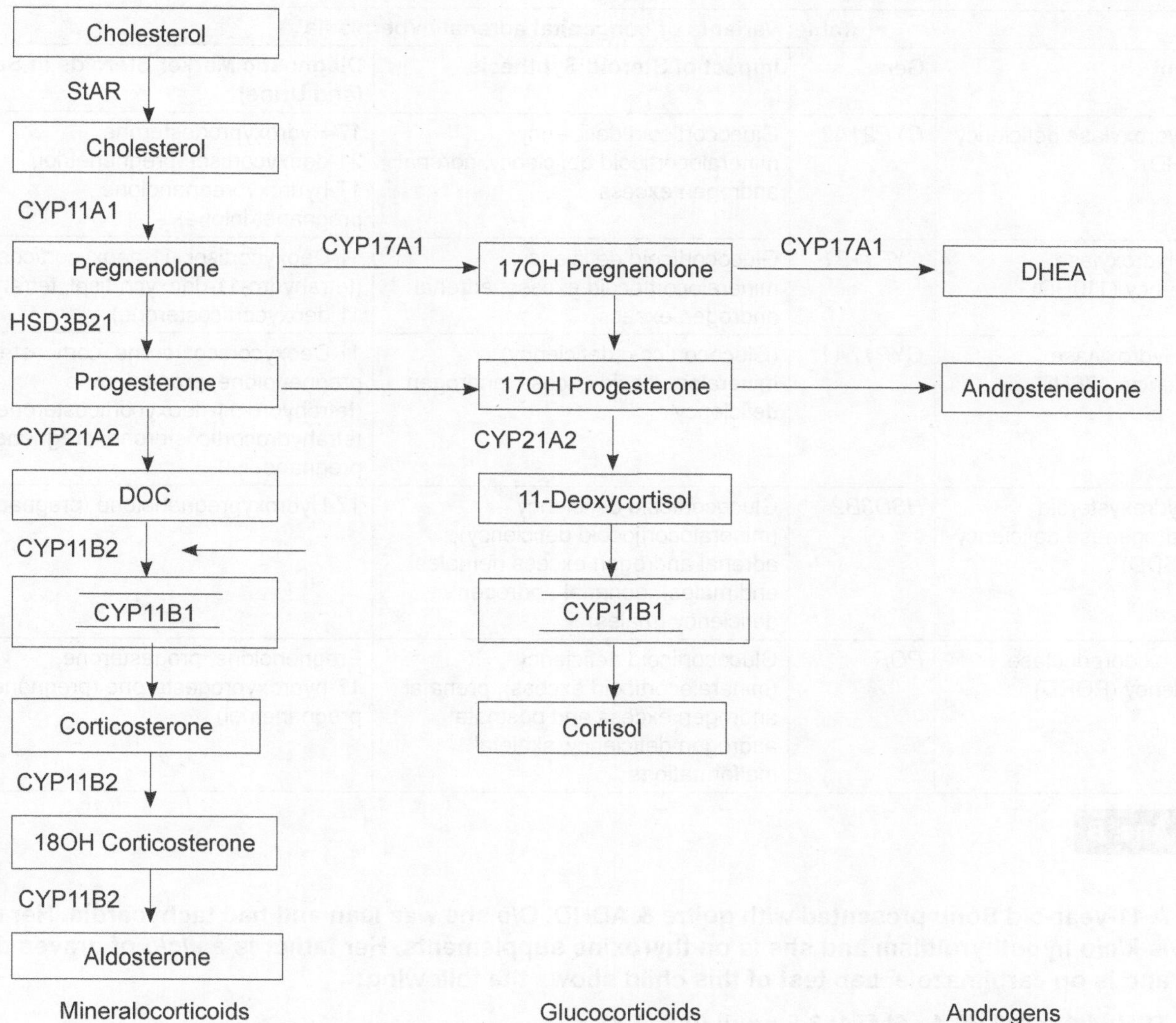

Figure: Congenital adrenal hyperplasia related to 11β-hydroxylase deficiency. The normal synthesis of cortisol is impaired, and adrenocorticotropic hormone (ACTH) levels increase because of the loss of normal negative feedback inhibition, which result in an increase in adrenal steroid precursors proximal to the block. The results are cortisol deficiency, mineralocorticoid excess related to excessive deoxycorticosterone (DOC) secretion, and excessive secretion of adrenal androgens CYP, cytochrome P450; *DHEA*, dehydro-epiandrosterone; HSD, hydroxysteroid dehydrogenase; StAR, steroidogenic acute regulatory protein

Sexual ambiguity); again, milder cases can manifest later in childhood or even young adulthood. The principal difference from 21-hydroxylase deficiency is hypertension, which is thought to be secondary to the mineralocorticoid effect of DOC excess. However, there is a poor correlation between DOC secretion and the presence of hypertension, and unexplained salt wasting has been reported in few patients during early life. On this clinical background, the diagnosis can be made by measuring a plasma synacthen-stimulated 11-deoxycortisol value, which will be greater than 52 nmol/l (>1800 ng/dl) and often much higher. Basal concentrations of 17 OHP are commonly increased but may be normal even during the first weeks of life.

Table: Variants of congenital adrenal hyperplasia			
Variant	**Gene**	**Impact of Steroid Synthesis**	**Diagnostic Marker Steroids in Serum (and Urine)**
21-Hydroxylase deficiency (21OHD)	*CYP21A2*	Glucocorticoid deficiency, mineralocorticoid deficiency, adrenal androgen excess	17-Hydroxyprogesterone, 21-deoxycortisol (pregnanetriol, 17-hydroxypregnanolone, pregnanetriolone)
11β-Hydroxylase deficiency (11OHD)	*CYP11B1*	Glucocorticoid deficiency, mineralocortiocoid excess, adrenal androgen excess	11-Deoxycortisol, 11-deoxycorticosterone (tetrahydro-11-deoxycortisol, tetrahydro-11-deoxycorticosterone)
17α-Hydroxylase deficiency (17OHD)	*CYP17A1*	(Glucocorticoid deficiency), mineralocorticoid excess, androgen deficiency	11-Deoxycorticosterone, corticosterone, pregnenolone, progesterone (tetrahydro-11-deoxycorticosterone, tetrahydrocorticosterone, pregnenediol, pregnanediol)
3β-Hydroxysteroid dehydrogenase deficiency (3bHSDD)	*HSD3B2*	Glucocorticoid deficiency (mineralocortiocoid deficiency), adrenal androgen excess (females and males), gonadal androgen deficiency (males)	17-Hydroxypregnanolone (pregnanetriol)
P450 oxidoreductase deficiency (PORD)	*POR*	Glucocorticoid deficiency (mineralocorticoid excess), prenatal androgen excess and postnatal androgen deficiency, skeletal malformations	Pregnenolone, progesterone, 17-hydroxyprogesterone (pregnanediol, pregnanetriol)

Ans. B

260. A 11-year-old Sonu presented with goitre & ADHD. O/e she was lean and had tachycardia. Her mother is k/c/o hypothyroidism and she is on thyroxine supplements. Her father is a k/c/o of graves disease and is on carbimazole. Lab test of this child shows the following:

TSH: 4.1 mIU/L (0.4 - 5) fT4: 3.8 ng/dl (0.8- 1.8)

Most likely condition the child is suffering from is:

A. Grave's disease
B. Inadvertent intake of LT4 by the child
C. Thyroid hormone resistance syndrome
D. Psychiatric illness

Explanation

- The child presented with complaints suggestive of hyperthyroidism, also her fT4 is elevated. TSH is within normal limits.
- Clue to the diagnosis is not elevated fT4, it is the normal TSH despite elevated fT4.
- In grave's disease and inadvertent intake of LT4 by the child TSH must have been suppressed.
- Therefore appropriate diagnosis here would be thyroid hormone resistance syndrome wherein the TSH remains non suppressed even with elevated T4 levels.
- D/d here would be a pituitary tumor.

Ans. C

261. A 29-year-old Inchara, a primigravida, with single live gestation came for follow up in 2nd trimester. Her Obstertrician orders 50 gm OGTT. One hour plasma sugar after 50 gm OGTT was 198 mg/dl. Considering the above value she was diagnosed to have GDM. Inchara is now concerned about the baby getting diabetes in the future. What will you advise her?

A. Assure her that her child is not at risk for diabetes in the future
B. Convey that her concern is true. Her child is at risk for diabetes in the future
C. If her husband is not diabetic then she need not worry
D. None of the above

Explanation:

Federation (IDF) estimated that one in seven pregnancies worldwide was affected by either GDM or pre-existing DM. Most women with GDM revert to normal glucose tolerance postpartum but have a substantial risk (35-60%) of developing DM in the next 10-20 years. **In addition, children born to a mother with GDM also have an increased risk of developing metabolic syndrome and type 2 DM later in life.** Currently, the ADA recommends that women with a history of GDM undergo lifelong screening for the development of diabetes or prediabetes at least every 3 years.

Ans. B

262. A 22-year-old lady presented to emergency with features of tetany and on evaluation she was found to have severe hypocalcemia (6.1 mg/dl) and hyperphosphatemia (7.5 mg/dl). Hypoparathyroidism was suspected. PTH levels were ordered which was found to be inappropriately low for the aforesaid serum calcium levels. Diagnosis of primary hypoparathyroidism was made. Which of the following is used in treatment of hypoparathyroidism?

A. Calcium
B. Calcitriol
C. Teriparatide
D. All of the above

Explanation:

- Hypoparathyroididm is one of the very few conditions in endocrinology wherein the patients are not replaced with the missing hormones but they are given calcium and calcitriol.
- However recently rPTH have been approved for the treatment.
- **Hypoparathyroidism is rare among endocrine disorder is not being treated with the missing hormone. Recent developments have changed that. Experimental use of PTH (1-34), the synthetic fragment used in treatment of osteoporosis showed promise. Subsequently, the full length molecule PTH (1-84) has been shown to be effective and is now FDA-approved for therapy of hypoparathyroidism.**

Ans. D

263. All are true about gonadotropin deficiency except:

A. Hypogonadism is the most common presenting feature of adult hypopituitarism even when other pituitary hormones are also deficient
B. Hypogonadotropic hypogonadism is a common presenting feature of hyperprolactinemia
C. Acquired forms of GnRH deficiency leading to hypogonadotropism are seen in association with anorexia nervosa, stress, starvation
D. GnRH testing adds little to the information gained from baseline evaluation of the hypothalamic-pituitary-gonadotrope axis in Kallmann syndrome

Explanation:

- Hypogonadism is the most common presenting feature of adult hypopituitarism even when other pituitary hormones are also deficient.
- It is often a harbinger of hypothalamic or pituitary lesions that impair GnRH production or delivery through the pituitary stalk.

- ***Hypogonadotropic hypogonadism is a common presenting feature of hyperprolactinemia.***
- Mutations in *GPR54, DAX1,* kisspeptin, the GnRH receptor, and the LHβ or FSHβ subunit genes also cause pituitary gonadotropin deficiency.
- Acquired forms of GnRH deficiency leading to hypogonadotropism are seen in association with anorexia nervosa, stress, starvation, and extreme exercise but also may be idiopathic.
- Hypogonadotropic hypogonadism in these disorders is reversed by removal of the stressful stimulus or by caloric replenishment.
- In premenopausal women, hypogonadotropic hypogonadism presents as diminished ovarian function leading to oligomenorrhea or amenorrhea, infertility, decreased vaginal secretions, decreased libido, and breast atrophy. In hypogonadal adult men, secondary testicular failure is associated with decreased libido and potency, infertility, decreased muscle mass with weakness, reduced beard and body hair growth, soft testes, and characteristic fine facial wrinkles. Osteoporosis occurs in both untreated hypogonadal women and men.
- GnRH testing usually adds little to the information gained from baseline evaluation of the hypothalamic-pituitary-gonadotrope axis except in cases of isolated GnRH deficiency (e.g., Kallmann syndrome).
- MRI examination of the sellar region and assessment of other pituitary functions usually are indicated in patients with documented central hypogonadism.

Ans. D

264. An infant presented with features of multiple episodes of diarrhea, and failure to thrive. One examination hepatosplenomegaly was observed. On routine abdominal ultrasound examination calcification of adrenal glands was noted. Possibility of Wolman disease was considered. All about Wolman's disease are true except:

A. Defective acid lipase
B. Cholesterol ester storage disorder
C. Lysosomal storage disorder
D. Sphingolipidosis

Explanation:

Wolman disease:

- Defective acid lipase: There will be elevated triacylglycerol and cholesterol esters in histiocytic foam cells.
- Cholesterol ester storage disorder
- Calcification of adrenal glands will be seen
- Lysosomal storage disorder
- It is not Sphingolipidosis.
- C/f: Watery diarrhea, failure to thrive, vomiting, HSM.
- Pathological examination shows TG and cholesterol accumuation in liver, spleen, intestinal lining, bone marrow and vasculature, as well as severe adrenal calcification

https://www.sciencedirect.com/topics/medicine-and-dentistry/wolman-disease

Lysosomal Acid Lipase Deficiency

- Wolman syndrome (now infantile-onset LALD) and cholesterol esterstorage disease (now childhood/adult-onset LALD) are caused by deficiency of lysosomal acid lipase due to autosomal recessive mutations in the *LIPA*. The enzyme is responsible for hydrolysis of cholesterol esters and triglycerides delivered to the lysosome via the LDLR pathway. Accumulation of these in the tissues leads to progressive organ dysfunction including liver disease, intestinal malabsorption, heart dysfunction, and other manifestations. The most severe form presents in early infancy with failure to thrive, vomiting, and hepatosplenomegaly. The infantile-onset LALD patients die without specific treatment by age 1 year (median age of death 3.7 months). Childhood/adult-onset LALD can have a variable age of initial presentation with nonspecific signs, but often involves elevated liver enzymes, non-alcoholic fatty liver disease, cryptogenic cirrhosis, and varying severities of hepatosplenomegaly. Disease progresses throughout life and may result in early (adolescence) liver cirrhosis and (early adulthood) atherosclerosis or early without treatment. Importantly, statins can decrease the hypercholesterolemia, but do not alter the basic progressive tissue (e.g., liver) pathology. Enzyme replacement therapy for LALD has major effects in reversing disease manifestations and was approved for patients at all ages by EMA, FDA and several other country agencies in 2015 and 2016.

Ans. D

265. Maximum number of oocytes seen in a female child during:

A. Puberty
B. 20 week of gestation
C. 16 week of gestation
D. At birth

Explanation:

Superimposed on oogonial mitosis. As a result of the combined impact of these processes, the number of germ cells peaks at 6 to 7 × 10^6 by 20 weeks of gestation. At this time, two-thirds of the total germ cells are intrameiotic primary oocytes; the remaining third can still be viewed as oogonial.

- **The primordial germ cells** are identified by 3rd week of gestation and they migrate towards the primitive gonad by 6 weeks of gestation.
- Oogonia enter prophase of first meiotic division during the intrauterine period to form primary oocytes.
- The oogonia number reaches a maximum of 7 million at 20 weeks of gestation.
- *At birth: 1 million germ cells are present.*
- This progressive loss of oocyte is due to oocyte atresia.
- Only 400 oocytes enter into ovulation during the entire reproductive life of female.

Ans. B

266. A 50-year-old male was diagnosed with chronic hypertension on multiple antihypertensives. On evaluation for resistant hypertension CT abdomen was ordered which reveals a large adrenal mass ~4.5 cm with density of 25HU and intense IV contrast enhancement indicative of pheochromocytoma. 24-hr urine metanephrines levels confirmed the diagnosis of pheochromocytoma. Triad of pheochromocytoma is all except:

A. Headache
B. Tachycardia
C. Sweating
D. Syncope

Explanation:

Clinical Features

Its clinical presentation is so variable that pheochromocytoma has been termed "the great masquerader" **Among the presenting manifestations, episodes of palpitation, headache, and profuse seating are typical, and these manifestations constitute a classic triad. The presence of all three manifestations in association with hypertension makes pheochromocytoma a likely diagnosis. However, a pheochromocytoma can be asymptomatic for years, and some tumors grow to a to a considerable size, before patients note symptoms.**

- Paroxysm lasts for 15-20 mins.
- Triad present only in 30% of patients.
- Specificity of this triad is around 90%.
- Paroxysms are precipitated by drugs like metaclopromide, phenothiazines, methyldopa, TCA, glucocorticoids, postural changes, anxiety and exercise.

Ans. D

267. 25 year old male with family history of multiple tumors presented to OPD with above lesion. The above lesion is seen in:

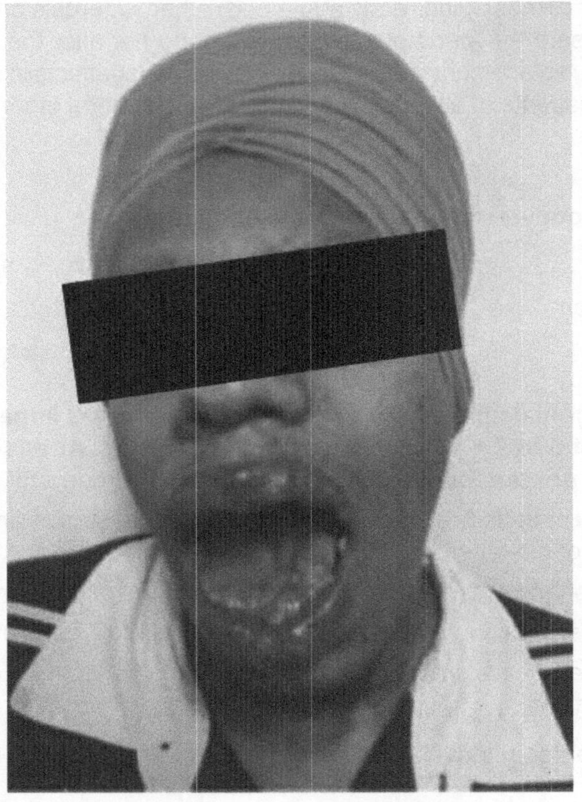

A. NF1
B. MEN2A
C. MEN2B
D. VHL

Explanation:

MEN2A (10 cen-10q11.2)	MTC (90%) Pheochromocytoma (50%) Parathyroid adenoma (20-30%)	*RET* 634, missense (e.g., Cys→Arg)
MEN3, also known as MEN2B (10 cen-10q11.2)	MTC (>90%) Pheochromocytoma (40-50%) Associated abnormalities (40-50%) Mucosal neuromas Marfanoid habitus Medullated corneal nerve fibers Megacolon	*RET* 918, Met→Thr

Ans. C

268. 8 year child presented with history of progressive bowing of bilateral lower limbs. On evaluation diagnosed to have rickets. However nutritional rickets was ruled out. Possibility of genetic forms of rickets was considered. True regarding Vit-D dependent type 1 rickets:

A. AD
B. Pseudo Vit-D deficiency rickets
C. Mutation of Vit-D receptor
D. Improves only with high doses of cholecalciferol.

Explanation:

Vitamin-D Dependent Type 1 Rickets

- AR Inheritance.
- VDDR1
- Also known as pseudo Vit-D deficiency rickets.
- Mutation in gene encoding 1 alpha hydroxylase causes this disease.
- Doesn't respond to cholecalciferol.
- Responds to calcitriol, hence the name pseudo Vit-D deficiency rickets.

Renal tubular disorders, or excess or ectopic production of FGF23, known to inhibit 1α-hydroxylase enzyme activity. **Genetic defect in the 25-hydroxyvitamin D 1α-hydroxylase enzyme, VDDR1A, or pseudo-vitamin D deficiency, is a rare autosomal recessive disorder due to mutations in the cytochrome P450 (*CYP27B1*) gene for the 1α -hydroxylase enzyme located on the chromosome 12q13.3, resulting in decreased serum levels of 1,25-dihydroxyvitamin D.**

Table: Relevant abnormalities in various type of vitamin D-related rickets and osteomalacia

Variable	Vitamin D Deficiency	Vitamin D Dependency Type 1B	Vitamin D Dependency Type 1A	Vitamin D Dependency Type 2	Hypophosphatemic Vitamin D Resistant[a]
Basic defect	Nutritional/ malabsorption	25-Hydroxylase defect	1α-Hydroxylase defect	VDR defect	Excess FGF 23
Gene locus	Not applicable	Chromosome 11p15.2	Chromosome 12q13.1	Chromosome 12q12-q14	Xp22.11
Enzyme defect	Not applicable	CYP2R1	CYP27B1	Receptor defect	*PHEX* gene defect
Serum calcium	Low/normal	Low	Low	Low	Normal/high
Serum phosphate	Normal/low	Normal/low	Normal/low	Normal/low	Very low
Alkaline phosphatase	High	High	High	High	High
Parathyroid hormone	High	High	High	High	Normal/high
25-Hydroxyvitamin D	Low	Low/very low	Normal	Normal	Normal
1,25-Dihydroxy vitamin D	Variable	Low/low normal	Low	High	Low
Urine calcium	Low	Low	Low	Low	Normal/high
Vitamin D dose required to heal/ cure rickets[b]	1000-2000 IU daily Few weeks to months	10,000 IU daily Lifelong	10,000 IU daily Lifelong	100,000 units daily Lifelong	100,000 units daily Lifelong
Calcitriol dose required to heal/ cure rickets	0.04 μg/kg per day Few weeks to months	0.04 μg/kg per day Lifelong	0.04 μg/kg per day Lifelong	1-2 μg/day Lifelong	1-2 μg/day and oral phosphate Lifelong

Ans. B

269. 75 year old female on routine DEXA imaging found to have osteoporosis. Drugs effective against both vertebral and non vertebral fracture is:

A. Calcitonin
B. Ibandronate
C. Raloxifene
D. Abaloparatide

Explanation:

- **Raloxifene reduces the occurrence of vertebral fracture by 30-50%, depending on the population; however, there are no data confirming that raloxifene can reduce the risk of nonvertebral fractures >8 years of observation.**
- **Ibandronate is the third amino-bisphosphonate approved in the United States. Ibandronate (2.5 mg/d) has been shown in clinical trials to reduce vertebral fracture risk by ~40% but with no overall effect on non-vertebral fractures. In a post hoc analysis of subjects with a femoral neck T-score of <-3, ibandronate reduced the risk of nonvertebral fracture by ~60%. In clinical trials, ibandronate doses**
- **Use limited. A nasal spray containing calcitonin (200 IU/d) is available for treatment of osteoporosis in postmenopausal women. One study suggests that nasal calcitonin produces small increments in bone mass and a small reduction in new vertebral fractures in calcitonin-treated patients (at one dose) versus those on calcium alone. There has been no proven effectiveness against nonvertebral fractures. Calcitonin is not indicated for prevention of osteoporosis and is not sufficiently potent to prevent bone loss in early post**
- **Teriparatide); in the total hip, BMP increments were slightly larger with abaloparatide (4.2% vs 3.3%). New vertebral fracture incidence was reduced by 86% with abaloparatide and 80% with teriparatide compared with placebo (both p<0.001). Nonvertebral fractures were reduced by 43% with abaloparatide (p=0.05) and 28% with TPTD (NS, p=0.22). The ACTIVE study is in an ongoing extension where**

Ans. D

270. 48 year old with history of multiple drug intake history even for minor aliments. He was diagnosed to have osteoporotic fracture. Which one of the following is a definitive risk factor for osteoporosis?

A. H2 blocker
B. Meglitinides
C. Lithium
D. Clozapine

Explanation:

Table: Drugs associated with an increased risk of generalized osteoporosis in adults	
Glucocorticoids Cyclosporine Cytotoxic drugs Anticonvulsants Aromatase inhibitors SSRIs	Excessive thyroxine Aluminum Gonadotropin-releasing hormone agonists Heparin Lithium Protein Pump Inhibitors Thiazolidinediones Androgen Deprivation Therapies

Ans. C

271. Treatment or trial may be indicated for subclinical hypothyroidism in all the below conditions except:

A. Pregnant lady
B. Positive TPO antibodies
C. Evidence of heart disease
D. Evicence of kidney disease

Explanation:

- By definition, subclinical hypothyroidism refers to biochemical evidence of thyroid hormone deficiency in patients who have few or no apparent clinical features of hypothyroidism.
- There are no universally accepted recommendations for management of subclinical hypothyroidism, but levothyroxine is recommended if patient is woman who wishes to conceive or is pregnant, or when TSH levels are >10 mIU/L.
- Otherwise, when TSH levels are below 10 mIU/L, a trial of treatment may be considered when patients have suggestive symptoms of hypothyroidism, positive TPO antibodies, or any evidence of heart disease.
- It is important to confirm that any elevation of TSH is sustained over a 3-month period before treatment is given.
- Treatment is administered by starting with a low dose of levothyroxine (25–50 μg/d) with the goal of normalizing TSH.
- If levothyroxine is not given, thyroid function should be evaluated annually.

Ans. D

272. 70 year old male presented to endocrinology to get routinely checked. DEXA was ordered which showed osteopenia. Indication for vertebral imaging are:

A. All women aged 60 and all men aged 70 if BMD T-score at the spine, total hip, or femoral neck is <1.0

B. Women aged from 65 to 69 and men aged from 70 to 79 if BMD Tscore at the spine, total hip, or femoral neck is <1.5

C. Both A + B

D. None of the above

Explanation:

Table: Indications for vertebral testing
Consider vertebral imaging tests for the following individuals[a] • All women aged ≥70 and all men aged ≥80 if BMD T-score at the spine, total hip, or femoral neck is <1.0 • Women aged from 65 to 69 and men aged from 70 to 79 if BMD T-score at the spine, total hip, or femoral neck is <1.5 • Postmenopausal women and men aged ≥50 with specific risk factors: – Low-trauma fracture during adulthood (aged ≥50) – Historical height loss of ≥1.5 in. (4 cm)[b] – Prospective height loss of >0.8 in. (2 cm)[c] – Recent or ongoing long-term glucocorticoid treatment
[a] If bone density testing is not available, vertebral imaging may be considered based on age alone. [b] Current height compared to peak height during childhood. [c] Cumulative height loss measured during interval medical assessment.

Ans. B

273. Patients most likely to relapse in Graves' disease when treatment stops include all except:

A. Males

B. Smokers

C. Large goiter

D. Older patients

Explanation:

- Maximum remission rates (up to 30–60% in some populations) are achieved by 12–18 months for the titration regimen and are higher in patients where TRAb levels are no longer detected, than in those with TRAb persistence.

- For unclear reasons, remission rates appear to vary in different geographic regions.
- Younger patients, males, smokers, and patients with a history of allergy, severe hyperthyroidism or large goiters are most likely to relapse when treatment stops, but outcomes are difficult to predict.
- All patients should be followed closely for relapse during the first year after treatment and at least annually thereafter.

Ans. D

274. 21 year old male presented with history of delayed onset of puberty with absent secondary sexual characteristics. On evaluation eunuchoid proportions. LS>US. With small firm testis was noted. With above clinical features Klinefelter's syndrome was considered.

Prevalence of Klinefelter's Syndrome is:

A. 0.2% men B. 0.3% men
C. 0.4% men D. 0.5% men

Explanation:

Disorder	Approx. prevalence in adults	Screening/testing recommendations
Klinefelter's syndrome	0.2%, men	Karyotype Testosterone
Vitamin D deficiency	10%	Measure serum 25-OH vitamin D Consider secondary causes
Turner's syndrome	0.03%, women	Karyotype Consider comorbid conditions

Ans. A

275. All are true about steroid synthesis except:

A. Mineralocorticoid synthesis occurring in the outer zona glomerulosa
B. 17α-hydroxylase enzyme is located in the mitochondrion
C. StAR protein shuttles cholesterol from the outer to the inner mitochondrial membrane
D. Adrenal androgen synthesis occurs in the inner zona reticularis

Explanation:

- Majority of steroidogenic enzymes are cytochrome P450 (CYP) enzymes, which are either located in the mitochondrion (side chain cleavage enzyme, CYP11A1; 11β-hydroxylase, CYP11B1; aldosterone synthase, CYP11B2) or in endoplasmic reticulum membrane (17α-hydroxylase, CYP17A1; 21-hydroxylase, CYP21A2; aromatase, CYP19A1).
- These enzymes require electron donation via specific redox cofactor enzymes, P450 oxidoreductase (POR), and adrenodoxin/adrenodoxin reductase (ADX/ADR) for the microsomal and mitochondrial CYP enzymes, respectively.
- In addition, short-chain dehydrogenase 3β-hydroxysteroid dehydrogenase type 2 (3β-HSD2), also termed Δ4, Δ5 isomerase, plays a major role in adrenal steroidogenesis.

Ans. B

276. Mr. Bob presents to you with uncontrolled diabetes. His BMI is 37 kg/m². He is also having OSA and hypertension. He is requesting for fitness for bariatric surgery and his surgeon wants documentation from an Endocrinologist. He is ready to pay you any amount you ask to let him undergo the surgery. Your answer is:

A. Give clearance to undergo surgery

B. Deny surgery as it is against guidelines

C. Ask him to wait till his BMI increases to 40 kg/m2 and then give clearance.

D. Refer him to senior Endocrinologist.

Explanation:

- The patient is a candidate for bariatric surgery as he has comorbidities along with obesity.
- The guidelines say that you need to do surgery only if BMI is more than 40 kg/m2.
- But relaxation is given for patients with BMI with 35 - 40 kg/m2 and if they have comorbidities, you can opt for surgery.
- Bariatric surgery is highly effective in curing diabetes & almost 50% of patients do not need drugs for initial 5 years after surgery.

Table: A guide to opting for treatment for obesity

Treatment	BMI Category (kg/m²)				
	25-26.9	27-29.9	30-34.9	35-39.9	≥ 40
Diet, exercise, behavioral therapy	With comorbidities	With comorbidities	+	+	+
Pharmacotherapy	–	With comorbidities	+	+	+
Surgery	–	–	–	With comorbidities	+

Source: From the National Heart, Lung and Blood Institute, North American Association for the Study of Obesity (2000).

Ans. A

277. 14 year old male child with generalized obesity with features suggestive of hypogonadism. Obesity hypogonadism syndrome was considered. All of these syndromes are associated with mental retardation except:

A. Prader-willi syndrome

B. Lawrence-Moon-Bidet syndrome

C. Carpenter syndrome

D. Alström syndrome

Explanation:

Table: A comparison of syndromes of obesity—Hypogonadism and mental retardation

Feature	Syndrome				
	Prader-Willi	Laurence-Moon-Biedl	Ahlstrom's	Cohen's	Carpenter's
Inheritance	Sporadic; two-thirds have defect	Autosomal recessive	Autosomal recessive	Probably autosomal recessive	Autosomal recessive
Stature	Short	Normal; infrequently short	Normal; infrequently short	Short or tall	Normal
Obesity	Generalized Moderate to severe Onset 1-3 years	Generalized Early onset, 1-2 years	Truncal Early onset, 2-5 years	Truncal Mid-childhood, age 5	Truncal, gluteal

Contd.

Contd.

Craniofacies	Narrow bifrontal diameter Almond-shaped eyes Strabismus V-shaped mouth High-arched palate	Not distinctive	Not distinctive	High nasal bridge Arched palate Open mouth Short philtrum	Acrocephaly Flat nasal bridge High-arched palate
Limbs	Small hands and feet Hypotonia	Polydactyly	No abnormalities	Hypotonia Narrow hands and feet	Polydactyly Syndactyly Genu valgum
Reproductive status	1° Hypogonadism	1° Hypogonadism	Hypogonadism in males but not in females	Normal gonadal function or hy-pogonadotropic hypogonadism	2° Hypogonadism
Other features	Enamel hypoplasia Hyperphagia Temper tantrums Nasal speech			Dysplastic ears Delayed puberty	
Mental retardation	Mild to moderate		**Normal intelligence**	Mild	Slight

Ans. D

278. 4 day old newborn was diagnosed to have type 1 DM. Neonate also had history suggestive of enteropathy. A diagnosis of IPEX syndrome was made. IPEX syndrome is due to mutation of:

A. FOXP3
B. FOXD3
C. FOXL2
D. FOXZ3

Explanation:

The only life-saving form of the therapy and can be fully curative by normalizing the imbalanced immune system found in the this disorder.

- **IPEX is caused by mutations in the *FOXP3* gene, which is also mutated in the Scurfy mouse**, an animal model that shares much of phenotype of IPEX patients. The FOXP3 transcription factor is expressed in regulatory T cells designated CD4+CD25+FOXP3+ (Treg).

Table: Rare polyendocrine disorders

Disorder	Clinical Features	Causes
Hirata disease (insulin resistance syndrome)	Hypoglycemia	Insulin autoantibodies Associated with methimazole
IPEX or **CD25 deficiecny**	**Type 1 diabetes** **Enteropathy**	**Mutations of FOXP3 for IPEX** **Mutations of IL2RA for CD25-deficiency**
Autoimmune lymphoproliferative syndrome type V	Autoimmune thyroiditis Autoimmune cytopenias Hypogammaglobulinemia	Mutations of CTLA4 resulting in haploinsufficiency
Infantile-onset autoimmune disease 1	Autoimmune cytopenias Autoimmune thyroiditis Type 1 diabetes Short stature	Dominant activating mutations of STAT3 in heterozygosity

Contd.

Contd.

Kearns-Sayre syndrome	Hypoparathyroidism Primary gonadal failure Nonautoimmune diabetes Hypopituitarism	Deletions of mitochondrial DNA
POEMS	Polyneuropathy Organomegaly Diabetes Primary gonadal failure	Plasma cell dyscrasia with production of M protein and cytokines
Thymic tumors	Myasthenia gravis Red blood cell hypoglobulinemia Autoimmune thyroid disease Adrenal insufficiency	Thymomas
Type B insulin resistance	Severe insulin resistance	Insulin receptor autoantibodies
Wolfram syndrome	Diabetes insipidus Nonautoimmune diabetes Bilateral optic atrophy Sensorinerual deafness	Mutations of WSF1, which encodes wolframin

Ans. A

279. 50 year old male presented with jaw tumor. On evaluation found to have hypercalcemia and hypophosphatemia. s/o parathyroid adenoma. Mutation causing hyperparathyroidism jaw tumor syndrome:

A. CDC 73 gene
B. HRPT2 gene
C. Both
D. None

Explanation:

HPT- JT Syndrome

- CDC 73 / HRPT2 GENE
- A/W
- Benign jaw tumors
- Parathyroid adenoma and carcinoma (15%)

Hyperparathyroidism–Jaw Tumor Syndrome
Clinical Manifestations: Hyperparathyroidism-jaw tumor (HPT-JT) syndrome is an autosomal dominant disorder characterised by the development of parathyroid tumors **(15% are carcinomas) and fibro-osseous jaw tumors. In addition, some patients may also develop Wilms' tumors, renal cysts, renal hamartomas, renal cortical adenomas, papillary RCCs, pancreatic adenocarcinomas, uterine tumors, testicular mixed germ cell tumors with a major seminoma component, and Hurthle cell thyroid adenomas.** The parathyroid tumors may occur in isolation and without any evidence of jaw tumors, and this may cause confusion with other hereditary hypercalcemic disorders, such as MEN 1. However, genetic testing to identify the causative mutation will help to establish the correct diagnosis. The investigation and treatment for HPT-JT–associated tumors are similar to those in non-HPT-JT patients, except that early parathyroidectomy is advisable because of the increased frequency of parathyroid carcinoma.
Genetic and Screening: The gene that causes HPT-JT is located on **Chromosome 1q31.2 and encodes a 531-amino acid protein, parafibromin (Table 381-2). Parafibromin is also referred to as cell division cycle protein 73 (CDC73)** and has a role in transcription. Genetic testing in families helps to identify mutation carriers who should be periodically screened for the development of tumors (Table 381-5).

Table: HPT-JT screening guidelines		
Tumor[a]	Test	Frequency[b]
Parathyroid	Serum Ca, PTH	6-12 months
Ossifying jaw fibroma	Panoramic jaw X-ray with neck shielding[c]	5 years
Renal	Abdominal MRI[c,d]	5 years
Uterine	Ultrasound (transvaginal or transabdominal) and additional imaging ± D&C if indicated[e]	Annual

[a] Screening for most common HPT-JT-associated tumors is considered. Assessment for other reported tumor types may be indicated (e.g., pancreatic, thyroid, testicular tumors).
[b] Frequency of repeating test after baseline tests performed.
[c] X-rays and imaging involving ionizing radiation should ideally be avoided to minimize risk of generating subsequent mutations.
[d] Ultrasound scan recommended if MRI unavailable.
[e] Such selective pelvic imaging should be considered after obtaining a detailed menstrual history.

Ans. C

280. Against which of the following autoantibodies of Type 1 DM are not produced?

A. Proinsulin
B. Zinc transporter
C. Glutamic acid decarboxylase
D. Preproinsulin

Explanation:

- Pancreatic islet molecules targeted by the autoimmune process include proinsulin, insulin, glutamic acid decarboxylase (GAD; biosynthetic enzyme for the neurotransmitter GABA), ICA-512/IA-2 (homology with tyrosine phosphatases), and a beta cell–specific zinc transporter (ZnT-8). Most of the autoantigens are not beta cell–specific, which raises question of how the beta cells are selectively destroyed.
- Current theories favor initiation of an autoimmune process directed at one beta cell molecule, which then spreads to other islet molecules as the immune process destroys beta cells and creates a series of secondary autoantigens.
- Stress pathways and processes arising within the beta cell may exacerbate autoimmunity through the development of modified proteins or "neoantigens" that serve as additional immune targets.

Ans. D

281. All are elevated in the type 2 DM except:

A. Adiponectin
B. IL-6
C. C-Reactive protein
D. Non esterified free fatty acids

Explanation:

- Obesity accompanying type 2 DM, particularly in a central or visceral location, is thought to be part of the pathogenic process.
- In addition to these white fat depots, humans now are recognized to have brown fat, which has much greater thermogenic capacity.
- Efforts are under way to increase the activity or quantity of brown fat.
- Increased adipocyte mass leads to increased levels of circulating free fatty acids and other fat cell products.
- For example, adipocytes secrete a number of biologic products (nonesterified free fatty acids, retinol-binding protein 4, leptin, TNF-α, resistin, IL-6, and adiponectin). In addition to regulating body weight, appetite, and energy expenditure, adipokines also modulate insulin sensitivity.

- Increased production of free fatty acids and some adipokines may cause insulin resistance in skeletal muscle and liver.
- Venous drainage of the visceral adipose beds is the portal circulation and this likely contributes to hepatic dysfunction.
- Free fatty acids also impair glucose utilization in skeletal muscle, promote glucose production by the liver, and impair beta cell function. In contrast, the production by adipocytes of adiponectin, an insulin-sensitizing peptide, is reduced in obesity, and this may contribute to hepatic insulin resistance.
- Adipocyte products and adipokines also produce an inflammatory state and may explain why markers of inflammation such as IL-6 and C-reactive protein are often elevated in type 2 DM. In addition, inflammatory cells have been found infiltrating adipose tissue.

Ans. A

282. All are the reason for the beta cell dysfunction in type 2 DM except:

A. Glucose toxicity
B. Amylin secretion
C. Lipotoxicity
D. Reduced GLP 1 secretion

Explanation:

- Reason(s) for decline in insulin secretory capacity in type 2 DM is unclear.
- Assumption is that a second genetic defect—superimposed upon insulin resistance—leads to defects in beta cell function, mass, and potentially cellular identity and differentiation status.
- Beta cell mass is decreased by ~50% in individuals with long-standing type 2 DM. Islet amyloid polypeptide or amylin, co-secreted by the beta cell, forms amyloid fibrillar deposits found in the islets of individuals with long-standing type 2 DM.
- Whether such islet amyloid deposits are a primary or secondary event is not known.
- Metabolic environment of diabetes also negatively impacts islet function. For example, chronic hyperglycemia paradoxically impairs islet function ("glucose toxicity") and leads to a worsening of hyperglycemia.
- Improvement in glycemic control is often associated with improved islet function.
- In addition, elevated levels of free fatty acids ("lipotoxicity"), and systemic and local elevations in pro-inflammatory cytokines from increased numbers of islet-associated macrophages, may also worsen islet function.
- Reduced GLP-1 action may contribute to the reduced insulin secretion. Only action is impaired , not the secretion.

Ans. D

283. Which of the following substances insulin secretion is not impaired at the onset of Type 2 DM?

A. Glucose
B. Arginine
C. Glycine
D. GLP 1

Explanation:

- Insulin secretion and sensitivity are interrelated.
- In type 2 DM, insulin secretion initially increases in response to insulin resistance to maintain normal glucose tolerance.
- Initially, insulin secretory defect is mild and selectively involves glucose-stimulated insulin secretion, including a greatly reduced first secretory phase.

- Response to other non glucose secretagogues, such as arginine and leucine is preserved, but overall beta cell function is reduced by as much as 50% at the onset of type 2 DM.
- Abnormalities in proinsulin processing are reflected by increased secretion of proinsulin in type 2 DM. Eventually, the insulin secretory defect is progressive.

Ans. B

284. Assertion(A): Starvation may cause hypoglycemia.
Reason(R): There is increased usage of lactate and pyruvates in Starvation.

A. Both (A) and (R) are correct and (R) explains (A)
B. Both (A) and (R) are correct but (R) doesn't explain (A)
C. (R) is correct But (A) is false
D. (A) is correct But (R) is false

Explanation:

- Hypoglycemia can be seen with starvation.
- Due to brain conversion and utilization of alternative substrates, such as lactate, pyruvate, and ketone bodies, there is only a modest counter regulatory neuroendocrine and autonomic nervous system response.
- During periods of prolonged starvation (fasting) plasma glucose levels are lower in women as compared to men; perhaps because of loss of whole-body fat stores and subsequent depletion of gluconeogenic precursors (e.g., amino acids), necessitating increased glucose utilization.

Ans. A

285. Most common cause of cushingoid features is:

A. Iatrogenic hypercortisolism
B. Cushing's disease
C. Cortisol-producing adrenal adenomas
D. Adrenal hyperplasia

Explanation:

- Pituitary corticotrope adenomas (Cushing's disease) account for 70% of patients with endogenous causes of Cushing's syndrome.
- However, it should be emphasized that iatrogenic hypercortisolism is the most common cause of cushingoid features.
- Ectopic tumor ACTH production, cortisol-producing adrenal adenomas, adrenal carcinoma, and adrenal hyperplasia account for other causes; rarely, ectopic tumor CRH production is encountered.

Ans. A

286. All are used to reduce serum cortisol in patients with Cushing's syndrome except:

A. Metyrapone
B. Mifepristone
C. Pasireotide
D. Ketoconazole

Explanation:

- Ketoconazole, an imidazole derivative antimycotic agent, inhibits several P450 enzymes and effectively lowers cortisol in most patients with Cushing's disease when administered twice daily (600–1200 mg/d). Elevated hepatic transaminases, gynecomastia, impotence, gastrointestinal upset, and edema are common side effects.
- Mifepristone (300–1200 mg/d), a glucocorticoid receptor antagonist, blocks peripheral cortisol action and is approved to treat hyperglycemia in Cushing's disease. Because the drug does not target the pituitary tumor, both ACTH and cortisol levels remain elevated, thus obviating a reliable circulating biomarker. Side effects are largely due to general antagonism of other steroid hormones and include hypokalemia, endometrial hyperplasia, hypoadrenalism, and hypertension.

- Metyrapone (2–4 g/d) inhibits 11β-hydroxylase activity and normalizes plasma cortisol in up to 75% of patients. Side effects include nausea and vomiting, rash, and exacerbation of acne or hirsutism.
- Mitotane (o,p′-DDD; 3–6 g/d orally in four divided doses) suppresses cortisol hypersecretion by inhibiting 11β-hydroxylase and cholesterol side-chain cleavage enzymes and by destroying adrenocortical cells. Side effects of mitotane include gastrointestinal symptoms, dizziness, gynecomastia, hyperlipidemia, skin rash, and hepatic enzyme elevation. It also may lead to hypoaldosteronism.
- Other agents include aminoglutethimide (250 mg tid), trilostane (200–1000 mg/d),cyproheptadine (24 mg/d), and IV etomidate (0.3 mg/kg/h). Glucocorticoid insufficiency is a potential side effect of agents used to block steroidogenesis.

Ans. B

287. All the following agents suppress TSH when administered in pharmacologic doses except:

A. Insulin
B. Glucocorticoid
C. Somatostatin
D. Dopamine

Explanation:

- TRH is the major positive regulator of TSH synthesis and secretion. Peak TSH secretion occurs ~15 min after administration of exogenous TRH.
- Dopamine, glucocorticoids, and somatostatin suppress TSH but are not of major physiologic importance except when these agents are administered in pharmacologic doses.
- Reduced levels of thyroid hormone increase basal TSH production and enhance TRH-mediated stimulation of TSH. High thyroid hormone levels rapidly and directly suppress TSH gene expression secretion and inhibit TRH stimulation of TSH, indicating that thyroid hormones are the dominant regulator of TSH production.

Ans. A

288. A 45-year-male patient has phenotypic feature of type 2 DM, Autoimmune markers, but don't have absolute insulin deficiency suggestive of:

A. Latent autoimmune diabetes of adults
B. Ketosis prone type 2 DM
C. Type 1 DM
D. Monogenic form

Explanation:

- Some individuals (5–10%) with the phenotypic appearance of type 2 DM do not have absolute insulin deficiency but have autoimmune markers (GAD and other ICA autoantibodies) suggestive of type 1 DM (termed *latent autoimmune diabetes of the adult*). Such individuals are more likely to be <50 years of age, thinner, and have a personal or family history of other autoimmune disease than individuals with type 2 DM. They are much more likely to require insulin treatment within 5 years.
- Monogenic forms of diabetes should be considered in those with diabetes onset in childhood or early adulthood and especially those diagnosed within the first 6 months of life, an autosomal pattern of diabetes inheritance, diabetes without typical features of type 1 or 2 diabetes, and stable mild fasting hyperglycemia. Genetic testing should be considered in individuals suspected of having a monogenic form of diabetes as this may guide therapy selection.
- Despite recent advances in the understanding of the pathogenesis of diabetes, it often remains difficult to categorize some patients unequivocally. Individuals who deviate from the clinical profile of type 1 and type 2 DM, or who have other associated defects such as deafness, pancreatic exocrine disease (type 3c DM), and other endocrine disorders, should be classified accordingly.

Ans. A

289. Most common dermatologic manifestation of Diabetes is:

A. Bullosa diabeticorum
B. Necrobiosis lipoidica
C. Xerosis & Pruritis
D. Acanthosis nigricans

Explanation:

- Most common skin manifestations of DM are xerosis and pruritus and are usually relieved by skin moisturizers.
- Protracted wound healing and skin ulcerations are also frequent complications. Diabetic dermopathy, sometimes termed pigmented pretibial papules, or "diabetic skin spots," begins as an erythematous macule or papule that evolves into an area of circular hyperpigmentation. These lesions result from minor mechanical trauma in the pretibial region and are more common in elderly men with DM.
- Bullous diseases, such as bullosa diabeticorum (shallow ulcerations or erosions in the pretibial region), are also seen.
- Necrobiosis lipoidica diabeticorum is an uncommon disorder, accompanying diabetes in predominantly young women. This usually begins in the pretibial region as an erythematous plaque or papules that gradually enlarge, darken, and develop irregular margins, with atrophic centers and central ulceration. They are often painful. Vitiligo occurs at increased frequency in individuals with type 1 DM.
- Acanthosis nigricans (hyperpigmented velvety plaques seen on the neck, axilla, or extensor surfaces) is sometimes a feature of severe insulin resistance and accompanying diabetes.
- Generalized or localized granuloma annulare (erythematous plaques on the extremities or trunk), lichen planus (violaceous papules on the cutaneous surface +/– erosions in the mouth and genitalia), and scleredema (areas of skin thickening on the back or neck at the site of previous superficial infections) are more common in the diabetic population.
- Lipoatrophy & lipohypertrophy can occur at insulin injection sites but are now unusual with use of human insulin, and avoided by rotating injection sites.

Ans. C

290. All are inherited multiple endocrine neoplasia except:

A. Carney's complex
B. McCune Albright syndrome
C. Cowden syndrome
D. Von Hippel Lindau syndrome

Explanation:

- Inheritance for these disorders is autosomal dominant, except MAS, which is due to mosaicism that results from the postzygotic somatic cell mutation of the GNAS1 gene, encoding Gsα unknown.

Table: Multiple endocrine and other organ neoplasia syndromes (MEONs)

Disease[a]	Gene Product	Chromosomal Location
Hyperparathyroidism-jaw tumor (HPT-JT)	Parafibromin	1q31.2
Carney complex		
• CNC1	PPKAR1A	17q24.2
• CNC2	?[b]	2p16
von Hippel-Lindau disease (VHL)	pVHL (elongin)	3p25
Neurofibromatosis type 1 (NF1)	Neurofibromin	17q11.2
Cowden's syndrome (CWS)		
• CWS1	PTEN	10q23.31
• CWS2	SDHB	1p36.13
• CWS3	SDHD	11q23.1
• CWS4	KLLN	10q23.31
• CWS5	PIK3CA	3q26.32
• CWS6	AKT1	14q32.33
• CWS7	SEC23B	20q11.23
McCune-Albright syndrome (MAS)	Gsα	20q13.32

Ans. B

291. A 35 year old male presented with history of severe headache and he was diagnosed to have accelrated hypertension. He was prescribed T. Telamasartan 40mg 1-0-1. He was referred to tertiary centre for further management. For evaluation of young onset hypertension. He was ordered ARR to rule out primary hyperaldosteronism. How does telmesartan affects ARR?

A. Decrease B. Increase

C. No effect D. Any of the above

Explanation:

- Beta blocker causes an increase in aldosterone levels and decrease in renin levels leading to increased ARR.
- ACEI / ARB causes a decrease in aldosterone levels and increase in renin levels, leading to decreased ARR.
- CCB – no effect on ARR.

Ans. A

292. A 55 year old gentleman with obesity and type 2 DM comes for review. He is on tab metformin 1g BD, Ramipril 10mg and amlodipine 10mg OD. PR- 70/min, BMI is 36. HbA1c – 8.4%. He is started on sitagliptin? What is the mode of action of sitagliptin?

A. DPP IV inhibitor B. GLP1 agonist

C. GLT2 inhibitor D. Sulphonylurea

Explanation:

- DPP IV inhibitors inhibit breakdown of naturally occurring peptides including GLP1, a gut peptide produced along with Gastric inhibitory peptide in incretin response.
- Incretin response occurs in response to a meal and results in increased insulin release, feeling of satiety and slowed gastric emptying. DPP IV inhibitors result in reduction of HBA1C of between 0.6 and 0.9%.

Ans. A

293. A 70 year old lady with type 2 DM comes for review. She is on mixed insulin twice daily, anxious about weight gain. Other comorbids include ischemic heart disease and renal impairment. Her BMI is 33, eGFR 27m/min. Which is the suitable agent to add?

A. Gliclazide B. Linagliptin

C. Metformin D. Pioglitazone

Explanation:

- Linagliptin is used in renal impairment patients even without dose adjustment. It is excreted in faeces. It can cause modest weight loss also.

Ans. C

294. A 40 year old lady who works on a permanent night shift comes to the hospital for review. She is a known case of type 2 diabetes mellitus, on metformin 1g BD and Gliclazide 160mg BD. She suffers from frequent hypoglycaemia, weight gain and BMI is 32. Her BP is 150/90 mm Hg, Pulse is 78/min, regular. What is the next step with response to diabetes therapy?

A. Change gliclazide to pioglitazone. B. Change gliclazide to sitagliptin

C. Reduce gliclazide D. Reduce metformin

Explanation:

- Patient has frequent episodes of hypoglycaemia and has weight gain.
- Most suitable option is to substitute sulphonylurea with DPPIV inhibitor which is weight neutral and does not result in hypoglycaemia.

Ans. B

295. A 25 year old man presents to diabetes clinic for review. He had recurrent balanitis and was found to have glycosuria. Family history revealed his father, one aunt, one uncle have had type 2 DM for more than 20 years. They had good glycemic control without complications. His BP 120/80 mm Hg and Pulse 80/min, regular. BMI is 20, HbA1c -5.9%, fasting plasma glucose – 140mg/dl. What is the diagnosis?

A. MODY 2
B. MODY 3
C. MODY 5
D. Type 1 diabetes

Explanation:

- MODY 2 is caused by mutations in glucokinase which acts as a glucose sensor for the beta cells. It increases the fasting plasma glucose. Microvascular complications are rare.

Ans. A

296. A 65 year old gentleman, long standing type 2 DM. His BMI is 28. Hba1c -8%, eGFR -29ml/min. He has a past history of ischemic heart disease and is on regular treatment for the same. He was prescribed long acting peakless insulin analog. What is the insulin prescribed?

A. Insulin glargine
B. NPH
C. Insulin Lispro
D. Insulin Aspart

Explanation:

- Short acting insulin analogs are aspart, lispro and glulysine. NPH is intermediate acting insulin, long acting insulin analogs are degludec, glargine, detemir. These long acting analogs are peakless and have decreased number of hypoglycemic episodes.

Ans. A

297. A 28 year old female post partum presented with history of headache, blurring of vision. On evaluation she was found to have mild hyperprolactinemia. MRI brain was ordered and showed adenoma. Blood investigation showed normal CBC, high ESR, rest of the routine evaluation was normal. Which is the best mode of treatment for this patient?

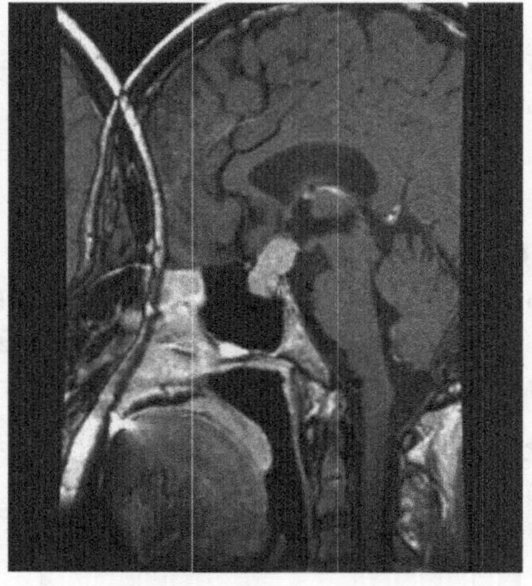

A. Bromocriptine
B. Trans nasal trans sphenoidal surgery
C. I.V. hydrocortisone
D. Cabergoline

Explanation:

- This is a case of Lymphocytic Hypophysitis.
- Affects Postpartum women & presents with hyperprolactinemia
- MRI evidence of a prominent pituitary mass that often resembles an adenoma, with mildly elevated PRL levels.
- Can be transient or permanent
- Erythrocyte sedimentation rate often is elevated
- MRI image may be indistinguishable from that of a pituitary adenoma.
- Hypophysitis should be considered in a postpartum woman with a newly diagnosed pituitary mass before an unnecessary surgical intervention.
- Inflammatory process often resolves after several months of glucocorticoid treatment.

Ans. C

298. Tests of exocrine pancreatic function are all except:

A. Secretin test
B. Fecal elastase
C. Qualitative stool fat determination
D. Endoscopic secretin test

Explanation:

Table: Tests of exocrine pancreatic function		
Direct stimulation of the pancreas with analysis of duodenal contents		
1. Secretin test	Secretin leads to increased output of pancreatic juice and HCO_3^-; pancreatic secretory response is related to the functional mass of pancreatic tissue	Sensitive enough to detect occult disease; involves duodenal intubation and fluoroscopic placement of gastroduodenal tube; poorly defined normal enzyme response; overlap in chronic pancreatitis; large secretory reserve capacity of the pancreas; currently done at only a few medical centers
2. Endoscopic secretin test	Replaces need for tube placement duodenum	Sensitive enough to detect occult disease; high negative predictive value; avoids intubation and fluoroscopy; requires sedation
Measurement of intraluminal digestion products		
1. Quantitative stool fat determination	Lack of lipolytic enzymes brings about impaired fat digestion	Reliable reference standard for defining severity of malabsorption does not distinguish between maldigestion malabsorption
Measurement of pancreatic enzymes in feces		
1. Fecal elastase	Pancreatic secretion of proteolytic enzymes; not degraded in intestine	Diagnostic accuracy best if value is < 100 μg/g performed on a solid stool

Ans. C

299. A type 2 DM patient is referred from CHC to your hospital. His 24 hour urine protein is 2.2 gm. His BP is 150/80 mm Hg. His HbAIC is 7.2%. Which one of the following indications are false for consideration of renal biopsy in Type 2 DM?

A. Nephrotic range proteinuria in absence of diabetic retinopathy

B. Nephrotic range proteinuria with duration of less than 10 years

C. Nephrotic range proteinuria with normal kidney function

D. Unexplained microscopic hematuria

Explanation:

- Natural history of diabetic nephropathy in patients with types 1 and 2 diabetes is similar.
- However, since the onset of type 1 diabetes is readily identifiable and the onset of type 2 diabetes is not, a patient newly diagnosed with type 2 diabetes may present with *advanced diabetic nephropathy*.
- At the onset of diabetes, renal hypertrophy and glomerular hyperfiltration are present. The degree of glomerular hyperfiltration correlates with the subsequent risk of clinically significant nephropathy.
- In the ~40% of patients with diabetes who develop diabetic nephropathy, the earliest manifestation is an increase in albuminuria detected by sensitive radioimmunoassay.
- Albuminuria in the range of 30–300 mg/24 h is called *microalbuminuria*.
- Microalbuminuria appears 5–10 years after onset of diabetes. It is currently recommended to test patients with type 1 disease for microalbuminuria 5 years after diagnosis of diabetes and yearly thereafter and, because the time of onset of type 2 diabetes is often unknown, to test type 2 patients at the time of diagnosis of diabetes and yearly thereafter.

Ans. B

300. A 42 year old male known case of CKD-5D presented to OPD with painful nodule on abdomen. He was on warfarin for Atrial fibrillation. What's your diagnosis?

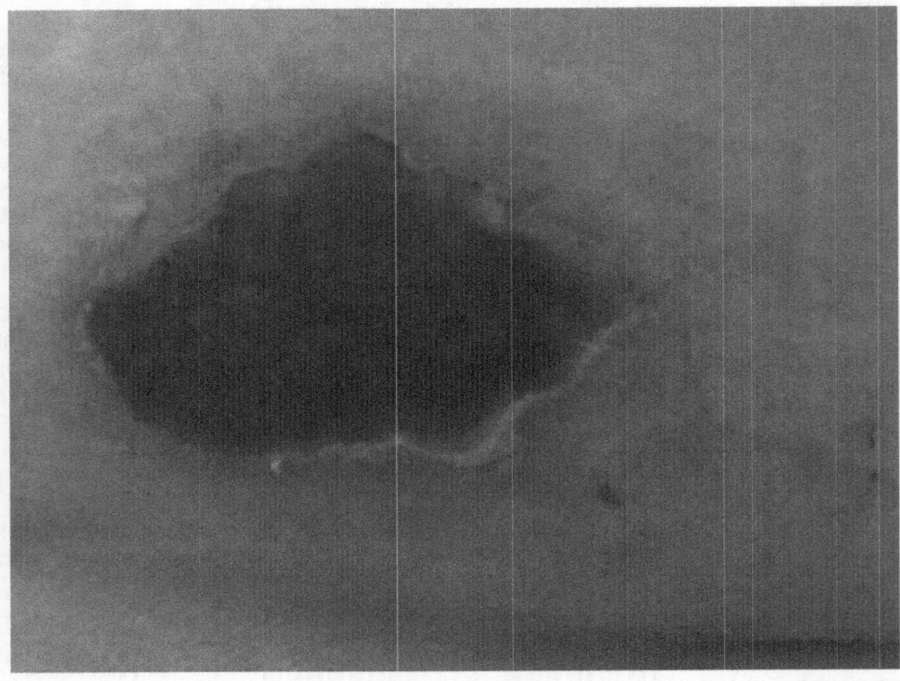

A. Tumor calcinosis

B. Dermatosis

C. Calciphylaxis

D. Steal syndrome

Explanation:

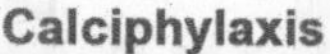

Calciphylaxis

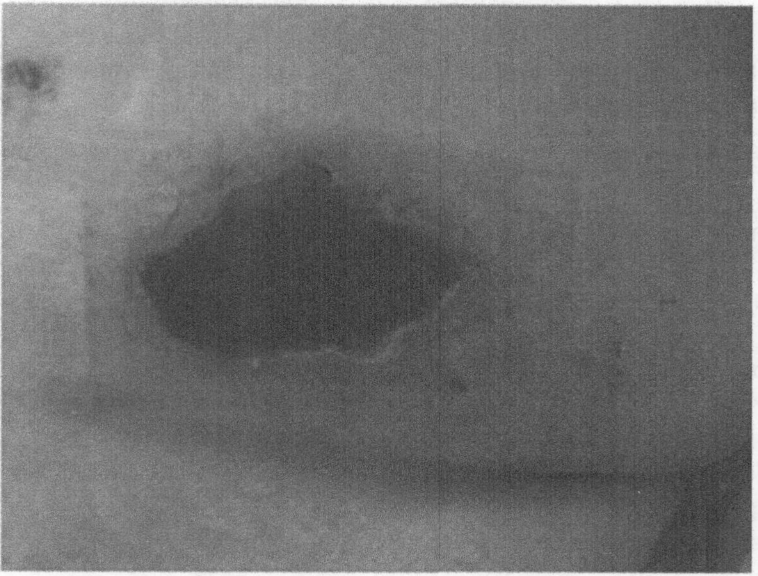

Figure: Calciphylaxis. This peritoneal dialysis patient was on chronic warfarin therapy for atrial fibrillation. She noticed a small painful nodule on the abdomen that was followed by progressive skin necrosis and ulceration of the anterior abdominal wall. She was treated with hyperbaric oxygen, intravenous thiosulfate, and discontinuation of warfarin, with slow resolution of the ulceration

Ans. C

301. Porphyrias are a group of disorders which occurs due to defect in heme biosynthesis. Few porphyrias doesn't have neurological manifestations. Which porphyria doesn't cause peripheral neuropathy?

A. Acute intermittent porphyria
B. Hereditary copro porphyria
C. Porphyria cutanea tarda
D. Variegate porphyria

Explanation:

- Three forms of porphyria are associated with peripheral neuropathy: acute intermittent porphyria (AIP), hereditary coproporphyria (HCP) and variegate porphyria (VP).

Ans. C

302. A 46 year old female presents with tiredness, dry skin, feeling cold, hair loss, weight gain with poor appetite, menorrhagia, impaired hearing and following facial features. Most likely diagnosis:

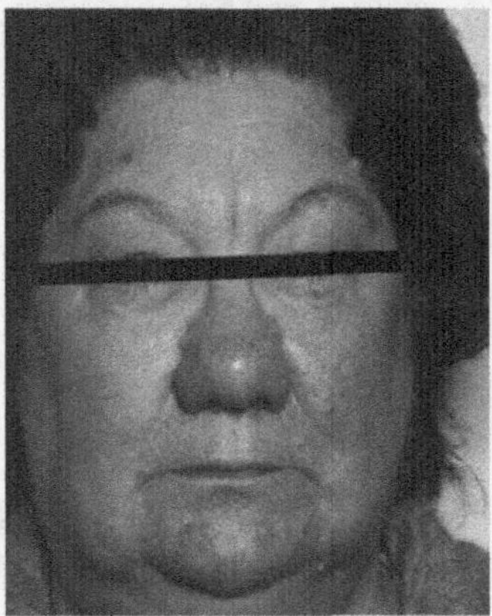

A. Hypothyroidism
B. Graves' disease
C. Cushing's syndrome
D. Addison's disease

Explanation:

- Tiredness, weakness, fatigue, dry skin, hair loss, weight gain and facial features of puffy eyes and thickened skin points towards hypothyroidism.

Table: Signs and symptoms of hypothyroidism (Descending order of frequency)	
Symptoms	**Signs**
• Tiredness, weakness • Dry skin • Feeling cold • Hair loss • Difficulty concentrating and poor memory • Constipation • Weight gain with poor appetite • Dyspnea • Hoarse voice • Menorrhagia (later oligomenorrhea or amenorrhea) • Paresthesia • Impaired hearing	• Dry coarse skin; cool peripheral extremities • Puffy face, hands and feet (myxedema) • Diffuse alopecia • Bradycardia • Peripheral edema • Delayed tendon reflex relaxation • Carpal tunnel syndrome • Serous cavity effusions

- Addison's disease: due to inadequate secretion of cortisol and aldosterone where fatigue, hypoglycaemic episodes, fall in BP, muscle cramps are seen.
- Cushing's syndrome presents with excessive body fat buffalo hump, fatigue, steroids abuse but menorrhagia, impaired hearing points more towards hypothyroidism here. Graves disease presents with excessive sweating, fatigue, palpations, insomnia, tremors & irritability.

Ans. A

303. Following features seen in:

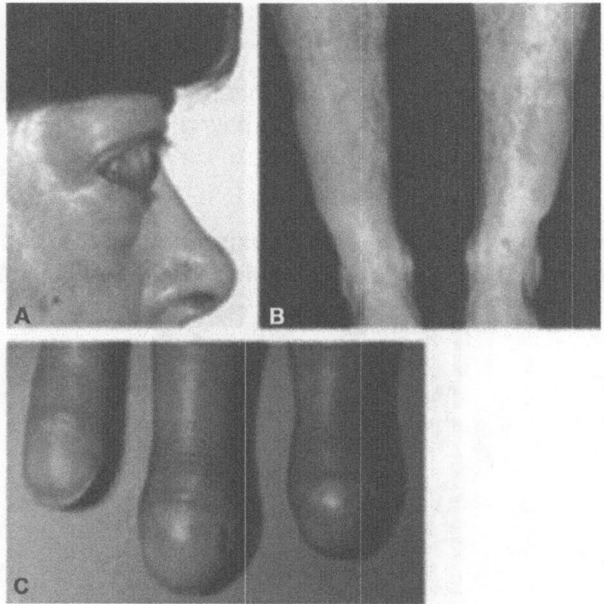

A. Hypothyroidism
B. Graves' disease
C. Cushing's syndrome
D. Addison's disease

Explanation:

- Ophthalmopathy, lid retraction, periorbital edema, conjunctival injection, proptosis, dermopathy over lateral aspect of shin, acropathy in favour of graves disease.
- **Hypothyroidism features:**

Table: Signs and symptoms of hypothyroidism (Descending order of frequency)	
Symptoms	**Signs**
• Tiredness, weakness • Dry skin • Feeling cold • Hair loss • Difficulty concentrating and poor memory • Constipation • Weight gain with poor appetite • Dyspnea • Hoarse voice • Menorrhagia (later oligomenorrhea or amenorrhea) • Paresthesia • Impaired hearing	• Dry coarse skin; cool peripheral extremities • Puffy face, hands and feet (myxedema) • Diffuse alopecia • Bradycardia • Peripheral edema • Delayed tendon reflex relaxation • Carpal tunnel syndrome • Serous cavity effusions

- **Cushing's syndrome:** Facial puffiness, fatigue, buffalo hump, hair loss, centripetal obesity, easy bruise are seen.
- **Addison's disease:** Fatigue, hypoglycaemic features, muscle weakness, fall in BP are seen.

Ans. B

304. Oogonia shown in following image are maximum with 5-7 million in number at:

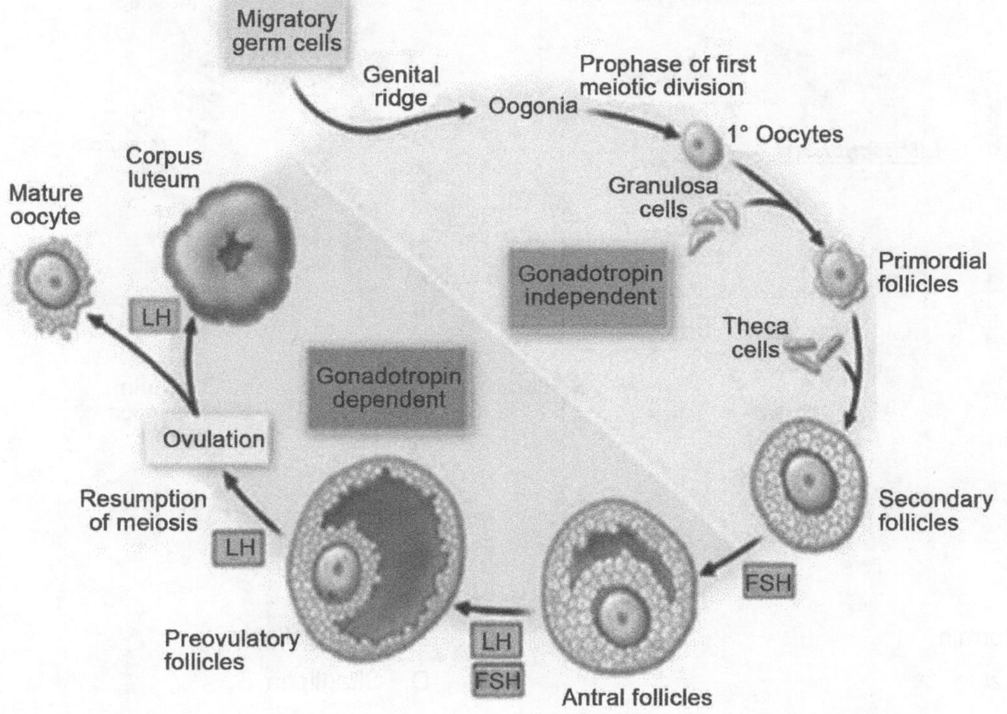

A. 20 weeks of gestation
B. At birth
C. Puberty
D. Adult life

Explanation:

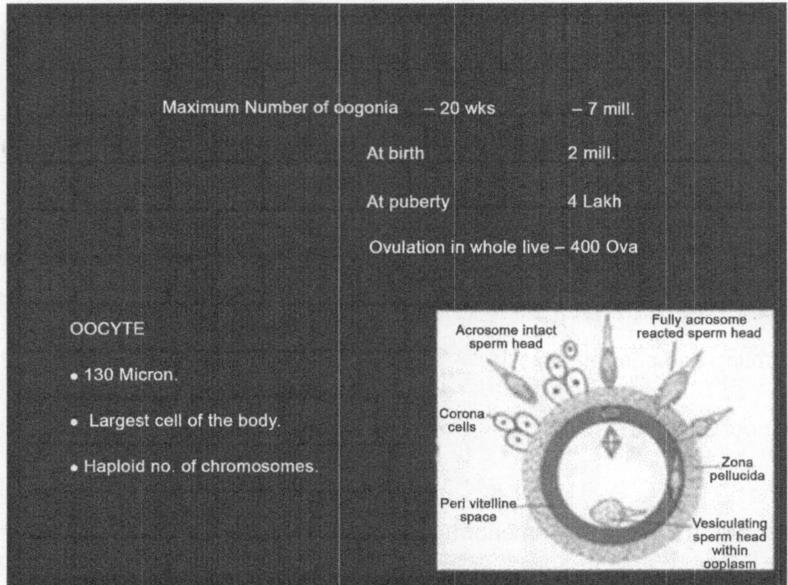

Ans. A

305. Drug that acts by inhibiting ATP sensitive K+ channel is:

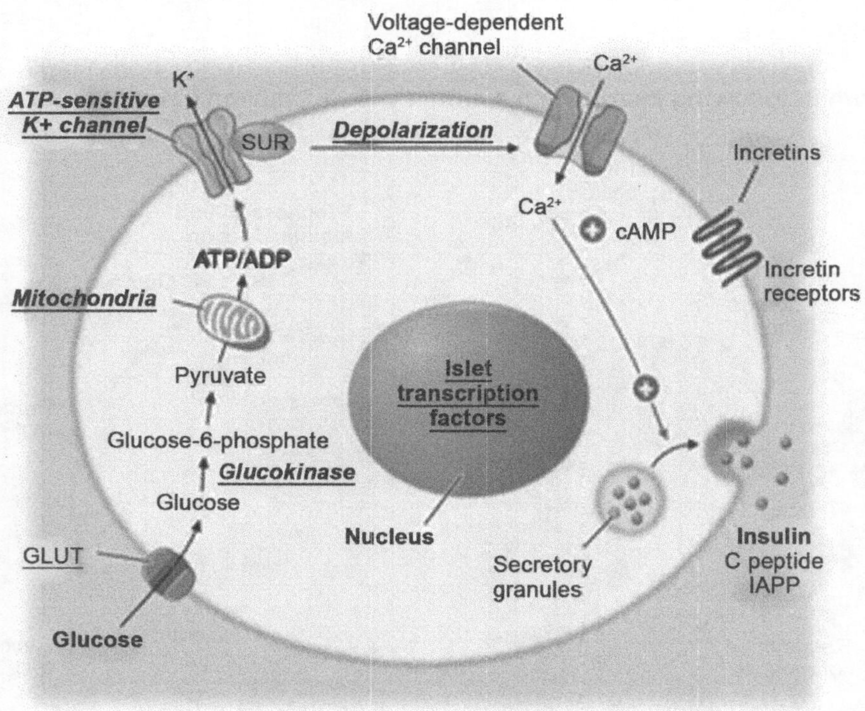

A. Metformin
B. Dapagliflozin
C. Glipizide
D. Sitagliptin

Explanation:

- Glipizide acts by inhibiting ATP K+ channel.

- Dapagliflozin acts by inhibiting sodium glucose co transport-2.
- Metformin is biguanide which is AMPk activator.
- Sitagliptin is an Dipetidyl peptiase-4 inhibitor.

Ans. C

306. Identify the X-ray of 60 year old women with backache:

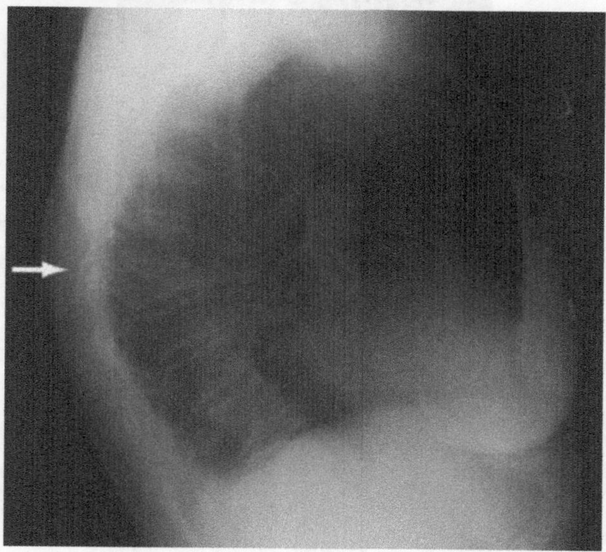

A. Paget's disease
B. Normal impression
C. Osteoporosis
D. Hemangioma

Explanation:

- Lateral spine X-ray shows severe osteopenia, wedge shaped deformity with anterior wedge compression so called codfish vertebrae in osteoporosis in an 60 year old woman.
- In Paget's disease cortical thickening of superior and inferior plate ends of vertebrae are seen results in picture frame vertebrae.

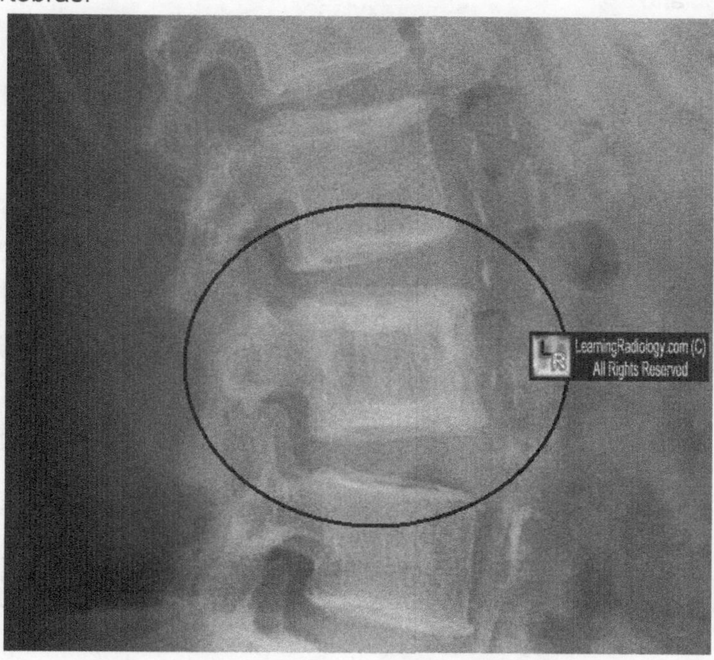

- In hemangioma corduroy appearance of vertebrae is seen.

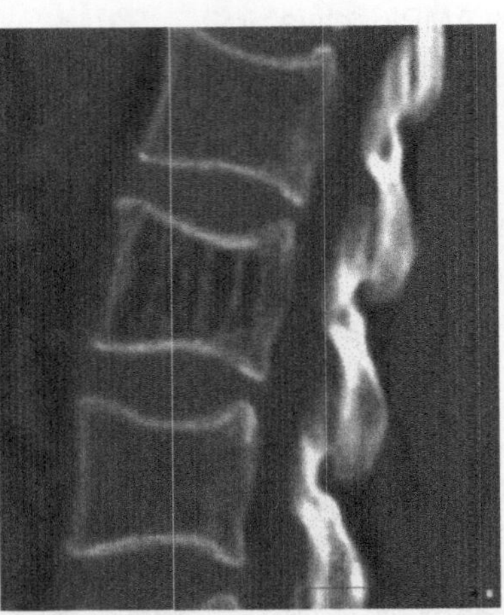

Ans. C

307. Hydroxalation required for mature hormone shown below occurs in:

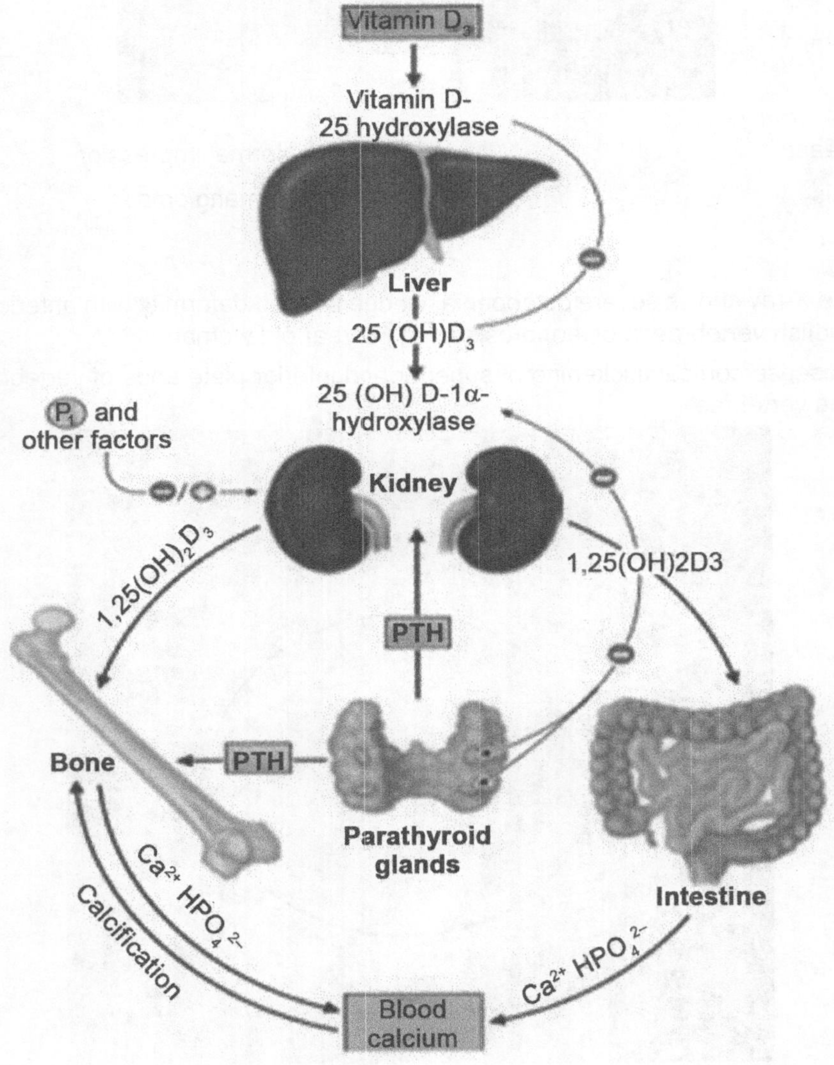

A. Liver
B. Kidney
C. Parathyroid
D. Intestine

Explanation:

- Vitamin D undergoes hydroxylation initially in liver that forms 25 hydroxycholecalciferol and then second hydroxylation occurs in kidney which forms 1alpha 25 dihydroxycholecalciferol (calcitriol) active form of vitamin D.

Ans. B

308. Treatment of sarcoidosis associated hypercalcemia with glucocorticoids acts on which of the following step:

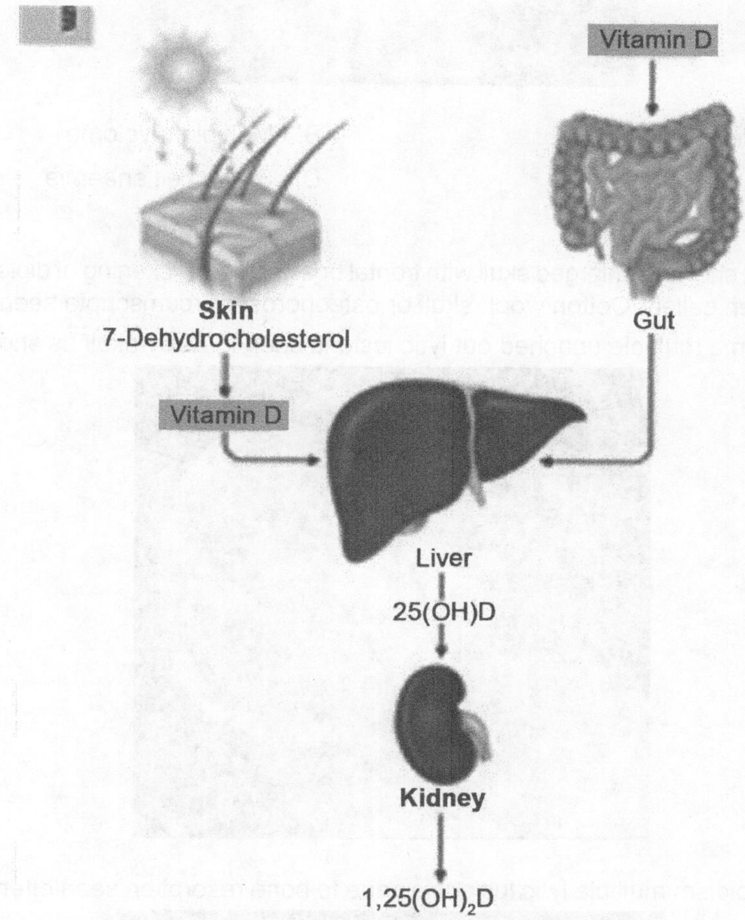

A. Decreases 7-Dehydrocholestrol
B. Decreases Vitamin D absorption in gut
C. Decreases 25 hydroxycholecalciferol
D. Decreases 1,25 dihydroxy cholecalciferol

Explanation:

- Decreases 1,25 dihydroxycholecalciferol production and decreases serum calcium so used in treatment of sarcoidosis associated hypercalcemia.
- Ketaconazole, chloroquine also acts by similar mechanism of action used in treatment of hypercalcemia associated with sarcoidosis.

Ans. D

309. Identify the image:

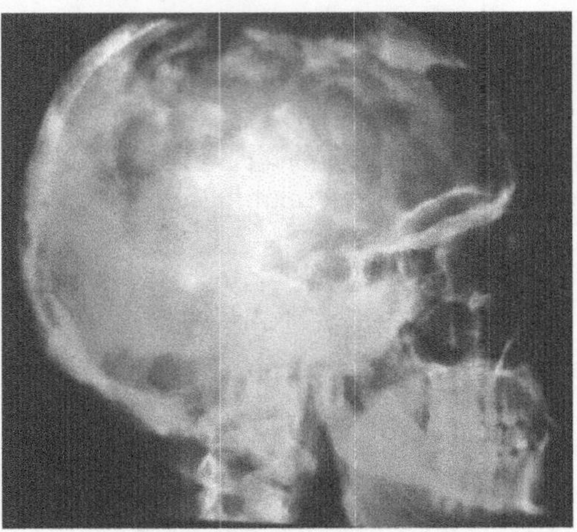

A. Hyperparathyroidism

B. Multiple myeloma

C. Paget's disease

D. Sickle cell anaemia

Explanation:

- Lateral X-ray skull showing enlarged skull with frontal bossing and thickening of diploic areas. Both resorption and sclerosis often called "Cotton wool" skull or osteoporosis circumscripta seen in Paget's disease.
- In multiple myeloma multiple punched out lytic lesions seen in X-ray skull as shown below:

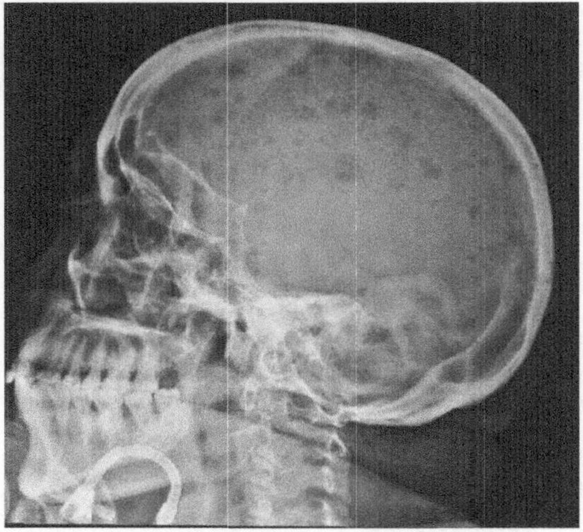

- In hyperparathyroidism multiple lytic luciencies due to bone resorption seen often called pepper pot skull.

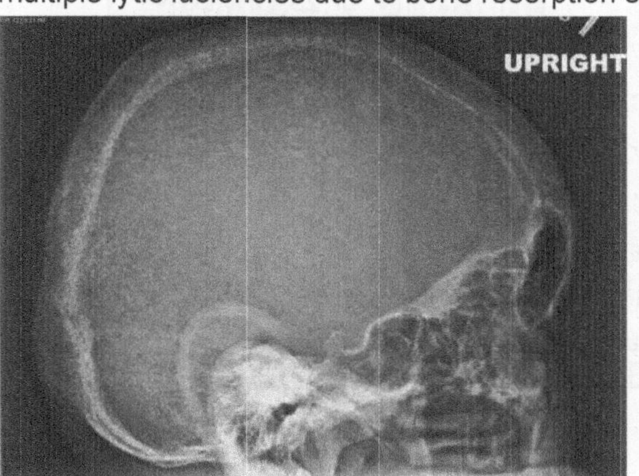

- In sickle cell anaemia hair on end appearence is seen due to bone marrow hyperplasia.

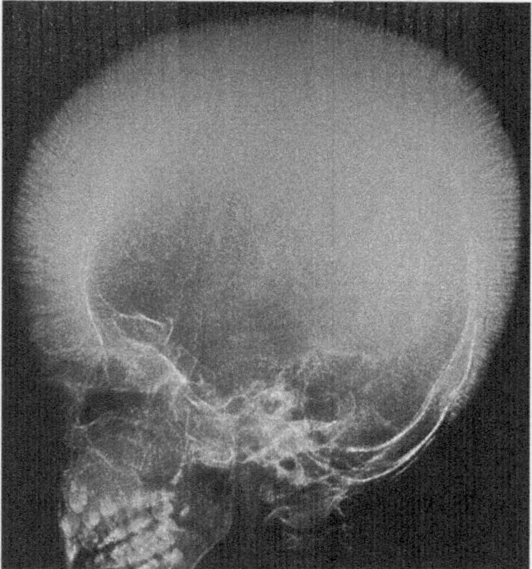

Ans. C

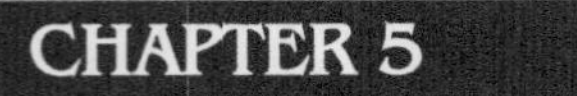

CENTRAL NERVOUS SYSTEM (CNS)

1. Stroke events are maximum following TIA within ____ days.

A. 2
B. 7
C. 21
D. 1

Explanation:

- TIAs are episodes of stroke symptoms that last only briefly; the standard definition of duration is <24 h, but most TIAs last <1 h.
- If a relevant brain infarction is identified on brain imaging, the clinical entity is now classified as stroke regardless of the duration of symptoms.
- The risk of stroke after a TIA is ~10–15% in the first 3 months, with most events occurring in the first 2 days.
- This risk can be directly estimated using the well-validated ABCD2 score

Table: Risk of stroke following transient ischemic attack: The ABCD[1] score	
Clinical Factor	**Score**
A: Age > 60 years	1
B: SBP > 140 mm Hg or DBP > 90 mm Hg	1
C: Clinical symptoms	
Unilateral weakness	2
Speech disturbance without weakness	1
D: Duration	
>60 min	2
10-59 min	1
E: Diabetes (oral medications or insulin)	1

Ans. A

2. A 23-year-old female presents to the clinic for evaluation of a headache. She is currently 14 weeks pregnant. She complains of a holocephalic headache for the last week, which is worsening in intensity. Headache is worse at night and causes blurry vision. Her neurological examination is remarkable for bilateral papilledema. Sagittal T1 magnetic resonance image (MRI) is shown here. Which of the following is the most likely diagnosis?

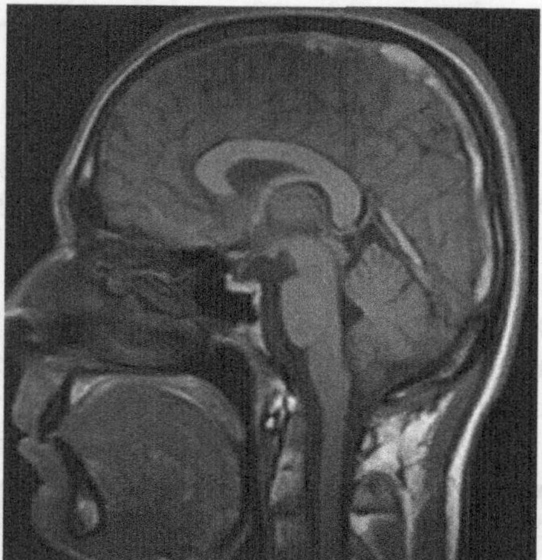

A. Pseudotumor cerebri
B. Meningioma
C. Venous sinus thrombosis
D. Preeclampsia

Explanation:

- This patient presents with worsening headaches and features of increased intracranial pressure with worsening headaches at night and papilledema.
- In pregnant patients, there should be immediate concern for venous sinus thrombosis (VST). Pregnancy-induced pseudotumor is possible, but VST must be ruled out first.
- Pregnant patients are at higher risk of VST because pregnancy creates a hypercoagulable state often worsened by dehydration. MRI and magnetic resonancevenography are the first-line tests for determining whether there is a VST because both can be done without contrast.
- Provided image is a noncontrast T1-weighted image. This demonstrates a hyperintense T1 signal in the sagittal sinus and the great vein of Galen, which is consistent with an acute VST.
- Papilledema could be seen additionally in preeclampsia and optic neuritis. The image provided does not show signs of optic neuritis because the optic nerves are not in the imaging plane. Optic neuritis would show hyperintense optic nerves on T2 imaging along with contrast enhancement. Preeclampsia has no radiographic findings. Meningiomas are not hyperintense on T1 imaging without contrast. However, they do homogeneously enhance with contrast.

Ans. C

3. **A 15-year-old male presents to your office with a complaint of falls. This has been occurring over the last several months. His examination demonstrates bilateral foot drop, loss of sensation to the midshin in both legs, absent reflexes, and high arched feet with atrophy in his feet. Nerve conduction studies demonstrate motor conduction velocities at 20 m/s in all nerves without conduction blocks and absent sensory responses. Electromyography shows neurogenic units in the distal leg. Which genetic mutation is most likely responsible for this patient's symptoms?**

A. PMP22 deletion on chromosome 17
B. MFN2 mutation on chromosome 3
C. PMP22 duplication on chromosome 17
D. SOD1 mutation on chromosome 21

Explanation:

- This patient has a hereditary, not acquired, demyelinating neuropathy, as evidenced by slow nerve conduction velocities without conduction block.
- Most common hereditary demyelinating neuropathy is Charcot-Marie-Tooth (CMT) type 1a, which is caused by a PMP22 duplication on chromosome 17.
- PMP22 deletion causes the syndrome of hereditary neuropathy with liability to pressure palsies. MFN2 is a common abnormality in CMT2a, which typically causes an axonal neuropathy more than a demyelinating neuropathy.

- SOD1 on chromosome 21 is involved in autosomal dominant motor neuron disease. GAA triplet repeat on chromosome 9 is involved in Friedrich ataxia.

Ans. C

4. **A 62-year-old woman presents with gradually progressive cognitive decline, along with stiffness, slowness, and intermittent jerks of her right upper extremity. Her speech has become monotone, slurred, and slow. On examination, she has dystonic posturing of the right arm with increased rigidity and bradykinesia. There is also intermittent myoclonus when the right arm is held up. When speaking, the patient's right arm will seemingly rise on its own accord, and she will use the left arm to pull it back down. Her family feels that she often neglects the right side of her body. The patient's MRI is shown in the figure below. Which of the following is typical of this diagnosis?**

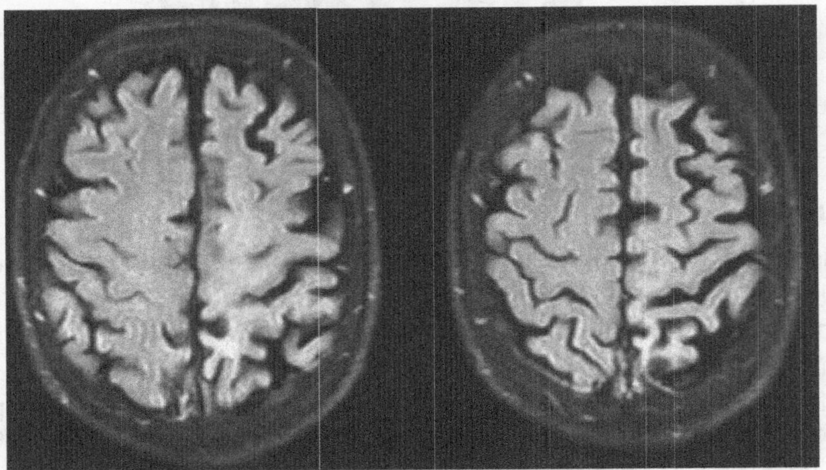

A. Tau deposition
B. Alpha-synuclein deposition
C. Levodopa-responsive rigidity
D. Autonomic dysfunction

Explanation:

- This case is a typical clinical scenario for corticobasal ganglionic degeneration (CBGD). This is a progressive neurodegenerative disease characterized by tau deposition and a number of clinical findings, including motor apraxia, cortical sensory loss, sensory neglect, myoclonus, tremor, rigidity and dystonia.
- Typically, the onset begins asymmetrically and may look clinically similar to idiopathic Parkinson disease (PD).
- However, CBGD is usually unresponsive to levodopa, and is associated with more cortical findings than is typical for idiopathic PD.
- Occasionally patients will have one limb that will slowly rise and "have a mind of its own," known as alien limb syndrome. Although CBGD may have some clinical overlap with progressive supranuclear palsy or frontotemporal dementia, magnetic resonance imaging will often differentiate with asymmetric parietal lobe atrophy.
- Alpha-synuclein deposits are commonly associated with multiple system atrophy (MSA), idiopathic PD, and dementia with Lewy bodies, but not with CBGD. Typically, autonomic dysfunction is found in MSA. Prominent hallucinations are found in dementia with Lewy bodies.

Ans. A

5. **A 63-year-old female presented to the emergency room with an acute aneurysmal subarachnoid hemorrhage (SAH) and underwent a clipping procedure on admission. She has since been recovering in the intensive care unit. On the tenth postoperative day, she was noted to have slurred speech, worsening right facial droop, and right arm weakness. She was more difficult to rouse. Noncontrast head computed tomography (CT) and four-vessel angiogram are shown. Which of the following is the best treatment for her condition?**

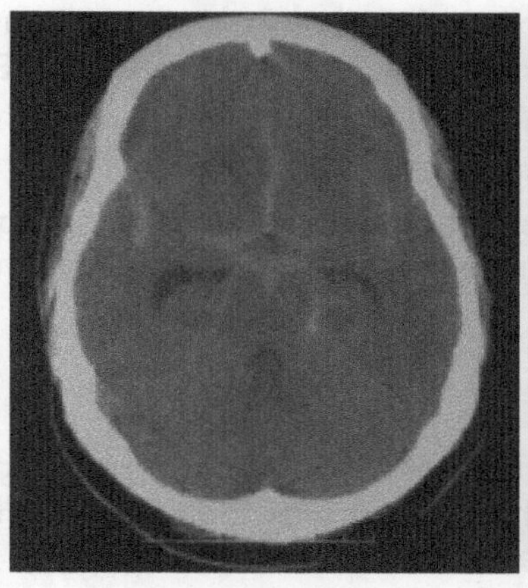

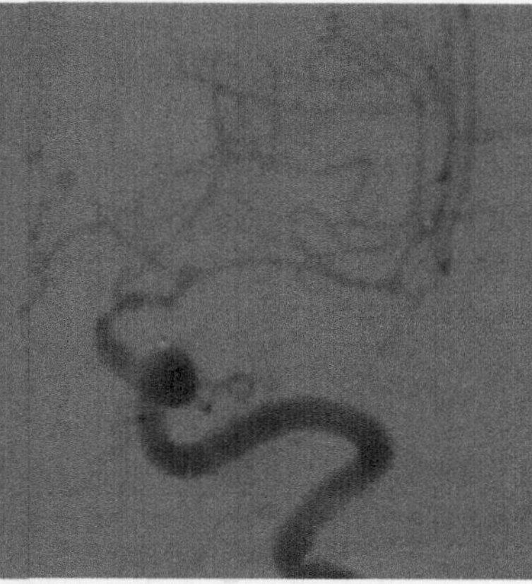

A. Intravenous (IV) tissue plasminogen activator (tPA)
B. Intraarterial calcium channel blockers
C. IV fosphenytoin load
D. Placement of extraventricular drain

Explanation:

- Patient is suffering from postsubarachnoid hemorrhage vasospasm. This is a common complication that can occur in the first 14 days after SAH, and can lead to further neurological deficits or even death if not quickly recognized and treated.
- Main emergent therapy remains intraarterial administration of calcium channel blockers and angioplasty.
- IV tPA would not be indicated, even if this patient had an ischemic stroke, because of her recent hemorrhage and cranial surgery. Although seizures are a possible cause of reduced level of alertness, new focal findings in the setting of an SAH should prompt an evaluation for vasospasm, which the angiogram shows.
- CT shown does not demonstrate hydrocephalus, so an extraventricular drain is not necessary. There is no indication of severe increased intracranial pressure, so mannitol is not necessary.

Ans. B

6. **A 9-year-old left-handed boy presents to the clinic with his parents due to concerns over school performance. He previously hit all milestones and was an average student in school. Over this past school year, he had progressive difficulty with reading, but did not display behavioral problems at school or at home. His neurological examination and mental status examination are normal and show that he is able to write a simple paragraph in clinic. An electroencephalogram (EEG) is normal in the awake and sleep states. Which of the following is the most likely diagnosis?**

A. Infarct of the splenium of corpus callosum & left occipital lobe
B. Landau-Kleffner syndrome
C. Developmental dyslexia
D. Mild intellectual disability

Explanation:

- Developmental dyslexia, also known as specific reading disorder, is an unexpected difficulty in learning to read despite normal intelligence.
- Usually associated with a normal neurological examination, and is without structural abnormalities on imaging. It is more common in left-handed males with a family history of dyslexia.
- An infarct of the splenium of corpus callosum and left occipital lobe could cause alexia without agraphia, but this should come on acutely, unlike the progressive course in this case.

- Landau-Kleffner syndrome is an acquired epileptic aphasia in which children slowly lose previous verbal language and can have electrographic status epilepticus of sleep seen on EEG.
- Mild intellectual disability involves deficits in language, reading, memory, social skills, and executive function, and is associated with an IQ between 50 and 70.
- Attention deficit/hyperactivity disorder can lead to school problems in this age group, but typically these patients present with complaints of inattention, hyperactivity, or impulsivity, which can result in disciplinary problems at school or home.

Ans. C

7. **A 17-year-old girl arrived to class immediately after cross-country running practice. While sitting at her desk, she felt sweaty, warm all over, and nauseated. She then slumped forward with fast, jerk like movements of her arms and legs. Her teacher rushed over to lower her to the floor, and she quickly began to rouse. She initially appeared confused but was able to answer questions appropriately. She had some urinary incontinence during the episode but no tongue trauma. She returned to her baseline mental status within a few minutes of the episode but was taken to the emergency room nonetheless. What is most likely the diagnosis?**

A. Complex partial seizure
B. Convulsive syncope
C. Nonepileptic spell
D. Absence seizure

Explanation:

- Case is consistent with convulsive syncope, based on the history of recent vigorous exercise, prodrome of nausea and diaphoresis, and loss of consciousness.
- Additional components of her presentation that suggest a syncopal etiology rather than seizure include the brevity of her loss of consciousness, the brevity of the postictal confusion, and the fast, jerk like movements that were likely myoclonus.
- Note that there was no mention of repetitive or stereotyped movement before losing consciousness that would suggest automatisms or tonic/clonic activity.
- There was a loss of bladder control during the episode, but this can occur with any alteration in consciousness.
- There is nothing in question stem that would indicate a nonepileptic spell.
- Diagnostic workup for syncope would generally include orthostatic vital signs, an electrocardiogram, Holter monitor, and/or transthoracic echocardiogram if there is a high suspicion of a cardiac etiology. If events are recurrent, an electroencephalogram may also be considered in case of an atypical seizure presentation.
- Treatment for the case presented would likely include volume resuscitation, with no other definitive therapy indicated unless there are abnormalities on evaluation.
- If the patient suffers recurrent syncope, both conservative measures (i.e. compression stockings, abdominal binders, liberalization of salt intake, moving legs before standing) and pharmacological measures (i.e. fludrocortisone, midodrine, droxidopa, pyridostigmine) may be considered.

Ans. B

8. **Miller fisher syndrome antibody formed against:**

A. GM1
B. GQ1b
C. GD1a
D. GM1b

Explanation:

- Miller fisher syndrome is a variant of GBS.
- Characterised by triad of Ophthalmoplegia, Ataxia, Areflexia without muscle weakness.
- More than 90 % of cases are positive for Anti GQ1b antibody.

Table: Principal antiglycolipid antibodies implicated in immune neuropathies		
Clinical Presentation	**Antibody Target**	**Usual Isotype**
Acute Immune Neuropathies (Guillain-Barré Syndrome)		
Acute inflammatory demyelinating polyneuropathy (AIDP)	No clear patterns GM1 most common	IgG (polyclonal)
Acute motor axonal neuropathy (AMAN)	GD1a, GM1, GM1b, GalNAc–GD1a (<50% for any)	IgG (polyclonal)
Miller Fisher syndrome (MFS)	GQ1b (>90%)	IgG (polyclonal)
Acute pharyngeal cervicobrachial neuropathy (APCBN)	GT1a (?most)	IgG (polyclonal)
Chronic Immune Neuropathies		
Chronic inflammatory demyelinating polyneuropathy (CIDP) (75%)	<10% to CNTN1 or NF155 and even more rare to PO, myelin P2 protein, or PMP22	IgG4 with CNTN1 and NF155
CIDP-M (MGUS associated) (25%)	Neural binding sites	IgG, IgA (monoclonal)
Chronic sensory > motor neuropathy	SPGP, SGLPG (on MAG) (50%)	IgM (monoclonal)
	Uncertain (50%)	IgM (monoclonal)
Multifocal motor neuropathy (MMN)	GM1, GalNAc-GD1a, others (25-50%)	IgM (polyclonal, monoclonal)
Chronic sensory ataxic neuropathy	GD1b, GQ1b, and other b-series gangliosides	IgM (monoclonal)

Ans. B

9. **A 63-year-old woman presents with left shoulder pain and gait difficulty for the last 1 year. Her husband states that she does not swing her left arm when she walks and has had difficulty using this hand to manipulate buttons. The patient also reports constipation and falling out of bed during vivid dreams for 6 years before the onset of gait difficulty. She denies history of tremor. What is the most likely diagnosis?**

A. Rotator cuff injury
B. Cervical myelopathy
C. Idiopathic Parkinson disease
D. Vascular parkinsonism

Explanation:

- Patient has shoulder pain and gait difficulty for last 1 year with decreased arm swing when walking and loss of dexterity in the left hand.
- These historical clues point toward bradykinesia and rigidity, two of the cardinal features of idiopathic Parkinson disease (PD).
- Note that tremor is not part of the diagnostic criteria of PD, as one can have the akinetic/rigid subtype.
- Physical examination would, of course, confirm these examination findings. It is not uncommon for patients to complain of joint pains likely from dystonia or rigidity, some of which persist after operations for orthopedic issues.
- Constipation and falling out of bed during vivid dreams (rapid eye movement [REM] sleep behavior disorder) are two nonmotor features of PD that often precede the diagnosis by up to 10 years, pointing further toward a neurodegenerative alphasynucleinopathy.
- Although shoulder injuries such as a rotator cuff injury could certainly cause decreased arm swing, other historical points with the constipation and REM sleep behavior disorder make this less likely. Same is also true for cervical myelopathy.
- Vascular parkinsonism would also not have these nonmotor features and would present predominately with lower extremity involvement and gait difficulty much more than asymmetric upper extremity involvement.
- Peripheral neuropathy is not likely given the constellation of other symptoms presented.

Ans. C

10. An 83-year-old male with a history of Parkinson disease presents to clinic for a follow-up appointment. His wife has noticed that he is not sleeping well. At night he appears restless, yells, and seems to be running in his sleep. She has been kicked on several occasions, so she sleeps in the next room. Which of the following is true of this condition?

A. First-line treatment is amitriptyline

B. Polysomnogram (PSG) shows rapid eye movement (REM) sleep without atonia

C. PSG shows an abrupt onset of motor activity during slow wave sleep

D. Genetic testing for mutations in CHRNA2 would be positive

Explanation:

- This patient presents with REM sleep behavior disorder (RBD). This is a disorder that generally starts in middle age or in the elderly and is more common in men.
- It is typically seen in association with neurodegenerative conditions like Parkinson disease, progressive supranuclear palsy, multiple system atrophy, and various dementias.
- This disorder involves he loss of REM atonia, resulting in patients acting out their dreams. This involves talking, yelling, kicking movements, arm movements, or walking. It can result in injury to the patient or the bed partner, as well as result in very vivid dreams often confused with hallucinations.
- PSG is not necessary for the diagnosis, although if performed, it would demonstrate increased electromyogram activity during REM sleep.
- PSG findings of an abrupt onset of motor activity during slow wave sleep are consistent with night terrors, not RBD. Amitriptyline, other tricyclics, sedative-hypnotics, and anticholinergics can cause or exacerbate this disorder. CHRNA2 mutations are common in autosomal-dominant frontal lobe epilepsy.
- RBD can be confused with frontal seizures due to the occurrence at night and odd behaviors.

Ans. B

11. An 8-year-old boy presents with frequent staring episodes while in class. Based on the electroencephalogram (EEG) shown, which of the following is the most appropriate medication for this patient?

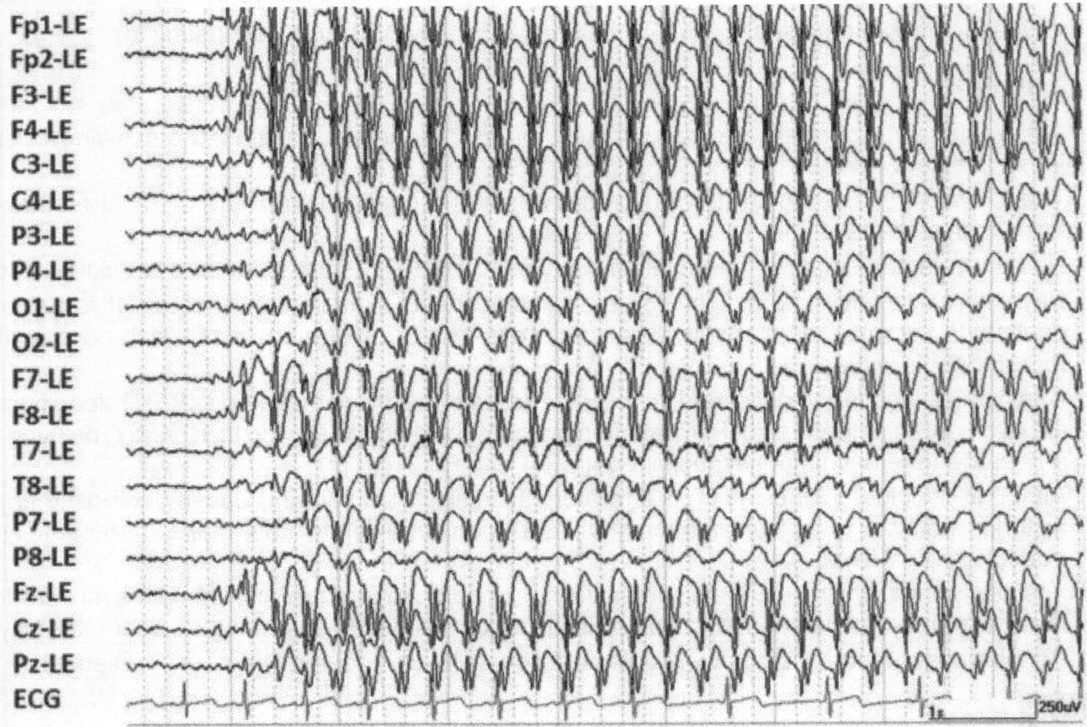

A. Valproic acid
B. Ethosuximide
C. Phenytoin
D. Levetiracetam

Explanation:

- EEG demonstrates the typical 3-Hz spike and wave pattern seen in absence epilepsy.
- Best medication for absence epilepsy is ethosuximide.
- Valproic acid is also used in absence epilepsy, but typically if there are generalized tonic-clonic seizures in addition to staring episodes.
- Phenytoin and carbamazepine have the potential to worsen generalized epilepsy.
- Levetiracetam is also good option for generalized epilepsy, but is not best choice listed.

Ans. B

12. A 72-year-old female smoker was active and independent, taking hormone replacement as her only medication. She spent all weekend in her yard pulling weeds in the warm summer sun. The next day, she complained of headaches, but declined an appointment with her physician. Her headache worsened, and she became confused then sleepy over the next 2 days. She passed away at home alone and was later found by her daughter. An image of her brain taken at autopsy is shown. Which of the following would have been appropriate therapy had she sought emergency care?

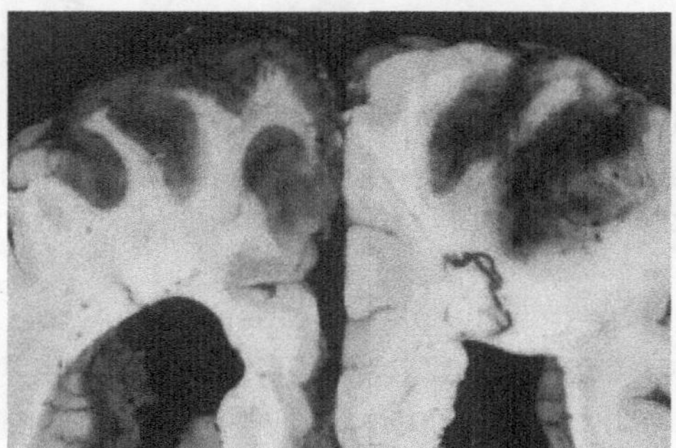

A. Triple H therapy
B. Intravenous tissue plasminogen activator therapy
C. Platelets and clotting factors
D. Unfractionated heparin and intravenous fluids

Explanation:

- Case and image are classic for cerebral venous thrombosis. The woman was prothrombotic due to smoking and estrogen use and likely became hypovolemic in the sun. The pathology image demonstrates thrombosed cortical veins as well as superficial hemorrhage. The best treatment for cerebral venous thrombosis is volume expansion and anticoagulation, usually with unfractionated heparin.
- Triple H therapy (hypertension, hypervolemia, hemodilution) is appropriate for subarachnoid hemorrhage. Platelets and clotting factors are appropriate for intracerebral hemorrhage if there is history of antiplatelet or anticoagulant use or laboratory evidence of clotting cascade insufficiency.
- Normotension and observation would not be appropriate for cerebral venous thrombosis.

Ans. D

13. A 60 year elderly male consumed excessive laxatives for his constipation, followed which he had multiple episodes of diarrhoea, suddenly developed seizures. Acute management of seizures includes all except:

A. Patient should be placed in semi prone position with head to the side to avoid aspiration.
B. Tongue blades or other objects should be forced between clenched teeth to prevent tongue bite

C. Oxygen should be given via face mask.
D. Reversible metabolic disorders should be promptly corrected.

Explanation:

Acute management of seizures

- Patient should be placed in semi prone position with head to the side to avoid aspiration.
- Tongue blades or other objects should not be forced between clenched teeth.
- Oxygen should be given via face mask.
- Reversible metabolic disorders (e.g., hypoglycemia, hyponatremia, hypocalcemia, and drug or alcohol withdrawal) should be promptly corrected.

Ans. B

14. A 42-year-old man develops vertical diplopia, which seems worst when watching television from bed. On examination, he has left hypertropia, which is exacerbated with downward gaze of an adducted left eye. If he tilts his head to the right, the vision improves. Which of the following is the affected cranial nerve?

A. Right oculomotor nerve
B. Left abducens nerve
C. Left trochlear nerve
D. Right trochlear nerve

Explanation:

- Trochlear nerve innervates the superior oblique muscle, whose job is to abduct, depress, and intort eye.
- With trochlear nerve palsy, patients generally have vertical diplopia that is worsened by looking down nose—watching television from bed or descending stairs. Resting gaze tends to have hypertropia ipsilateral to the affected eye.
- Bielschowsky head tilt test may also help localize the affected nerve, as tilting the head away from the affected eye leads to globe extorsion and correction of the diplopia.
- Individuals with chronic trochlear nerve palsy may have a chronic head tilt as an unconscious compensatory movement.

Ans. C

15. A 63-year-old male presents to the clinic with memory problems. Over the last several months he developed problems with his speech. He frequently calls objects by the wrong name or cannot come up with the words he wants to say. His neurological examination is normal, and magnetic resonance imaging (MRI) of his brain shows temporal lobe atrophy. On mental status examination he is alert and oriented. His speech is clear and he can repeat, but he has difficulty with naming objects. He frequently replaces words with either nonsensical words or the wrong words. He is able to remember three words at 3 minutes, draw intersecting pentagons, and draw a clock accurately. In 1 minute he was only able to name four animals. Which of the following is the most likely diagnosis?

A. Alzheimer disease
B. Dementia with Lewy bodies
C. Primary progressive aphasia
D. Mild cognitive impairment

Explanation:

- Primary progressive aphasia is a subclass of frontotemporal dementia that involves progressive loss of speech to the point of mutism. This patient presents with normal memory and orientation but has paraphasic errors.
- Memory and visuospatial function should be normal. Early in the disease this disorder may not be appreciated unless testing of verbal fluency is performed, including categorical fluency (naming as many animals as possible in 1 minute, or naming as many words starting with the letter "S" as possible in 1 minute) or more formal testing like the Boston Naming Test.
- Alzheimer disease would present with short-term memory loss and visuospatial dysfunction, in addition to anomic aphasia.

- Dementia with Lewy bodies presents with well-formed visual hallucinations, fluctuating levels of alertness, memory loss, and parkinsonism. Mild cognitive impairment is a disorder of mild memory impairment that is isolated and not significant enough to affect daily life.
- Although this patient's language dysfunction is isolated, the speech abnormalities are significant and abnormalities are noted on imaging.
- Vascular dementia is the second most common type of dementia and results from cerebral ischemia, usually progressing in a stepwise fashion, related to either large or small infarcts. This often results in poor short-term memory and slow processing, and can appear similar to Alzheimer disease except the MRI shows multiple ischemic lesions.
- This disorder should be recognized because with stroke risk reduction measures, the underlying process of this type of dementia can be slowed.

Ans. C

16. A 63-year-old man presents to the neurology clinic for burning pain in both feet, causing discomfort while walking. He also feels as if something is stuck in his shoe at times. His examination is notable for normal vibration, pinprick, and temperature sensation, although he complains of tenderness to palpation of his feet. His deep tendon reflexes are normal. Which of the following is not true?

A. Diagnosis is often made on skin biopsy

B. Nerve conduction studies are usually normal

C. Disorders of glucose dysregulation cause the majority of cases

D. Examination usually shows impaired proprioception and light touch

Explanation:

- This case discusses the most common scenario of an early peripheral polyneuropathy. He has a normal neurological examination with no evidence of largefiber nerve dysfunction, although he is symptomatic because his small peripheral nerve fibers are affected (myelinated Aδ and unmyelinated C-fibers).
- Given that he has normal vibration and pin prick on his examination, his A-alpha and A-beta fibers are likely unaffected. Typically, proprioception and light touch are also normal. Many patients report the feeling of a wrinkle in their sock or small pebbles in their shoe. They also may report coldlike pain, tingling, or pins and needles sensation with burning or allodynia. There are many causes of small-fiber neuropathy, but diabetes and insulin resistance are the most frequent causes, as indicated by an abnormal 2-hour glucose tolerance test or abnormal fasting glucose level. Other conditions that can lead to small-fiber neuropathy include human immunodeficiency virus, Guillain-Barré syndrome, hepatitis C, complex regional pain syndrome type 1, paraproteinemias, lupus, Sjögren syndrome, amyloidosis, and paraneoplastic syndromes.
- Diagnosis of small-fiber neuropathy is frequently made with a skin biopsy, which shows a reduction in the nerve fiber density.
- Electromyography and nerve conduction studies are normal, as these tests detect large-fiber pathology.

Ans. D

17. A 24-year-old woman with asthma has several years' history of recurrent headaches that are severe, pulsatile, and holocephalic in nature, with associated nausea. The headaches occur at least twice per week and tend to last about half a day, after which she feels "worthless" for the remainder of the day. She refused a trial of oral birth control pills due to religious beliefs. Based on the suspected headache diagnosis, which of the following would be appropriate first-line daily therapy?

A. Sumatriptan

B. Topiramate

C. Amitriptyline

D. Valproic acid

Explanation:

- Patient suffers from migraine without aura. Given the frequency of her headaches, daily preventive therapy is indicated.

- Amitriptyline is considered a first-line migraine therapy, and is safe both in case of pregnancy and with a history of asthma.
- Propranolol is also a preferred medication in migraineurs of childbearing potential, but is contraindicated with a history of asthma.
- Both valproic acid and topiramate may be efficacious for migraine, but are associated with teratogenicity; given the patient's refusal to use birth control, these would be less favored.
- Sumatriptan is useful for abortive therapy in case of migraine, but frequent use can result in rebound headaches.

Ans. C

18. A 55-year-old man presents with a 3-month history of progressive right hemiparesis. A contrast-enhanced magnetic resonance image of the brain was obtained in the emergency room and is shown here. What is the most likely diagnosis for the lesion shown?

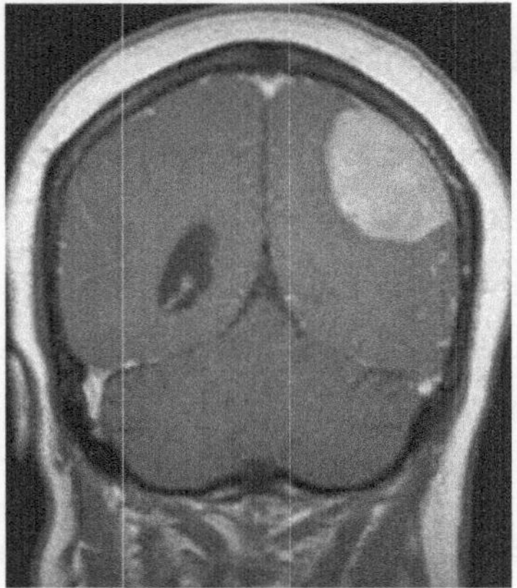

A. Meningioma B. Glioblastoma

C. Central nervous system (CNS) lymphoma D. Ependymoma

Explanation:

- Image most likely demonstrates a meningioma arising from the convexity.
- Most telling characteristics of the image include the lightbulb– bright, homogeneous enhancement pattern, extraparenchymal location, and the dural tail at superior margin.
- Glioblastoma would generally appear as an intraaxial, centrally necrotic mass with rim enhancement, substantial edema, and mass effect; it often extends to the corpus callosum.
- CNS lymphoma, although generally homogeneous in enhancement pattern among immunocompetent patients, is most commonly intraaxial, abuts the ventricular system, and demonstrates hypointensity on an apparent diffusion coefficient map related to restricted diffusion from high cellularity.
- Intracranial ependymomas are generally intraventricular tumors (either lateral ventricles or, more commonly, third or fourth ventricles), with heterogeneous enhancement.
- Metastasis is generally rim enhancing, often presenting with multiple lesions, with substantial edema and mass effect, and often in watershed distributions

Ans. A

19. A 53-year-old female presents to your outpatient clinic with 3 months of pain in the left arm. She describes a burning and tingling pain in the lateral aspect of her forearm and her left thumb. Examination reveals normal strength and normal cranial nerves. She has reduced sensation over the lateral aspect of her forearm and her entire left thumb, but no sensory loss in other parts of the hand. Her biceps and brachioradialis reflexes are reduced. Which of the following muscles would most likely show electromyography (EMG) abnormalities?

A. First dorsal interosseous and abductor pollicis brevis
B. Flexor pollicis longus and flexor carpi ulnaris
C. Brachioradialis and pronator teres
D. Triceps and extensor indicis proprius

Explanation:

- This patient has a C6 radiculopathy on the left side. She has dermatomal sensory loss in a pattern consistent with a C6 radiculopathy. The area of sensory loss is innervated by the lateral antebrachial cutaneous nerve, superficial radial sensory, and median nerve. The only area in which these nerves all meet is at the C6 root. EMG should show abnormalities in muscles with significant C6 innervation, like the biceps, brachioradialis, triceps, pronator teres and brachialis.

Ans. C

20. Familial hemiplegic migraine 2 is due to involvement of which of the following ion channels?

A. Sodium- Poatssium ATPase
B. SCN 1A
C. SCN 4A
D. SCN 5A

Explanation:

- Mutations involving the Cav2.1 (P/Q)–type voltage-gated calcium channel *CACNA1A* gene are now known to cause FHM 1; this mutation is responsible for about 50% of FHM cases.
- **Mutations in Na+- K+ ATPase *ATP1A2* gene, designated FHM 2, are responsible for about 20% of FHMs.**
- Mutations in the neuronal voltage-gated sodium channel *SCN1A* cause FHM 3.

Ans. A

21. A patient presents to the emergency department with acute horizontal binocular diplopia and left hemiparesis. Examination reveals mild ptosis and mydriasis on the right, as well as weakness of medial rectus, superior rectus, inferior rectus, and inferior oblique muscles on the right. Which of the following is the most likely location of this stroke?

A. Midbrain tegmentum
B. Lateral medulla
C. Cerebral peduncle
D. Angular gyrus

Explanation:

- Weber syndrome (ipsilateral oculomotor palsy, contralateral hemiparesis) localizes to the cerebral peduncle where the oculomotor fascicles and corticospinal tracts are adjacent to each other. This results from occlusion of branches from the posterior cerebral artery (PCA) or the top of the basilar. Claude syndrome (ipsilateral oculomotor palsy, contralateral ataxia) results from infarction in the midbrain tegmentum where the oculomotor fascicles and red nucleus are adjacent. Similarly, this results from occlusion of branches of the PCA or top of the basilar. Wallenberg syndrome (vertigo, nystagmus, dysphagia, ipsilateral ataxia, ipsilateral Horner syndrome, ipsilateral facial numbness, contralateral hemisensory loss to pain and temperature) results from lateral medullary lesions where the trigeminal nucleus, restiform body, vestibular nucleus, nucleus ambiguous, spinothalamic tract, and sympathetic tract are adjacent. This is generally related to occlusion of distal branches from the vertebral arteries. Gerstmann syndrome (agraphia, acalculia, finger agnosia, and left–right confusion) localizes to the dominant angular gyrus on the parietal lobe. This syndrome is often related to occlusion of the middle cerebral artery. Dejerine-Roussy syndrome (ipsilateral tongue weakness, contralateral weakness and sensory loss to vibration and proprioception) is related to a medial medullary lesion, where the hypoglossal nucleus, pyramidal tract, and medial lemniscus are adjacent. This generally results from occlusion of the anteromedial artery (off the vertebral artery) or from basilar artery perforators.

Ans. C

22. A 6-month-old was brought to the emergency room with eye movement abnormalities and head bobbing, which were thought to represent seizure. On examination, the patient appears to be comfortable and in no apparent distress. He has nystagmus, which is primarily horizontal, and head nodding. Additionally, his neck intermittently turns to the left. Brain imaging is normal, as is the remainder of the patient's neurological examination. Which of the following is the most likely diagnosis?

A. Congenital nystagmus
B. Seizure
C. Chiari malformation
D. Spasmus nutans

Explanation:

- Patient has spasmus nutans, which is a triad of pendular nystagmus, head nodding, and cervical dystonia. Most cases begin between 4 and 12 months of age and are sporadic, although rarely patients with spasmus nutans may be found to have structural causes such as tumors in the optic pathway. The nystagmus can be horizontal, vertical, or rotatory and is usually pronounced more in one eye than the other. Further, the nystagmus is almost never synchronized between the two eyes, and most often is associated with a disconjugate gaze. The head motion associated with spasmus nutans is usually oblique with both nodding and shaking and is usually a compensatory measure that suppresses nystagmus. The cervical dystonia is not always present, but occurs in up to 30% of the patients with spasmus nutans. Idiopathic spasmus nutans is considered self-limiting and transient, lasting only a few months to years. Alternatively, congenital nystagmus almost always begins at less than 6 months old and is not associated with head nodding or cervical dystonia. In addition, congenital nystagmus has a larger amplitude, slower frequency, and does not usually resolve. Seizures are typically associated with forced gaze deviation or head deviation rather than nystagmus or nodding. A Chiari malformation may have downward nystagmus but without the association of head nodding or cervical dystonia. Benign paroxysmal torticollis may have intermittent episodes of cervical dystonia, but does not have nystagmus.

Ans. D

23. A colleague presents to the office with her husband for an evaluation. He is a 56-year-old male cardiologist with no significant medical history whose wife is concerned about recent changes in his behavior, including gambling and inappropriate sexual comments at work. His wife has also noticed that he mixes up the names of medications, but he insists there is nothing wrong. His neurological examination is unremarkable, and he scores 28/30 on the mini mental state examination. He was able to name seven animals in 1 minute. Laboratory work is normal, including a complete blood count, metabolic panel, liver enzymes, urine drug screen, vitamin B12, thyroid stimulating hormone, and rapid plasma regain. Magnetic resonance imaging (MRI) of his brain is also unremarkable. Which of the following is true of this condition?

A. FDG-PET scan shows hypometabolism of posterior temporoparietal region
B. This is caused by buildup of amyloid protein
C. Lithium is commonly used for behavioral control
D. Obsessions and hoarding are common behaviors

Explanation:

- The patient presents with behavioral variant frontotemporal dementia (FTD), which is marked by early behavioral changes, including impulsivity, hypersexuality, obsessions, and compulsions. Other common features include difficulty with planning, early loss of speech, and apathy. MRI may show anterior temporal and frontal atrophy. FDG-PET scans show anterior temporal and frontal lobe hypometabolism, whereas posterior temporoparietal hypometabolism is seen in Alzheimer disease. FTD is caused by a buildup of tau protein, which can be seen histologically as Pick bodies, whereas neurofibrillary tangles are seen in Alzheimer disease. Frequently trazodone, selective serotonin reuptake inhibitors, and antipsychotics are used for behavioral control. Lithium is used in the treatment of bipolar disorder. Although he has some impulsivity and hypersexuality, the presence of memory loss and language dysfunction points to FTD rather than a manic episode.

Ans. D

24. Drug that maintains mini mental state examination score close to year in average patient is:

A. Anti cholinesterase inhibitor
B. Ginkgo biloba
C. Memantine
D. HMG CoA reductase inhibitors

Explanation:

- Average patient on an anticholinesterase inhibitor maintains his or her mini-mental state examination (MMSE) score for close to a year, whereas a placebo-treated patient declines 2–3 points over the same time period.
- Memantine, used in conjunction with cholinesterase inhibitors or by itself, slows cognitive deterioration and decreases caregiver burden for patients with moderate to severe AD, but is not approved for mild AD.
- Each of these compounds has only modest efficacy for AD.
- Cholinesterase inhibitors are relatively easy to administer, and their major side effects are gastrointestinal symptoms (nausea, diarrhea, cramps), altered sleep with unpleasant or vivid dreams, bradycardia (usually benign), and muscle cramps

Ans. B

25. A 45-year-old man has recently moved from Mexico. He suffers a focal seizure followed by secondary generalization. He denies symptoms of active infection and has not suffered any recent trauma. His neurological examination has returned to normal in the emergency room. A magnetic resonance image (MRI) of the brain is shown. Which of the following is the next best step in management?

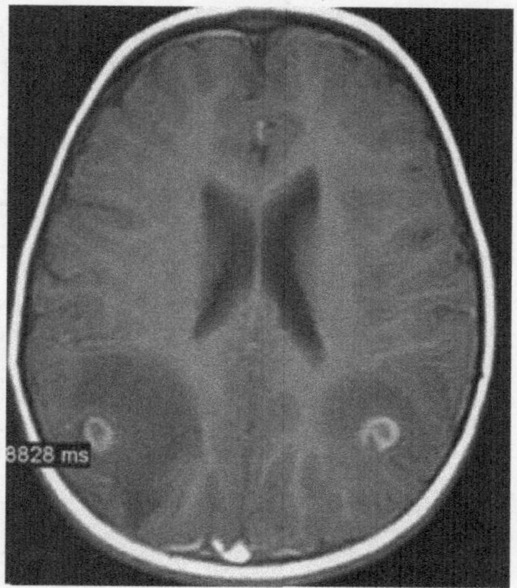

A. Levetiracetam and albendazole
B. Levetiracetam and acyclovir
C. Lacosamide and a biopsy of the largest lesion
D. Lacosamide, vancomycin and cefepime

Explanation:

- Clinical presentation and MRI findings are classic for neurocysticercosis, a tapeworm infection with Taenia solium, which is often related to ingestion of undercooked pork. This disease is commonly seen in individuals from Mexico and South America. Whereas treatment with an antihelminth may be safely avoided in cases of completely calcified cysts, the cysts on this patient's MRI appear active with a scolex, suggesting that treatment may be beneficial in reducing subsequent seizure risk. As such, treating with both levetiracetam and albendazole is warranted. Levetiracetam and acyclovir is not suggested, as there is no evidence of viral infection in the history or on MRI. Although lacosamide may also be used for focal seizures, neither a biopsy nor antibiotics would be warranted in this patient currently. Finally, methylprednisolone would not necessarily provide any therapeutic benefit for this patient in the absence of edema or inflammatory disease.

Ans. A

26. Coat hanger headache is most likely due to:

A. Migraine

B. Subarachnoid hemorrhage

C. Sinusitis

D. Neck muscle ischemia

Explanation:

- Neck pain, typically in suboccipital, posterior cervical, and shoulder region ("coat-hanger headache"), most likely due to neck muscle ischemia, may be only symptom.

Ans. D

27. A 57-year-old alcoholic was found unresponsive behind a gas station. A head computed tomography was negative for hemorrhage. Complete blood count and basic metabolic profile were normal. His examination demonstrates a somnolent male who wakes up briefly to painful stimulation, grunts, and moves all of his extremities equally. He is afebrile, and no nuchal rigidity is noted. The electroencephalogram (EEG) is shown here. Which of the following is the most likely diagnosis?

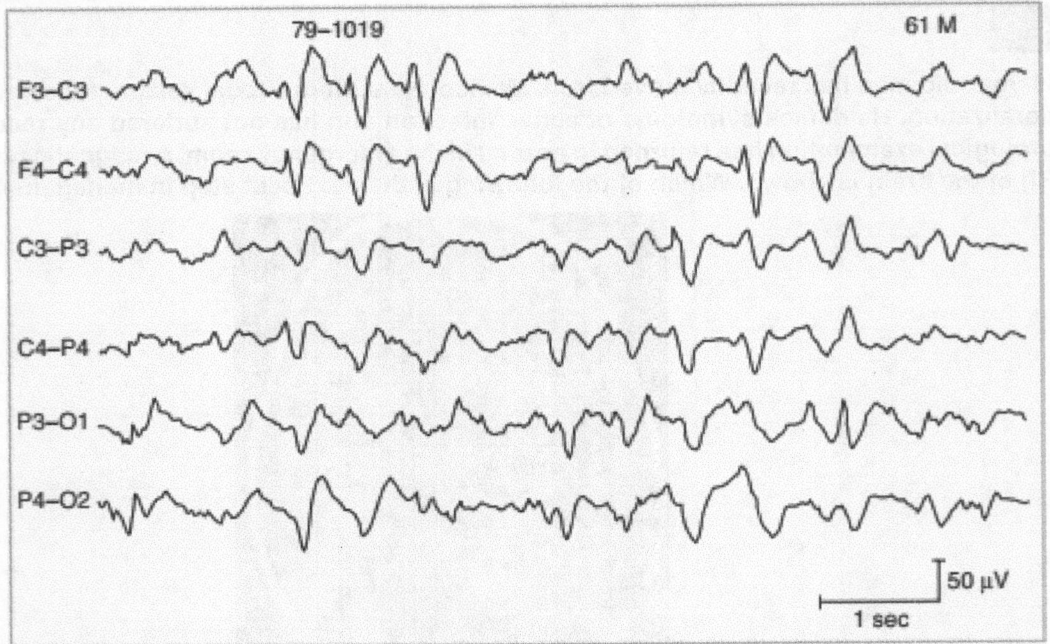

A. Herpes encephalitis

B. Nonconvulsive status epilepticus

C. Hepatic encephalopathy

D. Ischemic stroke

Explanation:

- EEG demonstrates triphasic waves, which are classically seen in hepatic encephalopathy, but they can be seen in other metabolic or toxic encephalopathies. The patient's history of alcoholism should also point to hepatic encephalopathy. The EEG in herpes encephalitis would show temporal periodic lateralized epileptiform discharges (PLEDs). The EEG in nonconvulsive status epilepticus would show rhythmic discharges with spikes and slow waves, which can be confused with triphasic waves. The EEG in acute strokes is frequently normal, but focal slowing or even focal PLEDs can be seen in some cases. Meningitis does not have any characteristic EEG findings, but seizures and various levels of encephalopathy can be seen

Ans. C

28. A 26-year-old man with a history of Tourette syndrome presents for new symptoms that are causing great distress with maintaining a job. He is often late for work because he feels the need to check the lock on his front door five times each morning. If he forgets or is distracted, he feels the need to start

over and recheck the door five times. Another example he provides includes stepping up on curbs three times and tapping the wall four times before walking through a doorway. What is the most likely diagnosis?

A. Manifestations of his Tourette syndrome

B. Panic disorder with agoraphobia

C. Obsessive-compulsive disorder (OCD)

D. Obsessive-compulsive personality disorder (OCPD)

Explanation:

- OCD often coexists with Tourette syndrome. Obsessions are recurring ideas or thoughts that are intrusive, causing great anxiety and stress. Compulsions are repetitive behaviors such as counting, checking, or repeating actions. Most patients realize that the obsessions or compulsions are unreasonable and excessive. OCD can be very time consuming, often affecting school or workplace performance. Treatment involves selective serotonin reuptake inhibitors, tricyclic antidepressants, and psychotherapy involving various forms of behavioral therapy. Imaging usually shows decreased caudate size and hypermetabolism in the frontal cortex. Although OCD can coexist with Tourette syndrome, there is no indication that these are motor tics, as there is no indication of preceding urge or sense of relief after. Panic disorder is less likely, as there is no mention of panic attacks. OCPD is incorrect, as the obsessions and compulsions in this case are seen as unhealthy and unwanted, which tend to go with OCD rather than OCPD. In OCPD, they are often rational and desirable. There is no indication of paranoia such as distrust or suspiciousness to suggest paranoid personality disorder.

Ans. C

29. A 32-year-old female who is 27 weeks pregnant presents to your office for evaluation of abnormal movements. She cannot sit still and is always fidgeting. Her husband says her arms always move but this stops when she goes to sleep. She has no urge to move and does not get a sense of relief with movements. There is no family history of movement disorders, and she is not taking any medications. Her neurological examination is normal except for abnormal movements of her arms that seem to flow from body part to body part. They do not interrupt her ability to reach for objects or keep her from walking. Laboratory work, including a complete blood count, metabolic panel, liver function tests, thyroid-stimulating hormone, and ceruloplasmin, were normal. Which of the following is true of this condition?

A. There is a high risk of recurrence with future pregnancies

B. Her child has a 50% chance of inheriting this disorder

C. Treatment with haloperidol is necessary

D. Slit lamp examination would demonstrate Kayser Fleischer rings

Explanation:

- This patient presents with movements concerning for chorea. These can be described as movements that flow from one part of the body to the next without interrupting overall movements. Patients are able to walk, but have a "lurching" gait. They can reach for objects, but may have extra movements on the way to that object. Chorea gravidarum is not uncommon and typically starts in the second to fifth month of pregnancy and typically resolves within a few months of delivery without needing treatment. There is a high risk of recurrence with future pregnancies. Low doses of haloperidol or similar dopamine antagonists can be useful if treatment is needed, but these are rarely required and not necessary in most patients. Without a family history and given her pregnancy status, an autosomal-dominant disorder like Huntington disease is less likely. Wilson disease would show Kayser Fleischer rings on slit lamp examination, but this patient's ceruloplasmin and liver function tests are normal. Her movements are not tics because there is no urge to move, no sense of relief with the movements, and cannot be suppressed. Clonidine is helpful with tics but not chorea.

Ans. A

30. After an 18-hour delivery, a 26-year-old woman with a history of relapsing remitting multiple sclerosis gives birth to her first child. After her epidural wears off, the patient goes for a walk in the hall and notices that both feet slap the floor more loudly than before. There is tingling on the lateral aspect of both lower legs, but otherwise intact strength and sensation throughout. Which is the most likely mechanism of her problem?

A. Side effect of oxytocin

B. Lumbosacral plexopathy resulting from pelvic trauma

C. Uhthoff phenomenon after strenuous labor

D. Compressive neuropathy of bilateral common peroneal (fibular) nerves

Explanation:

- The common peroneal (fibular) nerve passes over the fibular head superficially. In prolonged childbirth, if a woman holds back her legs around the knees or malpositions her legs in the stirrups, she may compress these nerves and lead to temporary peroneal neuropathy. Generally the symptoms of weakness and numbness will resolve spontaneously within weeks, although the patient may benefit from an ankle–foot orthotic to prevent falls as her strength returns. Neither oxytocin nor epidural anesthesia causes mononeuropathies. A lumbosacral plexopathy may result from pelvic trauma, but would present with more widespread symptoms. Although the risk of multiple sclerosis relapse is thought to increase during the first few postpartum months, there is little study of Uhthoff phenomenon after delivery. Further, although foot drop may be seen with either a multiple sclerosis flare or Uhthoff phenomenon (assuming prior symptom thereof), this is most likely to result from a central nervous system lesion and therefore would not have concurrent sensory loss in the same peripheral nerve distribution.

Ans. D

31. Anterior choroidal artery occlusion is characterized by:

A. Abulia

B. Homonymous hemianopia

C. Aphasia

D. Anosognosia

Explanation:

- This artery arises from internal carotid artery and supplies posterior limb of internal capsule & white matter posterolateral to it, through which pass some of geniculocalcarine fibers.
- Complete syndrome of anterior choroidal artery occlusion consists of contralateral hemiplegia, hemianesthesia (hypesthesia), and homonymous hemianopia.
- However, because this territory is also supplied by penetrating vessels of the proximal MCA and the posterior communicating and posterior choroidal arteries, minimal deficits may occur, and patients frequently recover substantially.
- Anterior choroidal strokes are usually the result of in situ thrombosis of the vessel, and the vessel is particularly vulnerable to iatrogenic occlusion during surgical clipping of aneurysms arising from the internal carotid artery.

Ans. B

32. A 25-year-old woman presents with a history of left arm automatisms and lip smacking, followed by a generalized convulsion. Her history is also remarkable for recurring headaches previously attributed as migraines. An axial magnetic resonance image (MRI) is shown. Which of the following is considered the most likely diagnosis?

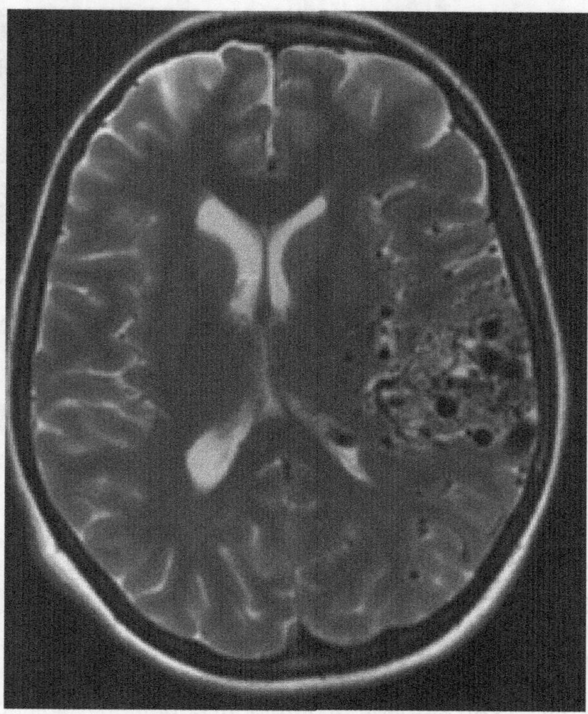

A. Developmental venous anomaly
B. Cavernous malformation
C. Cerebral aneurysm
D Arteriovenous malformation

Explanation:

- Most likely diagnosis is a complex partial seizure with secondary generalization from an arteriovenous malformation (AVM, seen in the MRI).
- AVMs are arteriovenous connections without capillary networks, usually with gliotic brain tissue within AVM. These often present with hemorrhages, headaches, or seizures. Typically, AVMs are observed if unruptured, but several factors are taken into consideration when determining whether or not to intervene: age, surgical risk, location, gender, and lifetime hemorrhage risk.
- Treatment options include surgical resection, radiosurgery, endovascular embolization, or a multimodal approach (especially if >3 cm).
- Spetzler-Martin grading system is a scale of 1–5 that helps estimate the risk of surgical repair of AVMs. A developmental venous anomaly is a congenital malformation of veins that drain normal brain and is considered one of the most common cerebral vascular malformations. On imaging, it appears as a curvilinear enhancing structure best seen on contrast sequences or susceptibility weighted imaging. A cavernous malformation is a collection of vessels without elastic tissue and has no normal brain parenchyma between the hyalinized vessels. They typically appear as a "popcorn kernel" on T2 imaging.
- An aneurysm is a weakening of a vessel wall that creates either a saccular aneurysm or a fusiform aneurysm.
- Capillary telangiectasias are capillary-sized vessels that have normal brain tissue in between them and are typically found in the pons. They often appear as ill-defined areas of focal enhancement.

Ans. D

33. A 33-year-old woman presents with an inability to sit still and difficulty sleeping, which have developed gradually over 3 years. On examination, there are subtle choreiform movements involving both the trunk and the distal upper extremities. She also has delayed initiation of saccades, as well as tongue impersistence. She is adopted, but knows that her mother committed suicide after years of abusing drugs. Her magnetic resonance image (MRI) is shown. What is the most likely diagnosis?

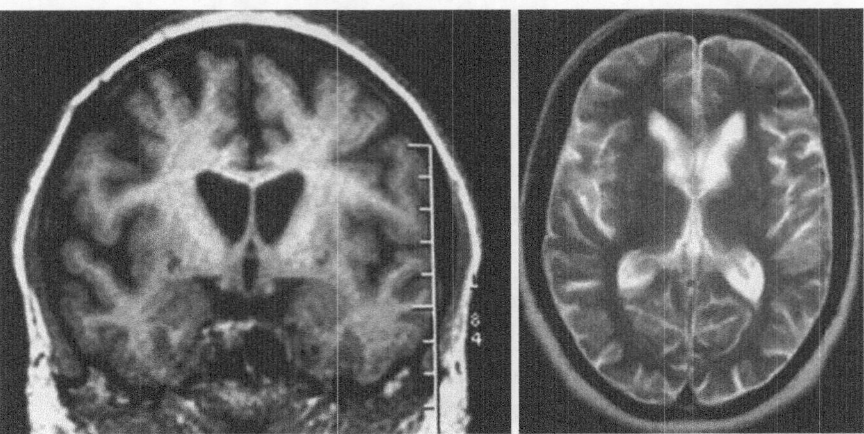

A. Stroke

B. Sydenham chorea

C. Anti–N-methyl-D-aspartate (anti-NMDA) encephalitis

D. Huntington disease

Explanation:

- Huntington disease (HD) is an autosomal dominant condition resulting from an expansion of CAG repeats of the HD gene on chromosome 4.
- Generally, HD appears with more than 40 CAG repeats and tends to be earlier onset with greater numbers of repeats, known as genetic anticipation.
- From a psychiatric perspective, patients can have depression, irritability, psychosis, obsessive-compulsive disorder, or even suicide. Many times, patients will complain of difficulty with sleep initiation as well.
- Examination will often show parkinsonism, especially in young onset HD. Other examination findings include dystonia and chorea (either facial, truncal, distal extremities, or generalized). Imaging will often show atrophy or absence of the caudate, resulting in "box-car ventricles."
- In this case, the gradual onset (rather than acute) of both motor and psychiatric symptoms in setting of family history of suicide and drug use makes HD high on the differential. Even if family history is unknown or reportedly negative, genetic testing should still be completed.
- A stroke of the subthalamic nucleus can also lead to choreiform movements, but the onset is usually acute and leads to unilateral chorea. There is nothing in the question stem indicating a recent streptococcal infection that would point toward Sydenham chorea. Anti-NMDA receptor encephalitis has been associated with chorea, but would not show an absence of caudate nuclei. Substance abuse resulting in dopamine release, such as cocaine intoxication, can also lead to chorea, but usually has an acute onset and would not have absent caudate nuclei.

Ans. D

34. A 17-year-old male presents to your office for evaluation of excessive sleepiness. He falls asleep frequently in class and even fell asleep while giving a speech in class. His mother notes that when he is angry, he will drop objects or become "weak in the knees." He will frequently wake in the morning but be unable to move or speak for 3 minutes before he can get out of bed. Which of the following would be seen in this condition?

A. Apnea-Hypopnea Index (AHI) of 15

B. Electroencephalogram (EEG) with continuous slow wave and spikes during sleep

C. Sleep latency of 20 minutes

D. Low cerebrospinal fluid hypocretin level

Explanation:

- This patient presents with signs and symptoms concerning for narcolepsy with cataplexy. This is disorder marked by sleep attacks, cataplexy, hypnogogic hallucinations, and sleep paralysis.
- Patients with this disorder typically have a hypocretin (also known as orexin) deficiency in the lateral hypothalamus. This can be tested with a lumbar puncture. Levels <200 pg/mL suggest narcolepsy, whereas levels <110 pg/mL are diagnostic.
- Sleep apnea can occur in narcolepsy, but an AHI of 15 would only prove there is sleep apnea, not narcolepsy.
- EEG showing continuous slow wave and spikes during sleep is seen with Landau-Kleffner syndrome, not narcolepsy. EEG in narcolepsy is normal and shows normal rapid eye movement (REM) during sleep attacks.
- Narcolepsy is associated with a short sleep latency, usually <5 minutes, and associated sleep-onset REM. Kleine-Levin syndrome is a syndrome of hypersomnolence associated with hyperphagia and hypersexuality, but no associated cataplexy, sleep attacks, or sleep paralysis.

Ans. D

35. Most efficacious agent for severe acute attack of migraine is:

A. Sumitriptan
B. Almotriptan
C. Rizatriptan
D. Zolmitriptan

Explanation:

- Rizatriptan and eletriptan are, on a population basis, the most efficacious of triptans currently available in the United States.
- Sumatriptan and zolmitriptan have similar rates of efficacy as well as time to onset, with an advantage of having multiple formulations, whereas almotriptan has a similar rate of efficacy to sumatriptan and is better tolerated, and frovatriptan and naratriptan are somewhat slower in onset and are also well tolerated.

Ans. C

36. A 16-year-old male suffers sharp, stabbing pain across his entire head each time he coughs. The pain is severe, but resolves quickly after coughing. Which of the following should be done?

A. Daily antihistamine
B. Amitriptyline
C. Pulmonary function tests
D. Cranial magnetic resonance imaging (MRI)

Explanation:

- Primary cough headache is most commonly associated with an underlying structural cause, including a Chiari I malformation or aneurysm.
- Patients may also have similar pain with other Valsalva maneuvers. MRI should be performed to identify such a cause. Doing nothing would not be prudent, as patient may have a serious structural defect.
- Although an antihistamine may reduce coughing and a pulmonary function test would identify any respiratory illness, neither would address the underlying intracranial problem.
- Amitriptyline would not be an appropriate first-line therapy for a secondary headache syndrome.

Ans. D

37. Freezing gait is seen in all except:

A. PSP
B. MSA
C. Frontal disorder
D. Corticobasal degeneration

Explanation:

- Freezing of gait is also common in other neurodegenerative disorders associated with parkinsonism, including progressive supranuclear palsy (PSP), multiple-system atrophy, and corticobasal degeneration.
- *Freezing* is defined as a brief, episodic absence of forward progression of the feet, despite the intention to walk.
- Freezing may be triggered by approaching a narrow doorway or crowd, may be overcome by visual cueing, & contributes to fall risk.
- Gait freezing is present in approximately one-quarter of Parkinson's patients within 5 years of onset, and its frequency increases further over time.
- In treated patients, an end-of-dose gait freezing is a common problem that may improve with more frequent administration of dopaminergic drugs, or with use of monoamine oxidase type B inhibitors such as rasagiline or selegiline

Ans. C

38. A 50-year-old man experiences frequent recurrent pain on the left side of his throat, near his tonsils. He says that this feels like a hot poker. Assuming a radiographic evaluation is unrevealing, which of the following is the appropriate first-line therapy?

A. Carbamazepine
B. Amitriptyline
C. Levetiracetam
D. Phenytoin
E. Oxycodone

Explanation:

- Carbamazepine is the first-line therapy for glossopharyngeal neuralgia (as in this case), as well as for trigeminal neuralgia. Phenytoin and amitriptyline may also be tried, but as salvage options.
- Levetiracetam is not generally considered in the treatment algorithm for this disorder.Oxycodone may provide temporary benefit, but will not control the disorder overall, and so is only used for emergency or last-resort scenarios.

Ans. A

39. A 6-year-old girl presents with involuntary jerking movements of her right arm. She had several episodes of this that would last for hours before stopping spontaneously. In the last 2 weeks, the patient's mother has noted that she seems unaware during parts of these episodes and may have had shaking in her right leg and right side of her face. Her speech has been regressing. Electroencephalogram reveals left hemispheric spikes. A magnetic resonance image (MRI) of her brain is shown. Which of the following is the best treatment for this condition?

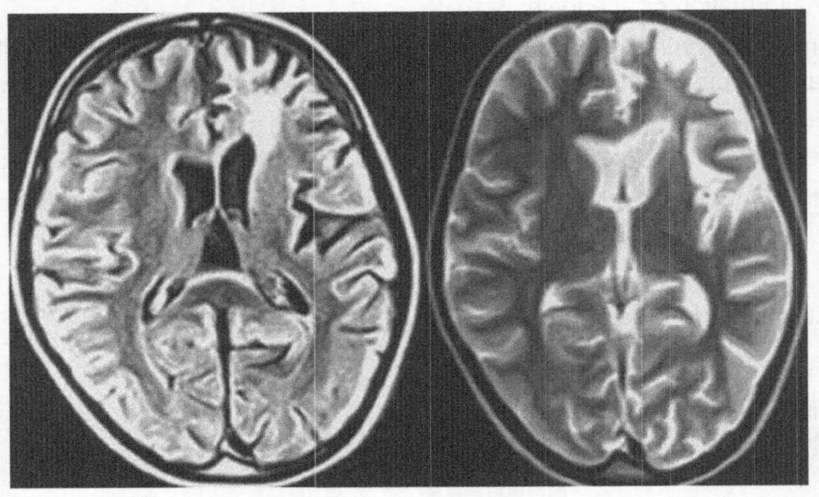

A. Carbamazepine
B. Hemispherectomy
C. Vagal nerve stimulator
D. Intravenous (IV) immunoglobulin

Explanation:

- This patient presents with Rasmussen encephalitis.
- This commonly presents with focal motor seizures, which can last for extended periods.
- Eventually these seizures progress to cause complex partial and generalized convulsion.
- Typically, epileptic discharges come from one hemisphere. Imaging can show atrophy of the affected hemisphere, as is shown in the MRI.
- Positron emission tomography will show hypometabolism of the affected hemisphere.
- Although some patients respond to IV immunoglobulin, definitive treatment is hemispherectomy.
- Both carbamazepine and valproic acid are good medications for partial-onset seizures and may be used in patients with Rasmussen encephalitis, but will not adequately control seizures.
- Vagal nerve stimulator can be used in refractory epilepsy; however, it is not the preferred surgical procedure to provide seizure relief in patients who have Rasmussen encephalitis.

Ans. B

40. Artery of percherone is branch of:

A. P1 segment
B. P2 segment
C. A1 segment
D. A2 segment

Explanation:

- *P1 syndrome*: Midbrain, subthalamic, and thalamic signs, which are due to disease of the proximal P1 segment of the PCA or its penetrating branches (thalamogeniculate, Percheron, and posterior choroidal arteries); and
- *P2 syndrome*: Cortical temporal and occipital lobe signs, due to occlusion of the P2 segment distal to the junction of the PCA with the posterior communicating artery.

Ans. A

41. A 6-year-old boy is brought to the emergency department by his parents for 3 weeks of headache, 2 weeks of increasing ataxia, and 2 days of headache and vomiting. A magnetic resonance image is obtained, and postcontrast T1 sagittal imaging is shown. Based on the most likely diagnosis, which of the following is the best first treatment?

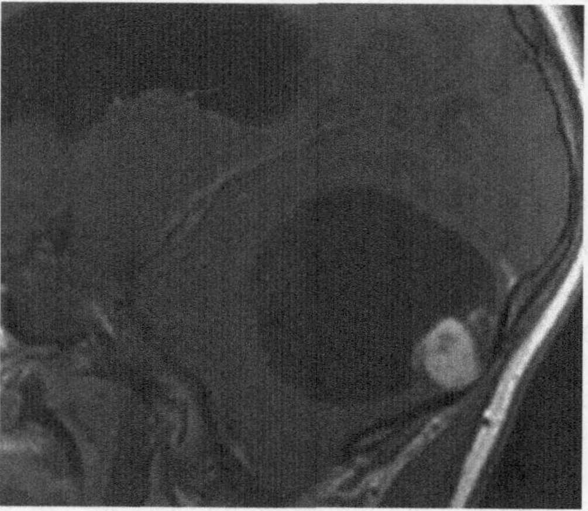

A. Intravenous antibiotics
B. Surgical resection
C. Embolization
D. Intravenous chemotherapy

Explanation:

- A cerebellar mass in a pediatric patient may represent abscess, pilocytic astrocytoma, ependymoma, hemangioblastoma, or medulloblastoma.
- Slow onset of symptoms in this patient argues against abscess.
- Appearance of an avidly enhancing mural nodule with large cystic component is most suggestive of pilocytic astrocytoma.
- As such, surgical resection is the best choice of therapy, which is often curative.
- Neither chemotherapy nor radiation is necessary for newly diagnosed pilocytic astrocytoma, and is rarely required at all if total resection is obtained.
- Embolization may be used for arteriovenous malformations or aneurysms, but is not routinely necessary for pilocytic astrocytomas.
- Finally, intravenous antibiotics would only be necessary if lesion were an abscess, along with surgical draining.

Ans. B

42. All are characteristic manifestations of Essential tremor except:

A. Typically manifests as mild high frequency (10-12 Hz)

B. Typically bilateral & symmetric but may begin on one side & remain asymmetric

C. Predominantly affects upper extremities

D. Usually neurologic examination is normal aside from tremor

Explanation:

- ET is the most common movement disorder, affecting ~5% of the population (an estimated 5–10 million persons in the United States or Western Europe). It can present in childhood but dramatically increases in prevalence in those aged >70 years.
- ET is characterized by a high frequency tremor (6–10 Hz) that predominantly affects the upper extremities.
- Tremor is most often manifest as a postural or action tremor and, in severe cases, can interfere with functions such as eating and drinking.
- It is typically bilateral and symmetric but may begin on one side and remain asymmetric. Patients with severe ET can have an intention tremor with overshoot and slowness of movement suggesting the possibility of a cerebellar origin. Tremor involves the head in ~30% of cases, voice in ~20%, tongue in ~20%, face/jaw in ~10%, and lower limbs in ~10%. Multiple body parts are involved in at least 50% of cases.
- Tremor is characteristically improved by alcohol and worsened by stress. Subtle impairment of coordination or tandem walking may be present, and disturbances of hearing, cognition, personality, mood, and olfaction have been described, but usually neurologic examination is normal aside from tremor.

Ans. A

43. A 26-year-old female patient is diagnosed with an astrocytoma. In childhood, she also suffered from osteosarcoma. Her family history is notable for several cancers in her maternal lineage, including both breast and brain tumors in her mother. Which of the following is the most likely underlying problem?

A. Li-Fraumeni syndrome

B. Neurofibromatosis 1

C. Retinoblastoma

D. Multiple endocrine neoplasia type 1

Explanation:

- Li-Fraumeni syndrome is an autosomal-dominant disorder caused by a loss of function mutation in the p53 tumor suppressor gene.

- Patients are at significantly increased risk of childhood sarcomas, early breast cancers, and brain tumors.
- Neurofibromatosis 1 (NF1) is an autosomal-dominant disorder caused by a loss of function mutation in the NF1 gene, the loss of which leads to constitutive activation of cellular growth pathways, including RAS/RAF/MEK/ERK.
- Individuals with NF1 are at increased risk of developing multiple nerve sheath tumors (neurofibromas), malignant peripheral nerve sheath tumors, gastrointestinal stromal tumors, and breast cancer.
- Retinoblastoma is a cancer of the retina that is associated with autosomal-dominant inactivation of the Rb tumor suppressor gene in 40% of patients. Other 60% of patients develop retinoblastoma spontaneously.
- Multiple endocrine neoplasia type 1 is a syndrome of cancers in the pituitary, parathyroid, and pancreas associated with autosomal-dominant mutation in the tumor suppressor gene MEN1. Von Hippel-Lindau is an autosomaldominant syndrome associated with mutations in VHL gene that leads to hemangioblastomas of the brain, clear cell carcinomas of the kidneys, and pancreatic neuroendocrine tumors.

Ans. A

44. Cremasteric reflex root value is:

A. L1 & L2
B. L3, L4 & L5
C. S1, S2 & S3
D. L4, L5 & S1

Explanation:

- Other useful cutaneous reflexes include the cremasteric (ipsilateral elevation of the testicle following stroking of the medial thigh; mediated by L1 and L2) and anal (contraction of the anal sphincter when the perianal skin is scratched; mediated by S2, S3, S4) reflexes.

Ans. A

45. A 4-month-old baby is brought to the emergency room by his grandmother, who is visiting for the weekend. He has been inconsolable for many hours. His general medical examination reveals a crying child, but is otherwise unrevealing. His neurological examination reveals slightly decreased movements in the right arm and leg compared with the left. Further, his ophthalmological examination is abnormal, shown here. A computed tomography (CT) on the head is performed and also shown here. Which of the following is the next most appropriate action?

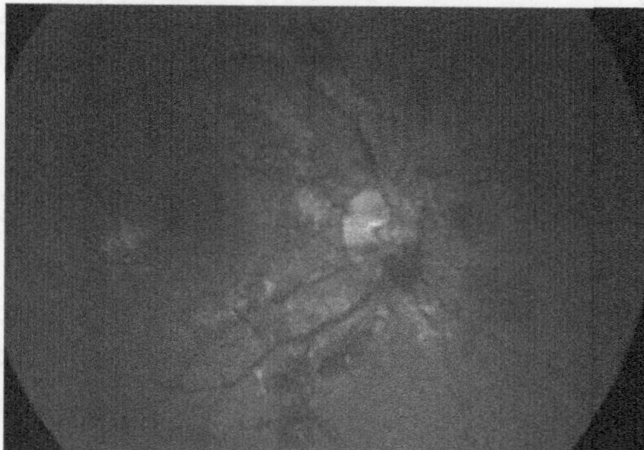
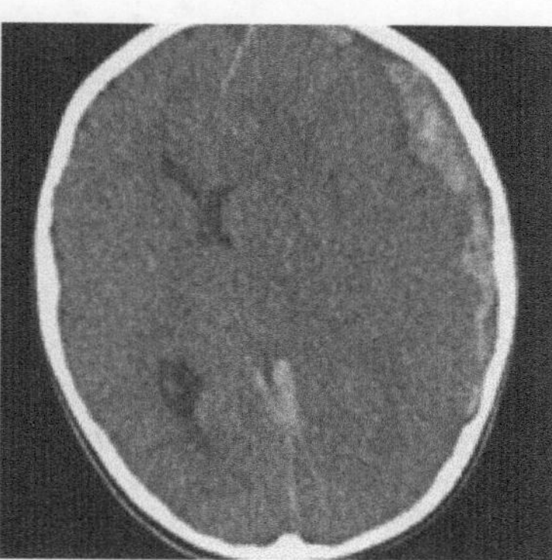

A. Renal consult for malignant hypertension
B. Neurosurgery consult for tumor resection
C. Genetics consult for Tay-Sachs disease
D. Child protective services notification for abuse

Explanation:

- Images demonstrate flame and blot retinal hemorrhages, and the CT shows a subdural hematoma.
- This is a classic pattern of findings for shaken baby syndrome.
- Child protective services should be contacted immediately upon suspicion of child abuse.

Ans. D

46. During resection of a right vestibular schwannoma, brainstem auditory evoked potentials (BAEPs) were monitored. Near the end of the surgery, there was loss of wave III and wave V, but wave I remained on the right side. These waves did not recover by the end of the surgery. BAEP on the left remained normal. What is the clinical significance of this change?

A. Significant right-sided hearing loss
B. Transient right-sided hearing loss
C. Right pontine infarct
D. Displacement of acoustic stimulator

Explanation:

- Brainstem auditory evoked potentials are useful during brainstem surgeries to monitor the cochlear nerve and brainstem for acute ischemia or injury.
- Pattern of a normal wave I and loss of wave III and V on the right and a normal BAEP on the left indicates a lesion at the next location after the cochlea, which is the cochlear nerve. With quick identification during surgery, the surgeon can quickly adjust the procedure to have the responses return.
- However, if waves III and V do not return, there is likely significant permanent hearing loss due to injury to the cochlear nerve.
- If waves III and V return, there could be transient hearing loss or no deficit at all.
- Preservation of waves I and III with bilateral loss of wave V would indicate a brainstem stroke.

Ans. A

47. Under normal circumstances which of the following structure in the spine is not pain sensitive?

A. Periosteum
B. Nucleus pulposus
C. Facet Joints
D. Longitudinal ligaments

Explanation:

- Pain sensitive structure of spine include Periosteum of vertebrae, deera, facet joints, arduous fibrosis, epidural veins and arteries and longitudral ligaments.
- Under normal circumstances nucleus pulposus of intervertebral disk is not pain sensitive.

Ans. B

48. Latency period of auto regulatory mechanism which maintains the cerebral blood flow is:

A. 0-5 Seconds
B. 5-10 Seconds
C. 10-15 Seconds
D. 15-20 Seconds

Explanation:

- In a normal patient the auto regulatory mechanism prevent the cerebral hypoperfusion when this mechanism fails Syncope will occur Latency period for this auto regulatory mechanism to get activated is 5-10 Seconds

Ans. B

49. A 36 years old patient with paramyotonia congenita can present with all of the features except:

A. Myotonia worsens with cold
B. Myotonia improves with exercise
C. Sodium channel mutation
D. Autosomal dominant

Explanation:

- Paramyotonia congenita attacks are coldinduced

- Myotonia is a prominent feature but worsens with muscle activity (paradoxical myotonia). This is in contrast to classic myotonia in which exercise alleviates the condition.
- It is inherited as an autosomal dominant condition; voltage-gated sodium channel mutations

Ans. B

50. Nature of headache in subarachnoid Hemorrhage is:

A. Mild Headache
B. Moderate Headache
C. Excruciating Headache
D. Thunder clapping Headache

Explanation:

- Headache is SAH in excruciating in nature and it will be sudden in onset The patient often calls the headache the worst headache in my life and it may be associated with neck stiffness and vomiting.
- Thunderclap Headache is a variant of migraine that simulates an SAH.

Ans. C

51. Ekiri syndrome is seen in:

A. Lyme's disease
B. Cat scratch disease
C. Neurosyphilis
D. Shigellosis

Explanation:

Shigellosis

- Fever and severe metabolic alterations are more often the major causes of altered consciousness than is meningitis.
- Ekiri syndrome (toxic encephalopathy) associated with bizarre posturing, cerebral edema, and fatty degeneration of viscera.
- This Syndrome was reported mostly in Japanese children. .

Ans. D

52. Segment of vertebral artery that circles around the arch of the atlas is:

A. V1
B. V2
C. V3
D. V4

Explanation:

- Vertebral artery, which arises from the innominate artery on the right and the subclavian artery on the left, consists of four segments.
- First (V1) extends from its origin to its entrance into the sixth or fifth transverse vertebral foramen.
- Second segment (V2) traverses the vertebral foramina from C6 to C2. The third (V3) passes through transverse foramen and circles around the arch of the atlas to pierce dura at the foramen magnum.
- Fourth (V4) segment courses upward to join the other vertebral artery to form the basilar artery, only the fourth segment gives rise to branches that supply brainstem and cerebellum.
- Posterior inferior cerebellar artery (PICA) in its proximal segment supplies the lateral medulla and, in its distal branches, the inferior surface of the cerebellum.

Ans. C

53. NCCT given below likely to be:

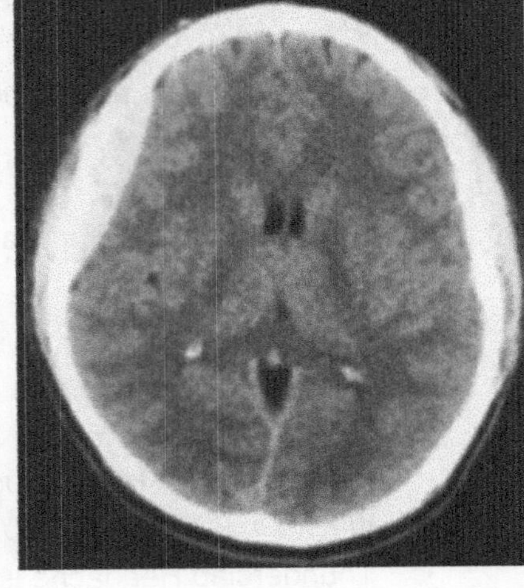

A. Subdural hemorrhage

B. Epidural hemorrhage

C. Subarachnoid hemorrhage

D. Intraparenchymal hemorrhage

Explanation:

- NCCT shows biconvex or lenticular shaped hemorrhage on NCCT due to middle meningeal artery bleed.
- Subdural haemorrhage shows concavo convex shaped bleed on NCCT, bleeding occurs due to bridging veins which is venous origin
- Subarachnoid hemorrhage shows blood in sylvian fissure on NCCT
- Intraparenchymal bleed: Blood is seen in parenchyma and ventricles.

Cerebral Hemorrhages

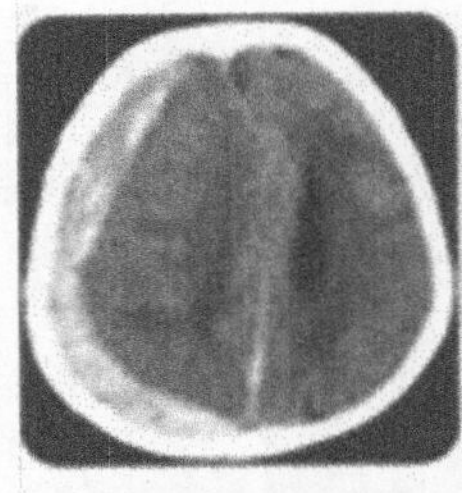

Subdural hematoma
- Crescent shaped
- Blood collection between dura and arachnoid matter
- Tear in bridging veins
- Alcoholics and elderly are prone

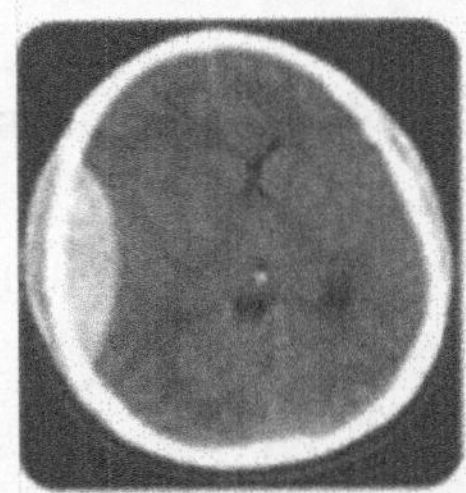

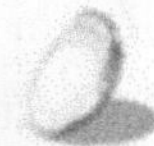

Epidural hematoma
- Biconvex (lens) shaped
- Blood between dura and skull
- Tearing of middle meningeal artery
- Adolescents and young adults (trauma)

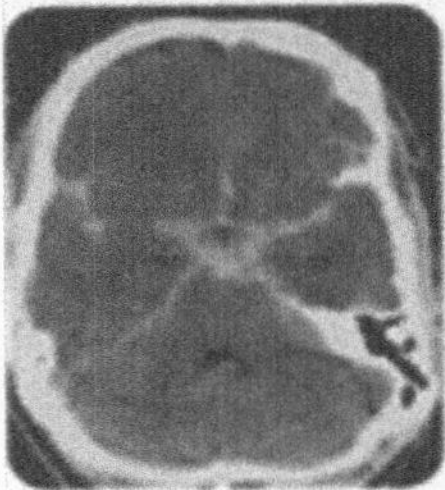

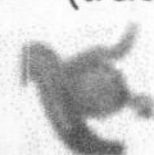

Subarachnoid hemorrhage
- Blood in circle of Willis, cisberns, and fissures
- Flupture of berry aneuryam
- Polycystic kidney disease (risk factor)

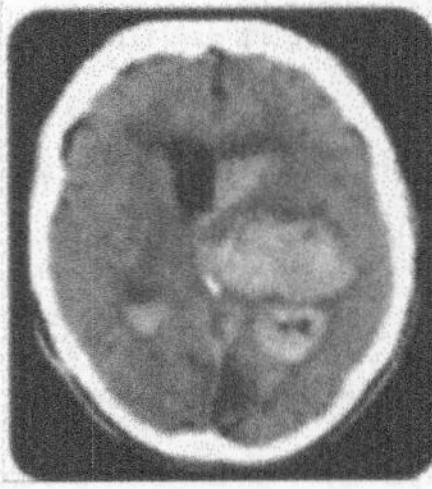

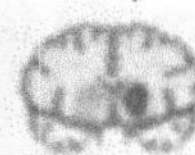

Intracerebral hemorrhage
- Blood in parenchyma and ventricles
- Hypertensive vasoulpathy
- Territory of penetrator arteries

Ans. B

54. Identify the MRI image-Axial T2 weighted:

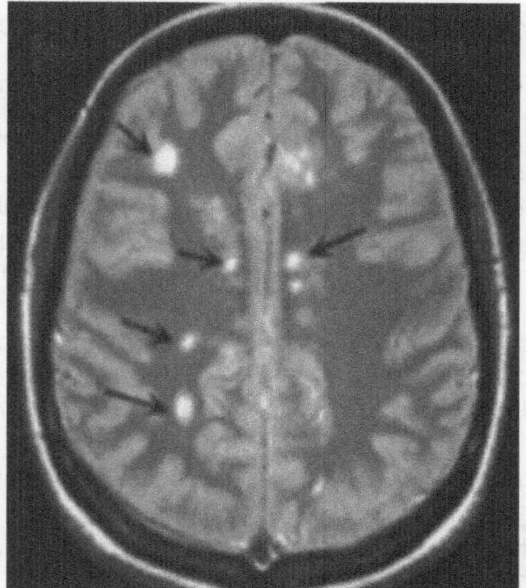

A. Multiple sclerosis
B. Wilson's disease
C. Multiple system atrophy
D. Hallervorden-Spatz disease

Explanation:

- Axial T2 weighted image with bright signal abnormality in white matter typical for multiple sclerosis.
- Wilson disease: Face of panda appearance on MRI
- Multiple system atrophy: Hot cross bun sign appearence on MRI.
- Hallervorden-Spatz disease: Eye of tiger on MRI.

Ans. A

55. Following MIDAS questionnaire used in:

*MIDAS Questionnaire	
Instructions: Please answer the following questions about ALL headaches you have had over the last 3 months. Write zero if you did not do the activity in the last 3 months.	.
1. On how many days in the last 3 months did you miss work or school because of your headaches?	...........days
2. How many days in the last 3 months was your productivity at work or school reduced by half or more because of your headaches *(do not include days you counted in question 1 where you missed work or school)?*	...........days
3. On how many days in the last 3 months did you **not** do household work because of your headaches?	...........days
4. How many days in the last 3 months was your productivity in household work reduced by half or more because of your headaches *(do not include days you counted in question 3 where you did not do household work)?*	...........days
5. On how many days in the last 3 months did you miss family, social, or leisure activities because of your headaches?	...........days
A. On how many days in the last 3 months did you have a headache *(If a headache lasted more than one day, count each day)?*	...........days
B. On a scale of 0-10, on average how painful were these headaches *(Where 0= no pain at all, and 10= pain as bad as it can be)?*	....

A. Subarachnoid hemorrhage
B. Tension headache
C. Migraine
D. Cluster headache

Explanation:

- MIDAS (Migraine disability assessment) questionnaire used in assessment of migraine headache.

*MIDAS Questionnaire	
Instructions: Please answer the following questions about ALL headaches you have had over the last 3 months. Write zero if you did not do the activity in the last 3 months.	
1. On how many days in the last 3 months did you miss work or school because of your headaches?	...........days
2. How many days in the last 3 months was your productivity at work or school reduced by half or more because of your headaches *(do not include days you counted in question 1 where you missed work or school)?*	...........days
3. On how many days in the last 3 months did you not do household work because of your headaches?	...........days
4. How many days in the last 3 months was your productivity in household work reduced by half or more because of your headaches *(do not include days you counted in question 3 where you did not do household work)?*	...........days
5. On how many days in the last 3 months did you miss family, social, or leisure activities because of your headaches?	...........days
A. On how many days in the last 3 months did you have a headache *(If a headache lasted more than one day, count each day)?*	...........days
B. On a scale of 0-10, on average how painful were these headaches *(Where 0= no pain at all, and 10= pain as bad as it can be)?*	....
*Migraine Disability Assessment Score (Questions 1-5 are used to calculate the MIDAS score) Grade I–Minimal or Infrequent Disability: 0-5 Grade II–Mild or Infrequent Disability: 6-10 Grade III–Moderate Disability: 11-20 Grade IV–Severe Disability: > 20	

Ans. C

56. A 60-year-old male patient presented to medicine OPD with gait ataxia and dysarthria, MRI done. Most likely diagnosis to be:

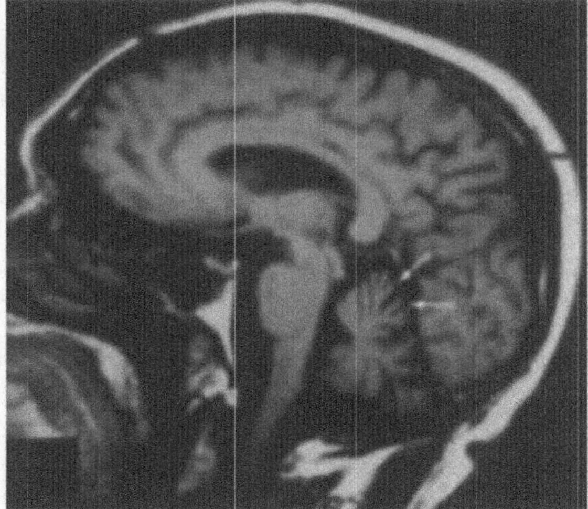

A. Wilson's disease
B. Prion's disease
C. Multiple system atrophy
D. Spinocerebellar ataxia

Explanation:

- A 60-year-old with gait ataxia and dysarthria with cerebellar degeneration on MRI points towards spinocerebellar degeneration.

- In Multiple system atrophy also ataxia, dysarthria seen with visual disturbances and hot cross bun sign on MRI.

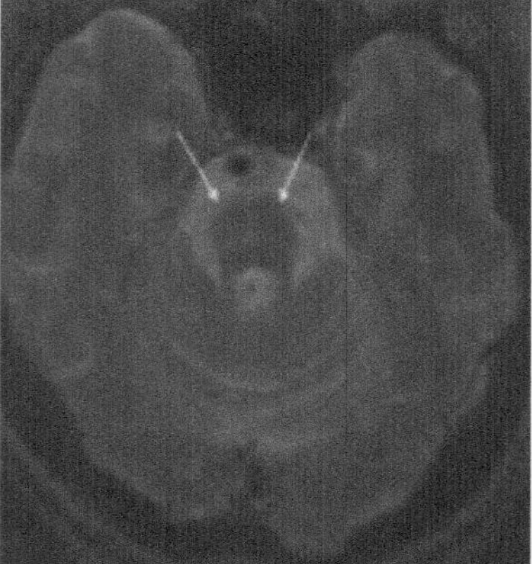

- Wilson's disease present with tremors, neuropsychiatric problems and face of panda on MRI.

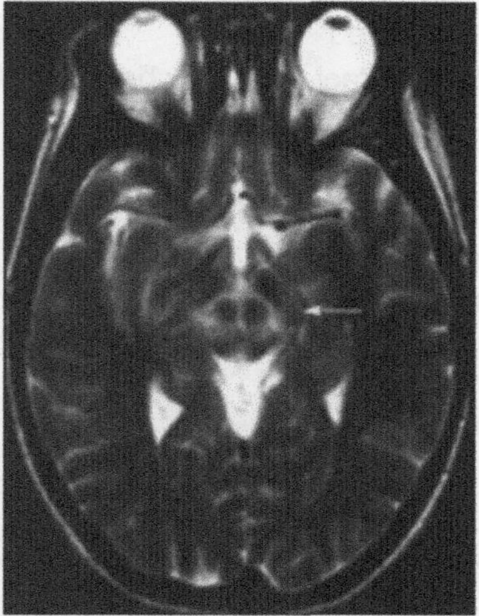

In prion's disease MRI reveals cortical ribboning with progressive myoclonus and apathy like features.

Ans. D

57. Which of the following is most common neuropathy in DM?

A. Distal symmetric polyneuropathy
B. Autonomic neuropathy
C. Mononeuropathy
D. Polyradiculopathy

Explanation:

- DSPN, the most common form of diabetic neuropathy, most frequently presents with distal sensory loss and pain, but up to 50% of patients do not have symptoms of neuropathy.
- Symptoms may include a sensation of numbness, tingling, sharpness, or burning that begins in the feet and spreads proximally.
- Hyperesthesia, paresthesia, and dysesthesia also may occur.
- Pain typically involves the lower extremities, is usually present at rest, and worsens at night.
- Both an acute (lasting <12 months) and a chronic form of painful diabetic neuropathy may occur.
- Acute form is sometimes treatment-related, occurring in the context of improved glycemic control.
- As diabetic neuropathy progresses, the pain subsides and eventually disappears, but a sensory deficit persists and motor defects may develop. Physical examination often reveals sensory loss (to 10-g monofilament and/or vibration), loss of ankle deep-tendon reflexes, abnormal position sense, and muscular atrophy or foot drop.

- Annual screening for DSPN should begin 5 years after diagnosis of type 1 DM and at the time of diagnosis of type 2 DM and is aimed at detecting loss of protective sensation (LOPS).
- LOPS and DSPN are major risk factors for foot ulceration & falls due to small & large fiber dysfunction.

Ans. A

58. Useless hand of Oppenheim is seen in:

A. Myasthenia gravis
B. Diabetic neuropathy
C. Myotonic dystrophy
D. Multiple sclerosis

Explanation:

- Useless hand devoid of proprioception*
- Seen in cases of multiple sclerosis*
- Classical, yet, uncommon** finding
- U/L or B/L presentation*
- Usually, demyelinating* plaque in posterior*column of cervical*spinal cord
- Motor** sensation is generally preserved
- Light touch** perception – relatively intact, but, may be altered depending upon number and location of lesions

Ans. D

59. During the attack of syncope, cessation of how much quantity of blood flow per 100g brain tissue will result in impairment of consciousness.

A. Less than 25 ml/min
B. Less than 30 ml/min
C. Less than 15 ml/min
D. Less than 10 ml/min

Explanation:

- Cessation of blood flow for 6-8 seconds will result in loss of consciousness, while impairment of consciousness ensues when blood flow decreases to 25 ml/min per 100g brain tissue.

Ans. A

60. Confusion after SAH fits into which grade of Hunt-Hess scale:

A. 1
B. 2
C. 3
D. 4

Explanation:

Table: Grading scales for subarachnoid hemorrhage

Grade	Hunt-Hess Scale	World Federation of Neurosurgical Societies (WFNS) Scale
1	Mild headache, normal mental status, no cranial nerve or motor findings	GCSa score 15, no motor deficits
2	Severe headache, normal mental status, may have cranial nerve deficit	GCS score 13-14, no motor deficits
3	Somnolent, confused, may have cranial nerve or mild motor deficit	GCS score 13-14, with motor deficits
4	Stupor, moderate to severe motor deficit, may have intermittent reflex posturing	GCS score 7-12, with or without motor deficits
5	Coma, reflex posturing of flaccid	GCS score 3-6, with or without motor deficits

Ans. C

61. Paresthesia caused by all except:

A. Thiamine B. Pyridoxine

C. Vitamin B12 D. Biotin

Explanation:

Mental status/nervous system examination	Mental and nervous system findings indicate certain nutrient deficiencies Ophthalmoplegia and foot drop: thiamine Paresthesia: thiamine, vitamin B_{12} and biotin Depressed vibratory and position senses: vitamin B_{12} Anxiety, depression and hallucinations: niacin Memory disturbance: vitamin B_{12} Hyporeflexia, loss of lower extremity deep tendon reflexes: thiamine and vitamin B_{12} Conduct formal cognitive and depression assessments as appropriate. Dementia and depression are common causes of malnutrition among older persons. Wernicke-Korsakoff syndrome may be observed with severe thiamine deficiency

Ans. B

62. Findings helpful to localize cerebral disorders include all except:

A. Cognitive impairment B. Seizures

C. Chorea D. Crossed weakness

Explanation:

Table: Findings helpful for localizations within the nervous system

	Signs
Cerebrum	Abnormal mental status or cognitive impairment Seizures Unilateral weakness[a] and sensory abnormalities including head and limbs Visual field abnormalities Movement abnormalities (e.g., diffuse incoordination, tremor, chorea)
Brainstem	Isolated cranial nerve abnormalities (single or multiple) "Crossed" weakness[a] and sensory abnormalities of head and limbs, e.g., weakness of right face and left arm and leg
Spinal cord	Back pain or tenderness Weakness[a] and sensory abnormalities sparing the head Mixed upper and lower motor neuron findings Sensory level Sphincter dysfunction
Spinal roots	Radiating limb pain Weakness[b] or sensory abnormalities following root distribution Loss of reflexes
Peripheral nerve	Mild or distal limb pain Weakness[b] or sensory abnormalities following nerve distribution "Stocking or glove" distribution of sensory loss Loss of reflexes
Neuromuscular junction	Bilateral weakness including face (ptosis, diplopia, dysphagia) and proximal limbs Increasing weakness with exertion Sparing of sensation
Muscle	Bilateral proximal or distal weakness Sparing of sensation

Ans. D

63. All are true statements except:

A. Spasticity due to corticospinal tract disease

B. Paratonia due to frontal lobe disease

C. Rigidity due to pyramidal disease

D. Cogwheel rigidity in Parkinsonism

Explanation:

- Increased tone may be evident as spasticity (resistance determined by the angle and velocity of motion; corticospinal tract disease), rigidity (similar resistance in all angles of motion; extrapyramidal disease), or paratonia (fluctuating changes in resistance; frontal lobe pathways or normal difficulty in relaxing). Cogwheel rigidity, in which passive motion elicits jerky interruptions in resistance, is seen in parkinsonism.

Ans. C

64. Structures lacking blood brain barrier include all except:

A. Pituitary gland

B. Choroid plexus

C. Dura

D. Cranial nerve nucleus

Explanation:

- Intravenous iodinated contrast is used to identify vascular structures and to detect defects in the blood-brain barrier (BBB) that are caused by tumors, infarcts, and infections. In the normal CNS, only vessels and structures lacking a BBB (e.g., the pituitary gland, choroid plexus, and dura) enhance after contrast administration. While helpful in characterizing mass lesions as well as essential for the acquisition of CTA studies, the decision to use contrast material should always be considered carefully as it carries a small risk of allergic reaction and adds additional expense.

Ans. D

65. All are true statements except:

A. Inability to recognize numbers or letters is termed agraphesthesia

B. In polyneuropathy the process is nerve length–dependent, and the deficit is often described as "stocking-glove" in type

C. Touch is involved variably (in small fibre polyneuropathy); when it is spared, the sensory pattern is referred to as exhibiting sensory dissociation

D. Large-fiber polyneuropathies are characterized by burning, painful dysesthesias with reduced pinprick and thermal sensation but with sparing of proprioception, motor function, and deep tendon reflexes

Explanation:

- Small-fiber polyneuropathies are characterized by burning, painful dysesthesias with reduced pinprick and thermal sensation but with sparing of proprioception, motor function, and deep tendon reflexes. Touch is involved variably; when it is spared, sensory pattern is referred to as exhibiting *sensory dissociation*.
- Sensory dissociation may occur also with spinal cord lesions.
- Large-fiber polyneuropathies are characterized by vibration and position sense deficits, imbalance, absent tendon reflexes, and variable motor dysfunction but preservation of most cutaneous sensation.
- Dysesthesias, if present at all, tend to be tingling or bandlike in quality.

Ans. D

66. Pellicle in the CSF or a cobweb-like clot on surface of the fluid is suggestive of:

A. Tuberculous meningitis

B. Cryptococcal meningitis

C. Fungal meningitis

D. Syphilitic meningitis

Explanation:

- Combination of unrelenting headache, stiff neck, fatigue, night sweats, and fever with a CSF lymphocytic pleocytosis and a mildly decreased glucose concentration is highly suspicious for tuberculous meningitis.
- Last tube of fluid collected at LP is the best tube to send for a smear for acid-fast bacilli (AFB).
- If there is a pellicle in the CSF or a cobweb-like clot on the surface of the fluid, AFB can best be demonstrated in a smear of the clot or pellicle.
- Positive smears are typically reported in only 10–40% of cases of tuberculous meningitis in adults.
- Cultures of CSF take 4–8 weeks to identify the organism and are positive in ~50% of adults.
- **Culture remains gold standard to make the diagnosis of tuberculous meningitis.**
- PCR for the detection of M. tuberculosis DNA should be sent on CSF if available, but the sensitivity and specificity on CSF have not been defined.
- CDC recommends the use of nucleic acid amplification tests for the diagnosis of pulmonary tuberculosis.

Ans. A

67. False about cerebellar infarction is:

A. These strokes may mimic labyrinthitis

B. Presence of head or neck pain should alert the physician to consider cerebellar stroke due to vertebral artery embolism

C. Even small amounts of cerebellar edema can acutely increase intracranial pressure

D. Suboccipital decompression is recommended in patients with cerebellar infarcts who demonstrate neurological deterioration

Explanation:

- Special vigilance is warranted for patients with cerebellar infarction.
- These strokes may mimic labyrinthitis because of prominent vertigo and vomiting; the presence of head or neck pain should alert physician to consider cerebellar stroke due to vertebral artery dissection.
- Even small amounts of cerebellar edema can acutely increase intracranial pressure (ICP) by obstructing cerebrospinal fluid (CSF) flow leading to hydrocephalus or by directly compressing the brainstem.
- Resulting brainstem compression can manifest as coma and respiratory arrest and require emergency surgical decompression.
- Suboccipital decompression is recommended in patients with cerebellar infarcts who demonstrate neurological deterioration and should be performed before significant brainstem compression occurs.

Ans. B

68. Biopsy of an enhancing region of the basal meninges shows most commonly:

A. Tuberculosis

B. Sarcoidosis

C. Metastatic adenocarcinoma

D. Syphilis

Explanation:

- MRI demonstrated meningeal enhancement in 47% of patients undergoing meningeal biopsy; biopsy of an enhancing region was diagnostic in 80% of cases, biopsy of non-enhancing regions was diagnostic in only 9%, and sarcoid (31%) and metastatic adenocarcinoma (25%) were the most common conditions identified.
- Tuberculosis is the most common condition identified in many reports from outside United States.

Ans. A

69. Akinetic mutism can result from damage in all the following regions except:

A. Medial thalamic nuclei
B. Medial frontal lobe
C. Ventral pons
D. Extreme hydrocephalus

Explanation:

- Akinetic mutism refers to a partially or fully awake state in which patient is able to form impressions and think, as demonstrated by later recounting of events, but remains virtually immobile and mute.
- Condition results from damage in the regions of the medial thalamic nuclei or the frontal lobes (particularly lesions situated deeply or on orbitofrontal surfaces) or from extreme hydrocephalus.
- Term abulia describes a milder form of akinetic mutism characterized by mental and physical slowness and diminished ability to initiate activity.
- It is also usually the result of damage to the medial frontal lobes and their connections.

Ans. C

70. Reactive and bilateral small but no pinpoint pupils are seen in all except:

A. Metabolic encephalopathies
B. Hydrocephalus
C. Thalamic hemorrhage
D. Frontal lobe infarct

Explanation:

- Reactive and bilaterally small (1–2.5 mm) but not pinpoint pupils are seen in metabolic encephalopathies or in deep bilateral hemispheral lesions such as hydrocephalus or thalamic hemorrhage.
- Even smaller reactive pupils (<1 mm) characterize narcotic or barbiturate overdoses but also occur with extensive pontine hemorrhage.
- Response to naloxone and the presence of reflex eye movements assist in distinguishing between these.
- Unilateral miosis in coma has been attributed to dysfunction of sympathetic efferents originating in the posterior hypothalamus and descending in the tegmentum of the brainstem to the cervical cord.
- It is an occasional finding in patients with a large cerebral hemorrhage that affects the thalamus.

Ans. D

71. All are true about craniopharyngiomas except:

A. Craniopharyngiomas are malignant suprasellar cystic masses that present with headaches visual field deficits
B. They are derived from Rathke's pouch and arise near the pituitary stalk commonly extending into the suprasellar cistern
C. MRI is generally superior to CT for evaluating cystic structure and tissue components of craniopharyngiomas
D. CT is useful to define calcifications and evaluate invasion into surrounding bony structures and sinuses

Explanation:

- *Craniopharyngiomas* are benign, suprasellar cystic masses that present with headaches, visual field deficits, and variable degrees of hypopituitarism.
- Derived from Rathke's pouch and arise near the pituitary stalk, commonly extending into the suprasellar cistern.
- Craniopharyngiomas are often large, cystic, and locally invasive.
- Many are partially calcified, exhibiting a characteristic appearance on skull X-ray and CT images.

- More than half of all patients present before age 20, usually with signs of increased intracranial pressure, including headache, vomiting, papilledema, and hydrocephalus.
- Associated symptoms include visual field abnormalities, personality changes and cognitive deterioration, cranial nerve damage, sleep difficulties, and weight gain.
- Hypopituitarism can be documented in ~90%, and diabetes insipidus occurs in ~10% of patients.
- About half of affected children present with growth retardation.
- MRI is generally superior to CT for evaluating cystic structure and tissue components of craniopharyngiomas.
- CT is useful to define calcifications and evaluate invasion into surrounding bony structures and sinuses

Ans. A

72. Catamenial epilepsy is:

A. Women with increased seizure frequency during menses

B. Increased seizure frequency during pregnancy

C. Increased seizure frequency in menopause

D. Increased seizure frequency in childhood

Explanation:

- Some women experience a marked increase in seizure frequency around the time of menses.
- This is believed to be mediated by either the effects of estrogen and progesterone on neuronal excitability or changes in antiepileptic drug levels due to altered protein binding or metabolism.
- Some patients may benefit from increases in antiepileptic drug dosages during menses.
- Natural progestins or intramuscular medroxyprogesterone may be of benefit to a subset of women.

Ans. A

73. Uncal transtentorial herniation, first sign is:

A. Coma

B. Ipsilateral ptosis

C. Ipsilateral enlargement of pupil

D. Contralateral enlargement of pupil

Explanation:

- Uncal transtentorial herniation refers specifically to impaction of anterior medial temporal gyrus (the uncus) into the tentorial opening just anterior to and adjacent to the midbrain.
- The uncus compresses the third nerve as the nerve traverses the subarachnoid space, causing enlargement of the ipsilateral pupil as first sign (the fibers subserving parasympathetic pupillary function are located peripherally in nerve).
- Coma that follows is due to compression of the midbrain (and therefore the RAS) against the opposite tentorial edge by the displaced parahippocampal gyrus.
- Lateral displacement of midbrain may compress the opposite cerebral peduncle against tentorial edge, producing a Babinski sign and hemiparesis contralateral to hemiparesis that resulted from mass (Kernohan-Woltman sign).

Ans. C

74. You are appointed as a cardiac epidemiologist advisor on an international committee setting global health policy. Your committee is assigned to predict health trends in a Pacific East Asian nation with a population and environment very similar to China. At this point in history, the nation is just moving

from the first classic stage in the epidemiologic transition ("pestilence and famine") to the second classic stage ("receding pandemics"). In regard to the anticipated patterns of cardiovascular disease (CVD) in this nation, which of the following is true?

A. As this nation enters the stage of receding pandemics, you would expect the majority of CVD morbidity and mortality to be due to cardiomyopathies secondary to infectious agents

B. Each nation or geographical location progresses through the five stages of epidemiologic transition identically in regard to CVD risk

C. In this nation, when CVD mortality peaks, you would expect stroke mortality to be greater than coronary heart disease mortality

D. One would expect a very homogeneous epidemiologic pattern of CVD risk throughout this nation over time

Explanation:

- Global rise in cardiovascular disease (CVD) is the result of an unprecedented transformation in the causes of morbidity and mortality during the 20th century. Known as the epidemiologic transition, this shift is driven by industrialization, urbanization, and associated lifestyle changes and is taking place in every part of the world among all races, ethnic groups, and cultures. The transition is divided into four basic stages: pestilence and famine, receding pandemics, degenerative and man-made diseases, and delayed degenerative diseases. A fifth stage, characterized by an epidemic of inactivity and obesity, is emerging in some countries.
- Stages of the epidemiologic transition are shown in the table given below.

Five Stages of the Epidemiologic Transition

Stage	Description	Deaths Related to CVD,	Predominant CVD Type
Pestilence and famine	Predominance of malnutrition and infectious diseases as causes of death; high rates of infant and child mortality: low mean life expectancy	<10	Rheumatic heart disease, cardio myopathies caused by infection and malnutrition
Receding pandemics	Improvements in nutrition and public health lead to decrease in rates of deaths related to mal nutrition and infection; precipitous decline in infant and child mortality rates	10-35	Rheumatic valvar disease, hyper tension, CHD, and stroke (pre dominantly hemorrhagic)
Degenerative and man-made diseases	Increased fat and caloric intake and decrease in physical activity lead to emergence of hypertension and atherosclerosis; with increase in life expectancy, mortality from chronic, non communicable diseases exceeds mortality from malnutrition and infectious disease	35-65	CHD and stroke (ischemic and hemorrhagic)

Contd.

Contd.

Delayed degenerative diseases	CVD and cancer are the major causes of morbidity and mortality: better treatment and prevention efforts help avoid deaths among those with disease and delay primary events; age adjusted CVD mortality declines: CVD affecting older and older individuals	40-50	CHD, stroke, and congestive heart failure
Inactivity and obesity	Overweight and obesity increase at alarming rate; diabetes and hypertension increase; decline in smoking rates levels off; a minority of the population meets physical activity recommendations	33	CHD, stroke, and congestive heart failure, peripheral vascular disease

- Note that CVD mortality peaks in the third stage and then tends to decline aided by preventive strategies such as smoking cessation programs and effective blood pressure control, acute hospital management, and technologic advances, such as the availability of bypass surgery. In the stage of receding pandemics, the majority of CVD risk tends to be due to coronary heart disease, stroke, and rheumatic heart disease.
- Although the stages of epidemiologic transition is a useful construct to generalize expectations regarding CVD epidemiology over time, every nation experiences these stages in unique fashion due to environmental, behavioral, and genetic differences.
- For example, in China and Japan, stroke causes more deaths than coronary heart disease in a ratio of about three to one, as we would expect for this hypothetical nation.

Ans. C

75. Ceftazidime is used for CNS infection with:

A. Neisseria meningitides
B. Streptococcus pneumonia
C. Listeria monocytogenes
D. Pseudomonas aeruginosa

Explanation:

- Ceftazidime or meropenem should be substituted for ceftriaxone or cefotaxime in neurosurgical patients and in neutropenic patients, because ceftriaxone and cefotaxime do not provide adequate activity against CNS infection with *P. aeruginosa*.
- Meropenem is a carbapenem antibiotic that is highly active in vitro against *L. monocytogenes*, has been demonstrated to be effective in cases of meningitis caused by *P. aeruginosa*, and shows good activity against penicillin-resistant pneumococci.
- In experimental pneumococcal meningitis, meropenem was comparable to ceftriaxone and inferior to vancomycin in sterilizing CSF cultures.

Ans. D

76. For management of ICH following statements are true except:

A. Idarucizumab is monoclonal antibody to dabigatran & administration of 2 doses reverses anticoagulation effect of dabigatran quickly

B. Evacuation of supratentorial hematomas doesn't appear to improve outcome for most patients

C. Glucorticoids are helpful for edema from intracerebral hematoma

D. Most cerebrallar hematomas >3cm diameter will require surgical evacuation

Explanation:

- Idarucizumab is a monoclonal antibody to dabigatran and the administration of two doses reverses the anticoagulation effect of dabigatran quickly.
- PCC may partially reverse the effects of oral factor Xa inhibitors and are reasonable to administer if available; targeted drugs to reverse Xa inhibitors are under clinical investigation. When ICH is associated with thrombocytopenia (platelet count <50,000/μL), transfusion of fresh platelets is indicated.
- Recent clinical trial of platelet transfusions in patients with ICH and without thrombocytopenia who are taking antiplatelet drugs suggested no benefit and possible harm.
- Hematomas may expand for several hours following the initial hemorrhage, even in patients without coagulopathy. However, precise mechanism is unclear.
- A phase 3 trial of treatment with recombinant factor VIIa reduced hematoma expansion; however, clinical outcomes were not improved, so use of this drug is not recommended.
- Blood pressure lowering has been considered due to theoretical risk of acutely elevated blood pressure on hematoma expansion, although recent clinical trials did not find a difference in hematoma expansion between the SBP targets of 140–180 mmHg.
- Evacuation of supratentorial hematomas does not appear to improve outcome for most patients.
- For cerebellar hemorrhages, a neurosurgeon should be consulted immediately to assist with the evaluation; most cerebellar hematomas >3 cm in diameter will require surgical evacuation. If the patient is alert without focal brainstem signs and if the hematoma is <1 cm in diameter, surgical removal is usually unnecessary.
- Patients with hematomas between 1 and 3 cm require careful observation for signs of impaired consciousness, progressive hydrocephalus, and precipitous respiratory failure.
- Hydrocephalus due to cerebellar hematoma requires surgical evacuation and should not be treated solely with ventricular drainage.
- Glucocorticoids are not helpful for the edema from intracerebral hematoma.

Ans. C

77. Non inflammatory myopathy that spares quadriceps is:

A. Acquired IBM

B. Hereditary IBM

C. Dermatomyositis

D. Polymyositis

Explanation:

Hereditary subset of IBM (Inclusion body myositis) spares quadriceps

Acquired IBM:

- Presence of atrophy and weakness of the flexor forearm muscles and quadriceps in a person aged >50 years is most likely IBM.
- IBM usually manifests in patients over the age of 50 years and is slightly more common in men than women. It is associated with slowly progressive weakness and muscle atrophy that has a predilection for early involvement of the wrist and finger flexors in the arms and quadriceps in the legs.
- Weakness is often asymmetric. Dysphagia is common and rarely can be the presenting feature. These clinical features can help distinguish IBM from PM and other forms of myopathy. The mean duration from onset of symptoms to use of wheelchair or scooter is ~15 years. There is no known increased risk of malignancy.

Ans. B

78. All are well established risk factors for Multiple sclerosis except:

A. Genetic predisposition
B. Vitamin D excess
C. EBV exposure
D. Cigarette smoking

Explanation:

- Well-established risk factors for MS include a genetic predisposition, vitamin D deficiency, Epstein-Barr virus (EBV) exposure after early childhood, and cigarette smoking.
- Vitamin D deficiency is associated with an increase in MS risk, and data suggest that ongoing deficiency also increases disease activity after MS begins. Immunoregulatory effects of vitamin D could explain these apparent relationships.
- Exposure of the skin to ultraviolet-B (UVB) radiation from the sun is essential for the biosynthesis of vitamin D, and this endogenous production is the most important source of vitamin D in most individuals.
- A diet rich in fatty fish represents another source of vitamin D.
- At high latitudes, the amount of UVB radiation reaching the earth's surface is often insufficient, particularly during winter months, and consequently, low serum levels of vitamin D are common in temperate zones.
- Common practice to avoid direct sun exposure and the widespread use of sun block would be expected to exacerbate any population-wide vitamin D deficiency (sun protection factor [SPF] 15 blocks 94% of incoming UVB radiation).

Ans. B

79. Which of the following is not true statement?

A. Third nerve palsy with contralateral ataxia is Claude's syndrome
B. Third nerve palsy with contralateral hemiplegia is Weber's syndrome
C. Sensory loss is seen with occlusion of artery of Percheron
D. Contralateral hemisensory loss is Dejerine Roussy syndrome

Explanation:

- Infarction usually occurs in the ipsilateral subthalamus and medial thalamus and in the ipsilateral cerebral peduncle and midbrain.
- Third nerve palsy with contralateral ataxia (Claude's syndrome) or with contralateral hemiplegia (Weber's syndrome) may result. Ataxia indicates involvement of the red nucleus or dentatorubrothalamic tract; the hemiplegia is localized to the cerebral peduncle. If the subthalamic nucleus is involved, contralateral hemiballismus may occur.
- **Occlusion of the artery of Percheron produces paresis of upward gaze and drowsiness and often abulia.**
- Extensive infarction in the midbrain and subthalamus occurring with bilateral proximal PCA occlusion presents as coma, unreactive pupils, bilateral pyramidal signs, and decerebrate rigidity.
- Occlusion of the penetrating branches of thalamic and thalamogeniculate arteries produces less extensive thalamic and thalamocapsular lacunar syndromes.
- ***Thalamic Déjérine-Roussy syndrome*** consists of contralateral hemisensory loss followed later by an agonizing, searing, or burning pain in the affected areas. It is persistent and responds poorly to analgesics.
- Anticonvulsants (carbamazepine or gabapentin) or tricyclic antidepressants may be beneficial.

Ans. C

80. All are true about preventive medications for migraine except:

A. Patients with attacks that are either unresponsive or poorly responsive to abortive treatments are good candidates for preventive agents

B. Preventive medication should be considered in patients with four or more attacks a month

C. Significant side effects are associated with the use of many of these agents

D. Most treatments must be taken daily and there is usually a lag of between 2 to 5 days before an effect is seen

Explanation:

- Patients with an increasing frequency of migraine attacks or with attacks that are either unresponsive or poorly responsive to abortive treatments are good candidates for preventive agents.
- In general, a preventive medication should be considered in patients with four or more attacks a month.
- Significant side effects are associated with use of many of these agents; furthermore, determination of dose can be difficult because the recommended doses have been derived for conditions other than migraine.
- Mechanism of action of these drugs is unclear; it seems likely that the brain sensitivity that underlies migraine is modified.
- Patients are usually started on a low dose of a chosen treatment; the dose is then gradually increased, up to a reasonable maximum, to achieve clinical benefit. Most treatments must be taken daily, and there is usually a lag of between 2 and 12 weeks before an effect is seen.
- Drugs that have been approved by the FDA for the preventive treatment of migraine include propranolol, timolol, sodium valproate, and topiramate.
- In addition, a number of other drugs appear to display preventive efficacy. This group includes amitriptyline, nortriptyline, flunarizine, phenelzine, and cyproheptadine.
- Placebo controlled trials of onabotulinum toxin type A in episodic migraine were negative, whereas, overall, placebo-controlled trials in chronic migraine were positive.

Ans. D

81. Structures lacking blood brain barrier include all except:

A. Pituitary gland
B. Choroid plexus
C. Dura
D. Cranial nerve nucleus

Explanation:

- Intravenous iodinated contrast is used to identify vascular structures and to detect defects in the blood-brain barrier (BBB) that are caused by tumors, infarcts, and infections.
- **In the normal CNS, only vessels and structures lacking a BBB (e.g., pituitary gland, choroid plexus, and dura) enhance after contrast administration.**
- While helpful in characterizing mass lesions as well as essential for the acquisition of CTA studies, the decision to use contrast material should always be considered carefully as it carries a small risk of allergic reaction and adds additional expense.

Ans. D

82. For all below brain conditions MRI with contrast is preferred except:

A. Infection/abscess
B. Trauma
C. Immunosuppressed with focal findings
D. Cranial neuropathy

Explanation:

Table: Guidelines for the use of CT, ultrasound and MRI	
Condition	**Recommended Technique**
Hemorrhage	
• Acute parenchymal	CT, MR
• Subacute/chronic	MRI
• Subarachnoid hemorrhage	CT, CTA, lumbar puncture→angiography
Aneurysm	Angiography > CTA, MRA
Ischemic infarction	
• Hemorrhagic infarction	'CT or MRI
• Bland infarction	MRI with diffusion > CT, CTA, angiography
• Carotid or vertebral dissection	MRI/MRA
• Vertebral basilar insufficiency	CTA, MRI/MRA
• Carotid stenosis	CTA, MRA > US
Suspected mass lesion	
• Neoplasm, primary or metastatic	MRI + contrast
• Infection/abscess	MRI + contrast
• Immunosuppressed with focal findings	MRI + contrast
Vascular malformation	MRI + angiography
White matter disorders	
• Demyelinating disease	MRI
Dementia	MRI + contrast
Trauma	MRI > CT
• Acute trauma	CT
• Shear injury/chronic hemorrhage	MRI + susceptibility-weighted imaging
Headache/migraine	CT/MRI
Seizure	
• First time, no focal neurologic deficits	MRI > CT
• Partial complex/refractory	MRI
Cranial neuropathy	MRI with contrast
Meningeal disease	MRI with contrast
Spine	
Low back pain	
• No neurologic deficits	MRI or CT after > 6 weeks
• With focal deficits	MRI > CT
Spinal stenosis	MRI or CT
Cervical spondylosis	MRI, CT, CT myelography
Infection	MRI + contrast, CT
Myelopathy	MRI + contrast
Arteriovenous malformation	MRI + contrast, angiography

Ans. B

83. Most common form of jerk nystagmus is:

A. Gaze evoked nystagmus
B. Vestibular nystagmus
C. Downbeat nystagmus
D. Upbeat nystagmus

GAZE-EVOKED NYSTAGMUS

- This is the most common form of jerk nystagmus. When the eyes are held eccentrically in the orbits, they have a natural tendency to drift back to primary position. The subject compensates by making a corrective saccade to maintain the deviated eye position. Many normal patients have mild gaze-evoked nystagmus. Exaggerated gaze-evoked nystagmus can be induced by drugs (sedatives, anticonvulsants, alcohol); muscle paresis; myasthenia gravis; demyelinating disease; and cerebellopontine angle, brainstem, and cerebellar lesions.

Ans. A

84. All are causes for headache on rising in the morning except:

A. Raised CSF pressure headache
B. Poorly controlled hypertension
C. Obstructive sleep apnea
D. Giant cell induced arteritis

Explanation:

- Headache on rising in the morning or nocturnal headache is also characteristic of obstructive sleep apnea or poorly controlled hypertension.

Ans. D

85. EMG and NCSs will be normal when:

A. Nerve plexus is the cause of pain
B. Sensory nerve root injury causes pain
C. Peripheral sensory nerve injury causes pain
D. Muscle is the cause of pain

Explanation:

- Sensory NCSs are normal when focal sensory loss confirmed by examination is due to nerve root damage because the nerve roots are proximal to the nerve cell bodies in the dorsal root ganglia.
- Injury to nerve tissue distal to the dorsal root ganglion (e.g., plexus or peripheral nerve) results in reduced sensory nerve signals.
- Needle EMG complements NCSs by detecting denervation or reinnervation changes in a myotomal (segmental) distribution.
- Multiple muscles supplied by different nerve roots and nerves are sampled; the pattern of muscle involvement indicates the nerve root(s) responsible for the injury.
- Needle EMG provides objective information about motor nerve fiber injury when clinical evaluation of weakness is limited by pain or poor effort.
- EMG and NCSs will be normal when sensory nerve root injury or irritation is the pain source.

Ans. B

86. Hypertensive hemorrhage is uncommon in:

A. Putamen
B. Frontal lobe
C. Thalamus
D. Cerebellar hemisphere

Explanation:

Table: Causes of intracranial hemorrhage		
Causes	**Location**	**Comments**
Head trauma	Intraparenchymal: frontal lobes, anterior temporal lobes; subarachnoid; extra-axial (subdural, epidural)	Coup and contrecoup injury during brain deceleration
Hypertensive hemorrhage	Putamen, globus pallidus, thalamus, cerebellar hemisphere, pons	Chronic hypertension produces hemorrhage from small (~30-100 μm) vessels in these regions
Transformation of prior ischemic infarction	Basal ganglion, subcortical regions, lobar	Occur in 1-6% ischemic stroke with predilection for large hemispheric infarctions
Metastatic brain tumor	Lobar	Lung, choriocarcinoma, melanoma, renal cell carcinoma, thyroid, atrial myxoma
Coagulopathy	Any	Risk for ongoing hematoma expansion
Drug	Any, lobar, subarachnoid	Cocaine, amphetamine
Arteriovenous malformation	Lobar, intraventricular, subarachnoid	Risk is ~2-3% per year for bleeding if previously unruptured
Aneurysm	Subarachnoid, intraparenchymal, rarely subdural	Mycotic and nonmycotic form of aneurysms
Amyloid angiopathy	Lobar	Degenerative disease of intracranial vessels; associated with dementia, rare in patients <60 years
Cavernous angioma	Intraparenchymal	Multiple cavernous angiomas linked to mutations in *KRIT1, CCM2* and *PDCD10 genes*
Dural arteriovenous fistula	Lobar, subarachnoid	Produces bleeding by venous hypertension
Capillary telangiectasias	Usually brainstem	Rare cause of hemorrhage

Ans. B

87. All are true about management of ICH patient except:

A. "Spot sign" is thought to represent ongoing bleeding

B. The presence of a spot sign is associated with an increased risk of hematoma expansion, increased mortality, and lower likelihood of favorable functional outcome

C. Evacuation of supratentorial hematomas appear to improve outcome for most patients

D. Most cerebellar hematomas >3 cm in diameter will require surgical evacuation

Explanation:

- Evacuation of supratentorial hematomas does not appear to improve outcome for most patients.
- International Surgical Trial in Intracerebral Haemorrhage (STICH) randomized patients with supratentorial ICH to either early surgical evacuation or initial medical management.
- No benefit was found in the early surgery arm, although analysis was complicated by the fact that 26% of patients in the initial medical management group ultimately had surgery for neurologic deterioration.
- Follow-up study STICH-II found that surgery within 24 h of lobar, supratentorial hemorrhage did not improve overall outcome, but might have a role in select severely affected patients.
- Therefore, existing data do not support routine surgical evacuation of supratentorial hemorrhages in stable patients.
- However, many centers still consider surgery for patients deemed salvageable and who are experiencing progressive neurologic deterioration due to herniation.

- Surgical techniques continue to evolve, and minimally invasive endoscopic hematoma evacuation is currently being investigated in clinical trials.

Ans. C

88. All are true about evaluation of acute ischemic stroke except:

A. Nearly 30% of strokes remain unexplained despite extensive evaluation

B. Hollenhorst plaques are due to cholesterol emboli

C. Brain imaging, prothrombin time (PT), partial thromboplastin time (PTT), capillary blood glucose are necessary prior to IV rtPA

D. Cardioembolism is responsible for ~20% of all ischemic strokes

Explanation:

- Clinical examination should focus on the peripheral and cervical vascular system (carotid auscultation for bruits and blood pressure), the heart (dysrhythmia, murmurs), extremities (peripheral emboli), and retina (effects of hypertension and cholesterol emboli [Hollenhorst plaques]).
- A complete neurologic examination is performed to localize the anatomic site of stroke. An imaging study of the brain is nearly always indicated and is required for patients being considered for thrombolysis; it may be combined with CT- or MRI-based angiography to visualize the vasculature of the neck and intracranial vessels.
- A chest X-ray, electrocardiogram (ECG), urinalysis, complete blood count, erythrocyte sedimentation rate (ESR), serum electrolytes, blood urea nitrogen (BUN), creatinine, blood glucose, serum lipid profile, prothrombin time (PT), and partial thromboplastin time (PTT) are often useful and should be considered in all patients.
- An ECG, and subsequent cardiac telemetry, may demonstrate arrhythmias or reveal evidence of recent myocardial infarction (MI).
- Of all these studies, only brain imaging and capillary blood glucose are necessary prior to IV rtPA; the results of other studies should not delay the rapid administration of IV rtPA if the patient is eligible.

Ans. C

89. Cauda equina syndrome most commonly occurs due to:

A. Lumbosacral spine fracture

B. Hematoma in the spinal canal

C. Ruptured intervertebral disc

D. Tumors

Explanation:

- Cauda equine syndrome is most commonly due to a large ruptured lumbosacral intervertebral disk, but other causes include lumbosacral spine fracture, hematoma within the spinal canal (sometimes following lumbar puncture in patients with coagulopathy), and tumor or other compressive mass lesions.
- Treatment is surgical decompression, sometimes on an urgent basis in an attempt to restore or preserve motor or sphincter function, or radiotherapy for metastatic tumors.

Ans. C

90. All are true about lower back pain except:

A. ALBP is defined as pain of <3 months in duration

B. There is good evidence to support the use of opioid analgesics or tramadol as first-line therapy for ALBP

C. Back pain is the most frequent reason for seeking complementary and alternative treatments

D. Term sciatica is used when the leg pain radiates posteriorly in a sciatic or L5/S1 distribution

Explanation:

- There is no good evidence to support the use of opioid analgesics or tramadol as first-line therapy for ALBP.
- Their use is best reserved for patients who cannot tolerate acetaminophen or NSAIDs and for those with severe refractory pain.
- As with muscle relaxants, these drugs are often sedating, so it may be useful to prescribe them at nighttime only.
- Side effects of short-term opioid use include nausea, constipation, and pruritus; risks of long-term opioid use include hypersensitivity to pain, hypogonadism and dependency.
- Falls, fractures, driving accidents, and fecal impaction are other risks. Clinical efficacy of opioids for chronic pain beyond 16 weeks of use is unproven.

Ans. B

91. Opening pressure of CSF always high with:

A. Viral meningitis
B. Bacterial meningitis
C. Encephalitis
D. Tuberculous meningitis

Explanation:

Table: Typical cerebrospinal fluid profiles for meningitis and encephalitis[a]

	Normal	Bacterial Meningitis	Viral Meningitis	Fungal Meningitis[b]	Parasitic Meningitis	Tuber-culous Meningitis	Encephalitis
WBC count (per μl)	<5	>1000	25-500	40-600	150-2000	25-100	50-500
Differential of WBC	60-70% lymphocytes, ≤ 30% monocytes/ macrophages	↑↑PMNs (≥ 80%)	Predominantly lymphocytes[c]	Lymphocytes or PMNs, depending on specific organism	↑↑Eosinophils (≥ 50%)[d]	Predominantly lymphocytes[e]	Predominantly[c]
Gram's stain	Negative	Positive (in >60% of cases)	Negative	Rarely positive	Negative	Occasion-ally positive[e]	Negative
Glucose (mg/dl)	40-85	<40	Normal	↓ to normal	Normal	<50 in 75% of cases	Normal
Protein (mg/dl)	15-45	>100	20-80	150-300	50-200	100-200	50-100
Opening pressure (mmH_2O)	50-180	>300	100-350	160-340	Normal	150-280	Normal to ↑
Common causes	–	*Streptococcus pneumoniae, Neisseria meningitidis*	Entero-viruses	*Candida, Cryptococcus, and Aspergillus spp.*	*Angiostrongylus cantonensis, Gnathostoma spinigerum, Baylisascaris*	*Mycobacterium tuberculosis*	Herpesviruses, enteroviruses, influenza virus, rabies virus

Ans. B

92. Least common in Bacterial meningitis:

A. Fever
B. Papilledema
C. Meningismus
D. Altered mental status

Explanation:

- Bacterial meningitis is one of the most common infectious disease emergencies involving the central nervous system. Although hosts with cell-mediated immune deficiency (including transplant recipients, diabetic patients, elderly patients, and cancer patients receiving certain chemotherapeutic agents) are at particular risk for *Listeria monocytogenes* meningitis, most cases in adults are due to *S. pneumoniae* (30–60%) and *N. meningitidis* (10–35%).

- The classic presentation of fever, meningismus, and altered mental status is seen in only one-half to two-thirds of patients. The elderly can present without fever or meningeal signs. Cerebral dysfunction is evidenced by confusion, delirium, and lethargy that can progress to coma.
- In some cases, the presentation is fulminant, with sepsis and brain edema; papilledema at presentation is unusual and suggests another diagnosis (e.g., an intracranial lesion).
- Focal signs, including cranial nerve palsies (IV, VI, VII), can be seen in 10–20% of cases; 50–70% of patients have bacteremia.
- Poor outcome is associated with coma, seizures, hypotension, a pneumococcal etiology, respiratory distress, a CSF glucose level of <0.6 mmol/L (<10 mg/dL), a CSF protein level of >2.5 g/L, a peripheral white blood cell count of <5000/µL, and a serum sodium level of <135 mmol/L.

Ans. B

93. If these fibres are cut ability to detect painful stimuli is completely abolished:

A. A-beta
B. A-delta and C
C. B
D. A-gamma

Explanation:

- Ability to detect painful stimuli is completely abolished when conduction in Aδ and C fiber axons is blocked.

Ans. B

94. First to impair in language in patients with Alzheimer's disease is:

A. Naming
B. Comprehension
C. Fluency
D. Repetition

Explanation:

- Cognitive changes of AD tend to follow a characteristic pattern, beginning with memory impairment and progressing to language and visuospatial deficits, followed by executive dysfunction.
- Yet, ~20% of patients with AD present with non-memory complaints such as word-finding, organizational, or navigational difficulty.
- In other patients, visual processing dysfunction (referred to as posterior cortical atrophy syndrome) or a progressive "logopenic" aphasia characterized by difficulties with naming and repetition are the primary manifestations of AD for years before progressing to involve memory and other cognitive domains.
- Still other patients may present with an asymmetric akinetic-rigid-dystonic ("corticobasal") syndrome or a dysexecutive/behavioral, i.e., "frontal" variant of AD

Ans. A

95. All are findings of Parkinson's disease except:

A. Rest tremor, rigidity (stiffness), bradykinesia (slowing)
B. Degeneration of dopaminergic neurons in the substantia nigra pars compacta (SNc)
C. Intraneuronal proteinaceous inclusions known as pick bodies are seen
D. Mutations of the LRRK2 gene are the most common known cause of familial PD

Explanation:

- Pathologically, the hallmark features of PD are degeneration of dopaminergic neurons in the substantia nigra pars compacta (SNc), reduced striatal dopamine, and intraneuronal proteinaceous inclusions known as Lewy bodies and Lewy neurites that primarily contain the protein α-synuclein.

Ans. C

96. All signs can differentiate between LMN lesion and myopathic lesions except:

A. Atrophy
B. Fasciculations
C. Distribution of weakness
D. Babinski sign

Explanation:

Table: Signs that distinguish the origin of weakness

Sign	Upper Motor Neuron	Lower Motor Neuron	Myopathic	Psychogenic
Atrophy	None	Severe	Mild	None
Fasciculations	None	Common	None	None
Tone	Spastic	Decreased	Normal/decreased	Variable/paratonia
Distribution of weakness	Pyramidal/regional	Distal/segmental	Proximal	Variable/inconsistent with daily activities
Muscle stretch reflexes	Hyperactive	Hypoactive/absent	Normal/hypoactive	Normal
Babinski sign	Present	Absent	Absent	Absent

Ans. D

97. Classic clinical triad of headache, fever and focal neurologic deficit is seen in:

A. Meningitis
B. Encephalitis
C. Brain abscess
D. Brain tumor

Explanation:

- Classic clinical triad of headache, fever, and a focal neurologic deficit is present in <50% of cases.
- Most common symptom in patients with a brain abscess is headache, occurring in >75% of patients.
- Headache is often characterized as a constant, dull, aching sensation, either hemicranial or generalized, and it becomes progressively more severe and refractory to therapy.
- Fever is present in only 50% of patients at the time of diagnosis, and its absence should not exclude the diagnosis.
- New onset of focal or generalized seizure activity is a presenting sign in 15–35% of patients.
- Focal neurologic deficits including hemiparesis, aphasia, or visual field defects are part of initial presentation in >60% of patients.

Ans. C

98. In comparison to PD, the atypical parkinsonism are characterized clinically by all except:

A. Early involvement of speech and gait
B. Absence of rest tremor
C. Presence of motor asymmetry
D. Poor or no response to levodopa

Explanation:

- Atypical parkinsonism refers to a group of neurodegenerative conditions that usually are associated with more widespread pathology than found in PD (potentially with degeneration of striatum, globus pallidus, cerebellum and brainstem as well as the SNc).

- These include Multiple System Atrophy (MSA), Progressive Supranuclear Palsy (PSP), and Corticobasal syndrome (CBS). As a group, they present with arkinsonism (rigidity and bradykinesia) but manifest clinical differences from PD reflecting the differences in their underlying pathology.
- In comparison to PD, atypical parkinsonisms are characterized clinically by early involvement of speech and gait, absence of rest tremor, lack of motor asymmetry, poor or no response to levodopa, and a more aggressive clinical course.
- In early stages, they may show a modest benefit from levodopa and can be difficult to distinguish from PD, but diagnosis becomes clearer with disease evolution.
- Pathologically, neurodegeneration involves the SNc (typically without Lewy bodies) and has more extensive neurodegeneration than occurs in PD
- Neuroimaging of the dopamine system is usually not helpful, as striatal dopamine depletion can be seen in both PD and atypical parkinsonism. By contrast, metabolic imaging of the basal ganglia/thalamus network (using 2-F-deoxyglucose) may be helpful, showing a pattern of decreased activity in the GPi with increased activity in the thalamus, the reverse of what is seen in PD.

Ans. C

99. Diplopia and impaired down gaze is suggestive of:

A. FTD B. MSA

C. PSP D. DLB

Explanation:

Table: Features suggesting an atypical or secondary causes of parkinsonism

Symptoms/Signs	Alternative Diagnosis to Consider
History	
Early speech and gait impairment (Lack of tremor, lack of motor asymmetry	Atypical parkinsonism
Exposure to neuroleptics	Drug-induced parkinsonism
Onset prior to age 40	Genetic from PD
Liver disease	Wilson's disease, non-Wilsonian hepatolenticular degeneration
Early hallucinations and dementia with later development of PD features	Dementia with Lewy bodies
Diplopia, impaired down gaze	PSP
Poor or no response to an adequate trial of levodopa	Atypical or secondary parkinsonism
Physical Examination	
Dementia as first or early feature	Dementia with Lewy bodies
Prominent orthostatic hypotension	MSP-p
Prominent cerebellar signs	MSA-c
Slow saccades with impaired down gaze	PSP
High-frequency (6-10 Hz) symmetric postural tremor with a prominent kinetic component	Essential tremor

Ans. B

100. All below findings are seen on side of lesion in lateral superior pontine syndrome except:

A. Horner's syndrome

B. Ataxia of limbs and gait, falling to side of lesion

C. Impaired touch, vibration, and position sense, more in leg than arm

D. Dizziness, nausea, vomiting; horizontal nystagmus

Explanation:

Lateral superior pontine syndrome (syndrome of superior cerebellar artery)

On side of lesion

- Ataxia of limbs and gait, falling to side of lesion: *Middle and superior cerebellar peduncles, superior surface of cerebellum, dentate nucleus*
- Dizziness, nausea, vomiting; horizontal nystagmus: *Vestibular nucleus*
- Paresis of conjugate gaze (ipsilateral): *Pontine contralateral gaze*
- Skew deviation: *Uncertain*
- Miosis, ptosis, decreased sweating over face (Horner's syndrome): Descending sympathetic fibers
- Tremor: Localization unclear—*Dentate nucleus, superior cerebellar peduncle*

On side opposite lesion

- Impaired pain and thermal sense on face, limbs, and trunk: *Spinothalamic tract*
- Impaired touch, vibration, and position sense, more in leg than arm (there is a tendency to incongruity of pain and touch deficits): *Medial lemniscus (lateral portion).*

Ans. C

101. Most common small-vessel stroke syndromes are the following except:

A. Pure motor hemiparesis

B. Pure sensory stroke

C. Ataxic hemiparesis

D. Paraparesis and dysarthria

Explanation:

- Most common small-vessel stroke syndromes are the following: (1) *Pure motor hemiparesis* from an infarct in the posterior limb of the internal capsule or the pons; the face, arm, and leg are almost always involved; (2) *pure sensory stroke* from an infarct in the ventral thalamus; (3) *ataxic hemiparesis* from an infarct in the ventral pons or internal capsule; (4) and *dysarthria and a clumsy hand* or arm due to infarction in the ventral pons or in the genu of the internal capsule.

Ans. D

102. All are true about spinal cord lesions except:

A. Quadriparetic patients exhibit both supine hypertension and OH after upward tilting

B. Autonomic dysreflexia describes a dramatic decrease in BP in patients with traumatic spinal cord lesions above the T6 level

C. Vasodilator drugs may be used to treat acute elevations in BP

D. Clonidine can be used prophylactically to reduce the hypertension resulting from bladder stimulation

Explanation:

- Spinal cord lesions from any cause can result in focal autonomic deficits or autonomic hyperreflexia (e.g., spinal cord transection or hemisection) affecting bowel, bladder, sexual, temperature-regulation, or cardiovascular functions.
- Quadriparetic patients exhibit both supine hypertension and OH after upward tilting.
- *Autonomic dysreflexia* describes a dramatic increase in BP in patients with traumatic spinal cord lesions above the T6 level, often in response to irritation of bladder, skin, or muscles.

- Triggers may be clinically silent because perception of painful sensations arising from structures innervated below the level of a spinal cord lesion is often blunted or absent.
- Distended bladder, often from an obstructed Foley catheter or a urinary infection, are common triggers of dysreflexia.
- Associated symptoms can include facial flushing, headache, hypertension, or piloerection.
- Potential complications include intracranial vasospasm or hemorrhage, cardiac arrhythmia, and death. Awareness of the syndrome, identifying the trigger, and careful monitoring of BP during procedures in patients with acute or chronic spinal cord injury are essential.
- In patients with supine hypertension, BP can be lowered by tilting the head upward or sitting the patient up.
- Vasodilator drugs may be used to treat acute elevations in BP. Clonidine can be used prophylactically to reduce hypertension resulting from bladder stimulation. Dangerous increases or decreases in body temperature may result from an inability to sense heat or cold exposure or control peripheral vasoconstriction or sweating below the level of the spinal cord injury.

Ans. B

103. 28 year old female post partum presented with history of headache, blurring of vision. On evaluation she was found to have mild hyperprolactinemia . MRI brain was ordered and showed adenoma . Blood investigation showed normal CBC, high ESR, rest of the routine evaluation was normal. Which is the best mode of treatment for this patient?

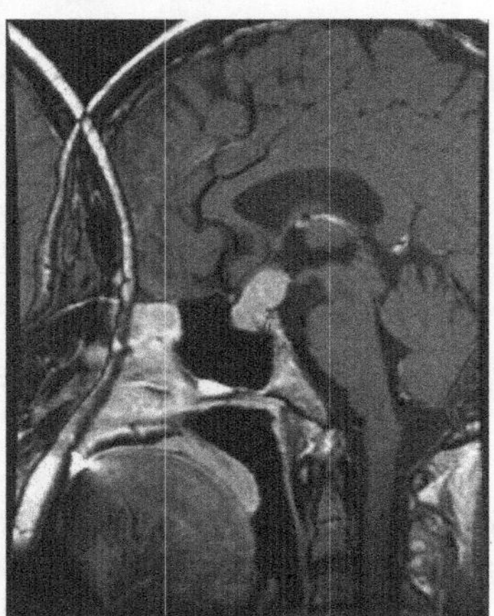

A. Bromocriptine
B. Trans nasal trans sphenoidal surgery
C. IV hydrocortisone
D. Cabergoline

Explanation:

- This is a case of **Lymphocytic Hypophysitis**
- Postpartum women
- presents with hyperprolactinemia
- MRI evidence of a prominent pituitary mass that often resembles an adenoma, with mildly elevated PRL levels.
- Transient or permanent
- The erythrocyte sedimentation rate often is elevated
- MRI image may be indistinguishable from that of a pituitary adenoma
- hypophysitis should be considered in a postpartum woman with a newly diagnosed pituitary mass before an unnecessary surgical intervention
- The inflammatory process often resolves after several months of glucocorticoid treatment

Ans. C

104. All are true statements except:

A. Fisher's syndrome, an ocular variant of Guillain-Barré, produces ophthalmoplegia with areflexia and ataxia

B. A patient with bilateral injury to the medial longitudinal fasciculus will have bilateral INO

C. Stroke is the most common cause for bilateral INO, although multiple sclerosis, trauma, or any brainstem process may be responsible

D. Distal basilar artery ischemia is the most common etiology for disorders of vertical gaze

Explanation:

Internuclear Ophthalmoplegia

- Results from damage to medial longitudinal fasciculus ascending from abducens nucleus in pons to oculomotor nucleus in midbrain (hence, "internuclear").
- Damage to fibers carrying the conjugate signal from abducens interneurons to the contralateral medial rectus motoneurons results in a failure of adduction on attempted lateral gaze.
- For example, a patient with a left internuclear ophthalmoplegia (INO) will have slowed or absent adducting movements of the left eye
- A patient with bilateral injury to the medial longitudinal fasciculus will have bilateral INO.
- Multiple sclerosis is the most common cause, although tumor, stroke, trauma, or any brainstem process may be responsible.
- *One-and-a-half syndrome* is due to a lesion of the medial longitudinal fasciculus combined with a lesion of either the abducens nucleus or paramedian pontine reticular formation on the same side.
- Patient's only horizontal eye movement is abduction of the eye on the other side

Ans. C

105. All below findings are seen on side of lesion in lateral midpontine syndrome except:

A. Ataxia of limbs

B. Paralysis of muscles of mastication

C. Impaired sensation over side of face

D. Impaired pain and thermal sense on limbs and trunk

Explanation:

Lateral midpontine syndrome (short circumferential artery)

On side of lesion

- Ataxia of limbs: *Middle cerebellar peduncle*
- Paralysis of muscles of mastication: *Motor fibers or nucleus of fifth nerve*
- Impaired sensation over side of face: *Sensory fibers or nucleus of fifth nerve*

On side opposite lesion

- Impaired pain and thermal sense on limbs and trunk: *Spinothalamic tract.*

Ans. D

106. All are true about Progressive multifocal leukoencephalopathy (PML) except:

A. Multifocal areas of demyelination of varying size distributed throughout the brain including spinal cord and optic nerves

B. There have been >700 reported cases of PML occurring in patients being treated for multiple sclerosis and inflammatory bowel disease with natalizumab

C. Astrocytes are enlarged and contain hyperchromatic, deformed, and bizarre nuclei and frequent mitotic figures

D. Oligodendrocytes have enlarged, densely staining nuclei that contain viral inclusions formed by crystalline arrays of JC virus (JCV) particles

Explanation:

- Diagnosis of PML is frequently suggested by MRI.
- MRI reveals multifocal asymmetric, coalescing white matter lesions located periventricularly, in the centrum semiovale, in parietal-occipital region, and in the cerebellum. These lesions have increased signal on T2 and FLAIR images and decreased signal on T1-weighted images.
- HIV-PML lesions are classically nonenhancing (90%), but patients with immunomodulatory drug-associated PML may have peripheral ring enhancement.
- PML lesions-not typically associated with edema/ass effect.
- CT scans, which are less sensitive than MRI for the diagnosis of PML, often show hypodense nonenhancing white matter lesions.
- CSF is typically normal, although mild elevation in protein and/or igg may be found. Pleocytosis occurs in <25% of cases, is predominantly mononuclear & rarely exceeds 25 cells/µl.
- PCR amplification of JCV DNA from CSF has become an important diagnostic tool.
- Presence of a positive CSF PCR for JCV DNA in association with typical MRI lesions in the appropriate clinical setting is diagnostic of PML, reflecting the assay's relatively high specificity (92–100%); however, sensitivity is variable, and a negative CSF PCR does not exclude the diagnosis.
- In HIV-negative patients and HIV-positive patients not receiv ng highly active antiviral therapy (HAART), sensitivity is likely 70–90%.
- In HAART-treated patients, sensitivity may be closer to 60% reflecting the lower JCV CSF viral load in this relatively more immunocompetent group.
- Patients with natalizumab-associated PML have highly variable amounts of JCV DNA in CSF.
- Some patients may have negative CSF pcrs performed in commercial laboratories where assay detection thresholds are typically >100 JCV DNA copies/µl, but positive results in reference laboratories using supersensitive techniques (detection of 10 JCV copies/µl or less).
- CSF studies with quantitative JCV PCR indicate that patients with low JCV loads (<100 copies/µl) have a generally better prognosis than those with higher viral loads. Patients with negative CSF PCR studies may require brain biopsy for definitive diagnosis.
- In biopsy or necropsy specimens of brain, JCV antigen and nucleic acid can be detected by immunocytochemistry, in situ hybridization, or PCR amplification.

Ans. A

107. Trial supporting endovascular therapy for stroke more than 6 hrs:

A. DAWN
B. DEFUSE-3
C. Both of the above
D. None of the above

Explanation:

- Extending time window beyond 6 h appears to be effective if patient has specific imaging findings demonstrating good vascular collaterals (CT perfusion or MR perfusion techniques) and can be treated within 24 h; Clinical Mismatch in the Triage of Wake Up and Late Presenting Strokes Undergoing Neurointervention With Trevo (DAWN) trial reported good outcomes more frequently with endovascular therapy than with medical care alone (47 vs 13%, p<0.0001). The Endovascular Therapy Following Imaging

Evaluation for Ischemic Stroke 3 (DEFUSE-3) trial confirmed these results (45 vs 17%, p<0.001) if treated up to 16 hours from stroke onset.

Ans. C

108. All are true about prevention of stroke with antiplatelets except:

A. Ticagrelor has not been found to be better than aspirin for stroke prevention

B. CAPRIE trial found that clopidogrel was only marginally more effective than aspirin in reducing risk of stroke

C. Long term use of clopidogrel in combination with aspirin is not recommended for stroke prevention

D. Short term combination of clopidogrel with aspirin may be effective in preventing the stroke

Explanation:

- Short-term combination of clopidogrel with aspirin may be effective in preventing second stroke, however.
- A trial of 5170 Chinese patients enrolled within 24 h of tia or minor ischemic stroke found that a clopidogrel-aspirin regimen (clopidogrel 300 mg load then 75 mg/d with aspirin 75 mg for the first 21 days) was superior to aspirin (75 mg/d) alone, with 90-day stroke risk decreased from 11.7 to 8.2% (p <.001) and no increase in major hemorrhage.
- This benefit was limited to those not carrying the cyp2c19 polymorphism associated with clopidogrel hypometabolism.
- An international nihsponsored trial of similar design is ongoing.

Ans. D

109. Most common cause of primary headache is:

A. Tension type

B. Migraine

C. Exertional

D. Cluster

Explanation:

- Most common are migraine, tension-type headache, and the TACs, notably cluster headache.

Table: Common causes of headache

Primary Headache		Secondary Headache	
Type	**%**	**Type**	**%**
Tension-type	69	Systemic infection	63
Migraine	16	Head injury	4
Idiopathic stabbing	2	Vascular disorders	1
Exertional	1	Subarachnoid hemorrhage	<1
Cluster	0.1	Brain tumor	0.1

Ans. A

110. All are true about presentation of posterior fossa brain tumors except:

A. Vomiting that precedes the appearance of headache by weeks

B. History of amenorrhea or galactorrhea

C. Head pain appearing abruptly after bending

D. Head pain appearing abruptly after coughing

Explanation:

- Approximately 30% of patients with brain tumors consider headache to be their chief complaint.

- Head pain is usually nondescript— an intermittent deep, dull aching of moderate intensity, which may worsen with exertion or change in position and may be associated with nausea and vomiting.
- This pattern of symptoms results from migraine far more often than from brain tumor.
- Headache of brain tumor disturbs sleep in about 10% of patients. Vomiting that precedes appearance of headache by weeks is highly characteristic of posterior fossa brain tumors.
- History of amenorrhea or galactorrhea should lead one to question whether a prolactin-secreting pituitary adenoma (or the polycystic ovary syndrome) is the source of headache.
- Headache arising de novo in a patient with known malignancy suggests either cerebral metastases or carcinomatous meningitis, or both.
- Head pain appearing abruptly after bending, lifting, or coughing can be due to a posterior fossa mass, a Chiari malformation, or low cerebrospinal fluid (CSF) volume.

Ans. B

111. Biopsy of an enhancing region of the basal meninges shows most commonly:

A. Tuberculosis
B. Sarcoidosis
C. Metastatic adenocarcinoma
D. Syphilis

Explanation:

- In one series, MRI demonstrated meningeal enhancement in 47% of patients undergoing meningeal biopsy; biopsy of an enhancing region was diagnostic in 80% of cases, biopsy of non-enhancing regions was diagnostic in only 9%, and sarcoid (31%) and metastatic adenocarcinoma (25%) were the most common conditions identified.
- ***Tuberculosis is the most common condition identified in many reports from outside the United States.***

Ans. A

112. Episodic generalized weakness caused by all except:

A. Hypocalcemia
B. Hypernatremia
C. Hyponatremia
D. Hypophosphatemia

Explanation:

Table: Causes of episodic generalized weakness
1. Electrolyte disturbances, e.g., hypokalemia, hyperkalemia, hypercalcemia, hypernatremia, hypophosphatemia, hypermagnesemia
2. Muscle disorders
a. Channelopathies (periodic paralyses)
b. Metabolic defects of muscle (impaired carbohydrate or fatty acid utilization; abnormal mitochondrial function)
3. Neuromuscular junction disorders
a. Myasthenia gravis
b. Lambert-Eaton myasthenic syndrome
4. Central nervous system disorders
a. Transient ischemic attacks of the brainstem
b. Transient global cerebral ischemia
c. Multiple sclerosis
5. Lack of voluntary effort
a. Anxiety
b. Pain of discomfort
c. Somatization disorder

Ans. A

113. Not a cause of secondary Parkinson's disease is:

A. Aluminium hydroxide
B. Carbon monoxide
C. Hexane
D. Manganese

Explanation:

Table: Differential diagnosis of parkinsonism

Parkinson's Disease	Atypical Parkinsonism	Secondary Parkinsonism	Neurodegenerative Disorders and other forms of Parkinsonism
• Sporadic • Genetic Dementia with Lewy bodies	• Multiple-system atrophy (MSA) – Cerebellar type (MSA-c) – Parkinson type (MSA-p) • Progressive supranuclear palsy – Parkinsonism – Richardson variant Corticobasal syndrome Frontotemporal dementia	• Drug-induced • Tumor • Infection • Vascular • Normal-pressure hydrocephalus • Tramua • Liver failure • Toxins (e.g., carbon monoxide, manganese, MPTP, cyanide, hexane, methanol, carbon disulfide)	• Wilson's disease • Huntington's disease • Neurodegeneration with brain iron accumulation • SCA 3 (spinocerebellar ataxia) • Fragile X-associated ataxia-tremor-parkinsonism • Prion disease • X-linked Dystonia-parkinsonism • Alzheimer's disease with parkinsonism • Dopa-Responsive Dystonia

Ans. A

114. Which of the following is not a lower motor neuron MND only?

A. Kennedy disease
B. Amyotropic lateral sclerosis
C. Spinal muscular atrophy
D. Adult tay sachs disease

Explanation:

- **Selected lower motor neuron MND-** Kennedy disease, Spinal muscular atrophy, Adult tay sachs disease & Multifocal motor neuropathy with conduction block
- **Selected upper motor neuron MND-** Primary lateral sclerosis & Hereditary spastic paraplegia
- **Amyotropic lateral sclerosis-** Has features of both.

Ans. B

115. Not true regarding Balint syndrome is:

A. Bilateral visual association area lesions
B. Palinopsia
C. Asimultanagnosia
D. Abulia

Explanation:

- Bilateral infarction in the distal PCAs produces cortical blindness (blindness with preserved pupillary light reaction).
- Patient is often unaware of the blindness or may even deny it (*Anton's syndrome*).
- Tiny islands of vision may persist, and the patient may report that vision fluctuates as images are captured in the preserved portions.
- Rarely, only peripheral vision is lost and central vision is spared, resulting in "gun-barrel" vision.

- Bilateral visual association area lesions may result in *Balint's syndrome*, a disorder of the orderly visual scanning of the environment, usually resulting from infarctions secondary to low flow in the "watershed" between the distal PCA and MCA territories, as occurs after cardiac arrest.
- Patients may experience persistence of a visual image for several minutes despite gazing at another scene (*palinopsia*) or an inability to synthesize the whole of an image (*asimultanagnosia*).

Ans. D

116. For chronic tension type headache only proven treatment is:

A. Amytriptillin
B. Nortryptillin
C. Sumitriptan
D. NSAIDS

Explanation:

- Pain of TTH can generally be managed with simple analgesics such as acetaminophen, aspirin, or NSAIDS.
- Behavioral approaches including relaxation can also be effective.
- Clinical studies have demonstrated that triptans in pure TTH are not helpful, although triptans are effective in TTH when the patient also has migraine.
- For chronic TTH, amitriptyline is the only proven treatment; other tricyclics, selective serotonin reuptake inhibitors, and the benzodiazepines have not been shown to be effective.
- There is no evidence for the efficacy of acupuncture. Placebo-controlled trials of onabotulinum toxin type A in chronic TTH were negative.

Ans. A

117. Mutation associated with multiple small vessel strokes with hemorrhagic transformation:

A. NOTCH 1
B. COL4A1
C. GATA 4
D. SPINK

Explanation:

- *CADASIL* (cerebral autosomal dominant arteriopathy with subcortical infarcts and leukoencephalopathy) is an inherited disorder that presents as small-vessel strokes, progressive dementia, and extensive symmetric white matter changes often including the anterior temporal lobes visualized by MRI.
- Approximately 40% of patients have migraine with aura, often manifest as transient motor or sensory deficits.
- Onset is usually in the fourth or fifth decade of life. This autosomal dominant condition is caused by one of several mutations in *Notch-3*, a member of a highly conserved gene family characterized by epidermal growth factor repeats in its extracellular domain.
- Other monogenic ischemic stroke syndromes include cerebral autosomal recessive arteriopathy with subcortical infarcts and leukoencephalopathy (CARASIL) and hereditary endotheliopathy, retinopathy, nephropathy, and stroke (HERNS).
- Fabry's disease also produces both a large-vessel arteriopathy and small-vessel infarctions. The COL4A1 mutation is associated with multiple small vessel strokes with hemorrhagic transformation.

Ans. B

118. Hereditary ataxia with neuropathy seen in:

A. Krabbe disease
B. Fabry disease
C. Bassen Kornzweig disease
D. Cerebrotendinous xanthomatosis

Explanation:

Table: Hereditary ataxias with neuropathy
Friedreich's ataxia
Vitamin E deficiency
Spinocerebellar ataxia
Abetalipoproteinemia (Bassen-Kornzweig disease)

Ans. C

119. Form of Porphyria is not associated with Peripheral neuropathy:

A. Acute intermittent prophyria

B. Hereditary coproporphyria

C. Porphyria cutanea trada

D. Variegate porphyria

Explanation:

Table: Rare hereditary neuropathies
Hereditary Disorders of Lipid Metabolism
Metachromatic leukodystrophy
Krabbe's disease (globoid cell leukodystrophy)
Fabry's disease
Adrenoleukodystrophy/adrenomyeloneuropathy
Refsum's disease
Tangier disease
Cerebrotendinous xanthomatosis
Hereditary Ataxias with Neuropathy
Friedreich's ataxia
Vitamin E deficiency
Spinocerebellar ataxia
Abetalipoproteinemia (Bassen-Kornzweig disease)
Disorder of Defective DNA Repair
Ataxia-telangiectasia
Cockayne's syndrome
Giant Axonal Neuropathy
Porphyria
Acute intermittent porphyria (AIP)
Hereditary coproporphyria (HCP)
Variegate porphyria (VP)
Familial Amyloid Polyneuropathy (FAP)
Transthyretin-related
Gelsolin-related
Apolipoprotein A1-related

Ans. C

120. 5 year old child brought to the OPD with the above skull X-ray which was done for other purpose. Child was diagnosed with as hand Schuller Christian disease. Hand Schuller Christian disease include all except:

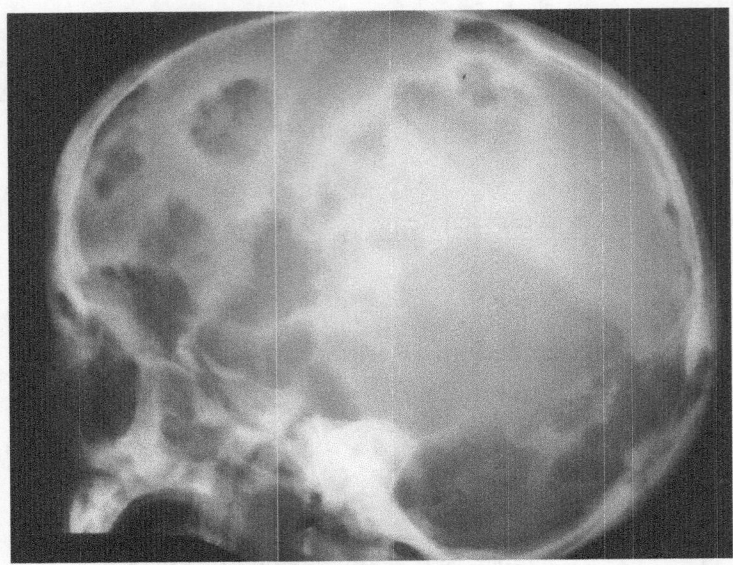

A. DI
B. DM
C. Exophthalmos
D. Punched out lytic lesion

Explanation:

Hand Schuller Christian disease

- DI
- Exophthalmos
- Punched out lytic lesion
- Axillary skin rash

Ans. B

121. Most common cause of headache due to persistent low CSF volume is:

A. Spontaneous CSF leaks
B. CSF leak following LP
C. Vigorous Valsalva maneuver
D. Clearing the eustachian tubes in an airplane

Explanation:

- Most common cause of headache due to persistent low CSF volume is CSF leak following LP. Post-LP headache usually begins within 48 h but may be delayed for up to 12 days.
- Its incidence is between 10 and 30%.
- Beverages with caffeine may provide temporary relief. Besides LP, index events may include epidural injection or a vigorous Valsalva maneuver, such as from lifting, straining, coughing, clearing eustachian tubes in an airplane, or multiple orgasms.
- Spontaneous CSF leaks are well recognized, and the diagnosis should be considered whenever the headache history is typical, even when there is no obvious index event.
- As time passes from the index event, the postural nature may become less apparent; cases in which the index event occurred several years before the eventual diagnosis have been recognized.
- Symptoms appear to result from low volume rather than low pressure: although low CSF pressures, typically 0–50 mm CSF, are usually identified, a pressure as high as 140 mm CSF has been noted with a documented leak.

Ans. B

122. All are true statements except:

A. Aggregates of amyloid fibrils are deposited outside neurons in the form of neuritic plaques in AD

B. Among the causes of familial AD are mutations in genes involved in β-amyloid production, including APP and presenilin 1 and 2

C. About 50–55% of ALS cases are familial

D. A CAG length of 40–60 repeats produces adult onset HD, while repeats of ≥60 produce juvenile onset disease

Explanation:

- First application of stem cell-derived motor neurons to study ALS involved the use of mouse motor neurons generated from transgenic mice expressing a mutation in SOD1 gene, most common mutation responsible for familial ALS.
- Only 5–10% of ALS cases are familial, but the known mutations provide a useful entry point to tease apart the causative pathophysiology.
- Mutations in SOD1 produce ALS through a toxic gain of function for which the mechanism remains unclear, despite use of multiple transgenic animal and iPSC models.
- Use of mouse ESC-derived motor neurons, however, demonstrated that toxic factors secreted by SOD1 astrocytes contribute to the death of motor neurons.

Ans. C

123. Theta waves are seen during:

A. Normal awake with eyes closed

B. Awake with eyes open

C. Drowsiness

D. Light sleep

Explanation:

- During drowsiness, the alpha rhythm is also attenuated; **with light sleep**, slower activity in theta (4–7 Hz) and delta (<4 Hz) ranges becomes more conspicuous.
- Rhythmic activity normally recorded represents the postsynaptic potentials of vertically oriented pyramidal cells of the cerebral cortex and is characterized by its frequency.
- In normal awake adults lying quietly with the eyes closed, an 8- to 13-Hz alpha rhythm is seen posteriorly in the EEG, intermixed with a variable amount of generalized faster (beta) activity (>13 Hz); the alpha rhythm is attenuated when the eyes are opened.

Ans. D

124. All are presentations of distal PCA involvement except:

A. Blindness with preserved pupillary light reaction

B. Only peripheral vision is lost and central vision is spared

C. Persistence of a visual image for several minutes despite gazing at another scene

D. Sudden onset of bilateral signs, including ptosis, pupillary asymmetry or lack of reaction to light, and somnolence

Explanation:

- Bilateral infarction in the distal PCAs produces cortical blindness (blindness with preserved pupillary light reaction).

- Patient is often unaware of the blindness or may even deny it (*Anton's syndrome*). Tiny islands of vision may persist, and the patient may report that vision fluctuates as images are captured in the preserved portions.
- Rarely, only peripheral vision is lost and central vision is spared, resulting in "gun-barrel" vision.
- Bilateral visual association area lesions may result in *Balint's syndrome*, a disorder of the orderly visual scanning of the environment usually resulting from infarctions secondary to low flow in the "watershed" between the distal PCA and MCA territories, as occurs after cardiac arrest.

Ans. D

125. All below findings are seen on side of lesion in medial superior pontine syndrome except:

A. Cerebellar ataxia
B. Paralysis of face, arm, and leg
C. Internuclear ophthalmoplegia
D. Myoclonic syndrome

Explanation:

1. Medial superior pontine syndrome (paramedian branches of upper basilar artery)

   On side of lesion

   - *Cerebellar ataxia (probably):* Superior and/or middle cerebellar peduncle
   - *Internuclear ophthalmoplegia:* Medial longitudinal fasciculus
   - *Myoclonic syndrome, palate, pharynx, vocal cords, respiratory apparatus, face, oculomotor apparatus, etc.:* Localization uncertain–central tegmental bundle, dentate projection, inferior olivary nucleus

   On side opposite lesion

   - *Paralysis of face, arm and leg:* Corticobulbar and corticospinal tract
   - *Rarely touch, vibration and position are affected:* Medial lemniscus

2. Lateral superior pontine syndrome (syndrome of superior cerebellar artery)

   On side of lesion

   - *Ataxia of limbs and gait, falling to side of lesion:* Middle and superior cerebellar peduncles, superior surface of cerebellum, dentate nucleus
   - *Dizziness, nausea, vomiting; horizontal nystagmus:* Vestibular nucleus
   - *Paresis of conjugate gaze (ipsilateral):* Pontine contralateral gaze
   - *Skew deviation:* Uncertain
   - *Miosis, ptosis, decreased sweating over face (Horner's syndrome):* Descending sympathetic fibers
   - *Tremor:* Localization unclear–Dentate nucleus, superior cerebellar peduncle

   On side opposite lesion

   - *Impaired pain and thermal sense on face, limbs and trunk:* Spinothalamic tract
   - *Impaired touch, vibration and position sense, more in leg than arm (there is a tendency to incongruity of pain and touch deficits):* Medial lemniscus (lateral portion)

Ans. B

126. A 60 year old patient came with behavioural disturbances of 1 year duration and was found to have fronto temporal dementia. Which of the following pathogenesis is not related to fronto temporal dementia?

A. Tau
B. TDP 43
C. FUS
D. Synuclein

Explanation:

Table: The molecular basis for degenerative dementia				
Dementia	**Molecular Basis**	**Causal Genes (Chromosome)**	**Susceptibility Genes**	**Pathologic Findings**
AD	Aβ/tau	*APP* (21), *PS*-1 (14), *PS*-2 (1) (<2% carry these mutations, most often in *PS-1*)	*Apo* ε4 (19)	Amyloid plaques, neurofibrillary tangles and neuropil threads
FTD	Tau	*MAPT* exon and intron mutations (17) (about 10% of familial cases)	H1 *MAPT* haplotype	Tau neuronal and glial inclusions varying in morphology and distribution
	TDP-43	*GRN* (10% of familial cases), *C90RF72* (20-30% of familial cases), rare *VCP*, very rare *TARDBP, TBK1, TIA1*		TDP-43 neuronal and glial inclusions varying in morphology and distribution
	FUS	Very rare *FUS*		FUS neuronal and glial inclusions varying in morphology and distribution
DLB	α-Synuclein	Very are *SNCA* (4)	Unknown	α-Synuclein neuronal inclusions (Lewy bodies)

Ans. D

127. A 70 year old came with sudden onset language disturbances. His examination was suggestive of nonfluent transcortical aphasia. His MRI showed acute infarct in deep frontal white matter. which of the following findings are not suggestive of non fluent transcortical aphasia?

A. Preserved comprehension
B. Preserved repetition
C. Preserved naming
D. Impaired fluency

Explanation:

Table: Clinical features of aphasias and related conditions commonly seen in cerebrovascular accidents				
	Comprehension	**Repetition of Spoken Language**	**Naming**	**Fluency**
Wernicke's	Impaired	Impaired	Impaired	Preserved or increased
Broca's	Preserved (except grammar)	Impaired	Impaired	Decreased
Global	Impaired	Impaired	Impaired	Decreased
Conduction	Preserved	Impaired	Impaired	Preserved
Nonfluent (anterior) transcortical	Preserved	Preserved	Impaired	Impaired
Fluent (posterior) transcortical	Impaired	Preserved	Impaired	Preserved
Isolation	Impaired	Echolalia	Impaired	No purposeful speech
Anomic	Preserved	Preserved	Impaired	Preserved except for word-finding pauses
Pure word deafness	Impaired only for spoken language	Impaired	Preserved	Preserved
Pure alexia	Impaired only for reading	Preserved	Preserved	Preserved

Ans. C

128. A 60 year old engineer had sudden onset difficulty in reading. His vision is normal and he could write whatever is being told. This occurs due to lesion in?

A. Left occipital cortex and splenium

B. Left superior temporal gyrus and splenium

C. Right parietal and splenium

D. Left inferior frontal gyrus and splenium

Explanation:

- **Patient has Pure Alexia without Agraphia**
- The lesions (usually a combination of damage to the left occipital cortex and to a posterior sector of the corpus callosum—the splenium) interrupt the flow of visual input into the language network

Ans. A

129. A 60 year old has acute stroke involving bilateral parieto occipital infarcts and has Balints syndrome. Which of the following is not feature of Balints syndrome?

A. Oculomotor apraxia

B. Optic ataxia

C. Simultanagnosia

D. Extinction

Explanation:

Balint's syndrome involves

- Deficits in the orderly visuomotor scanning of the environment (oculomotor apraxia)
- Accurate manual reaching toward visual targets (optic ataxia)
- Ability to integrate visual information in the center of gaze with more peripheral information (simultanagnosia)
- Palinopsia-persistence of a visual image for several minutes despite gazing at another

Ans. D

130. A 20 year old patient has sleep disorder and found to have narcolepsy on polysomnography. Which of these findings on polysomnography are not suggestive of narcolepsy?

A. Sudden muscle weakness without loss of consciousness

B. Sleep paralysis

C. REM sleep disturbance

D. NREM sleep disturbance

Explanation:

- **REM sleep is characterized by:**
  - Sudden muscle weakness without a loss of consciousness, which is usually triggered by strong emotions
  - Hallucinations at sleep onset (hypnagogic hallucinations) or upon awakening (hypnopompic hallucinations)
  - Muscle paralysis upon awakening (sleep paralysis)
- Caused by loss of the hypothalamic neurons that produce
- The orexin neuropeptides (also known as hypocretins)
- Loss of orexin signaling results in frequent intrusions of sleep during the usual waking episode, with REM sleep and fragments of REM sleep at any time of day

Ans. D

131. All trials in stroke used rtPA except:

A. PROACT II
B. NINDS
C. ECASS III
D. All of the above

Explanation:

- National Institute of Neurological Disorders and Stroke (NINDS) rtPA Stroke Study showed a clear benefit for IV rtPA in selected patients with acute stroke. The NINDS study used IV rtPA (0.9 mg/kg to a 90-mg maximum; 10% as a bolus, then the remainder over 60 min) versus placebo in ischemic stroke within 3 h of onset. One-half of the patients were treated within 90 min. Symptomatic intracranial hemorrhage occurred in 6.4% of patients on rtPA and 0.6% on placebo. In the rTPA group, there was a significant 12% absolute increase in the number of patients with only minimal disability (32% on placebo and 44% on rtPA) and a nonsignificant 4% reduction in mortality (21% on placebo and 17% on rtPA). Thus, despite an increased incidence of symptomatic intracranial hemorrhage, treatment with IV rtPA within 3 h of the onset of ischemic stroke improved clinical outcome
- Three subsequent trials of IV rtPA did not confirm this benefit, perhaps because of the dose of rtPA used, the timing of its delivery, and small sample size. When data from all randomized IV rtPA trails were combined, however, efficacy was confirmed in the <3-h time window, and efficacy likely extended to 4.5 h and possibly to 6 h. Based on these combined results, the European Cooperative Acute Stroke Study (ECASS) III explored the safety and efficacy of rtPA in the 3- to 4.5-h time window. Unlike the NINDS study, patients aged >80 years and diabetic patients with a previous stroke were excluded. In this 821-patient randomized study, efficacy was again confirmed, although the treatment effect was less robust than in the 0- to 3-h time window. In the rtPA group, 52.4% of patients achieved a good outcome at 90 days, compared to 45.2% of the placebo group (odds ratio [OR] 1.34, $p = .04$). The symptomatic intracranial hemorrhage rate was 2.4% in the rtPA group and 0.2% in the placebo group ($p = .008$).

Ans. A

132. All are true about Atherosclerotic cause of ischemic stroke except:

A. Atherosclerosis within the carotid artery occurs most frequently within the common carotid bifurcation
B. Greater degrees of arterial narrowing are generally associated with a higher risk of stroke and those with near occlusions are at highest risk
C. Male gender, older age, smoking, hypertension, diabetes, and hypercholesterolemia are risk factors for carotid disease
D. Carotid atherosclerosis produces an estimated 10% of ischemic stroke

Explanation:

- Greater degrees of arterial narrowing are generally associated with a higher risk of stroke, except that those with near occlusions are at lower risk of stroke.

Ans. B

133. A 50 year suffering from REM sleep parasomnias undergone polysomnography. Which of the following disorder can be seen in his polysomnography?

A. Somnambulism
B. Sleep terrors
C. Night mares
D. Sleep enuresis

Explanation:

- NREM parasomnias
  - Somnambulism

  - Sleep terrors
  - Enuresis, bruxism
- REM
  - RBD (REM sleep behavior disorder) – Night mares

Ans. C

134. A 2 year old child was diagnosed as Lennox gastaut syndrome. Which of the following features are not suggestive of LGS?

A. Multiple seizure types

B. EEG showing slow (<3 Hz) spike-and-wave discharges

C. Impaired cognitive function

D. Good response to treatment

Explanation:

- Triad constitutes
  - Multiple seizure types (usually including generalized tonicclonic, atonic, and atypical absence seizures)
  - EEG showing slow (<3 Hz) spike-and-wave discharges
  - Impaired cognitive function
- Patients with LGS have refractory epilepsy but it is not a part of triad.
- Occurs in people with diffuse neuronal dysfunction such as developmental abnormalities, perinatal hypoxia/ischemia, trauma, infection, and few denovo mutations.
- Seizures are usually refractory and prognosis is poor.

Ans. D

135. A 65 year old patient developed anterior choroidal artery infarction during surgical clipping of internal carotid artery. He is not likely to have which symptoms?

A. Hemiparesis

B. Hemi anaesthesia

C. Homonomous hemianopia

D. Ataxia

Explanation:

Anterior Choroidal Artery

- Arises from the internal carotid artery
- Supplies posterior limb of the internal capsule and the white matter posterolateral to it, through which geniculocalcarine fibers pass
- Contralateral hemiplegia, hemianesthesia, homonymous hemianopia.
- Minimal deficits occur, and patients frequently recover substantially.
- The vessel is particularly vulnerable to iatrogenic occlusion during surgical clipping of aneurysms arising from the internal carotid artery

Ans. D

136. A patient suffering from lateral medullary syndrome has which of the following symptom?

A. Contralateral Facial loss of pain
B. Contralateral Ataxia
C. Contralateral Taste
D. Contralateral loss of pain and temperature

Explanation:

Lateral Medullary Syndrome

- Ipsilateral- FAT VH 9,10
  - Facial loss of pain
  - Ataxia
  - Taste
  - Vertigo
  - Horners
  - 9, 10 cranial palsies
- Contralateral
  - Spinothalamic- loss of pain and temperature
- Occlusion of vertebral, PICA, superior, middle, or inferior lateral medullary arteries

Anatomical Location	Presenting Symptoms
Spinothalamic tract	Contralateral loss of pain and temperature sensation
Spinal trigeminal nucleus	Ipsilateral facial loss of pain and temperature
Nucleus ambiguus	Supplies vagus and glossopharyngeal nerves; dysphagia/ dysphonia/diminished gag reflex
Inferior vestibular nucleus	Vertigo/diplopia/nystagmus/vomiting
Sympathetic fibres	Ipsilateral Horners syndrome
Central trigeminal tract	Palatal clonus
Inferior cerebellar peduncle	Ataxia

Ans. D

137. An elderly male who is a known diabetic had ischemic stroke and is in locked state. Which part of his brain is likely involved?

A. Ventral pons
B. Dorsal pons
C. Ventral medulla
D. Dorsal medulla

Explanation:

- Locked-in-state

  Involvement of ventral pons

  Consciousness is intact

  Extraocular movement- vertical movements spared Quadriplegia

Ans. A

138. CT myelography superior in all below except:

A. Lateral recess of the spinal canal
B. Bony abnormalities
C. Definition of soft tissue structures
D. All of the above

Explanation:

- A lumbar spine MRI scan or CT myelogram can often confirm location and type of pathology. Spine MRIs yield exquisite views of intraspinal and adjacent soft tissue anatomy, whereas bony lesions of lateral recess or intervertebral foramen are optimally visualized by CT myelography.
- Correlation of neuroradiologic findings to clinical symptoms, particularly pain, is not simple.
- Contrast-enhancing tears in the annulus fibrosus or disk protrusions are widely accepted as common sources of back pain; however, studies have found that many asymptomatic adults have similar findings.
- Entirely asymptomatic disk protrusions are also common, occurring in up to one-third of adults, and these may also enhance with contrast.
- Furthermore, in patients with known disk herniation treated either medically or surgically, persistence of the herniation 10 years later had no relationship to the clinical outcome.
- In summary, MRI findings of disk protrusion, tears in the annulus fibrosus, or hypertrophic facet joints are common incidental findings that, by themselves, should not dictate management decisions for patients with back pain.

Ans. C

139. Regarding Neurogenic claudication, all are true except:

A. Pain in Buttock
B. Pain on standing and walking
C. Pain on walking but not while standing
D. Relieved on sitting

Explanation:

- Neurogenic claudication consists of pain, typically in the back and buttock or leg, that is brought on by walking or standing and relieved by sitting.
- Symptoms in the legs are usually bilateral. Unlike vascular claudication, symptoms are often provoked by standing without walking.
- Unlike lumbar disk disease, symptoms are usually relieved by sitting.
- Patients with neurogenic claudication can often walk much farther when leaning over a shopping cart and can pedal a stationary bike with ease while sitting.
- These flexed positions increase the anteroposterior spinal canal diameter and reduce intraspinal venous hypertension, producing pain relief.
- Focal weakness, sensory loss, or reflex changes may occur when spinal stenosis is associated with neural foraminal narrowing and radiculopathy.
- Severe neurologic deficits, including paralysis and urinary incontinence, occur only rarely.

Ans. C

140. In a patient with amyloid angiopathy, which of the following is prone to hemorrhage?

A. Putamen
B. Cerebellum
C. Pons
D. Lobar

Explanation:

Table: Causes of intracranial hemorrhage		
Cause	**Location**	**Comments**
Head trauma	Intraparenchymal; frontal lobes, anterior temporal lobes; subarachnoid; extra-axial (subdural, epidural)	Coup and contrecoup injury during brain deceleration
Hypertensive hemorrhage	Putamen, globus pallidus, thalamus, cerebellar hemisphere, pons	Chronic hypertension produces hemorrhage from small (~30-100 μm) vessels in these regions
Transformation of prior ischemic infarction	Basal ganglion, subcortical regions, lobar	Occurs in 1-6% ischemic strokes with predilection for large hemispheric infarctions
Metastatic brain tumor	Lobar	Lung, choriocarcinoma, melanoma, renal cell carcinoma, thyroid, atrial myxoma
Coagulopathy	Any	Risk for ongoing hematoma expansion
Drug	Any, lobar, subarachnoid	Cocaine, amphetamine
Arteriovenous malformation	Lobar, intraventricular, subarachnoid	Risk is ~2-3% per year for bleeding if previously unruptured
Aneurysm	Subarachnoid, intraparenchymal, rarely subdural	Mycotic and nonmycotic form of aneurysms
Amyloid angiopathy	Lobar	Degenerative disease of intracranial vessels; associated with dementia, rare in patients <60 years
Cavernous angioma	Intraparenchymal	Multiple cavernous angiomas linked to mutations in *KRIT1, CCM2* and *PDCD10 genes*
Dural arteriovenous fistula	Lobar, subarachnoid	Produces bleeding by venous hypertension
Capillary telangiectasias	Usually brainstem	Rare cause of hemorrhage

Ans. D

141. A young patient is suffering from episodic cluster headache. Which of the following cannot used as prophylaxis for him?

A. Verapamil
B. Topiramate
C. Carbamazapine
D. Lithium

Explanation:

Table: Preventive management of cluster headache	
Short-Term Prevention	**Long-Term Prevention**
Episodic cluster headache	**Episodic cluster headache and prolonged chronic cluster headache**
Prednisone 1 mg/kg up to 60 mg qd, tapering over 21 days Verapamil 160-960 mg/d Greater occipital nerve injection	Verapamil 160-960 mg/d Topiramate[a] 100-400 mg/d nVNS[b] 6 to 24 stimulations/d Lithium 400-800 mg/d Melatonin[a] 9-12 mg/d Gabapentin[a] 1200-3600 mg/d

Ans. C

142. A 50 year old person whose father was suffering Alzheimers disease got evaluated and was diagnosed as Prodromal AD. Which of the following is not true about the patient?

A. Symptomatic memory loss

B. PET showing hypometabolism in medial temporal and parietal lobes

C. Decreased CSF levels of A-beta 42

D. Increased CSF levels of P-tau

Explanation:

- "Prodromal AD" refers to a person with biomarker evidence of AD (amyloid imaging positive with positron emission tomography (PET) or low cerebrospinal Aβ42 and mildly elevated tau) in the absence of symptoms

Ans. A

143. Alzheimer's is the most common form of dementia and is caused due to many gene abnormalities. However, which of the following genes were not implicated in causation of Alzheimer's disease?

A. APP gene

B. Presenilin-1

C. Apo E gene

D. C9ORF72

Explanation:

- **Genes implicated in causation of Alzheimer's disease**
  - APP – CHROMOSOME 21
  - PRESENILIN1 (PSEN1)- CHROMOSOME 14
  - PRESENILIN 2 (PSEN2)- CHROMOSOME 1
  - APO E – CHROMOSOME 19

Ans. D

144. First-line agents for trigeminal neuralgia is:

A. Newer anticonvulsants

B. Opioids

C. NSAIDs

D. Antidepressants

Explanation:

- Phenytoin (Dilantin) and carbamazepine (Tegretol) were first shown to relieve the pain of trigeminal neuralgia. This pain has a characteristic brief, shooting, electric shock-like quality.
- In fact, anticonvulsants seem to be particularly helpful for pains that have such a lancinating quality.
- Newer anticonvulsants, the calcium channel alpha-2-delta subunit ligands gabapentin (Neurontin) and pregabalin (Lyrica), are effective for a broad range of neuropathic pains.
- Furthermore, because of their favorable side effect profile, these newer anticonvulsants are often used as first-line agents.

Ans. A

145. A 65 year old engineer, interested in politics, came with decreased interest in politics, couldn't even tell prime minister name. He is suffering from which disease?

A. Bevioural variant FTD

B. Semantic variant of PPA

C. Non fluent variant of PPA

D. Logopenic variant of PPA

Explanation:

- Patient has loss of semantics (knowledge). Suffering from semantic dementia which is a type of FTD

Ans. B

146. All are used for treatment of Vasospasm of SAH except:

A. NTG
B. Nimodipine
C. Aggressive IV fluid administration
D. Phenylephrine

Explanation:

- Subarachnoid hemorrhage may occur secondary to aneurysm rupture and is often complicated by cerebral vasospasm, re-bleeding, and hydrocephalus.
- Vasospasm can be detected by either transcranial Doppler assessment or cerebral angiography; it is typically treated with the calcium channel blocker nimodipine, aggressive IV fluid administration, and therapy aimed at increasing blood pressure, typically with vasoactive drugs such as phenylephrine.
- IV fluids and vasoactive drugs (hypertensive hypervolemic therapy) are used to overcome the cerebral vasospasm.
- Early surgical clipping or endovascular coiling of aneurysms is advocated to prevent complications related to re-bleeding.
- Hydrocephalus, typically heralded by a decreased level of consciousness, may require ventriculostomy drainage

Ans. A

147. A 60 year old man suffering from frontotemporal dementia. He is not likely to show which of the following mutation?

A. C9ORF72- chromosome 9
B. GRN- chromosome 17
C. MAPT- chromosome 17
D. PSEN-1- chromosome 14

Explanation:

- PSEN1 is associated with Alzheimer's disease

Ans. D

148. A 60 year old patient presented with magnetic gait, dementia mainly executive dysfunction and urinary incontinence. His MRI showed enlarged lateral ventricles with wide open sylvian fissures. His most likely diagnosis is:

A. Normal pressure hydrocephalus
B. Vascular dementia
C. Alzheimer's dementia
D. Prion diseases

Explanation:

- NPH clinical triad includes an abnormal gait (ataxic or apractic), dementia (usually mild to moderate, with an emphasis on executive impairment), and urinary urgency or incontinence.
- Neuroimaging reveals enlarged lateral ventricles (hydrocephalus) with little or no cortical atrophy, although the sylvian fissures may appear propped open (so-called "box carring") and crowding of dorsal frontal-parietal gyri.

Ans. A

149. A 40 year old man who is a chronic alcoholic is suffering from Wernicke's encephalopathy. His memory loss correlates with damage to:

A. Dorsomedial thalamus
B. Mammillary bodies
C. Periaqueductal gray matter
D. Midline cerebellum

Explanation:

- Wernicke's encephalopathy presents with confusion, ataxia, and diplopia resulting from inflammation and necrosis of periventricular midline structures, including dorsomedial thalamus, mammillary bodies, midline cerebellum, periaqueductal gray matter, and trochlear and abducens nuclei.
- Damage to the dorsomedial thalamus correlates most closely with the memory loss.

Ans. A

150. An elderly lady suffering from DLB (Diffuse Lewy Body) dementia suffering from behavioural problems. Which of the following is false about her?

A. Visual hallucinations
B. Fluctuating alertness
C. REM sleep behavioural disorder
D. Drug of choice for behavioural symptoms–Neuroleptics

Explanation:

Dementia with Lewy Bodies

- DLB clinical syndrome- visual hallucinations, parkinsonism, fluctuating alertness, falls, and rapid eye movement (REM) sleep behavior disorder (RBD)
- Neuropathologic feature in DLB is the presence of Lewy bodies and Lewy neurites
- MIBG cardiac scintigraphy and PET/SPECT
- Treatment- AChIs
- Neuroleptics are contraindicated–causes severe parkinsonism and delirium

Ans. D

151. Accumulation of alpha synuclein causes many degenerative diseases. Which of the following disease is not caused due to accumulation of synuclein?

A. Parkinson's Disease
B. Multi system atrophy
C. Dementia with Lewy Body Disease
D. Progressive supra nuclear palsy

Explanation:

TAU pathies	Synucleopathies
FTD PSP CBD	PD MSA DLBD

Ans. D

152. All are true except:

A. Interruption of spinothalamic pathway produces permanent deficits in pain and temperature discrimination

B. Even the suggestion that a treatment will relieve pain can have a significant analgesic effect is called placebo effect

C. Suggestion that pain will worsen following administration of an inert substance can increase its perceived intensity is called nocebo effect

D. Hyperpathia, a greatly exaggerated pain response to innocuous or mild nociceptive stimuli, especially when applied repeatedly, is characteristic of somatic pain

Explanation:

- Neuropathic pain typically has an unusual burning, tingling, or electric shock-like quality and may occur spontaneously, without any stimulus, or be triggered by very light touch. These features are rare in other types of pain.
- On examination, a sensory deficit is characteristically present in the area of the patient's pain.
- Hyperpathia, a greatly exaggerated pain response to innocuous or mild nociceptive stimuli, especially when applied repeatedly, is also characteristic of neuropathic pain; patients often complain that the very lightest moving stimulus evokes exquisite pain (allodynia). In this regard, it is of clinical interest that a topical preparation of 5% lidocaine in patch form is effective for patients with postherpetic neuralgia who have prominent allodynia.

Ans. D

153. A 60 year old patient came with asymmetric rest tremors, rigidity, and bradykinesia. He showed good response to levodopa. His disease is due to degeneration of:

A. Substantia nigra pars compacta (SNc)

B. Substantia nigra pars reticulata (SNr)

C. Midbrain tectum

D. Subthalamic nucleus

Explanation:

- Parkinsons is caused due to Degeneration of dopaminergic neurons in the substantia nigra pars compacta (SNc)
- Cholinergic neurons of the nucleus basalis of Meynert (NBM)
- Norepinephrine neurons of the locus coeruleus (LC)
- Serotonin neurons in the raphe nuclei of the brainstem, and neurons of the olfactory system, cerebral hemispheres, spinal cord, and peripheral autonomic nervous system

Ans. A

154. All are true about brain abscess except:

A. 70% patients have headache

B. 50% have focal neurological signs

C. Almost all have fever

D. 25% have papilledema

Explanation:

- Brain abscess often occurs without systemic signs. Almost half of patients are afebrile, and presentations are more consistent with a space-occupying lesion in brain; 70% of patients have headache and/or altered mental status, 50% have focal neurologic signs, and 25% have papilledema.
- Abscesses can present as single or multiple lesions resulting from contiguous foci or hematogenous infection like endocarditis, or after surgery or trauma.
- Infection progresses over several days from cerebritis to an abscess with a mature capsule.
- More than half of infections are polymicrobial, with an etiology consisting of aerobic bacteria (primarily streptococcal species) and anaerobes.
- Abscesses arising hematogenously are especially apt to rupture into ventricular space, causing a sudden and severe deterioration in clinical status and a high mortality rate.

Ans. C

155. All are true statements except:

A. Disorders of deep sensation arising from muscle spindles, tendons, and joints affect proprioception

B. Imbalance, clumsiness of precision movements, and unsteadiness of gait, which are referred to collectively as sensory ataxia

C. Romberg sign is positive, which means that the patient sways markedly or topples when asked to stand with feet close together and eyes open

D. Continuous involuntary movements of the outstretched hands and fingers occur, particularly with eyes closed is called pseudoathetosis

Explanation:

- Romberg sign is positive, which means that patient sways markedly or topples when asked to stand with feet close together and eyes closed. In severe states of deafferentation involving deep sensation, patient cannot walk or stand unaided or even sit unsupported.
- Continuous involuntary movements (*pseudoathetosis*) of outstretched hands and fingers occur, particularly with eyes closed.

Ans. C

156. All can differentiate between frontal gait and sensory gait except:

A. Base of support

B. Velocity

C. Initiation

D. Falls

Explanation:

Table: Features of cerebellar ataxia, sensory ataxia and frontal gait disorders

Feature	Cerebellar Ataxia	Sensory Ataxia	Fontal Gait
Base of support	Wide-based	Narrow base, looks down	Wide-based
Velocity	Variable	Slow	Very slow
Stride	Irregular, lurching	Regular with path deviation	Short, shuffling
Romberg test	+/–	Unsteady, falls	+/–
Heel→shin	Abnormal	+/–	Normal
Initiation	Normal	Normal	Hesitant
Turns	Unsteady	+/–	Hesitant, multistep
Postural instability	+	+++	++++ Poor postural synergies rising from a chair
Falls	Late event	Frequent	Frequent

Ans. D

157. Genetic form of Parkinson's disease is caused due to many gene mutations and these are named as PARK. One of those genes is SNCA which codes for alpha synuclein. It causes which of the following disease?

A. PARK 1

B. PARK 2

C. PARK 3

D. PARK 4

Explanation:

Classical PD				
PARK-*SNCA*	Gene Reviews http://ww.ncbi.nlm.nih.gov/books/NBK1223/OMIM168601	Missense mutations cause classical parkinsonism. Duplication or triplication mutations in this gene cause early onset parkinsonism with prominent dementia	AD	PARK1
PARK-*LRRK2*	GeneReviews *http://www.ncbi.nlm.nih.gov/books/NBK1208/*OMIM 607060	Clinically typial PD	AD	PARK8
PARK-VPS35	GeneReviews *http://www.ncbi.nlm.nih.gov/books/NBK1223/*OMIM 614203	Clinically typical PD	AD	PARK17
Early-Onset PD				
PARK-*Parkin*	GeneReviews *http://www.ncbi.nlm.nih.gov/books/NBK1155/*OMIM 600116	Often presents with dystonia, typically in a leg	AR	PARK2
PARK-*PINK1*	GeneeReviews *http://.www.ncbi.nlm.nih.gov/books/NBK1223/*OMIM 605909	Often presents with psychiatric features	AR	PARK6
PARK-*DJ1*	GeneReviews *http://www.ncbi.nlm.nih.gov/books/NBK1223/*OMIM 606324		AR	PARK7
Parkinsonism				
PARK-*ATP13A2*	GeneReviews *http://www.ncbi.nlm.nih.gov/books/NBK1223/*OMIM 606693	Kufor-Rakeb syndrome with parkinosonism and dystonia; additional features: Supranuclear gaze palsy, spasticity/pyramidal signs, dementia, facial-faucial-finger mini-myoclonus, dysphagia, dysarthria, olfactory dysfunction	AR	PARK9
PARK-*FBX07*	GeneReviews *http://www.ncbi.nlm.nih.gov/books/NBK1223/*OMIM: 260300	Early onset parkinsonism with pyramidal signs	AR	PARK15
PARK-*DNAJC6*	GeneReviews: n/a OMIM 615528	May present with mental retardation and seizures	AR	PARK19
PARK-*SYNJ1*	Gene Reviews: n/a OMIM 615530	May have seizures, cognitive decline, abnormal eye movements and dystonia	AR	PARK20

Ans. A

158. Parkinson's disease is due to loss of dopaminergic neurons. Dopamine is metabolised by an enzyme MAO-B, the inhibition of which can improve symptoms in Parkinson's. Which of the following is MAO-B inhibitor?

A. Rasagiline
B. Carbidopa
C. Entacapone
D. Pramipixole

Ans. A

159. All statements are true except:

A. CT is better than MRI for demonstrating abscesses in early cerebritis stages

B. MRI is better than CT for identifying abscesses in posterior fossa

C. Cerebritis appears as an area of low signal intensity on T1 weighted images

D. Cerebritis appears as an area of increased signal intensity on T2 weighted images

Explanation:

- Diagnosis of Brain abscess is made by neuroimaging studies.
- MRI is better than CT for demonstrating abscesses in the early (cerebritis) stages and is superior to CT for identifying abscesses in the posterior fossa.
- Cerebritis appears on MRI as an area of low-signal intensity on T1-weighted images with irregular postgadolinium enhancement and as an area of increased signal intensity on T2-weighted images.
- Cerebritis is often not visualized by CT scan, but when present, appears as an area of hypodensity.
- On CECT scan, a mature brain abscess appears as a focal area of hypodensity surrounded by ring enhancement with surrounding edema (hypodensity).
- On contrast-enhanced T1-weighted MRI, a mature brain abscess has a capsule that enhances surrounding a hypodense center and surrounded by a hypodense area of edema.
- On T2-weighted MRI, there is a hyperintense central area of pus surrounded by a well-defined hypointense capsule and a hyperintense surrounding area of edema.
- It is important to recognize that CT and MRI appearance, particularly of the capsule, may be altered by treatment with glucocorticoids.
- Distinction between a brain abscess and other focal CNS lesions such as primary or metastatic tumors may be facilitated by use of diffusion-weighted imaging sequences on which a brain abscess typically shows increased signal due to restricted diffusion of abscess cavity with corresponding low signal on apparent diffusion coefficient images.

Ans. A

160. Many atypical Parkinson diseases has characteristic imaging features on MRI. Which of these features doesn't correlate with its respective diseases?

A. MSA-P- Putaminal rim sign

B. MSA-C- Hot cross bun sign

C. PSP- Humming bird sign

D. PD- Mickey mouse sign

Explanation:

Ans. D

161. A 10 year old child has dystonia of lower limbs followed by upper limb onset. Her genetic testing was suggestive of Dopamine Responsive Dystonia. Which of the following is false regarding the disease?

A. GTP cyclohydrolase enzyme defective

B. Symptoms are severe in morning

C. Common in children

D. Responsive to Levodopa

Explanation:

- GTP cyclohydrolase enzyme defective
- Symptoms are less in morning and worsens as day progresses- Diurnal variation
- Symptoms start in Lower limbs and ascend to upper limbs later
- Common in children
- Responsive to Levodopa

Ans. B

162. A 20 year old presented with tremors of upper limbs which occurs while drinking tea. There are no other extrapyramidal features. He was diagnosed as essential tremors. Which is not true regarding his disease?

A. Bilateral and symmetric

B. Increased with alcohol

C. 50% cases autosomal dominant inheritance

D. Cerebellum and inferior olive are tremor pacemakers

Explanation:

Essential Tremors

- ET- characterized by a high-frequency tremor (6–10 Hz)
- Predominantly affects the upper extremities
- Postural or action (kinetic) tremor
- Bilateral and symmetric
- Characteristically improved by alcohol and worsened by stress
- 50% of cases have a positive family history with an autosomal dominant pattern
- Cerebellum and inferior olives have been implicated as possible sites of a tremor pacemaker

Ans. B

163. CADASIL occurs due to defect of which of the following gene?

A. NOTCH 1

B. NOTCH 2

C. NOTCH 3

D. NOTCH 4

Explanation:

- *CADASIL* (cerebral autosomal dominant arteriopathy with subcortical infarcts and leukoencephalopathy) is an inherited disorder that presents as small-vessel strokes, progressive dementia, and extensive symmetric white matter changes often including the anterior temporal lobes visualized by MRI.
- Approximately 40% of patients have migraine with aura, often manifest as transient motor or sensory deficits.
- Onset is usually in the fourth or fifth decade of life.
- This autosomal dominant condition is caused by one of several mutations in *Notch-3*, a member of a highly conserved gene family characterized by epidermal growth factor repeats in its extracellular domain.
- Other monogenic ischemic stroke syndromes include cerebral autosomal recessive arteriopathy with subcortical infarcts and leukoencephalopathy (CARASIL) and hereditary endotheliopathy, retinopathy, nephropathy and stroke (HERNS).
- Fabry's disease also produces both a large-vessel arteriopathy and small-vessel infarctions. The COL4A1 mutation is associated with multiple small vessel strokes with hemorrhagic transformation.

Ans. C

164. A 20 year old presented with myoclonus, which improves with alcohol. He showed SGCE mutations. He is suffering from which disease?

A. Dopa responsive dystonia

B. Lubag dystonia

C. Myoclonic dystonia

D. Lesh nyhan syndrome

Explanation:

Myoclonic Dystonia

- Occurs due to mutation in SGCE gene (Sarcoglycan epsilon)
- Myoclonus decreased by alcohol
- Occurs in childhood or adolescence
- Predominantly affects head
- Cognitive decline
- Psychiatric- OCD, panic and phobia disorders

Ans. C

165. A 30 year old man presented with progressive chorea, behavioural problems and cognitive decline. Similar illness in father at 40 years of age and he committed suicide. He is most likely to suffer from which gene mutation?

A. Presenilin gene
B. c9ORF72
C. Huntingtin gene
D. Epsilon sarcoglycan gene

Explanation:

Huntington's disease

- Autosomal dominant
- Onset between the ages of 25 and 45 years
- Motor, behavioural, cognitive dysfunction
- In early stages, chorea tends to be focal or segmental, but progresses over time to involve multiple body regions
- Dysarthria, gait disturbance, oculomotor abnormalities, behavioral disturbance, cognitive impairment, dementia
- Advanced disease- reduction in chorea and the emergence of dystonia, rigidity, bradykinesia, and myoclonus
- Diabetes mellitus and neuroendocrineth abnormalities

Ans. C

166. A 40 year old patient presenting with severe chorea, dystonia. He was told to have neuroacanthocytosis. False about neuroacanthocytosis:

A. VPS13A gene mutation
B. Acanthocytes on peripheral smear
C. Autosomal dominant pattern
D. Self mutilating behaviour

Explanation:

- Neuroacanthocytosis
  - Autosomal recessive
  - Chorea, self mutilating behavior, dystonia, tics, seizures, polyneuropathy
  - Mutations in *VPS13A* gene encoding chorein

Ans. C

167. A 10 year old girl presented with choreiform movements. She has history of rheumatic fever. Other work up for childhood chorea was negative. Which is false regarding her disease?

A. Common in childhood

B. Associated with group A streptococcal infections

C. Poor prognosis

D. Treated with valproate or carbamazepine or dopamine blockers

Explanation:

Syndenham chorea

- St. Vitus's dance
- Common in girls
- 5–15 years
- Associated with group A streptococcal infections
- Good prognosis
- Treated with valproate or carbamazepine or dopamine blockers

Ans. C

168. Metastatic tumors commonly associated with ICH are all except:

A. Choriocarcinoma

B. Malignant melanoma

C. HCC

D. Renal cell carcinoma

Explanation:

- Hemorrhage into a *brain tumor* may be the first manifestation of neoplasm. Choriocarcinoma, malignant melanoma, renal cell carcinoma, and bronchogenic carcinoma are among the most common metastatic tumors associated with ICH. Glioblastoma multiform in adults and medulloblastoma in children may also have areas of ICH.

Ans. C

169. A patient presented with uneasy sensation in legs which are precipitated by rest and improves with walking, which are more common in night time. False about the disease is:

A. Low dose dopamine agonists are used

B. Iron excess can precipitate it

C. Can be caused by renal failure

D. Genetic cause is seen in few patients

Explanation:

Restless Leg Syndrome

- 4 core symptoms
  - An urge to move the legs
  - Accompanied by an unpleasant sensation in legs
  - Symptoms worsen with rest
  - Relief by movement
- Worsening during the evening or night

- Seen with iron deficiency.
- Other factors include renal failure, peripheral neuropathy

Ans. B

170. Most common cause of epidemic encephalitis is:

A. La crosse virus
B. West nile virus
C. CMV
D. HSV1

Explanation:

- Most commonly identified viruses causing sporadic cases of acute encephalitis in immunocompetent adults are herpesviruses (herpes simplex virus [HSV], varicella-zoster virus [VZV], Epstein-Barr virus [EBV]).
- Epidemics of encephalitis are caused by arboviruses, which belong to several different viral taxonomic groups including *Alphaviruses* (e.g., eastern equine encephalitis [EEE] virus), *Flaviviruses* (e.g., West Nile virus [WNV], St. Louis encephalitis virus, Japanese encephalitis virus, Powassan virus), and *Bunyaviruses* (e.g., California encephalitis virus serogroup, La Crosse virus).

Ans. B

171. All are features of multiple sclerosis except:

A. Autoimmune disease of CNS
B. Weakness of UMN type & tendon reflex never lost
C. Bilateral INO is particularly suggestive of MS
D. Facial weakness in MS is usually not associated with ipsilateral loss of taste sensation or retroauricular pain

Explanation:

- Weakness of the limbs may manifest as loss of strength, speed, or dexterity, as fatigue, or as a disturbance of gait. Exercise-induced weakness is a characteristic symptom of MS. Weakness is of the upper motor neuron type and is usually accompanied by other pyramidal signs such as spasticity, hyperreflexia, and Babinski signs. Occasionally, a tendon reflex may be lost (simulating a lower motor neuron lesion) if an MS lesion disrupts the afferent reflex fibers in the spinal cord.
- Facial weakness due to a lesion in the pons may resemble idiopathic Bell's palsy.
- Unlike Bell's palsy, facial weakness in MS is usually not associated with ipsilateral loss of taste sensation or retroauricular pain.

Ans. B

172. A patient presented with progressive dystonia and parkinsonism and was diagnosed as PKAN. False about PKAN (Panthothenate Kinase Associated Neurodegeneration)

A. PANK2 mutation
B. Accumulation of manganese in basal ganglia
C. Parkinsonism and dystonia common
D. MRI shows eye of tiger appearance

Explanation:

- NBIA represents a group of inherited disorders characterized by iron accumulation in the basal ganglia.
- Clinically, they can manifest as a progressive neurologic disorder with parkinsonism, dystonia, neuropsychiatric abnormalities, and retinal degeneration
- PKAN formerly known as Hallervorden-Spatz disease is caused by a mutation in the PANK2 gene, and is the most common form of NBIA accounting for about 50%

- MRI shows a characteristic low signal abnormality in the center of the globus pallidus on T2-weighted scans caused by iron accumulation known as the "eye of the tiger" sign

Ans. B

173. A patient presented with paroxysmal episodes of ataxia, nystagmus was evaluated and found to have Episodic ataxia type 1. Which of the following is false?

A. episodes of ataxia, myokymia, nystagmus lasts few seconds to a minute

B. Sudden movement induces attacks

C. Mutation of Calcium channel

D. Treated with acetazolamide

Explanation:

EA Type 1	EA Type 2
• KCNA1	• CACNA1A
• Ataxia, myokymia, nystagmus	• Ataxia, nystagmus
• Lasts minutes	• Hours or days
• Startle, sudden change in posture, exercise induce	• Stress, exercise, or excessive fatigue
• Acetazolamide, anticonvulsants	• Acetazolamide

Ans. C

174. A 18 year old presented with ataxia, scoliosis, foot deformities, cardiomyopathy, and extensor plantar response. Which is false regarding his illness?

A. Chromosome 9q

B. Frataxin gene mutation

C. CAG repeats

D. Usually onset before 25 years of age

Explanation:

Friedreich's ataxia

- Chromosome 9q
- Gene frataxin
- GAA triplet repeats
- Usually onset before 25 years of age
- Clinical features- Ataxia, dysarthria, nystagmus
- Absence of deep tendon reflexes, Extensor plantar responses
- Loss of vibratory and proprioceptive
- Scoliosis, foot deformity
- Cardiomyopathy- hypertrophy, murmurs, and conduction defects
- Diabetes mellitus 20%

Ans. C

175. Not true about clinical feature of GBS is:

A. Ascending paralysis

B. Deep tendon reflexes attenuate or disappear

C. Cutaneous sensory deficints are usually relatively mild

D. Large sensory fibers are not affected

Explanation:

- Fever and constitutional symptoms are absent at the onset and, if present, cast doubt on diagnosis.
- Deep tendon reflexes attenuate or disappear within first few days of onset.
- Cutaneous sensory deficits (e.g., loss of pain and temperature sensation) are usually relatively mild, but functions subserved by large sensory fibers, such as deep tendon reflexes and proprioception, are more severely affected.
- Bladder dysfunction may occur in severe cases but is usually transient. If bladder dysfunction is a prominent feature and comes early in the course or there is a sensory level on examination, diagnostic possibilities other than GBS should be considered, particularly spinal cord disease.

Ans. D

176. A 30 year presented with flaccid dysarthria, bulbar weakness, limb weakness and atrophy, gynaecomastia and infertility. He is likely inherited this disease in which mode?

A. X-linked

B. Autosomal dominant

C. Autosomal recessive

D. Mitochondrial

Explanation:

X-Linked Spinobulbar Muscular Atrophy (Kennedy's disease)

- X-linked
- Begins in males, mid-adult life
- LMN
- Progressive weakness and wasting of limb and bulbar muscles
- Androgen insensitivity- gynaecomastia and reduced fertility
- Expanded trinucleotide repeat (-CAG-) in the first exon of the androgen receptor gene on the X chromosome

Ans. A

177. Essential tremor improved by:

A. Stress

B. Alcohol

C. Valproate

D. Anxiety

Explanation:

- Essential tremor is characteristically improved by alcohol and worsened by stress. Subtle impairment of coordination or tandem walking may be present, and disturbances of hearing, cognition, personality, mood, and olfaction have been described, but usually the neurologic examination is normal aside from tremor.

Ans. B

178. Winking owl sign is earliest radiologic finding of vertebral tumor due to:

A. Erosion of pedicles

B. Enlargement of pedicles

C. Paravertebral extension

D. Canal narrowing

Explanation:

- Erosion of the pedicles (the "winking owl" sign) is the earliest radiologic finding of vertebral tumor.

- Other radiographic changes include increased intrapedicular distance, vertebral destruction, lytic or sclerotic lesions, scalloped vertebral bodies, and vertebral body collapse.
- Vertebral collapse is not a reliable indicator of the presence of tumor; ~20% of cases of vertebral collapse, particularly those in older patients and postmenopausal women, are due not to cancer but to osteoporosis.
- Also, a normal appearance on plain films of the spine does not exclude the diagnosis of cancer. The role of bone scans in the detection of cord compression is not clear; this method is sensitive but less specific than spinal radiography.

Ans. A

179. A 5 month old baby was brought to hospital and examination showed floppy baby with hypotonia. Genetic studies revealed SMN gene mutation and diagnosed as Spino muscular atrophy type 1. Which is false?

A. Mutation of SMN gene, chromosome 5
B. Known as Werdnig Hoffman disease
C. Onset in late childhood
D. Poor prognosis

Explanation:

Spinal Muscular Atrophy

- SMN gene- survival motor neuron
- *Infantile SMA* (SMA I, Werdnig-Hoffmann disease)
  - Earliest onset and most rapidly fatal course
  - Decreased fetal movements
  - Weak and floppy (hypotonic) and lack muscle stretch reflexes
  - Death before 1 year of age

Ans. C

180. A 50 year old presented with rigidity, myoclonus and altered sensorium and was diagnosed as CJD on basis of all except:

A. MRI showing cortical ribboning and basal ganglia hyperintensity
B. CSF- 14-3-3 elevation
C. EEG- short interval periodic discharges
D. MRI showing white matter periventricular changes

Explanation:

- Profound dementia- memory loss, impaired judgment, Myoclonus, Visual impairment or cerebellar gait and coordination deficits
- Extrapyramidal dysfunction- rigidity, masklike facies
- Pyramidal signs (usually mild), seizures, psychiatric symptoms
- CSF- elevated 14-3-3
- MRI- Cortical ribboning and basal ganglia hyperintensity
- vCJD- inverted hockey stick sign
- EEG- short interval periodic discharges

Ans. D

181. Drug available in multiple formulation in migraine is:

A. Sumitriptan
B. Frovatriptan
C. Almotriptan
D. Eletriptan

Explanation:

- Each drug in the triptan class has similar pharmacologic properties but varies slightly in terms of clinical efficacy. Rizatriptan and eletriptan are, on a population basis, the most efficacious of the triptans currently available in the United States.
- Sumatriptan and zolmitriptan have similar rates of efficacy as well as time to onset, with an advantage of having multiple formulations, whereas almotriptan has a similar rate of efficacy to sumatriptan and is better tolerated, and frovatriptan and naratriptan are somewhat slower in onset and are also well tolerated.

Ans. A

182. Which of the following is not a cardinal motor feature of parkinson's disease?

A. Bradykinesia
B. Rest tremor
C. Freezing
D. Postural instability

Explanation:

- Clinically, PD is characterized by rest tremor, rigidity (stiffness), bradykinesia (slowing), and gait dysfunction with postural instability.
- These are known as the "cardinal features" of the disease. Additional clinical features can include freezing of gait, speech difficulty, swallowing impairment, autonomic disturbances, and a series of nonmotor features that include sensory alterations, mood disorders, sleep dysfunction, cognitive impairment, and dementia.

Ans. C

183. Drug that causes Autoimmune myasthenia gravis is:

A. Sulfonamide
B. Penicillamine
C. Aminoglycoside
D. Procainamide

Explanation:

- Other conditions that cause weakness of the cranial and/or somatic musculature include the nonautoimmune congenital myasthenia, drug-induced myasthenia, Lambert-Eaton myasthenic syndrome (LEMS), neurasthenia, hyperthyroidism (Graves' disease), botulism, intracranial mass lesions, oculopharyngeal dystrophy, and mitochondrial myopathy (Kearns-Sayre syndrome, progressive external ophthalmoplegia).
- Treatment with penicillamine (used for scleroderma or rheumatoid arthritis) and check point inhibitors for cancer may also result in autoimmune MG.
- Aminoglycoside antibiotics or procainamide can cause exacerbation of weakness in myasthenic patients; very large doses can cause neuromuscular weakness in normal individuals

Ans. B

184. A 30 year old came with weakness of lower limbs with paresthesias, spasticity and brisk deep tendon reflexes. His symptoms cannot be attributed to which of the following?

A. Multiple sclerosis
B. Vitamin B12 deficiency
C. Copper deficiency
D. Thiamine deficiency

Explanation:

- Patient has myelopathy features.
- Thiamine deficiency causes peripheral neuropathy and not myelopathy

Ans. D

185. Prodromal symptoms suggest location of progressively enlarging unruptured aneurysm & third cranial nerve palsy indicate:

A. Cavarnous sinus aneurysm

B. Anterior communicating artery or MCA Bifurcation

C. Aneurysm at junction of PCA & ICA

D. Expanding supraclinoid carotid or ACA aneurysm

Explanation:

- Occasionally, prodromal symptoms suggest the location of a progressively enlarging unruptured aneurysm.
- 3rd cranial nerve palsy, particularly when associated with pupillary dilation, loss of ipsilateral (but retained C/L) light reflex, and focal pain above or behind eye, may occur with an expanding aneurysm at junction of posterior communicating artery and the internal carotid artery.
- Sixth nerve palsy may indicate an aneurysm in the cavernous sinus, and visual field defects can occur with an expanding supraclinoid carotid or anterior cerebral artery (ACA) aneurysm.
- Occipital and posterior cervical pain may signal a posterior inferior cerebellar artery or anterior inferior cerebellar artery aneurysm.

Ans. C

186. A patient came to emergency department with gun shot injury to conus medullaris. He doesn't have which of the following?

A. Saddle anaesthesia

B. Bowel, bladder involvement

C. Absent bulbocavernous reflex

D. Paraplegia

Explanation:

Conus Medullaris syndrome

- Saddle anaesthesia- S3-5
- Bowel, bladder involvement- S2-4
- Absent bulbocavernous reflex- S2-4

Ans. D

187. An army officer was brought with cord injury and diagnosed as Brown Sequard Syndrome. He manifests with all symptoms except:

A. Ipsilateral weakness

B. Ipsilateral loss of joint position

C. Ipsilateral loss of vibration

D. Ipsilateral loss of pain

Explanation:

Brown Sequard syndrome

- Ipsilateral

  - Weakness (corticospinal tract)
  - Loss of JPS, vibration (posterior column)
- Contralateral
  - Loss of pain and temperature (spinothalamic tract) one or two levels below

Ans. D

188. A 30 year with chronic chickpeas ingestion came spastic paraparesis. Which is likely agent responsible for his symptoms?

A. Beta N-Oxalyl Amino L-Alanine
B. Nitrous oxide
C. HTLV 1
D. Anti Hu antibodies

Explanation:

Lathyrism

- Ingestion of chickpeas
- Excitotoxin- β-N-oxalylamino-l-alanine (BOAA)
- Spastic paraparesis

Ans. A

189. Not consider a 2nd tier therapies for refractory elevated ICP is:

A. Decompressive craniectomy
B. High dose barbiturate therapy
C. Hypothermia to 33ºC
D. Hyperventilation

Explanation:

Table: Stepwise approach to treatment to elevated intracranial pressure (ICP)[a]
Insert ICP monitor—ventriculostomy versus parenchymal device
General goals: Maintain ICP < 20 mm Hg and CPP ≥ 60 mm Hg. For ICP > 20-25 mm Hg for > 5 min:
1. Elevate head of the bed; midline head position
2. Drain CSF via ventriculostomy (if in place)
3. Osmotherapy—mannitol 25-100 g q4h as needed (maintain serum osmolality < 320 mosmol) or hypertonic saline (30 ml, 23.4% NaCl bolus)
4. Glucocorticoids—dexamethasone 4 mg q6h for vasogenic edema from tumor, abscess (avoid glucocorticoids in head trauma, ischemic and hemorrhagic stroke)
5. Sedation (e.g., morphine, propofol, or midazolam); add neuromuscular paralysis if necessary (patient will require endotracheal intubation and mechanical ventilation at this point, if not before)
6. Hyperventilation—to $PaCO_2$ 30-35 mm Hg (short-term use or skip this step)
7. Pressor therapy—phenylephrine, dopamine, or norepinephrine to maintain adequate MAP to ensure CPP ≥ 60 mm Hg (maintain euvolemia to minimize deleterious systemic effects of pressors). May adjust target CPP in individual patients based on autoregulation status
8. Consider second-tier therapies for refractory elevated ICP a. Decompressive craniectomy b. High-dose barbiturate therapy ("pentobarb coma") c. Hypothermia to 33°C

Ans. D

190. Kernohan Woltman sign is due to:

A. Compression of 3rd nerve

B. Compression of opposite cerebral peduncle

C. Compression of anterior & posterior cerebral arteries

D. Compression of upper midbrain

Explanation:

- Lateral displacement of the midbrain may compress the opposite cerebral peduncle against the tentorial edge, producing a Babinski sign and hemiparesis contralateral to hemiparesis that resulted from mass (Kernohan-Woltman sign).
- Herniation may also compress anterior and posterior cerebral arteries as they pass over the tentorial reflections, with resultant brain infarction.
- These distortions may also entrap portions of the ventricular system, resulting in hydrocephalus

Ans. B

191. A patient with recurrent falls with patch of hair over low back was diagnosed as tethered cord syndrome. False about tethered cord syndrome:

A. Radicular pains in upper limbs

B. Deformities of foot

C. MRI shows low lying conus

D. Treatment is surgical release

Explanation:

- Tethered cord syndrome is a developmental disorder of the lower spinal cord and nerve roots that rarely presents in adulthood as low back pain accompanied by a progressive lower spinal cord and/or nerve root syndrome.
- Some patients have a small leg or foot deformity
- MRI demonstrates a low-lying conus medullaris and thickened filum terminale
- Treatment is with surgical release.

Ans. A

192. Glasgow coma scale is widely used for assessing sensorium of the patient. Which of the following is not a component of Glasgow Coma Scale

A. Eye opening

B. Verbal response

C. Motor response

D. Eye movements

Explanation:

Table: Glasgow coma scale

Eye Opening (E)		Verbal Response (V)	
Spontaneous	4	Oriented	5
To speech	3	Confused	4
To pressure	2	Words	3
None	1	Sounds	2
		None	1

Contd.

Contd.

Best Motor Response (M)			
Obeying commands	6		
Localizing	5		
Normal flexion	4		
Abnormal flexion	3		
Extension	2		
None	1		

Ans. D

193. A person suffered a road traffic accident and altered sensorium. His brain imaging showed extra dural hemorrhage. Which is false regarding extra dural haemorrhage?

A. Injury to meningeal artery
B. Biconvex shaped bleed
C. Usually has cortical damage
D. Good prognosis if treated early

Ans. C

194. Multiple sclerosis is a type of demyelinating disease. It has multiple forms. Which is most common form of Multiple Sclerosis?

A. Relapsing Remitting MS
B. Secondary progressive MS
C. Primary Progressive MS
D. Optico spinal form of MS

Ans. A

195. Risk factor for aneurysmal rupture in brain circulation is:

A. >7mm in diameter
B. At top of basilar artery
C. At origin of posterior communicating artery
D. At origin of anterior communicating artery

Explanation:

- Saccular aneurysms occur at the bifurcations of the large- to medium-sized intracranial arteries; rupture is into the subarachnoid space in the basal cisterns and sometimes into parenchyma of the adjacent brain. Approximately 85% of aneurysms occur in the anterior circulation, mostly on the circle of Willis. About 20% of patients have multiple aneurysms, many at mirror sites bilaterally. As an aneurysm develops, it typically forms a neck with a dome. The length of the neck and the size of the dome vary greatly and are important factors in planning neurosurgical obliteration or endovascular embolization. The arterial internal elastic lamina disappears at the base of the neck. The media thins, and connective tissue replaces smooth-muscle cells. At the site of rupture (most often the dome), wall thins, and the tear that allows bleeding is often ≤0.5 mm long. Aneurysm size and site are important in predicting risk of rupture. Those >7 mm in diameter and those at the top of the basilar artery and at the origin of the posterior communicating artery are at greater risk of rupture.

Ans. D

196. A 20 year old with relapsing remitting neurological illness was diagnosed as multiple sclerosis. Which of the following investigations were not suggestive of MS?

A. Periventricular lesions
B. Long segment transverse myelitis
C. Abnormal evoked potentials
D. Oligoclonal bands in CSF

Ans. B

197. The prevalence of multiple sclerosis is steadily increasing for the past 50 years. All of the following are risk factors for developing multiple sclerosis except:

A. Vitamin D deficiency
B. EBV exposure
C. Cigarette smoking
D. Alcoholism

Explanation:

- Risk factors for MS include a genetic predisposition, vitamin D deficiency, EpsteinBarr virus (EBV) exposure after early childhood, and cigarette smoking

Ans. D

198. A patient was diagnosed as multiple sclerosis based on MRI which is lesions consistent with MS and followed dissemination in time and space. Which of the following findings were not consistent with her diagnosis?

A. Dawson's fingers
B. Black holes
C. Long segment transverse myelitis
D. Infratentorial lesions

Explanation:

- Lesions are frequently oriented perpendicular to the ventricular surface, corresponding to the pathologic pattern of perivenous demyelination (Dawson's fingers).
- Lesions are multifocal within the brain, brainstem, and spinal cord.
- MS typically has short segment lesions in spinal cord. Long segment lesions are seen in NMO.

Ans. C

199. Natalizumab is a drug that is used for multiple sclerosis and is given monthly once. It acts by which mechanism?

A. Binding to α4β1 integrin
B. Decreased lymphocyte production
C. Sequestration of lymphocytes in lymphoid organs
D. Preventing entry of lymphocytes into CNS

Ans. A

200. Ocrelizumab, the only drug which is approved for treatment of primary progressive multiple sclerosis acts by binding to

A. CD20
B. CD52
C. CD115
D. A4β1 integrin

Ans. A

201. Not a goal for treatment of raised ICP is:

A. ICP <20 mm Hg
B. CPP >/= 60 mm Hg
C. Maintain serum osmolality <320 mosmol
D. None of the above

Explanation:

Table: Stepwise approach to treatment of elevated intracranial pressure (ICP)[a]
Insert ICP monitor–ventriculostomy versus parenchymal device
General goasls: Maintain ICP < 20 mm Hg and CPP ≥ 60 mm Hg. For ICP > 20–25 mm Hg for > 5 min:
1. Elevate head of the bed; midline head position
2. Drain CSF via ventriculostomy (if in place)
3. Osmotherapy–mannitol 25-100 g q4h as needed (maintain serum osmolality < 320 mosmol) or hypertonic saline (30 ml, 23.4% NaCl bolus)
4. Glucocorticoids–dexamethasone 4 mg q6h for vasogenic edema from tumor, abscess (avoid glucocorticoids in head trauma, ischemic and hemorrhagic stroke)
5. Sedation (e.g., morphine, propofol, or midazolam); add neuromuscular paralysis if necessary (patient will require endotracheal intubation and mechanical ventilation at this point, if not before)
6. Hyperventilation–to $PaCO_2$ 30–35 mm Hg (short-term use or skip this step)
7. Pressor therapy–phenylephrine, dopamine, or norepinephrine to maintain adequate MAP to ensure CPP ≥ 60 mm Hg (maintain euvolemia to minimize deleterious systemic effects of pressors). May adjust target CPP in individual patients based on autoregulation status
8. Consider second-tier therapies for refractory elevated ICP
a. Decompressive craniectomy
b. High-dose barbiturate therapy ("pentobarb coma")
c. Hypothermia to 33°C
[a] Throughout ICP treatment algorithm, consider repeat head computed tomography to identify mass lesions amenable to surgical evacuation. May alter order of steps based on directed treatment to specific cause of elevated ICP.

Ans. D

202. A 15 year old child presented with altered sensorium and seizures. His MRI brain was consistent with acute disseminated encephalomyelitis. Which is true regarding his illness?

A. Majority of people will get recurrent episodes

B. Follows an infection or vaccination

C. Poor response to steroids

D. Anti aquaporin antibodies are seen

Explanation:

- ADEM has a monophasic course and is most frequently associated with an antecedent infection (postinfectious encephalomyelitis
- Autoantibodies to MBP and to other myelin antigens have been detected in the CSF from some patients

Ans. B

203. Disorders in which increased capillary pressure dominates pathophysiology in posterior reversible encephalopathy syndrome?

A. Preeclampsia/Eclampsia

B. Calcineurin inhibitor toxicity

C. Chemotherapeutic agent toxicity

D. HELLP Syndrome

Explanation:

Table: Common etiologies of posterior reversible encephalopathy syndrome
Disorders in which increased capillary pressure dominates the pathophysiology
• Hypertensive encephalopathy, including secondary causes such as renovascular hyptertension, pheochromocytoma, cocaine use, etc.
• Postcarotid endarterectomy syndrome
• Preeclampsia/eclampsia
Disorders in which endothelial dysfunction dominates the pathophysiology
• Calcineurin-inhibitor toxicity (e.g., cyclosporine, tacrolimus)
• Chemotherapeutic agent toxicity (e.g., cytarabine, azathioprine, 5-fluorouracil, cisplatin, methotrexate, tumor necrosis factor α antagonists)
• HELLP syndrome (hemolysis, elevated liver enzyme levels, low platelet count)
• Hemolytic-uremic syndrome (HUS)

Ans. A

204. Neuromyelitis optica is a form of autoimmune disease which is common in young adults. Which is not true about neuromyelitis optica?

A. Antibodies against aquaporin

B. It's a demyelinating disease

C. It is an astrocytopathy

D. In majority of people, it is monophasic

Explanation:

- NMO is an autoimmune disease associated with a highly specific autoantibody directed against aquaporin-4 (AQP4)
- AQP4 is localized to the foot processes of astrocytes
- NMO is prone for recurrences.

Ans. D

205. Wingerchuk developed criteria for diagnosis of neuromyelitis optica. Which of the following is not core clinical feature of NMO according to this criteria?

A. Optic neuritis

B. Myelitis

C. Area postrema syndrome

D. Juxtacortical lesions on MRI

Explanation:

NMO-core clinical features

1. Optic neuritis
2. Acute myelitis
3. Area postrema syndrome
4. Acute brainstem syndrome
5. Symptomatic narcolepsy or diencephalic clinical syndrome
6. Symptomatic cerebral syndrome with NMOSD-typical brain lesions

Ans. D

206. A 30 year old lady came with altered sensorium and focal neurological deficits. Her investigations showed anti MOG antibodies. False about anti MOG associated demyelination?

A. Can be associated with acute disseminated encephalo myelitis

B. Papillitis may be seen

C. Longitudinally extensive myelitis can be present

D. Majority patients show poor response to steroids

Explanation:

- MOG found to be associated with cases of acute disseminated encephalomyelitis (ADEM)
- Papillitis seen by funduscopy or orbital MRI
- **Spinal cord lesions can be longitudinally** extensive or short
- Demyelination associated with anti-MOG antibodies is sometimes monophasic, as in ADEM, but can also be recurrent.
- Acute episodes are managed with high dose glucocorticoids followed by a prednisone taper and sometimes by plasmapheresis

Ans. D

207. Most common form of hereditary neuropathy is charcot marie tooth disease. In these, which most common form of CMT?

A. CMT1

B. CMT2

C. CMT3

D. CMT4

Ans. A

208. CMT 3 was originally described by Dejerine and Sottas as hereditary sensory motor neuropathy. Which is false about dejerine sotta syndrome?

A. Causes axonal neuropathy

B. Presents during early childhood

C. Weakness is usually severe

D. Can be caused due to PMP22 mutations

Explanation:

- CMT3 was originally described by Dejerine and Sottas as a hereditary demyelinating sensorimotor polyneuropathy presenting in infancy or early childhood.
- Affected children are severely weak.
- Motor NCVs are markedly slowed, typically ≤ 5–10 m/s.
- Most cases of CMT3 are caused by point mutations in the genes for PMP-22, MPZ, or ERG2

Ans. A

209. Hereditary neuropathy with liability to pressure palsies is an autosomal dominant disorder. Its manifestations are different though the gene affected is same as CMT1. Which is false about hereditary neuropathy with liability to pressure palsies?

A. Occurs due to PMP22 deletion

B. Manifests in infancy or early childhood

C. Multiple mononeuropathies occur

D. Triggered by trivial compressions

Explanation:

- HNPP is an autosomal dominant disorder
- HNPP is caused by deletion of PMP-22 gene.
- Patients usually manifest in the second or third decade of life
- Mononeuropathy or multiple mononeuropathies can occur
- Precipitated by trivial compression of nerve(s) as can occur with wearing a backpack, leaning on the elbows, or crossing one's legs for even a short period of time.

Ans. B

210. A patient presented with scapular pain with weakness and sensory loss involving right upper limb. His elder brother has similar episodes and was diagnosed as hereditary neuralgic amyotrophy. Which is false about Hereditary Neuralgic Amyotrophy?

A. Recurrent attacks involving brachial plexus
B. Mutation in septin 9 gene (SEPT9)
C. Triggered by stress
D. Autosomal recessive

Explanation:

- HNA is an autosomal dominant disorder characterized by recurrent attacks of pain, weakness, and sensory loss in the distribution of the brachial plexus often beginning in childhood.
- Attacks may occur in the postpartum period, following surgery, or at other times of stress.
- HNA is genetically heterogeneous but can be caused by mutations in septin 9 (SEPT9).

Ans. D

211. A patient presented with loss of pain and temperature sensation since childhood with multiple ulcerations, charcot joints. He was diagnosed as HSAN1 on genetic testing. Which of the gene is affected in this patient?

A. MFN2
B. GDAP1
C. SPTLC1
D. PMP22

Ans. C

212. A patient with hereditary neuropathy presented with asymmetric neuropathy and orange tonsils. Which of the following is false regarding this disease?

A. Mutations in ABC1 gene
B. Multiple mononeuropathies
C. Decreased HDL levels
D. Decreased triacylglycerol levels

Explanation:

- Tangier disease-can present as (1) asymmetric multiple mononeuropathies, (2) a slowly progressive symmetric polyneuropathy predominantly in the legs, or (3) a pseudo-syringomyelia pattern
- **The tonsils may appear swollen** and yellowish-orange in color
- Tangier disease is caused by mutations in the ATP-binding cassette transporter 1 (ABC1) gene
- Reduced levels of high-density lipoprotein (HDL) cholesterol levels, whereas triacylglycerol levels are increased.

Ans. D

213. Familial amyloid polyneuropathy are rare disorders which can cause peripheral neuropathies due to amyloid deposition. These disorders occurs due to all of the following except:

A. Transthyretin (TTR) mutation
B. Apolipoprotein A1
C. Gelsolin
D. Multiple myeloma

Explanation:

- Familial amyloid polyneuropathy (FAP) is caused by mutations in the genes for transthyretin (TTR), apolipoprotein A1, or gelsolin
- Multiple myeloma causes aquired amylodosis

Ans. D

214. A patient presented with paraesthesias and burning. He has been taking less amount of diet for weight loss. His examination was suggestive of neuropathy. Which of the following vitamin deficiency doesn't cause his symptoms?

A. Thiamine
B. Riboflavin
C. Pyridoxine
D. Cobalamine

Ans. B

215. Mean cerebral blood flow in ml per 100 gm/min is:

A. 30
B. 55
C. 65
D. 75

Explanation:

- Cerebral neurons are fully dependent on cerebral blood flow (CBF) and the delivery of oxygen and glucose.
- CBF is ~75 mL per 100 g/min in gray matter and 30 mL per 100 g/min in white matter (mean ~55 mL per 100 g/min); oxygen consumption is 3.5 mL per 100 g/min, and glucose utilization is 5 mg per 100 g/min.
- Brain stores of glucose are able to provide energy for ~2 min after blood flow is interrupted, and oxygen stores last 8–10 s after the cessation of blood flow. Simultaneous hypoxia and ischemia exhaust glucose more rapidly.
- Electroencephalogram (EEG) rhythm in these circumstances becomes diffusely slowed, typical of metabolic encephalopathies, and as substrate delivery worsens, eventually brain electrical activity ceases.

Ans. B

216. A 20 year old male, presented with acute onset symmetrical lower limb followed by upper limb weakness. The symptoms were preceded by fever. His examination showed hypotonia with areflexia. CSF examination showed increased protein with normal cell count. What is most probable diagnosis?

A. Guillain Barre syndrome
B. Myasthenia gravis
C. Infectitious myelitis
D. Acute disseminated encephalo myelitis

Explanation:

- GB syndrome has acute onset symmetrical limb and facial weakness with csf showing albumino cytological disassociation. Usually occurs after infection
- Myasthenia has fluctuating weakness that improves with rest
- ADEM has features of encephalopathy including altered sensorium, seizures, focal neurological deficits
- Myelopathy has weakness along with sensory and bladder involvement with brisk reflexes.

Ans. A

217. A 30 year old man was diagnosed as Miller Fisher syndrome. His anti GQ1b antibodies were positive. He is least likely to present with which symptom?

A. Ataxia
B. Areflexia
C. Paraesthesias
D. Ophthalmoplegia

Ans. C

218. A 65 year old lady presented with burring and paraesthesias of bilateral feet and legs. She is a known case of multiple myeloma. Which of the following is false regarding her neuropathy?

A. Usually demyelinating
B. often respond to radiation therapy or removal of the primary lesion
C. May be associated with POEMS syndrome
D. Decreased VEGF levels

Explanation:

- Neuropathy associated with multiple myeloma is usually demyelinating
- Respond to radiation therapy or removal of the primary lesion
- Associated with different monoclonal proteins and light chains
- POEMS syndrome may be seen
- Levels of vascular endothelial growth factor (VEGF) are increased in the serum, and this factor is thought to somehow play a pathogenic role in this syndrome. Treatment of the neuropathy is best directed at the osteosclerotic myeloma

Ans. D

219. Disorders in which increased capillary pressure dominates pathophysiology in posterior reversible encephalopathy syndrome is:

A. Preeclampsia/Eclampsia
B. Calcineurin inhibitor toxicity
C. Chemotherapeutic agent toxicity
D. HELLP Syndrome

Explanation:

Table: Common etiologies of posterior reversible encephalopathy syndrome
Disorders in which increased capillary pressure dominates the pathophysiology
• Hypertensive encephalopathy, including secondary causes such as renovascular hyptertension, pheochromocytoma, cocaine use, etc.
• Postcarotid endarterectomy syndrome
• Preeclampsia/eclampsia
Disorders in which endothelial dysfunction dominates the pathophysiology
• Calcineurin-inhibitor toxicity (e.g., cyclosporine, tacrolimus)
• Chemotherapeutic agent toxicity (e.g., cytarabine, azathioprine, 5-fluorouracil, cisplatin, methotrexate, tumor necrosis factor α antagonists)
• HELLP syndrome (hemolysis, elevated liver enzyme levels, low platelet count)
• Hemolytic-uremic syndrome (HUS)

Ans. A

220. A 70 year old patient was diagnosed as myasthenia gravis on the basis anti acetyl choline esterase antibodies. Which of the following statements is false regarding the disease?

A. Fluctuating weakness
B. Anti AchR antibody seen in 85% of generalised myasthenia gravis
C. Tensilon test is used
D. Treated with anti cholinergics

Explanation:

- Myasthenia gravis (MG) is a neuromuscular junction (NMJ) disorder characterized by weakness and fatigability of skeletal muscles.
- It is due to antibodies against acetylcholine receptors (AChRs) at NMJs
- Tensilon test is administration of edrophhonium which relieves symptoms
- Treatment is immunomodulation with anti choline esterases

Ans. D

221. A patient with lung carcinoma developed Lambert Eaton myasthenia which is a type of presynaptic myasthenia. It occurs due to antibody against:

A. AChR
B. P/Q type Calcium channel
C. Sodium channel
D. Chloride channel

Explanation:

- *LEMS is a presynaptic disorder of the NMJ that can cause weakness* similar to that of Myasthenia
- The proximal muscles of the lower limbs are most commonly affected
- Cranial nerve findings, including ptosis of the eyelids and diplopia, occur in up to 70% of patients
- LEMS is caused by autoantibodies directed against P/Q-type calcium channels at the motor nerve terminals
- These autoantibodies impair the release of ACh from nerve terminals.
- In older adults, most LEMS is associated with malignancy, most commonly small-cell lung cancer (SCLC)

Ans. B

222. A patient with myasthenia was admitted in a hospital with sepsis. Which of the following drugs can be safely given in this patient?

A. Aminoglycosides
B. Macrolides
C. Quinolines
D. Beta lactams

Explanation:

Table: Drugs with interactions in myasthenia gravis (MG)
Drugs That May Exacerbate MG
Antibiotics
Aminoglycosides: e.g., streptomycin, tobramycin, kanamycin
Quinolones: e.g., ciprofloxacin, levofloxacin, ofloxacin, gatifloxacin
Macrolides: e.g., erythromycin, azithromycin
Nondepolarizing muscle relaxants for surgey
D-Tubocurarine (curare), pancuronium, vecuronium, atracurium
Beta-blocking agents
Propranolol, atenolol, metoprolol
Local anesthetics and related agents
Procaine, Xylocaine in large amounts
Procainamide (for arrhythmias)

Contd.

Contd.

Botulinum toxin
Botox exacerbates weakness
Quinine derivatives
Quinine, quinidine, chloroquine, mefloquine (Lariam)
Magnesium
Decreases acetylcholine release
Penicillamine
May cause MG
Check point inhibitors
May cause MG and other autoimmune neuromuscular disorders (e.g., myositis, inflammatory neuropathy)

Ans. D

223. A 6 year old patient with difficulty walking was diagnosed as Duchenne muscular dystrophy on basis of genetic testing. Which of the following is not true about Duchenne muscular dystrophy?

A. Caused to mutation in dystrophin gene
B. Common in girls
C. Hypertrophy of calf muscles
D. Cardiac involvement

Explanation:

- DMD is X-linked recessive disorder. Common in boys

Ans. B

224. Limb girdle muscular dystrophy can be caused by either autosomal dominant or recessive. Which gene mutation doesn't cause autosomal dominant LGMD?

A. Myotilin
B. Caveolin
C. Lamin A/C
D. Calpain

Explanation:

- A systematic classification of LGMD is based on autosomal dominant (LGMD1) and autosomal recessive (LGMD2) inheritance
- Calpain mutation is LGMD type 2A which is autosomal recessive

Ans. D

225. A patient with progressive muscle weakness was diagnosed as fascio scapulo humeral dystrophy. Which of the following is false regarding this patient?

A. *DUX4 gene* mutation
B. Facial weakness is initial manifestation
C. Scapular winging seen
D. Cardiomyopathy is common

Explanation:

- FSHD -In most cases, facial weakness is the initial manifestation
- Loss of scapular stabilizer muscles makes arm elevation difficult

- Scapular winging becomes apparent with attempts at abduction and forward movement of the arms.
- The heart is not involved
- Cardiomyopathy is seen in DMD, emery dreifuss

Ans. D

226. A patient presented with features suggestive of myotonia and muscle weakness. His father has suffered from similar disease and excess CTG trinucleotide repeats in DMPK gene. Which is false regarding his disease?

A. Proximal muscle weakness

B. Hatched facies due to temporalis and massetter atrophy

C. Cardiac conduction block

D. Cataract

Explanation:

- Myotonic dystrophy type 1 causes distal weakness whereas type 2 causes proximal weakness

Ans. A

227. A patient presented with recurrent episodes progressive quadriparesis of 1 day duration with retained deep tendon reflexes. His investigations showed serum potassium levels of 1.7 (normal range 3.5 to 5.5). There is family history of similar illness. Which is false regarding His disease?

A. Autosomal recessive

B. Na/Ca channel mutation

C. Provoked by high carbohydrate meal

D. Respiratory muscles spared

Explanation:

- Autosomal dominant disorder
- HypoKPP type 1 is the most common form, and is caused by mutations in the voltage-sensitive, skeletal muscle calcium channel gene, CALCL1A3. Approximately 10% of cases are HypoKPP type 2, arising from mutations in the voltage-sensitive sodium channel gene (SCN4A).
- Attacks are often provoked by meals high in carbohydrates or sodium

Ans. A

228. Myopathies can be caused due to various mutations involving ion channels known as channelopathies. Which of the combination is false regarding channelopathies?

A. Paramyotonia congenita- sodium channel mutation

B. Andersen tawil syndrome- potassium channel mutation

C. Hyperkalemic periodic paralysis- Chloride channel mutation

D. Hypokalemic periodic paralysis- calcium channel mutation

Explanation:

- Hyperkalemic periodic paralysis- sodium channel mutation
- Chloride channel mutation is seen in thomsen and becker disease

Ans. C

229. A 11 year boy was brought with breif unresponsiveness lasting few seconds and there were multiple episodes per day. His EEG was showing following features. Treatment of choice is:

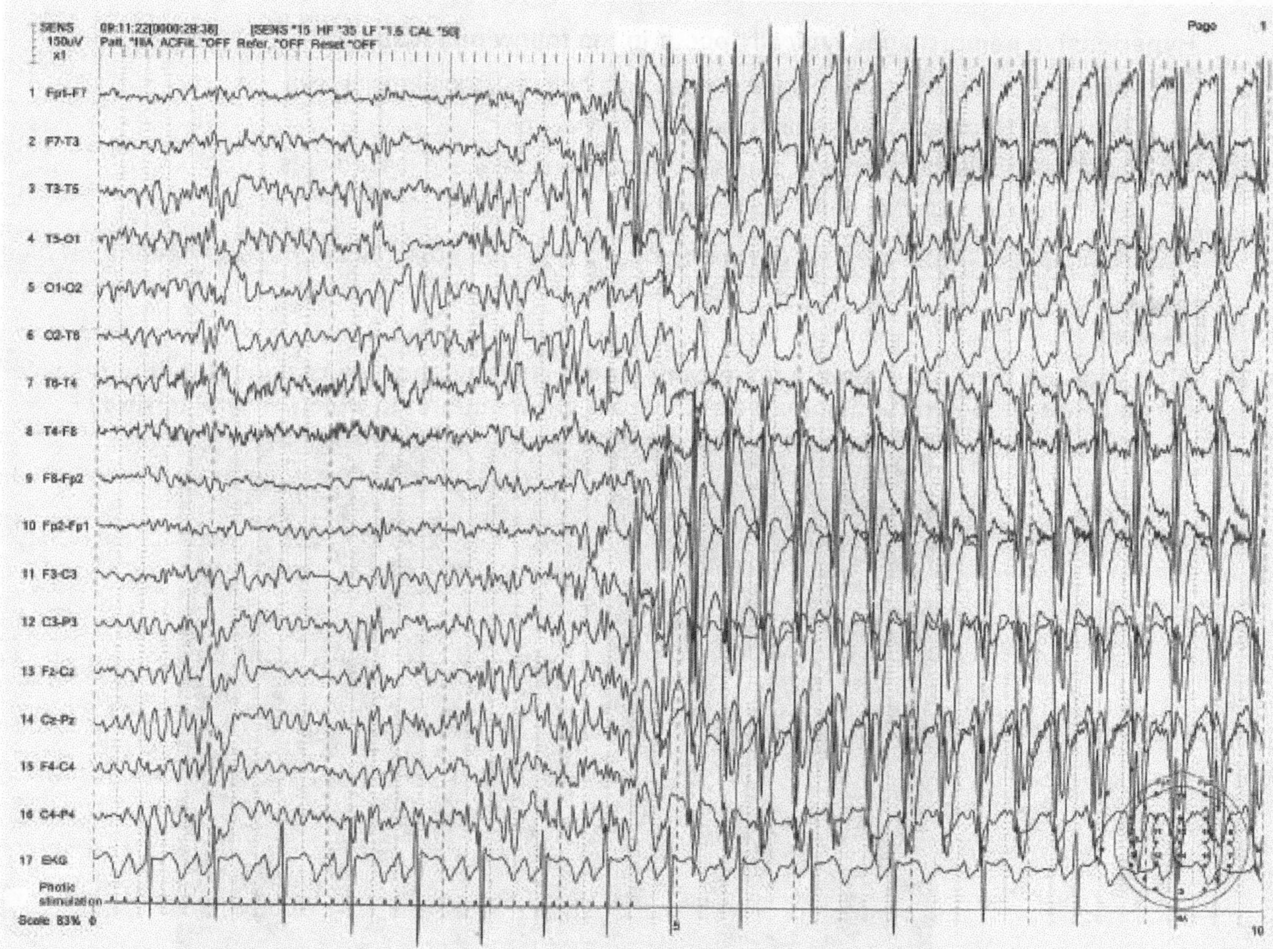

A. Phenytoin
B. Carbamazepine
C. Valpraote
D. Phenobarbitone

Explanation:

- EEG was suggestive of 3 Hz spike and wave. Patient is suffering from absence epilepsy and valproate is used in absence epilepsy

Ans. C

230. A 68 year old male who is a known case of hypertension for the last 20 years but has not taken his medication for the past 5 days because of a foreign trip comes to the Emergency room that half of his vision had disappeared suddenly while watching television 11 hours earlier and had not returned. He also reported a pounding headache located at the back of his head. It had started around the same time as the vision loss and gotten progressively worse. Other positive symptoms included gradual weakness of left sided limbs over the past 2 days. The patient probably has:

A. Right Homonymous hemianopia
B. Right Heteronymous Hemianopia
C. Bitemporal Hemianopia
D. Right homonymous scotoma

Explanation:

- Etiologies for intracranial hemorrhage are diverse but hypertension is the most common cause.

Hypertensive hemorrhages typically occur in the following locations:

- *Putamen:* Contralateral hemiparesis often with homonymous hemianopia
- *Thalamus:* Hemiparesis with prominent sensory deficit
- *Pons:* Quadriplegia, "pinpoint" pupils, impaired horizontal eye movements
- *Cerebellum:* Headache, vomiting, gait ataxia

Neurologic deficit that evolves gradually over 30–90 min strongly suggests intracerebral bleeding.

Ans. A

231. A 60 year old man has recently undergone surgical clipping of internal carotid aneurysm following which he developed right hemiparesis. CT brain shows infarct in which arterial territory?

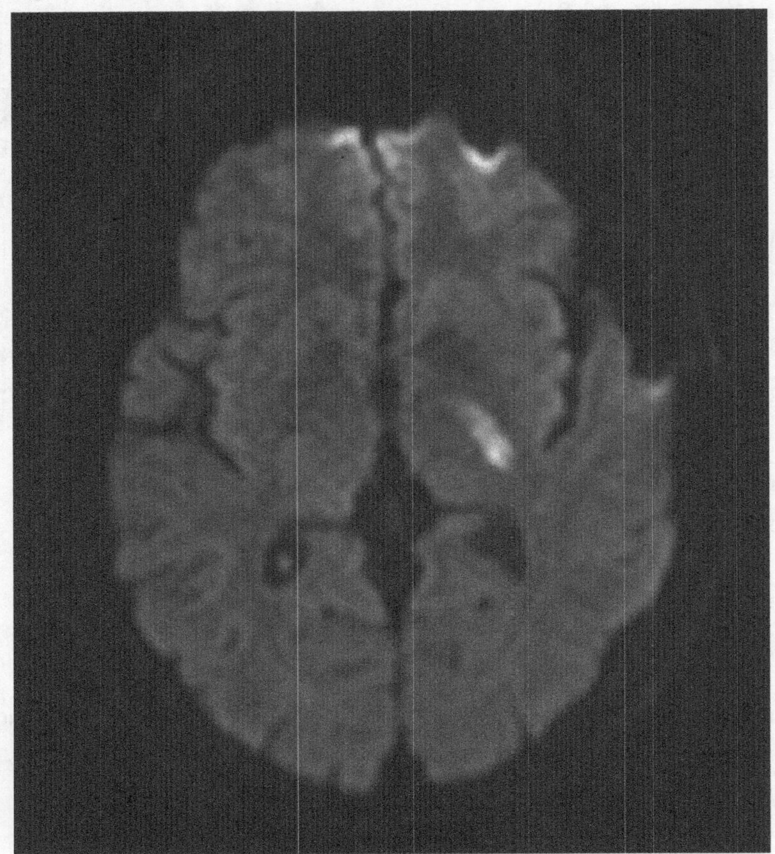

A. Anterior choroidal artery
B. Posterior choroidal artery
C. Artery of percheron
D. Lacunar infarct

Ans. A

232. A 20 year old lady came with 2 days history of paraesthesias of right lower limb and right facial weakness. MRI showed periventricular lesions perpendicular to corpus callosum and spine showed short segment lesion. CSF showed positive oligoclonal bands. Which of the following drugs can be given?

A. Interferon alpha
B. Aspirin and clopidogrel
C. Warfarin
D. Interferon beta

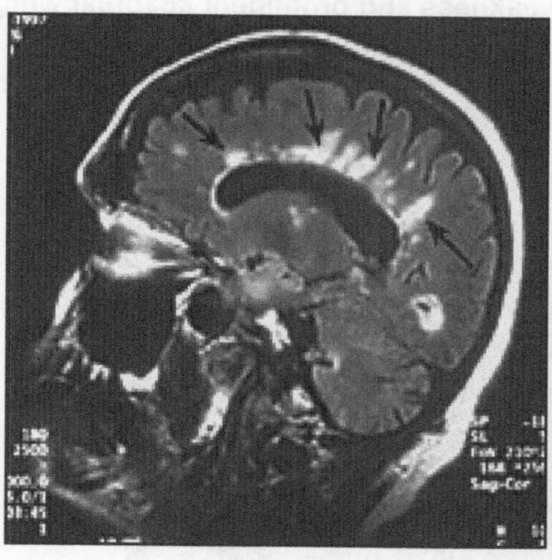
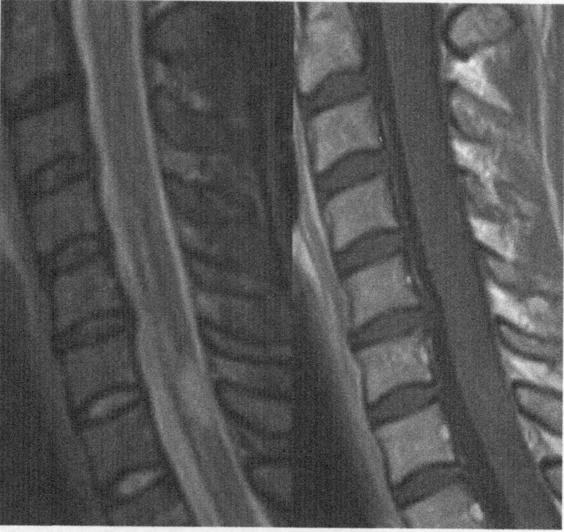

- The patient is suffering from multiple sclerosis. Interferon beta is used in MS

Ans. D

233. 20 year old man presented with fever, visual hallucinations and altered sensorium. MRI showing hyperintensities in medial temporal lobe, cingulate. What is possible diagnosis?

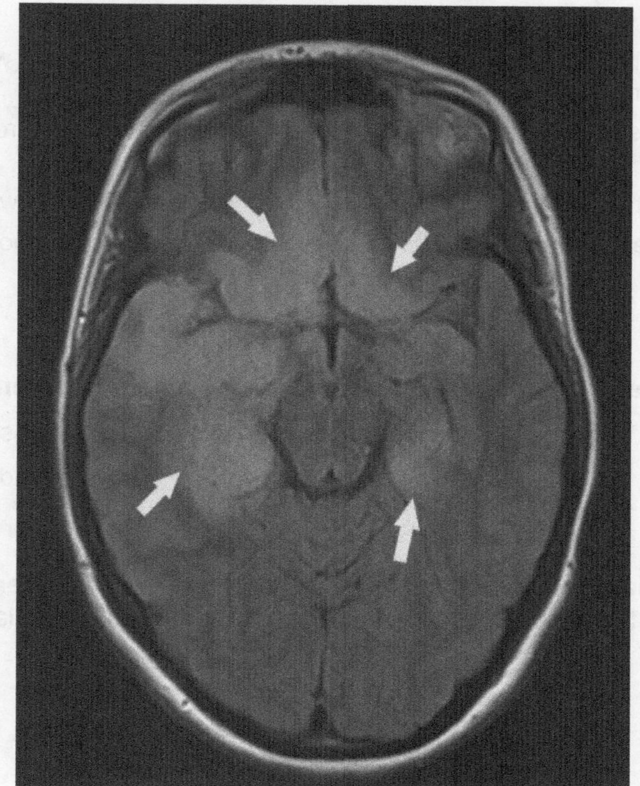

A. Herpes encephalitis
B. Japanese encephalitis
C. West nile encephalitis
D. Dengue encephalitis

- Herpes encephalitis- characteristically involves medial temporal lobe, cingulate, basifrontal lobe and insular cortex

Ans. A

234. A 14 year old male patient presented with facial weakness and prominent scapular winging as shown is likely to be:

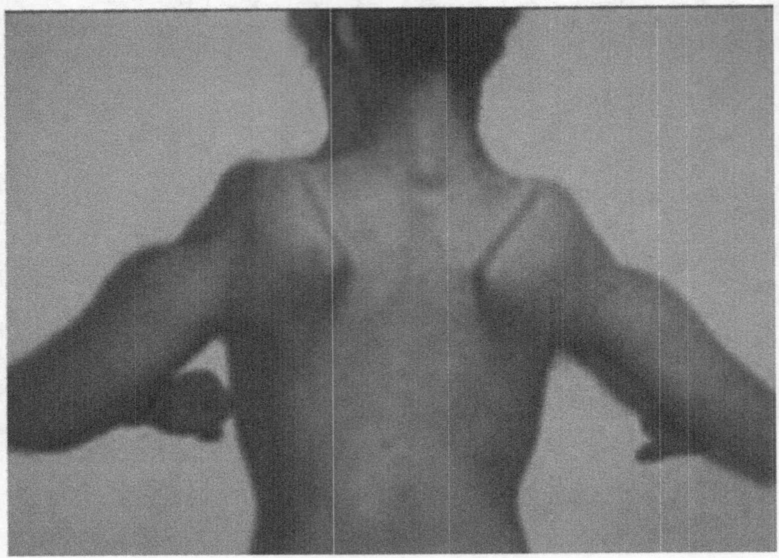

A. Myotonic dystrophy
B. Guillain-Barré syndrome
C. Fascioscapulohumeral dystrophy
D. Myasthenia gravis

Explanation:

- Fascioscapulohumeral dystrophy where facial palsy with limb muscle weakness and prominent winging of scapula is seen.
- In Guillain-Barré syndrome progressive ascending paralysis seen where lower limb involvement involved initially.
- Myotonic dystrophy calf muscle involvement is seen with weakness in lower limb and hip muscle weakness.
- In Myasthenia gravis jaw muscles involved with ptosis is seen. autoantibodies against Acetylcholinesterase are common.

Ans. C

235. Latency period of auto-regulatory mechanism which maintains cerebral blood flow is:

A. 0-5 Seconds
B. 5-10 Seconds
C. 10-15 Seconds
D. 15-20 Seconds

Explanation:

- In a normal patient the auto-regulatory mechanism prevent the cerebral hypo-perfusion when this mechanism fails Syncope will occur Latency period for this auto-regulatory mechanism to get activated is 5-10 Seconds.

Ans. B

CHAPTER 6

CONNECTIVE TISSUE DISORDERS AND IMMUNE DISORDERS (CTD)

1. A 55-year-old female presents to your office with a complaint of weakness which came on gradually over the last several months. She has difficulty raising her arms and walking up stairs. Her examination demonstrates significant proximal arm and leg weakness with forearm flexors spared. Creatine kinase is 2500. She has a rash around her eyes and on her knuckles. Electromyography demonstrates small motor units with ample fibrillations and positive sharp waves seen in proximal muscles and paraspinal muscles. What pattern of abnormalities would be expected on this patient's muscle biopsy?

A. Endomysial inflammatory infiltrate with CD8 T-cells

B. Endomysial inflammatory infiltrates with cytoplasmic inclusions and rimmed vacuoles

C. Nests of angular atrophic muscle fibers with fiber type grouping

D. Perimysial infiltrate with perifascicular atrophy

Explanation:

- Dermatomyositis (DM) is differentiated from polymyositis (PM) clinically by the presence of a rash, although in darker-skinned patients the rash may be difficult to see. On biopsy, DM involves perimysial infiltrates with perifascicular atrophy.
- PM involves endomysial inflammation with CD8 cells. Inclusion body myositis (IBM) has a different pattern of weakness than PM or DM, involving the forearm flexors and quads before other weakness developing. On biopsy, IBM has inclusions and rimmed vacuoles. Angular atrophic fibers with fiber type grouping would be seen in a neuropathic, not myopathic, condition.
- Ragged red fibers in combination with a COX− and SDH+ stain is highly suggestive of a mitochondrial disorder.

Ans. D

2. What is the initial line of treatment for Sydenham's Chorea?

A. Haloperidol

B. Valproate

C. Warfarin

D. Risperidone

Explanation:

Initial line of treatment for Sydenham's Chorea is Valproic acid

SYDENHAM'S CHOREA (SC)/CHOREA MINOR/RHEUMATIC CHOREA (RC)/ST. VITUS'S DANCE

- ***Late neurological manifestation in Rheumatic fever***
- Sydenham's chorea occurs in fewer than 10% patients with rheumatic fever.
- Occurs primarily in children and is rare after age of 20 years.

- Major diagnostic criteria for rheumatic disease
- Most common acquired chorea during childhood
- Characterized by rapid, involuntary, purposeless non repetitive & uncoordinated jerking movements primarily affecting the face, hands and feet.

> - Facial movements include grimaces, grins and frowns.
> - When the tongue is protruded, it resembles a 'bag of worms' and speech is jerky and staccato.
> - Handwriting becomes illegible and patient may stumble when attempting to walk. When the hands are extended, dorsum assumes a 'spoon' or 'dish' configuration due to flexion of wrist and hyperextension of metacarpophalangeal joints.
> - ***When raising the hands above the head, the patient may pronate one or both hands ('pronator sign').***

- ***Anticonvulsants are drug of 1st choice***

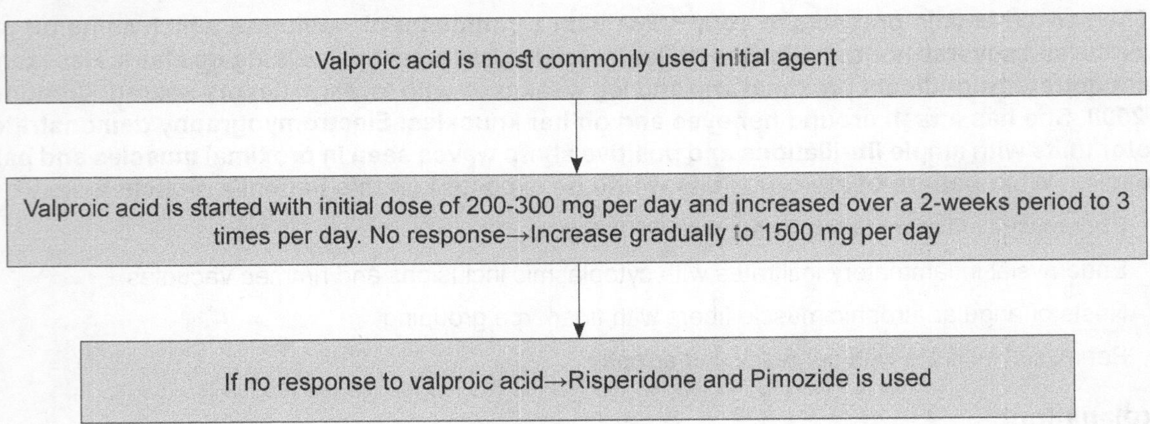

> - ***Neuroleptics are 1st choice of treatment in patients with chorea paralytica.***
> - Patients with Sydneham chorea has higher risk of drug induced parkinsonism & dystonia
> - So, D2 receptor blockers should be used in caution.
> - ***Tetrabenazine is another drug used in Symptomatic Sydneham chorea.***
> - **STEROIDS–** *Reserved for persistent disabling chorea refractory to other agents*
> - **IVIG/Plasmapheresis–** *Treatment of last resort.*

Ans. B

Version 2:	**Version 3:**
Drug of choice for refractory/resistant rheumatic chorea A. Haloperidol B. Risperidone C. Valproate D. Phenytoin **Ans. B**	**Treatment of choice for drug resistant rheumatic chorea is** A. Haloperidol B. IVIG C. Valproate D. Phenytoin **Ans. B**

CHOREA

- Sydenham's chorea (usually children, often with a history of rheumatic fever).
- Huntington's chorea (autosomal dominant condition affecting patients in middle life, associated with progressive dementia).
- Chorea of pregnancy (usually with first pregnancy).
- Chorea in patients on oral contraceptives.
- Senile or arteriosclerotic chorea (occurs in the elderly, with sudden onset and with other evidence of degenerative vascular disease).
- Chorea in primary polycythaemia.

Table: Diseases characterized by chorea

Inherited/Degenerative	Huntington's disease
	Wilson's disease
	Neuroacanthocytosis
	Benign hereditary chorea
Autoimmune (post-infection)	Systemic lupus erythematosus
	Antiphospholipid syndrome
	Hashimoto's chorea
	Sydenham's chorea
Infections	HIV Encephalopathy
	Creutzfeldt-Jakob disease (CJD)
Drugs	Dopamine receptor blockers
	Levodopa
	Oral contraceptives
	Anticonvulsants
Structural Lesions	Basal ganglia (caudate) lesions
Metabolic	Hyperthyroidism
	Hyperglycemia
	Sodium disturbances
	Calcium, manganese and iron deposition disorders

3. All are risk factors for SLE except:

A. Alcohol
B. Smoking
C. Silica exposure
D. UV light

Explanation:

Several environmental stimuli may influence the development of SLE.

Increased risk of SLE

1. Exposure to ultraviolet light

2. EBV infection
3. Drugs
4. Current tobacco smoking
5. Prolonged occupational exposure to crystalline silica (e.g., inhalation of soap powder dust or soil in farming activities)

Decreased risk of lupus:

Drinking alcohol (2 glasses of wine a week or ½ of an alcoholic drink daily) reduces the risk of SLE.

Ans. A

4. Most common hematologic problem in sarcoidosis is:

A. Lymphocytosis
B. Lymphopenia
C. Anemia
D. Thrombocytopenia

Explanation:

- Most common hematologic problem is lymphopenia in patients with Sarcoidosis
- This reflects sequestration of lymphocytes into areas of inflammation

Ans. B

5. Most common ocular manifestation of Sarcoidosis is:

A. Retinitis
B. Pars planitis
C. Anterior uveitis
D. Optic neuritis

Explanation:

- Most common ocular manifestation in sarcoidosis is anterior uveitis
- Retinitis & Pars planitis can also occur with sarcoidosis

Ans. C

6. Mauskopf facies is seen in:

A. Systemic sclerosis
B. SLE
C. MCTD
D. Sjögren's syndrome

Explanation:

- In established SSc, face assumes a characteristic "mauskopf" facies appearance with taut and shiny skin, loss of wrinkles, and occasionally an expressionless facies due to reduced mobility of the eyelids, cheeks, and mouth.
- Reduced oral aperture (microstomia) interferes with eating and oral hygiene.
- The nose assumes a pinched, beak-like appearance.

Ans. A

7. How long the disease to be in remission for renal transplantation in SLE patients?

A. 3 months
B. 6 months
C. 24 months
D. 1 month

Explanation:

- Renal transplantation in renal failure from lupus, usually performed after ~6 months of inactive disease.
- Leading causes of death in the first decade of disease are renal failure, and infections.

Ans. B

8. **All the following inflammatory causes of extremely elevated ESR except:**

A. SLE
B. RA
C. Giant cell arteritis
D. Takayasu arteritis

Explanation:

Table: Causes of an extremely elevated erythrocyte sedimentation rate (> 100 mm/h)

Etiologic Category (% of Cases)	Specific Causes
Infectious diseases (35-40)	Subacute bacterial endocarditis Abscesses Osteomyelitis Tuberculosis Urinary tract infection
Inflammatory diseases (15-20)	Giant cell arteritis Rheumatoid arthritis Systemic lupus erythematosus
Malignancies (15-20)	Multiple myeloma Leukemias Lymphomas Carcinomas
Other (20-35)	Drug hypersensitivity reaction (drug fever) Ischemic tissue injury/trauma Renal diseases

Ans. D

9. **Drug induced lupus is not seen with:**

A. Disopyramide
B. Propylthiouracil
C. Chlorthalidone
D. Lovastatin

Explanation:

- Drug induced lupus is a syndrome of positive ANA associated with symptoms such as fever, malaise, arthritis or intense arthralgias/myalgias, serositis, and/ or rash.
- Syndrome appears during therapy with certain medications and biologic agents, is predominant in whites, has less female predilection than SLE, rarely involves kidneys or brain, is rarely associated with anti-dsDNA, is commonly associated with antibodies to histones, and usually resolves over several weeks after discontinuation of offending medication.
- List of substances that can induce lupus like disease is long.
- ***Among the most frequent are the antiarrhythmics procainamide, disopyramide, and propafenone; the anti-hypertensive hydralazine; several angiotensin-converting enzyme nhibitors and beta blockers; the antithyroid propylthiouracil; antipsychotics chlorpromazine and lithium; the anticonvulsants carbamazepine and phenytoin; the antibiotics isoniazid, minocycline, and***

nitrofurantoin (Macrodantin); the antirheumatic sulfasalazine; the diuretic hydrochlorothiazide; the antihyperlipidemics lovastatin and simvastatin.

- Biologics that can cause drug-induced lupus (DIL) include inhibitors of IFNs and TNF. In DIL, ANA usually appears before symptoms; however, many of the medications mentioned above induce ANA in patients who never develop symptoms of drug-induced lupus. It is appropriate to test for ANA at the first hint of relevant symptoms and to use test results to help decide whether to withdraw the suspect agent.

Ans. C

10. All are true regarding pathogenesis of Ankylosing spondylitis except:

A. Enteric bacteria plays a role

B. Exogenous agents mainly trigger

C. Reverse interferon gene expression signature in antigen presenting cells

D. TNF alpha is known inducer of DKK 1

Explanation:

- No specific event or exogenous agent that triggers onset of disease has been identified, although overlapping features with ReA and IBD and involvement of the IL-23/IL-17 pathway suggest that enteric bacteria may play a role, and microdamage from mechanical stress at enthesial sites has also been implicated.

Ans. B

11. Psoriatric arthropathy is characterized by:

A. Arthritis tends to affect primarily lower extremities

B. Associated with mouth ulcers & bowel symptoms

C. Gradual onset

D. More association with periarthritis

Explanation:

- Reactive Arthritis shares many features in common with psoriatic arthropathy.
- However, PsA is usually gradual in onset; the arthritis tends to affect primarily the upper extremities; and there are usually no associated mouth ulcers, urethritis, or bowel symptoms.

Ans. C

12. Extravascular granuloma is seen in:

A. Wegeners granulomatosis

B. Chrug strauss syndrome

C. PAN

D. Microscopic polyangitis

Explanation:

- Eosinophilic granulomatosis with polyangiitis (Churg-Strauss) was described in 1951 by Churg and Strauss and is characterized by asthma, peripheral and tissue eosinophilia, **extravascular granuloma formation** and vasculitis of multiple organ systems.

Ans. B

13. Idiopathic cutaneous vasculitis presents most commonly due to involvement of:

A. Arterioles

B. Capillaries

C. Post capillary venules

D. All of the above

Explanation:

- Typical histopathologic feature of cutaneous vasculitis is the presence of vasculitis of small vessels.
- Postcapillary venules are the most commonly involved vessels; capillaries and arterioles may be involved less frequently.
- This vasculitis is characterized by a *leukocytoclasis*, a term that refers to the nuclear debris remaining from the neutrophils that have infiltrated in and around vessels during the acute stages.
- In the subacute or chronic stages, mononuclear cells predominate; in certain subgroups, eosinophilic infiltration is seen.
- Erythrocytes often extravasate from the involved vessels, leading to palpable purpura.
- *Cutaneous arteritis* can also occur, which involves slightly larger-sized vessels within the dermis.

Ans. C

14. False regarding drug induced vasculitis is:

A. Presents usually as palpable purpura

B. Generalized or limited to lower extremities

C. Signs & symptoms limited to skin predominantly

D. Drug causing vasculitis is associated with antimyeloperoxidase ANCA is Allopurinol

Explanation:

- Vasculitis associated with drug reactions usually presents as palpable purpura that may be generalized or limited to the lower extremities or other dependent areas; however, urticarial lesions, ulcers, and hemorrhagic blisters may also occur.
- Signs and symptoms may be limited to skin, although systemic manifestations like fever, malaise, and polyarthralgias may occur.
- Although the skin is the predominant organ involved, systemic vasculitis may result from drug reactions.
- **Drugs that have been implicated in vasculitis include allopurinol, thiazides, gold, sulfonamides, phenytoin, and penicillin**.

An increasing number of drugs have been reported to cause vasculitis associated with antimyeloperoxidase ANCA. Of these, best evidence of causality exists for hydralazine & propylthiouracil.

- Clinical manifestations in ANCA-positive drug-induced vasculitis can range from cutaneous lesions to glomerulonephritis and pulmonary hemorrhage.
- Outside of drug discontinuation, treatment should be based on severity of the vasculitis.
- Patients with immediately life-threatening small-vessel vasculitis should initially be treated with glucocorticoids and cyclophosphamide as described for granulomatosis with polyangiitis (Wegener's).
- Following clinical improvement, consideration may be given for tapering such agents along a more rapid schedule

Ans. D

15. Most common pulmonary disease in Sarcoidosis is:

A. Restrictive

B. Obstructive

C. Both pattern in same frequency

D. Early restrictive & later obstructive

Explanation:

- Approximately one-half of sarcoidosis patients present with obstructive disease, reflected by a reduced ratio of forced vital capacity expired in 1 second (FEV1/FVC).

- Cough is a very common symptom.
- Airway involvement causing varying degrees of obstruction underlies the cough in most sarcoidosis patients.
- Airway hyper reactivity, as determined by methacholine challenge, will be positive in some of these patients.

Ans. B & C

16. Not a part of new 2010 ACR-EULAR Classification criteria is:

A. Acute phase reactants
B. Rheumatoid nodule
C. Erosion on X-ray
D. Both B & C

Explanation:

- Application of the newly revised criteria yields a score of 0–10, with a score of ≥6 fulfilling the equirements for definite RA. The new classification criteria differ in several ways from the older criteria set. The new criteria include as an item a positive test for serum anti-CCP antibodies (also termed ACPA, anti-citrullinated peptide antibodies), which carries greater specificity for the diagnosis of RA than a positive test for RF.
- The newer classification criteria also do not take into account whether the patient has rheumatoid nodules or radiographic joint damage because these findings occur rarely in early RA.
- It is important to emphasize that the new 2010 ACR-EULAR criteria are "classification criteria" as opposed to "diagnostic criteria" and serve to distinguish patients at the onset of disease who have a high likelihood of evolution to chronic disease with persistent synovitis and joint damage.
- Presence of radiographic joint erosions or subcutaneous nodules may inform the diagnosis in the later stages of the disease

Ans. D

17. Which of the following is a feature of PAN?

A. Pulmonary artery mainly involved
B. Venules involved
C. Bronchial vessels not involved
D. Lesions are segmental

Explanation:

- Multisystem, necrotizing vasculitis of small- and medium-sized muscular arteries in which involvement of the renal and visceral arteries is characteristic.
- Polyarteritis nodosa does not involve pulmonary arteries, although bronchial vessels may be involved; granulomas, significant eosinophilia, and an allergic diathesis are not observed.
- ***Lesions are segmental and tend to involve bifurcations and branchings of arteries.***
- They may spread circumferentially to involve adjacent veins.
- However, involvement of venules is not seen in polyarteritis nodosa and, if present, suggests microscopic polyangiitis

Ans. D

18. Active SLE in pregnant woman should be controlled initially with:

A. Hydroxychloroquine
B. Prednisone
C. Azathioprine
D. Rituximab

Explanation:

- Active SLE in pregnant women should be controlled with hydroxychloroquine and, if necessary, prednisone/ prednisolone at lowest effective doses for the shortest time required.
- Azathioprine may be added if these treatments do not suppress disease activity.

- Adverse effects of prenatal glucocorticoid exposure (primarily betamethasone, which is not recommended) on offspring may include low birth weight, developmental abnormalities in the CNS, and predilection toward adult metabolic syndrome.
- It is likely that each of these glucocorticoids and immunosuppressive medications gets into breast milk, at least in low levels; patients should consider not breastfeeding if they need therapy for SLE.

Ans. A

19. Blau's syndrome is characterized by all except:

A. Granulomatous dermatitis
B. Uveitis
C. Arthritis
D. Predispose to Ulcerative colitis

Explanation:

- *Blau's syndrome* is caused by mutations in *CARD15* (also known as *NOD2*), which regulates nuclear factor κB activation.
- Blau's syndrome is characterized by granulomatous dermatitis, uveitis, and arthritis; distinct *CARD15* variants predispose to Crohn's disease.

Ans. D

20. Eosinophilic fasciitis is characterized by:

A. Rare idiopathic disorder of children associated with abrupt skin induration
B. Skin characteristically shows peau d orange appearance
C. Skin involvement involves fingers
D. Internal organs are involved frequently

Explanation:

Eosinophilic Fasciitis (Diffuse Fasciitis with Eosinophilia)

- Eosinophilic fasciitis is a rare idiopathic disorder of adults associated with abrupt skin induration.
- **Skin characteristically shows a coarse cobblestone "peau d'orange" appearance.**
- In contrast to SSc, Raynaud's phenomenon and SSc-associated internal organ involvement and autoantibodies are absent.
- Furthermore, skin involvement spares the fingers.
- Full-thickness biopsy of the lesional skin reveals fibrosis of subcutaneous fascia, with variable inflammation and eosinophil infiltration.
- In the acute phase of the illness, peripheral blood eosinophilia may be prominent.
- MRI appears to be a sensitive tool for diagnosis of eosinophilic fasciitis.
- Eosinophilic fasciitis can occur in association with, or preceding, various myelodysplastic syndromes or multiple myeloma.
- Although glucocorticoids cause prompt resolution of eosinophilia, skin shows slow and variable improvement.
- Prognosis of patients with eosinophilic fasciitis who do not develop hematological complications is generally good.

Ans. B

21. Team SSc scleroderma is used for:

A. Raynauds phenomenon & characteristic clinical & laboratory features of SSc occur in absence of detectable skin thickening

B. Raynauds phenomenon & characteristic clinical & laboratory features of SSc occur with detectable skin thickening
C. Raynauds phenomenon & characteristic clinical & laboratory features of SSc occur before detectable skin thickening
D. Raynauds phenomenon & characteristic clinical & laboratory features of SSc occur after detectable skin thickening

Explanation:

- Diffuse cutaneous SSc (dcSSc) is typically associated with extensive skin induration starting in the fingers (sclerodactyly) and ascending from distal to proximal limbs and the trunk.
- In these patients, interstitial lung disease (ILD) and acute renal involvement develop relatively early.
- In contrast, in patients with limited cutaneous SSc (lcSSc), Raynaud's phenomenon generally precedes other disease manifestations, sometimes by years. In these patients, skin involvement remains confined to the fingers, distal limbs, and face, while the trunk is spared.
- Constellation of calcinosis cutis, Raynaud's phenomenon, esophageal dysmotility, sclerodactyly, and telangiectasia, was historically termed *CREST syndrome*.
- In lcSSc, visceral organ involvement tends to show insidious progression, and digital ischemic ulcers, pulmonary arterial hypertension (PAH), hypothyroidism, and primary biliary cirrhosis may occur as late complications.
- In some patients, Raynaud's phenomenon and characteristic clinical and laboratory features of SSc occur in the absence of detectable skin thickening. This syndrome has been termed *SSc sine scleroderma.*

Ans. A

22. **All are true regarding IgA Vasculitis (Henoch-Schönlein) except:**
A. Seasonal variation with peak incidence in spring
B. More common in males
C. Polyarthralgia with frank arthritis
D. GI involvement is seen in almost 70% of pediatric patients

Explanation:

- *IgA vasculitis (Henoch-Schönlein)* is a small-vessel vasculitis characterized by palpable purpura (most commonly distributed over buttocks and lower extremities), arthralgias, gastrointestinal signs and symptoms and glomerulonephritis.

Incidence and Prevalence

- IgA vasculitis (Henoch-Schönlein) is usually seen in children; most patients range in age from 4 to 7 years; however, the disease may also be seen in infants and adults. It is not a rare disease; in one series it accounted for between 5 and 24 admissions per year at a pediatric hospital.
- Male-to-female ratio is 1.5:1. A seasonal variation with a peak incidence in spring has been noted.

Pathology and Pathogenesis

- Presumptive pathogenic mechanism for IgA (Henoch-Schönlein) vasculitis is immune-complex deposition. A number of inciting antigens have been suggested including upper respiratory tract infections, various drugs, foods, insect bites, and immunizations.
- IgA is the antibody class most often seen in the immune complexes and has been demonstrated in the renal biopsies of these patients.

Clinical and Laboratory Manifestations

- In pediatric patients, palpable purpura is seen in virtually all patients; most patients develop polyarthralgias in the absence of frank arthritis.
- Gastrointestinal involvement, which is seen in almost 70% of pediatric patients, is characterized by colicky abdominal pain usually associated with nausea, vomiting, diarrhea, or constipation, and is frequently accompanied by passage of blood and mucus per rectum; bowel intussusception may occur.
- Renal involvement occurs in 10–50% of patients and is usually characterized by mild glomerulonephritis leading to proteinuria and microscopic hematuria, with red blood cell casts in the majority of patients; it usually resolves spontaneously without therapy. Rarely, a progressive glomerulonephritis will develop.
- In adults, presenting symptoms are most frequently related to the skin and joints, while initial complaints related to the gut are less common.
- Although certain studies have found that renal disease is more frequent and more severe in adults, this has not been a consistent finding.
- However, the course of renal disease in adults may be more insidious and thus requires close follow-up. Myocardial involvement can occur in adults but is rare in children.
- Laboratory studies generally show a mild leukocytosis, a normal platelet count, and occasionally eosinophilia.
- Serum complement components are normal, and IgA levels are elevated in about one-half of patients.

Diagnosis

- Diagnosis of IgA vasculitis (Henoch-Schönlein) is based on clinical signs and symptoms.
- Skin biopsy specimen can be useful in confirming leukocytoclastic vasculitis with IgA and C3 deposition by immunofluorescence.
- Renal biopsy is rarely needed for diagnosis but may provide prognostic information in some patients

Ans. C

23. Drug contraindicated in RA with pregnancy is:

A. Prednisolone
B. Hydroxychloroquine
C. Leflunomide
D. Sulfasalazine

Explanation:

- Up to 75% of female RA patients will note overall improvement in symptoms during pregnancy, but often will flare after delivery.
- Flares during pregnancy are generally treated with low doses of prednisone; hydroxychloroquine and sulfasalazine are probably the safest DMARDs to use during pregnancy.
- Methotrexate and leflunomide therapy are contraindicated during pregnancy due to their teratogenicity in animals and humans.
- Experience with biologic agents has been insufficient to make specific recommendations for their use during pregnancy. Ideally, their use should be avoided, but controlling active RA during pregnancy may take precedence in some cases

Ans. C

24. Which of the following is true regarding Juvenile onset Spondyloarthritis?

A. Peripheral arthritis & enthesitis is rare
B. Axial symptoms supervening in early adolescence
C. Seen in developing countries
D. All of the above

Explanation:

- In juvenile onset spondyloarthritis, peripheral arthritis and enthesitis predominate, with axial symptoms supervening in late adolescence.
- Initially, axial physical findings mirror the inflammatory process.
- Most specific findings involve loss of spinal mobility, with limitation of anterior and lateral flexion and extension of the lumbar spine and of chest expansion.
- Limitation of motion is usually out of proportion to the degree of bony ankylosis and is thought to possibly reflect muscle spasm secondary to pain and inflammation.
- Pain in the sacroiliac joints may be elicited either with direct pressure or with stress on the joints.
- In addition, there is commonly tenderness upon palpation of the posterior spinous processes and other sites of symptomatic bony tenderness.

Ans. C

25. A 12-year-old boy presents to the office for evaluation of weakness. With exercise, he gets cramps and fatigue in his legs to the extent that he is unable to keep up with his peers during gym class. Cramps usually occur within minutes of starting exercise, and he seems to get a "second wind" if he is able to rest for a few minutes after the cramps begin. He denies dark urine. His neurological examination is normal. Serum creatine kinase (CK) level is elevated at 650 IU/L (normal is usually 50–200 IU/L). An exercise forearm test is performed and shows a normal rise in ammonia, but no rise in the lactate. The patient's most likely diagnosis is caused by which of the following?

A. Alpha-glucosidase deficiency
B. Myophosphorylase deficiency
C. PMP22 duplication
D. Absence of muscular dystrophin

Explanation:

- McArdle disease, also known as myophosphorylase deficiency or type V glycogenosis, is an autosomalrecessive disorder resulting in a deficiency of myophosphorylase. This is the most common disorder of carbohydrate metabolism. Patients typically present in childhood with exercise intolerance, cramps, and pain induced by brief intense activity. CK may be elevated. Often a phenomenon known as second wind is seen with McArdle disease, which involves a return of strength and reduction in pain after a short rest due to mobilization of blood glucose as a muscle energy source rather than relying on breakdown of glycogen. An exercise forearm test can identify a disorder of glycogen metabolism by measuring levels of ammonia and lactate. In this test, baseline ammonia and lactate levels are drawn, followed by intense exercise of the hand with levels of ammonia and lactate drawn at serial intervals. Glycogen metabolism disorders show a normal elevation of ammonia, but a lack of rise in lactate. The diagnosis is confirmed with a muscle biopsy that shows a lack of uptake to a myophosphorylase stain. Alpha-glucosidase deficiency is also known as Pompe disease. The most common form of this condition presents in childhood with hypotonia, cardiomegaly and hepatomegaly.
- Juvenile form presents with progressive proximal muscle weakness, lumbar lordosis, and a waddling gait, which can appear similar to Duchenne muscular dystrophy (DMD). An adult form presents in the 40s, with proximal muscle weakness similar to polymyositis.
- Pompe's disease is diagnosed with an assay for alpha glucosidase activity or muscle biopsy. PMP22 duplication is the genetic defect seen in Charcot-Marie-Tooth disease type 1A, which is an autosomal-dominant hereditary demyelinating neuropathy. Absence of dystrophin on muscle biopsy makes a diagnosis of DMD, which presents with progressive weakness, pseudohypertrophy of gastrocnemius, and a Gower's sign typically in young males. There is no "second wind" phenomenon in DMD. Debranching enzyme deficiency is a rare glycogenosis that presents in the third to fourth decade and causes severe weakness and atrophy of muscles, often mimicking amyotrophic lateral sclerosis. Liver failure can also occur, but there is no "second wind" phenomenon.

Ans. B

26. **Not true about microscopic polyangiitis is:**

A. More common in males
B. Glomerulonephritis is very common
C. Immune complex play role in pathogenesis
D. Upper airway disease and pulmonary nodules are not typically found

Explanation:

- Glomerulonephritis is very common in microscopic polyangiitis, and pulmonary capillaritis often occurs.
- Absence of granulomatous inflammation in microscopic polyangiitis is said to differentiate it from granulomatosis with polyangiitis (Wegener's).

Ans. C

27. **Identify the condition in which following image finding is seen?**

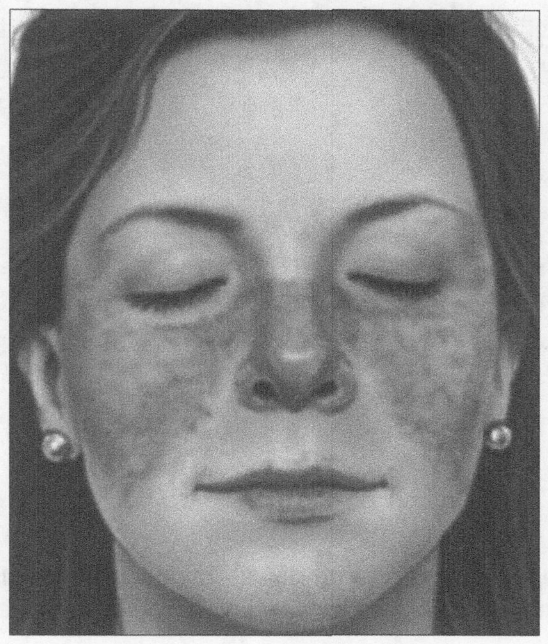

A. Systematic lupus erythematosus
B. Sarcoidosis
C. Rhinophyma
D. Psoriasis

Explanation:

- Specific complex of involvement of bridge of nose, area beneath the eye and cheeks known as lupus pernio seen in chronic form of sarcoidosis.
- Systemic lupus erythematosus involves cheeks and bridge of nose typically sparing nasolabial folds called butterfly rash.
- Rhinophyma is benign hyperplasia of sebaceous glands of nose.
- In psoriasis silvery mica scales, crusting is seen.

Ans. A

28. **A 30 year old female presents to the OPD with 3 months history of lethargy and increasing dyspnoea. Chest radiograph shows diffuse shadowing with bilateral hilar lymphadenopathy. Which one of the following investigations would be most useful in guiding the diagnosis?**

A. Serum amylase

B. Troponin I

C. Angiotensin converting enzyme

D. Serum magnesium

Explanation:

- Sarcoidosis is a multisystem disorder of unknown etiology that is characterized pathologically by the presence of noncaseating granuloma. Laboratory abnormalities seen in sarcoidosis include raised angiotensin converting enzyme, hypercalcemia and hypercalciuria.

Ans. C

29. Following kidney lesion of an systemic lupus erythematosus belongs to which class under classification of lupus nephritis?

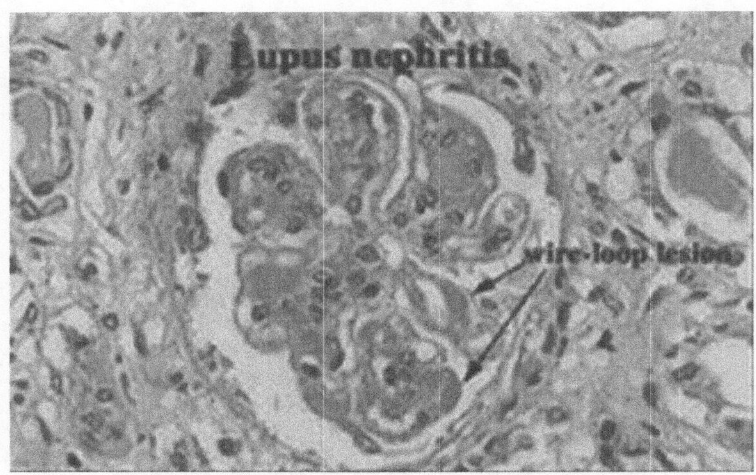

A. Class 1

B. Class 2

C. Class 3

D. Class 4

Explanation:

- In the image diffuse nephritis is seen with diffuse endocapillary proliferation with focal subendothelial immune deposits, mild mesangial alterations and wire loop lesions are also seen.

Classification of lupus nephritis:

Table: Classification for lupus nephritis		
Class I	Minimal mesangial	Normal histology with mesangial deposits
Class II	Mesangial proliferation	Mesangial hypercellularity with expansion of the mesangial matrix
Class III	Focal nephritis	Focal endocapillary + extracapillary proliferation with focal subendothelial immune deposits and mild mesangial expansion
Class IV	Diffuse nephritis	Diffuse endocapillary + extracapillary proliferation with diffuse subendothelial immune deposits and mesangial alterations
Class V	Membranous nephritis	Thickened basement membranes with diffuse subepithelial immune deposits; may occur with class III or IV lesions and is sometimes called mixed membranous and proliferative nephritis
Class VI	Sclerotic nephritis	Global sclerosis of nearly all glomerular capillaries

Ans. D

30. Most common rheumatological disorder associated with Relapsing Polychondritis?

A. SLE
B. Systemic vasculitis
C. Rheumatoid arthritis
D. Behcet's disease

Explanation:

- Relapsing polychondritis is an uncommon disorder of unknown cause characterized by inflammation of cartilage predominantly affecting ears, nose & laryngo tracheobronchial tree.
- Other manifestations include scleritis, neuro sensory hearing loss, polyarthritis, cardiac abnormalities, skin lesions and glomerulonephritis.
- Approximately 30% of patients with relapsing polychondritis will have another rheumatologic disorder, most frequent being systemic vasculitis, followed by rheumatoid arthritis & SLE.
- Non-rheumatic disorders have also been associated with relapsing polychondritis.

Ans. B

31. A 55 year old male has complaints of chronic fever, cough, breathing difficulty and an erythematous tender nodule over bilateral shins. There is also an acute onset of migratory poly arthritis. Chest radiograph reveals bilateral pulmonary infiltrates and bilateral hilar lymphadenopathy. What is the diagnosis?

A. Lofgren's syndrome
B. Heerfordt's syndrome
C. Behcet's syndrome
D. HenochSchönlein purpura

Explanation:

- Lofgren's syndrome is seen in sarcoidosis. It presents with fever, erythema nodosum, arthralgia and bilateral hilar lymphadenopathy.
- Heerfordt's syndrome also seen in sarcoidosis and presents with uveo-parotid fever (uveitis with parotid gland swelling).

Ans. A

32. A 49 year old patient presents with epistaxis and recurrent sinusitis. He suddenly developed palpable purpuric lesions and haemoptysis. CT chest revealed multiple cavitatory lesions. What is the most likely diagnosis?

A. Tuberculosis
B. Sarcoidosis
C. Granulomatosis with polyangiitis
D. Metastasis

Explanation:

- Granulomatous vasculitis of upper and lower respiratory tracts together with glomerulonephritis; upper airway lesions affecting the nose and sinuses can cause purulent or bloody nasal discharge, mucosal ulceration, septal perforation, and cartilaginous destruction (saddlenose deformity). Lung involvement may be asymptomatic or cause cough, hemoptysis, dyspnea; eye involvement may occur; glomerulonephritis can be rapidly progressive and asymptomatic and can lead to renal failure.

Ans. C

33. Bilateral skin thickening is a characteristic feature of:

A. Scleroderma
B. Dermatomyositis
C. Peyronie's disease
D. Sticker Syndrome

Explanation:

- Bilateral symmetrical skin thickening is the hallmark of SSc that distinguishes it from other connective tissue diseases.
- Skin involvement starts in the fingers and characteristically advances from distal to proximal extremities in an ascending fashion.
- Some patients note diffuse taming in the absence of sun exposure as a very early manifestation. In dark skinned individuals, vitiligo like hypopigmentation may occur.
- Because pigment loss spares the perifollicular areas, the skin may have "salt and pepper" appearance, most prominently on the scalp, upper back, and Chest.

Ans. A

34. **First line therapy for paget's disease is:**

A. Zoledronic acid
B. Calcitonin
C. Teriparatide
D. Denosumab

Explanation:

Paget's disease

- Bisphosphonates are the mainstay of pharmacologic therapy of Paget's disease.
- Among them, zoledronic acid is currently recommended as the first choice, particularly for those who have severe disease or need rapid normalization of bone turnover (neurologic symptoms, severe bone pain due to a lytic lesion, risk of an impending fracture, or pre-treatment prior to elective surgery in an area of active disease).

Ans. A

35. **Following clinical finding not seen in:**

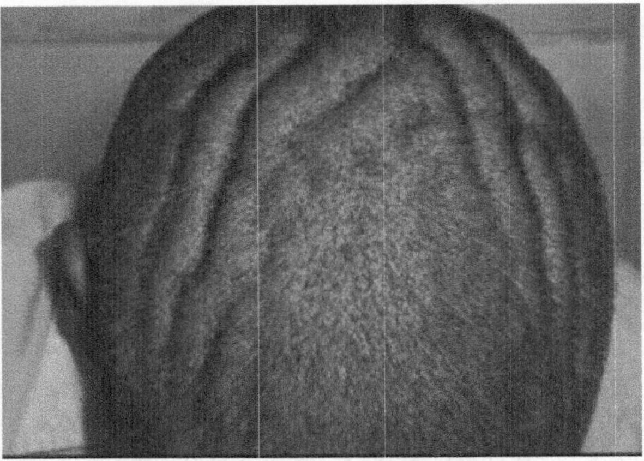

A. Scleroderma
B. Type 2 Diabetes mellitus
C. Syphilis
D. Primary hypertrophic osteoarthropathy

Explanation:

- **Image is showing a presentation of Cutis Verticis Gyrata**
- Progressive dermatological condition showing excessive skin folds in scalp, resembling surface of brain
- Most common in males
- Divided in to 2 types , PRIMARY & SECONDARY

Among the secondary causes – Primary hypertrophic osteoarthropathy is common

- Noonan syndrome
- Syphilis
- Type 2 DM
- Klinefelter syndrome
- Ehler danlos syndrome
- Hypothyroidism
- Acromegaly
- Turner syndrome
- Leukemia
- Amyloidosis
- T/t – Mild cases – treating Skin changes
- Severe case – Scalp reduction Surgery
- Secondary cases – Treatment of underlying causes

Ans. A

36. **Identify the image:**

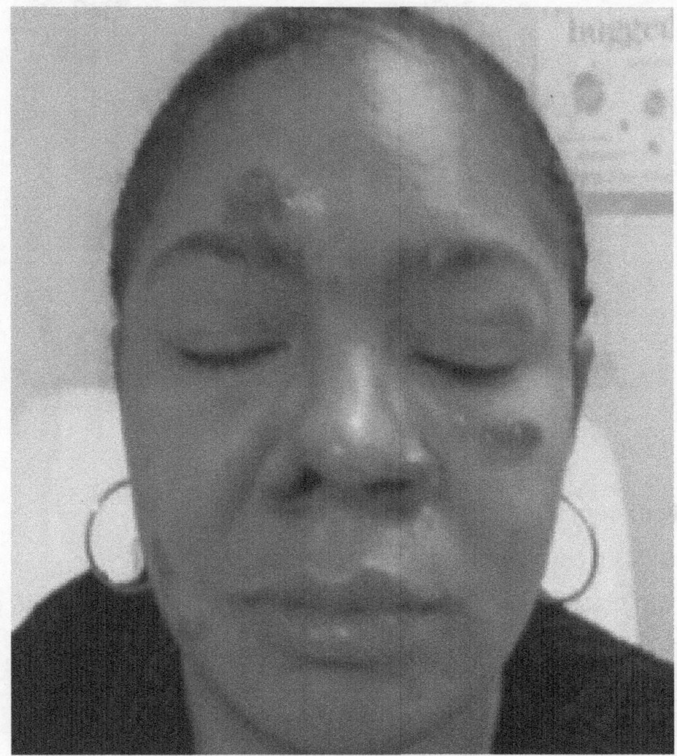

A. Systematic lupus erethymatosus
B. Sarcoidosis
C. Rhinophyma
D. Psoriasis

Explanation:

Specific complex of involvement of bridge of nose, area beneath the eye and cheeks known as lupus pernio seen in chronic form of sarcoidosis. Systemic lupus erythematosus involves cheeks and bridge of nose typically sparing nasolabial folds called butterfly rash.

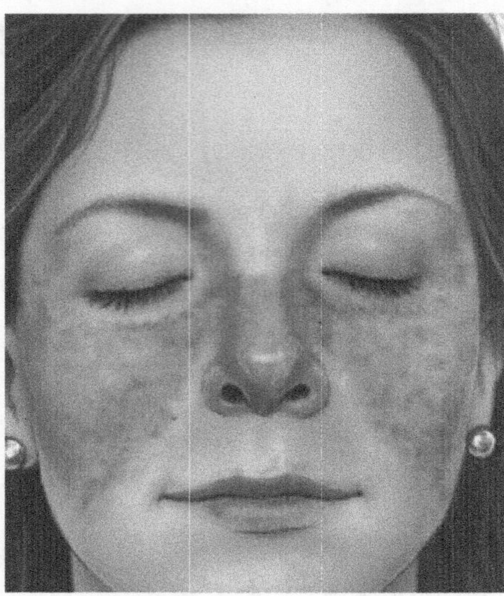

Rhinophyma is benign hyperplasia of sebaceous glands of nose. In psoriasis silvery mica scales, crusting is seen.

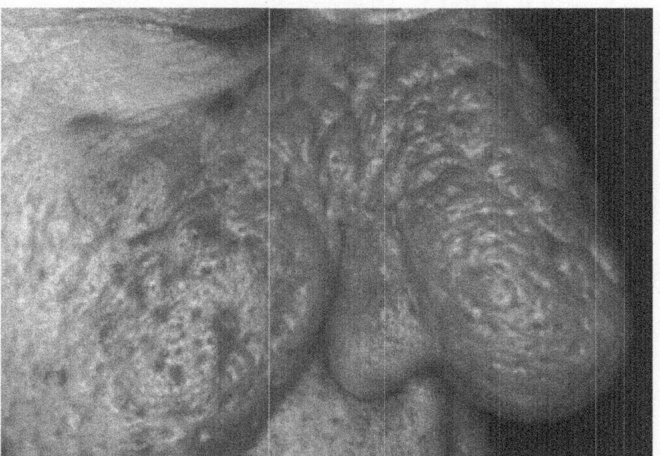

Ans. B

37. All are true about PAN except:

A. Involvement of renal & visceral arteries is characteristic

B. Pathology in kidney in classic polyarteritis nodosa is that of arteritis without glomerulonephritis

C. Hairy cell leukemia can be associated with PAN

D. Death usually occurs due to renal complication

Explanation:

- Multisystem, necrotizing vasculitis of small- and medium-sized muscular arteries in which involvement of the renal and visceral arteries is characteristic.
- Polyarteritis nodosa does not involve pulmonary arteries, although bronchial vessels may be involved; granulomas, significant eosinophilia, and an allergic diathesis are not observed.
- Vascular lesion in polyarteritis nodosa is a necrotizing inflammation of small- and medium-sized muscular arteries.

- Lesions are segmental and tend to involve bifurcations and branchings of arteries.
- They may spread circumferentially to involve adjacent veins.
- However, involvement of venules is not seen in polyarteritis nodosa and, if present, suggests microscopic polyangiitis.
- In the acute stages of disease, polymorphonuclear neutrophils infiltrate all layers of vessel wall and perivascular areas, which results in intimal proliferation and degeneration of the vessel wall.
- Mononuclear cells infiltrate area as the lesions progress to the subacute and chronic stages.
- Fibrinoid necrosis of the vessels ensues with compromise of lumen, thrombosis, infarction of the tissues supplied by involved vessel, and, in some cases, hemorrhage. As the lesions heal, there is collagen deposition, which may lead to further occlusion of the vessel lumen.
- Aneurysmal dilations up to 1 cm in size along the involved arteries are characteristic of polyarteritis nodosa. Granulomas and substantial eosinophilia with eosinophilic tissue infiltrations are not characteristically found and suggest eosinophilic granulomatosis with polyangiitis (Churg-Strauss).
- Multiple organ systems are involved, and the clinicopathologic findings reflect the degree and location of vessel involvement and resulting ischemic changes. As mentioned above, pulmonary arteries are not involved in polyarteritis nodosa, and bronchial artery involvement is uncommon.
- Pathology in the kidney in classic polyarteritis nodosa is that of arteritis without glomerulonephritis.
- In patients with significant hypertension, typical pathologic features of glomerulosclerosis may be seen. In addition, pathologic sequelae of hypertension may be found elsewhere in the body.
- Presence of a polyarteritis nodosa–like vasculitis in patients
- with hepatitis B together with the isolation of circulating immune complexes composed of hepatitis B antigen and immunoglobulin and demonstration by immunofluorescence of hepatitis B antigen, IgM, and complement in the blood vessel walls strongly suggest the role of immunologic phenomena in the pathogenesis of this disease.
- Polyarteritis nodosa–like vasculitis has also been reported in patients with hepatitis C. Hairy cell leukemia can be associated with polyarteritis nodosa; the pathogenic mechanisms of this association are unclear.

Ans. D

38. SAPHO Syndrome include all except:

A. Arthritis
B. Synovitis
C. Pustulosis
D. Hyperostosis

Explanation:

- Syndrome of synovitis, acne, pustulosis, hyperostosis, and osteitis (SAPHO) is characterized by a variety of skin and musculoskeletal manifestations.
- Dermatologic manifestations include palmoplantar pustulosis, acne conglobata, acne fulminans, and hidradenitis suppurativa.
- Main musculoskeletal findings are sternoclavicular and spinal hyperostosis, chronic recurrent foci of sterile osteomyelitis, and axial or peripheral arthritis.
- Cases with one or a few manifestations are probably the rule.
- ESR and/or CRP are usually mildly to moderately elevated, occasionally dramatically.

Ans. A

39. Anticardiolipin Antibody in APLA is detected by:

A. ELISA
B. Aptt
C. Kaolin clotting time
D. Dilute russell viper venom test

Explanation:

Table: Classification and nomenclature of antiphospholipid antibodies

Name	Assay for Their Detection	Comments
Antibodies against cardiolipin (aCl)	Enzyme-linked immunosorbent assay (ELISA) using as antigen cardiolipin (CL), a negatively charged phospholipid	aCL from patients with APS recognize β2GPI existing in the human serum as well as in bovine serum, which is used to block the nonspecific binding sites on the ELISA plate. CL simply stabilizes β2GPI at high concentration on the polystyrene surface
Antibodies against β2GPI (anti-β2GPI)	ELISA using as antigen affinity purified or recombinant β2GPI in the absence of PL	Antibodies recognized β2GPI bound the the absence of CL to an oxidized polystyrene surface, where oxygen atoms in the moieties C–O or C=O were introduced by γ-irradiation
Lupus anticoagulant (LA)	Activated partial thromboplastin time (aPTT) Karolin clotting time (KCT) Dilute Russel viper venom test (DRVVT)	Antibodies recognize β2GPI or prothrombin (PT) and elongate aPTT, implying that they interfere with the generation or thrombin by prothrombin, Prolongation of the clotting times is an in vitro phenomenon, and LA induces thromboses in vivo

Ans. A

40. A 48-year-old married mother presents with inability to lift shoulders due to pain. She noticed stiffness in both hands in the morning that lasted longer and longer. Stiffness now lasted more than 1 hour every morning and included hands, wrists and ankles. She also had increasing difficulty standing for long periods at work or at home due to foot and ankle pain. She began taking ibuprofen 800mg 3 times daily and found it helped her get through her day with less pain and stiffness. What is the diagnosis?

A. Rheumatoid arthritis
B. Osteoarthritis
C. Gouty arthritis
D. Synovitis

Explanation:

- Incidence of RA increases between 25 and 55 years of age, after which it plateaus until the age of 75 and then decreases.
- Presenting symptoms of RA typically result from inflammation of the joints, ten dons and bursae.
- Patients often complain of early morning joint stiff ness lasting more than 1 h that eases with physical activity.
- Earliest involved joints are typically the small joints of hands and feet.Some patients with inflammatory arthritis will present with too few affected joints to be classified as having RA-so called undifferentiated inflammatory arthritis.
- Those with an undifferentiated arthritis who are most likely to be diagnosed later with RA have a higher number of tender and swollen joints, test positive for serum rheumatoid factor (RF) or anti CCP antibodies, and have higher scores for physical disability.
- Once the disease process of RA is established, the wrists, metacarpophalangeal (MCP), and proximal interphalangeal (PIP) joints stand out as the most frequently involved joints.
- Distal interphalangeal (DIP) joint involvement may occur in RA, but it usually is a manifestation of coexistent osteoarthritis.
- Flexor tendon tenosynovitis is a frequent hallmark of RA and leads to decreased range of motion, reduced grip strength and "trigger" fingers.

Ans. A

41. Opsonization is mechanism of tissue damage in which Autoimmune disease?

A. Good pasture syndrome
B. SLE
C. RA
D. Autoimmune thrombocytopenic purpura

Explanation:

Table: Mechanisms of tissue damage in autoimmune disease			
Effector	**Mechanism**	**Target**	**Disease**
Autoantibody	Blocking of inactivation	α chain of the nicotinic acetylcholine receptor	Myasthenia gravis
		Phospholipid-β_2-glycoprotein I complex	Antiphospholipid syndrome
		Insulin receptor	Insulin-resistant diabetes mellitus
		Intrinsic factor	Pernicious anemia
	Stimulation	TSH receptor (LATS)	Graves' disease
		Proteinase-3 (ANCA)	Granulomatosis with polyangiitis
		Epidermal cadherin	Pemphigus vulgaris
		Desmoglein 3	
	Complement activation	α_3 Chain of collagen IV	Goodpasture's syndrome
	Immune complex formation	Double-stranded DNA	Systemic lupus erythematosus
		Immunoglobulin	Rheumatoid arthritis
	Opsonization	Platelet GpIIb:IIIa	Autoimmune thrombocytopenic purpura
		Rh angigens, I antigen	Autoimmune hemolytic anemia
	Antibody-dependent cellular cytotoxicity	Thyroid peroxidase, thyroglobulin	Hashimoto's thyroiditis
T cells	Cytokine production		Rheumatoid arthritis, multiple sclerosis, type 1 diabetes mellitus
	Cellular cytotoxicity		Type 1 diabetes mellitus

Ans. D

42. Not a true about lab investigation of HSP is:

A. Leucocytosis
B. Thrombocytopenia
C. Eosinophilia
D. Complement level normal

Explanation:

- In pediatric patients, palpable purpura is seen in virtually all patients; most patients develop polyarthralgias in the absence of frank arthritis.
- Gastrointestinal involvement, which is seen in almost 70% of pediatric patients, is characterized by colicky abdominal pain usually associated with nausea, vomiting, diarrhea, or constipation, and is frequently accompanied by the passage of blood and mucus per rectum; bowel intussusception may occur.
- Renal involvement occurs in 10–50% of patients and is usually characterized by mild glomerulonephritis leading to proteinuria and microscopic hematuria, with red blood cell casts in the majority of patients; it usually resolves spontaneously without therapy.
- Rarely, a progressive glomerulonephritis will develop. In adults, presenting symptoms are most frequently related to skin and joints, while initial complaints related to the gut are less common.
- Although certain studies have found that renal disease is more frequent and more severe in adults, this has not been a consistent finding.
- However, the course of renal disease in adults may be more insidious and thus requires close follow-up.
- Myocardial involvement can occur in adults but is rare in children.

- ***Laboratory studies generally show a mild leukocytosis, a normal platelet count, and occasionally eosinophilia.***
- ***Serum complement components are normal, and IgA levels are elevated in about one-half of patients.***

Ans. B

43. Biopsy from an following lesion shown on CT reveals typical necrotizing granulomatous vasculitis likely diagnosis:

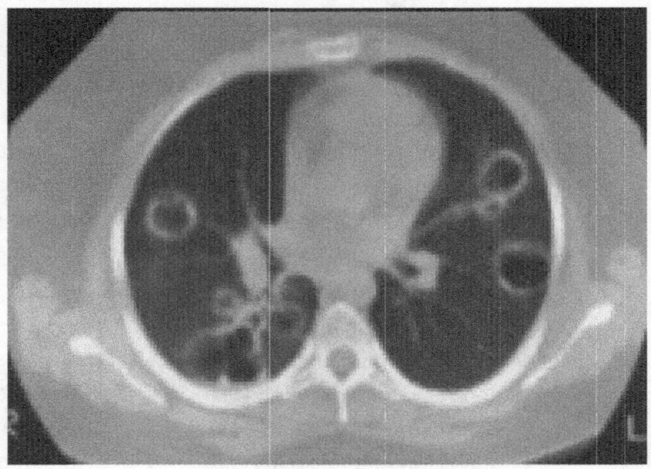

A. Tuberculosis
B. Secondaries
C. Wegeners granulomatosis
D. Sarcoidosis

Explanation:

- CT shows multiple, bilateral cavitatory lesions along with histological features of typical necrotizing granulomatous vasculitis diagnosing as Wegener's granulomatosis.
- In Tuberculosis histology of cavitatory lesions reveals caseous necrosis.
- In sarcoidosis histology of cavitatory lesions reveals non caseating granulomatous calcific nodules.
- Secondary's will reveal abnormal tumor cells.

Ans. C

44. Identify the condition based on histopathology slide shown below:

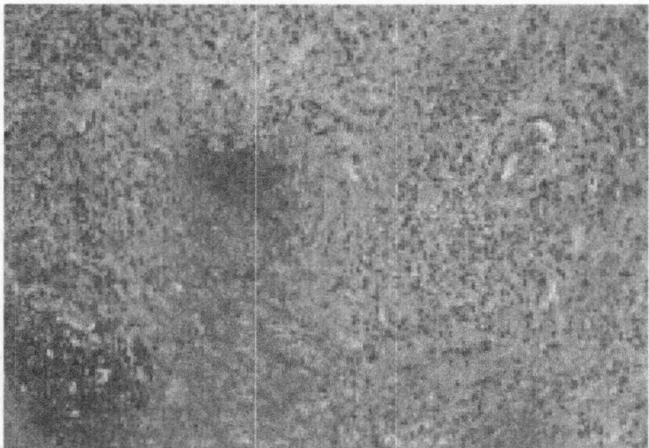

A. Sarcoidosis
B. Tuberculosis
C. Wegener's granulomatosis
D. Firinoid necrosis

Explanation:

- Geographic necrosis has serpiginous border of histiocytes and giant cells surrounding central necrotic zone. Vasculitis with neutrophils and lymphocytes in a wall of arterioles. In tuberculosis caseous necrosis along with giant cells, granuloma are seen.

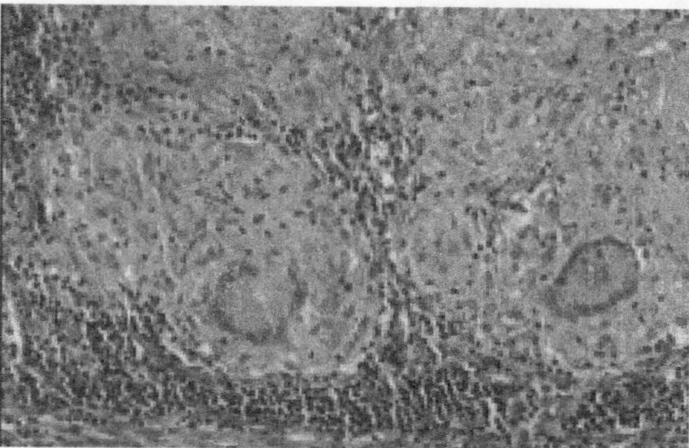

- In sarcoidosis non caseating granulomas with epitheloid cells and giant cells seen.
- In fibrinoid necrosis amorphous esinophilic material made up of fibrin is seen.

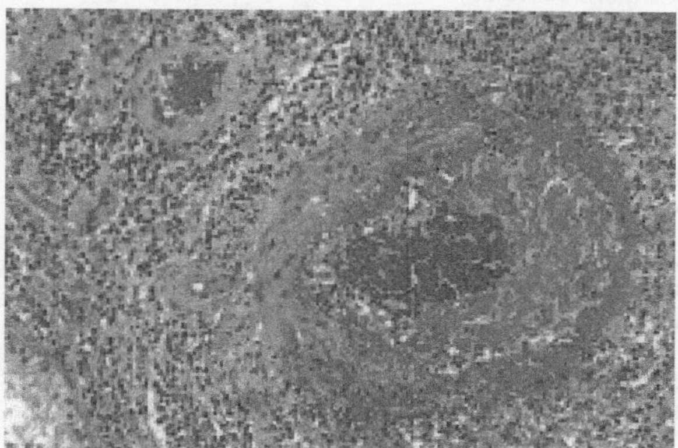

Ans. C

45. A 72-year-old woman, has been complaining of low-grade fever and dyspnea for 2 weeks. She has a 10-year history of scleroderma with involvement of the digits and esophagus. She has a 30-pack-year history of cigarette smoking but quit 8 years ago. On chest radiograph, she has a nodular infiltrate in the right lower lobe. Positron emission tomography (PET)/CT shows the right lower lobe lesion to be 3 cm in diameter with nodular infiltrate characteristics and enhanced fluorodeoxyglucose (FDG) uptake. Which of the following statements is most accurate regarding this condition of patient?

A. Additional diagnostic studies are indicated.

B. Findings on PET/CT make infection very likely.

C. Findings on PET/CT make infection very unlikely.

D. Findings on PET/CT make malignancy very likely

Explanation:

- This patient is at risk of infection and malignancy.
- Findings on positron emission tomography (PET)/CT are consistent with either diagnosis. Her risk of infection, particularly aspiration pneumonia, is related to her scleroderma-induced esophageal dysfunction, history of low-grade fever, and location.
- Most aspiration pneumonias involve the right lower lobe, particularly superior segment.

- They may appear as consolidation or nodular infiltrates. Given her history of smoking, she is also at risk of primary lung malignancies.
- Fluorodeoxyglucose (FDG)-PET can often differentiate benign from malignant lesions as small as 1 cm.
- However, false-positive results are seen in inflammatory conditions, such as pneumonia or granulomatous diseases.
- False-negative findings can occur in lesions with low metabolic activity such as carcinoid tumors and bronchioloalveolar cell carcinomas.

Ans. A

46. Drug toxicity that can mimic vasculitis include all except:

A. Cocaine
B. Methysergide
C. Arsenic
D. Lead

Explanation:

Table: Conditions that can mimic vasculitis
Infectious Diseases
• Bacterial endocarditis • Disseminated gonococcal infection • Pulmonary histoplasmosis • Coccidioidomycosis • Syphilis • Lyme disease • Rocky Mountain spotted fever • Whipple's disease
Coagulopathies/Thrombotic Microangiopathies
• Antiphospholipid syndrome • Thrombotic thrombocytopenic purpura
Neoplasma
• Atrial myxoma • Lymphoma • Carcinomatosis
Drug Toxicity
• Cocaine • Levamisole • Amphetamines • Ergot alkaloids • Methysergide • Arsenic
Other
• Sarcoidosis • Atheroembolic disease • Antiglomerular basement membrane disease (Goodpasture's syndrome) • Amyloidosis • Migraine • Fibromuscular dysplasia • Heritable disorders of connective tissue • Segmental arterial mediolysis (SAM) • Reversible cerebral vasoconstrictive syndrome

Ans. D

47. HBsAg in serum of patients with polyarteritis nodosa is:

A. 5%
B. 10%
C. 15%
D. 20%

Explanation:

- Glomerulonephritis with the nephrotic syndrome is observed occasionally; HBsAg, immunoglobulin, and C3 deposition has been found in the glomerular basement membrane. Whereas generalized vasculitis (polyarteritis nodosa) develops in considerably <1% of patients with chronic HBV infection, 20–30% of patients with polyarteritis nodosa have HBsAg in serum

Ans. D

48. Rheumatoid like arthritis with erosions and fulfill criteria for both RA and SLE:

A. Lupus
B. Arthus
C. Rhupus
D. Lupus rheumatoid

Explanation:

- Some individuals have rheumatoid-like arthritis with erosions and fulfill criteria for both RA and SLE ("rhupus").

Ans. C

49. All are true about Ankylosing spondylitis except:

A. Severe disease may show an elevated alkaline phosphatase
B. Elevated IgE levels are common
C. RF, Anti CCP & ANA are largely absent
D. ANA's may appear with anti TNF therapy

Explanation:

- No laboratory test is diagnostic of AS. In most ethnic groups, HLAB27 is present in 75–90% of patients.
- Erythrocyte sedimentation rate (ESR) and C-reactive protein (CRP) are often, but not always, elevated.
- Mild anemia may be present. Patients with severe disease may show an elevated alkaline phosphatase level.
- Elevated serum IgA levels are common.
- Rheumatoid factor, anti-cyclic citrullinated peptide (CCP), and antinuclear antibodies (ANAs) are largely absent unless caused by a coexistent disease, although ANAs may appear with anti-TNF therapy.
- Circulating levels of CD8 + T cells tend to be low, and serum matrix metalloproteinase 3 levels correlate with disease activity.
- Synovial fluid from peripheral joints in AS is nonspecifically inflammatory.
- Restricted chest wall motion causes decreased vital capacity, but ventilatory function is usually well maintained.

Ans. B

50. Not considered a true DMARD's in RA:

A. Hydroxychloroquine
B. Tofacitinib
C. Rituximab
D. Methotrexate

Explanation:

- DMARDs are so named because of their ability to slow or prevent structural progression of RA.

- Conventional DMARDs include hydroxychloroquine, sulfasalazine, methotrexate, and leflunomide; they exhibit a delayed onset of action of ~6–12 weeks.
- Methotrexate is the DMARD of choice for the treatment of RA and is the anchor drug for most combination therapies. It was approved for the treatment of RA in 1988 and remains the benchmark for the efficacy and safety of new disease-modifying therapies.
- At the dosages used for the treatment of RA, methotrexate has been shown to stimulate adenosine release from cells, producing an anti-inflammatory effect.
- Clinical efficacy of leflunomide, an inhibitor of pyrimidine synthesis, appears similar to that of methotrexate; it has been shown in well-designed trials to be effective for treatment of RA as monotherapy or in combination with methotrexate and other DMARDs.
- Although similar to other DMARDs in its slow onset of action, hydroxychloroquine has not been shown to delay radiographic progression of disease & thus is not considered to be true DMARD.
- In clinical practice, hydroxychloroquine is generally used for treatment of early, mild disease or as adjunctive therapy in combination with other DMARDs. Sulfasalazine is used in a similar manner and has been shown in randomized, controlled trials to reduce radiographic progression of disease.
- Minocycline, gold salts, penicillamine, azathioprine & cyclosporine have all been used for the treatment of RA with varying degrees of success; however, they are used sparingly now due to their inconsistent clinical efficacy or unfavorable toxicity profile.

Ans. A

51. In APLA with SLE, INR recommended for patients with arterial clotting particularly in CNS is:

A. 1.5-2 B. 2-2.5
C. 2.5-3 D. 3-3.5

Explanation:

- With warfarin, a target international normalized ratio (INR) of 2.0–2.5 is recommended for patients with one episode of venous clotting; an INR of 3.0–3.5 is recommended for patients with recurring clots or arterial clotting, particularly in the CNS.

Ans. D

52. Ankylosing spondylitis is characterized by all except:

A. Primarily affects axial skeleton B. Usually begins in 2nd/3rd decade
C. More common in females D. Concordance rate in identical twins is about 65%

Explanation:

- AS is an inflammatory disorder of unknown cause that primarily affects the axial skeleton; peripheral joints and extraarticular structures are also frequently involved.
- Disease usually begins in the second or third decade.
- AS is present in 1–6% of adults inheriting B27, whereas prevalence is 10–30% among B27+ adult first-degree relatives of AS probands.
- Concordance rate in identical twins is about 65%.
- Susceptibility to AS is determined largely by genetic factors, with B27 estimated to comprise about 20% of the genetic component.
- Genome-wide single-nucleotide polymorphism (SNP) analysis has identified over 100 additional non-HLA susceptibility alleles.

Ans. C

53. Most common disorder associated with relapsing polychondritis is:

A. Systemic vasculitis
B. Rheumatoid arthritis
C. Systemic lupus erythematosus
D. Overlapping connective tissue disease

Explanation:

- Systemic vasculitis is the most common association, followed by rheumatoid arthritis and systemic lupus erythematosus **associated with relapsing polychondritis**

Ans. A

54. Most common abnormality of liver function in sarcoidosis is an elevation of:

A. Transaminase levels
B. Alkaline phosphatase level
C. Bilirubin level
D. Hepatomegaly

Explanation:

- Using biopsies to detect granulomatous disease, liver involvement can be identified in over one-half of sarcoidosis patients.
- However, using liver function studies, only 20–30% of patients will have evidence of liver involvement.
- Most common abnormality of liver function is an elevation of the alkaline phosphatase level, consistent with an obstructive pattern. In addition, elevated transaminase levels can occur.
- An elevated bilirubin level is a marker for more advanced liver disease.

Ans. B

55. All are true regarding Ankylosing spondylitis except:

A. HLA –B27 is diagnostic of AS
B. ESR/CRP is elevated
C. Mild anemia is present
D. Serum IgA levels are elevated

Explanation:

- No laboratory test is diagnostic of AS. In most ethnic groups, HLAB27 is present in 75–90% of patients. Erythrocyte sedimentation rate (ESR) and C-reactive protein (CRP) are often, but not always, elevated.
- Mild anemia may be present. Patients with severe disease may show an elevated alkaline phosphatase level. Elevated serum IgA levels are common. Rheumatoid factor, anti-cyclic citrullinated peptide (CCP), and antinuclear antibodies (ANAs) are largely absent unless caused by a coexistent disease, although ANAs may appear with anti-TNF therapy.
- Circulating levels of CD8+ T cells tend to be low, and serum matrix metalloproteinase 3 levels correlate with disease activity. Synovial fluid from peripheral joints in AS is nonspecifically inflammatory. Restricted chest wall motion causes decreased vital capacity, but ventilatory function is usually well maintained.

Ans. A

56. Behcet's syndrome all are true except:

A. Skin involved in 80% of the patients
B. Eye involvement is common in males
C. Cerebral brain thrombosis is more common in females
D. GI involvement is more common in Asians

Explanation:

- Skin involvement is observed in 80% of patients and includes folliculitis, erythema nodosum, acne-like rashes, and, infrequently, vasculitis, Sweet syndrome, and pyoderma gangrenosum. Nonspecific skin inflammatory reactivity to scratch or intradermal saline injection (pathergy test) is a specific manifestation.

- Eye involvement with scarring and bilateral panuveitis is the most dreaded complication, since it occasionally progresses rapidly to blindness. Uveitis occurs in 10–15% of patients, primarily in males. It is usually present at the onset but may also develop within the first few years. In addition to iritis, posterior uveitis, retinal vessel occlusions, and optic neuritis can be rarely seen in some patients.
- Non-deforming arthritis/arthralgias are seen in 50% of patients and affect mostly knees and ankles. Enthesopathy, avascular necrosis, myalgia, and myositis can be also seen.
- Superficial or deep peripheral vein thrombosis is seen in 30% of patients. Pulmonary emboli are a rare complication. The superior vena cava is obstructed occasionally. Arterial involvement occurs in <1–5% of patients and presents with aortitis or peripheral arterial aneurysm and arterial thrombosis. Pulmonary artery vasculitis presenting with dyspnea, cough, chest pain, hemoptysis, and infiltrates on chest roentgenograms has been reported in <1% of patients and should be differentiated from thromboembolic disease since it warrants immunosuppressive and not thrombolytic therapy.
- Neurologic involvement (5–10%) appears mainly in the parenchymal form (80%); it is associated with brainstem involvement and has a grave prognosis (*central nervous system [CNS]-Behçet's syndrome*). Cerebral brain thrombosis is more common in female patients. IL-6 is persistently raised in cerebrospinal fluid of these patients. Cerebral venous thrombosis is most frequently observed in the superior sagittal and transverse sinuses and is associated with headache and increased intracranial pressure. Magnetic resonance imaging (MRI) and/or proton magnetic resonance spectroscopy (MRS) are very sensitive and should be employed if CNS-Behçet's syndrome is suspected.
- Gastrointestinal involvement is seen more frequently in patients from Japan and consists of mucosal ulcerations of the gut, resembling Crohn's disease.

Ans. D

57. All are findings on histology of IgG4-related disease except:

A. Lymphoplasmacytic infiltrate
B. Granuloma formation
C. Storiform pattern of fibrosis
D. Obliterative phlebitis

Explanation:

- IgG4-related disease is a potential cause of aortitis and periaortitis that is histologically differentiated from Takayasu arteritis by a dense lymphoplasmacytic infiltrate rich in IgG4-positive plasma cells, a storiform pattern of fibrosis, and obliterative phlebitis.

Ans. B

58. Characteristic of polyarteritis nodosa is:

A. Multiple stenosis of medium sized arteries
B. Aneurysm up to 1 cm of involved arteries
C. Isolated stenosis of large artery
D. Isolated aneurysm of large artery

Explanation:

- Vascular lesion in polyarteritis nodosa is a necrotizing inflammation of small- and medium-sized muscular arteries.
- Lesions are segmental and tend to involve bifurcations and branchings of arteries.
- They may spread circumferentially to involve adjacent veins. However, involvement of venules is not seen in polyarteritis nodosa and, if present, suggests microscopic polyangiitis.
- In the acute stages of disease, polymorphonuclear neutrophils infiltrate all layers of vessel wall and perivascular areas, which results in intimal proliferation and degeneration of the vessel wall.
- Mononuclear cells infiltrate area as lesions progress to the subacute and chronic stages.
- Fibrinoid necrosis of vessels ensues with compromise of lumen, thrombosis, infarction of the tissues supplied by the involved vessel, and, in some cases, hemorrhage.
- As the lesions heal, there is collagen deposition, which may lead to further occlusion of the vessel lumen.
- Aneurysmal dilations up to 1 cm in size along the involved arteries are characteristic of polyarteritis nodosa.

- Granulomas and substantial eosinophilia with eosinophilic tissue infiltrations are not characteristically found and suggest eosinophilic granulomatosis with polyangiitis (Churg-Strauss)

Ans. B

59. All combinations are correct except:

A. Hyperextension of the PIP joint with flexion of the DIP joint is swan-neck deformity

B. Flexion of the PIP joint with hyperextension of the DIP joint is boutonnière deformity

C. Subluxation of the first MCP joint with hyperextension of the first interphalangeal (IP) joint is Z-line deformity

D. Inflammation about the radial styloid and tenosynovitis of the extensor carpi radialis may cause subluxation of the distal radius, resulting in a "piano-key movement" of the radial styloid

Explanation:

- Once the disease process of RA is established, the wrists, metacarpophalangeal (MCP), and proximal interphalangeal (PIP) joints stand out as most frequently involved joints
- Distal interphalangeal (DIP) joint involvement may occur in RA, but it usually is a manifestation of coexistent osteoarthritis.
- Flexor tendon tenosynovitis is a frequent hallmark of RA and leads to decreased range of motion, reduced grip strength, and "trigger" fingers.
- Progressive destruction of the joints and soft tissues may lead to chronic, irreversible deformities.
- Ulnar deviation results from subluxation of the MCP joints, with subluxation, or partial dislocation, of the proximal phalanx to the volar side of the hand.
- Hyperextension of the PIP joint with flexion of the DIP joint ("swan-neck deformity"), flexion of the PIP joint with hyperextension of the DIP joint ("boutonnière deformity"), and subluxation of the first MCP joint with hyperextension of the first interphalangeal (IP) joint ("Z-line deformity") also may result from damage to the tendons, joint capsule, and other soft tissues in these small joints.
- Inflammation about the ulnar styloid and tenosynovitis of the extensor carpi ulnaris may cause subluxation of distal ulna, resulting in a "piano-key movement" of ulnar styloid.
- Although metatarsophalangeal (MTP) joint involvement in the feet is an early feature of disease, chronic inflammation of the ankle and midtarsal regions usually comes later and may lead to pes planovalgus ("flat feet").
- Large joints, including the knees and shoulders, are often affected in established disease, although these joints may remain asymptomatic for many years after onset.

Ans. D

60. Cranial nerve involved in Sjögrens syndrome is:

A. 3 B. 4

C. 5 D. 6

Explanation:

- Dry eyes and dry mouth (sicca complex) are common in SSC.
- Biopsy of the minor salivary glands shows fibrosis rather than focal lymphocytic infiltration characteristic of primary Sjögren's syndrome.
- Hypothyroidism resulting from Graves' or Hashimoto's disease is common, particularly in lcSSc, and may be under-recognized.
- Whereas the central nervous system is generally spared, unilateral or bilateral sensory trigeminal neuropathy can occur.
- Erectile dysfunction is a frequent, and occasionally initial, disease manifestation.
- Inability to attain or maintain penile erection is due to vascular insufficiency and fibrosis of corporeal smooth muscle.

- Sexual performance is also adversely affected in women. While fertility is not impaired in SSc, pregnancy is associated with higher risk of adverse fetal outcomes. Furthermore, cardiopulmonary involvement may worsen during pregnancy, and new onset of scleroderma renal crisis has been described.

Ans. C

61. Autoantibodies to Ro/SS-A and La/SS-B antigens in Sjögren's syndrome are associated with all except:

A. Usually present prior to diagnosis
B. Longer disease duration
C. More intense lymphocytic infiltration of major salivary glands
D. Extraglandular (systemic) manifestations

Explanation:

- Sera from patients with Sjögren's syndrome often contain autoantibodies to non-organ-specific antigens such as immunoglobulins (rheumatoid factors) and extractable nuclear and cytoplasmic antigens (Ro/ SS-A, La/SS-B). Ro/SS-A autoantigen consists of two polypeptides (52 and 60 kDa, respectively) in conjunction with cytoplasmic RNAs, whereas the 48-kDa La/SS-B protein is bound to RNA III polymerase transcripts.
- Autoantibodies to Ro/SS-A and La/SS-B antigens are usually present prior to diagnosis and are associated with earlier disease onset, longer disease duration, salivary gland enlargement, extraglandular (systemic) manifestations, and more intense lymphocytic infiltration of minor salivary glands.

Ans. C

62. Most common pulmonary manifestation of SSc is:

A. ILD
B. Pulmonary hypertension
C. Pleural effusion
D. Pleural thickening

Explanation:

- ILD is the most common pulmonary manifestation of SSc. ILD occurs in about 50% of SSc patients with diffuse disease and in about 30% of patients with limited disease.
- Pulmonary hypertension can occur separately or concomitantly with ILD and is more frequent in patients with limited SSc.

Ans. A

63. DD of Sjögren syndrome include all except:

A. HIV
B. SICCA syndrome
C. Sarcoidosis
D. Hypothyroidism

Explanation:

Table: Differential diagnosis of Sjögren's syndrome

HIV Infection and SICCA Syndrome	Sjögren's Syndrome	Sarcoidosis
Predominant in young males	Predominant in middle-aged women	No age or sex preference
Lack of autoantibodies to Ro/SS-A and/ or La/SS-B	Presence of autoantibodies	Lack of autoantibodies to Ro/SS-A and/or La/SS-B
Lymphoid infiltrates of salivary glands by CD8+ T lymphocytes	Lymphoid infiltrates of salivary glands by CD4+ T lymphocytes	Granulomas in salivary glands
Association with HLA-DR5	Association with HLA-DR3 and DRw52	Unknown
Positive serologic tests for HIV	Negative serologic tests for HIV	Negative serologic tests for HIV

Ans. D

64. Nucleolar immunofluorescence pattern may indicate antibodies to all of the below except:

A. U3-RNP (fibrillarin)
B. Th/To
C. PM/Scl
D. RNA polymerase III

Explanation:

- Antinuclear autoantibodies are detected in almost all patients with SSc.
- Anti-topoisomerase I (Scl-70) and anti-centromere antibodies are mutually exclusive and each is highly specific for SSc.
- Topoisomerase I antibodies are associated with increased risk of ILD and poor outcomes.
- Anticentromere antibodies are associated with PAH, but only infrequently with significant cardiac, pulmonary, or renal involvement.
- Nucleolar immunofluorescence pattern may indicate antibodies to U3-RNP (fibrillarin), Th/To, or PM/Scl, whereas speckled immunofluorescence indicates antibodies to RNA polymerase III

Ans. C

65. All are true about hematological manifestations of RA except:

A. A normochromic, normocytic anemia often develops in patients with RA and is the most common hematologic abnormality
B. Platelet counts may also be elevated in RA as an acute-phase reactant
C. Felty's syndrome incidence appears to be declining in the face of more aggressive treatment of the joint disease
D. T cell large granular lymphocyte leukemia (T-LGL) typically occurs in the late stages of severe RA and is more common in whites than other racial groups

Explanation:

- *Felty's syndrome* is defined by the clinical triad of neutropenia, splenomegaly, and nodular RA and is seen in <1% of patients, although its incidence appears to be declining in the face of more aggressive treatment of the joint disease.
- It typically occurs in the late stages of severe RA and is more common in whites than other racial groups.
- T cell large granular lymphocyte leukemia (T-LGL) may have a similar clinical presentation and often occurs in association with RA.
- T-LGL is characterized by a chronic, indolent clonal growth of LGL cells, leading to neutropenia and splenomegaly.
- As opposed to Felty's syndrome, T-LGL may develop early in the course of RA.
- Leukopenia apart from these disorders is uncommon and most often a side effect of drug therapy.

Ans. D

66. Enthesis is seen in all except:

A. Rheumatoid arthritis
B. Ankylosing spondylitis
C. Reactive arthritis
D. Psoriatic arthritis

Explanation:

- Inflammation in the fibrocartilaginous *enthesis*, the region where a tendon, ligament, or joint capsule attaches to bone, is a characteristic lesion in AS and other SpAs, both at axial and peripheral sites.

- Enthesitis is associated with prominent edema of adjacent bone marrow and is often characterized by erosive lesions that eventually undergo ossification.

Ans. A

67. Drugs useful in Scleroderma renal crisis include all except:

A. ACEI
B. ARB
C. Diuretics
D. CCB

Explanation:

- Scleroderma renal crisis is a medical emergency.
- Since the outcome is largely determined by the extent of renal damage at the time that aggressive therapy is initiated, prompt recognition of impending or early scleroderma renal crisis is essential, and efforts should be made to avoid its occurrence.
- High-risk SSc patients with early disease, extensive and progressive skin involvement, tendon friction rubs, and anti-RNA polymerase III antibodies should be instructed to monitor their blood pressure daily and report significant alterations immediately.
- Potentially nephrotoxic drugs should be avoided, and glucocorticoids should be used only when absolutely necessary and at low doses.
- Patients presenting with scleroderma renal crisis should be immediately hospitalized.
- Once other causes of renal diseases are excluded, treatment should be started promptly with titration of short-acting ACE inhibitors, with the goal of achieving rapid normalization of the blood pressure.
- In patients with persistent hypertension, addition of angiotensin II receptor blockers, calcium channel blockers, endothelin-1 receptor blockers, prostacyclins, and direct renin inhibitors should be considered.
- Up to two thirds of patients with scleroderma renal crisis will require dialysis.
- Substantial renal recovery can occur, and dialysis can be discontinued in 30–50% of the patients.
- Kidney transplantation is appropriate for patients unable to discontinue dialysis after 2 years.
- Survival of transplanted SSc patients is comparable to that of other diseases, and recurrence of renal crisis is rare.

Ans. C

68. Caplan syndrome is associated with:

A. Seropositive rheumatoid arthritis
B. Seronegative rheumatoid arthritis
C. Seropositve SLE
D. Seronegative SLE

Explanation:

- *Caplan syndrome* first described in coal miners but subsequently in patients with silicosis, is the combination of pneumoconiotic nodules and seropositive rheumatoid arthritis.
- Silica is often present in anthracitic coal dust and its presence may contribute to risk of PMF.

Ans. A

69. All are HLA B27 positive spondyloarthropathies except:

A. Juvenile arthritis pauciarticular
B. Reactive arthritis
C. Acute anterior uveitis
D. Psoriatric spondylitis

Explanation:

	Marker	Gene
Spondyloarthropathies		
Ankylosing spondylitis	B27	*B*27:02,–04, –05*
Reactive arthritis (Reiter's)	B27	
Acute anterior uveitis	B27	
Reactive arthritis *(Yersinia, Salmonella, Shigella, Chlamydia)*	B27	
Psoriatic spondylitis	B27	
Collagen Vascular Disease		
Juvenile arthritis, pauciarticular	DR8	
	DR5	
Rheumatoid arthritis	DR4	*DRB1*04:01, –04, –05*
Sjögren's syndrome	DR3	
Systemic lupus erythematosus		
White	DR3	
Japanese	DR2	
Autoimmune Gut and Skin		
Gluten-sensitive enteropathy (celiac disease)	DQ2	*DQA1 *05:01*
Chronic active hepatitis	DR3	*DQB1 *02:01*
Dermatitis herpetiformis	DR3	
Psoriasis vulgaris	Cw6	
Pemphigus vulgaris	DR4	*DRB1 *04:02*
	DQ1	*DQB1 *05:03*
Bullous pemphigoid variant	DQ7	*DQB1 *03:01*

Ans. A

70. Extra-articular manifestations in RA patients include all except:

A. Develop during clinical course of RA upto 40% of patients

B. Less common in patients who have history of cigarette smoking

C. Tests +ve for serum RF or anti CCP antibodies

D. Subcuatenous nodules, secondary sjögrens syndrome, interstitial disease, pulmonary nodules & anemia are most frequent

Explanation:

- Extra-articular manifestations may develop during the clinical course of RA in up to 40% of patients, even prior to the onset of arthritis.
- Patients most likely to develop extra-articular disease have a history of cigarette smoking, have early onset of significant physical disability, and test positive for serum RF or anti-CCP antibodies.
- Subcutaneous nodules, secondary Sjögren's syndrome, interstitial lung disease (ILD), pulmonary nodules, and anemia are among the most frequently observed extra-articular manifestations.
- Recent studies have shown a decrease in the incidence and severity of at least some extra-articular manifestations, particularly Felty's syndrome and vasculitis.

Ans. B

71. Which clinical manifestation is not used for diagnosis of SLE?

A. Oral or nasal ulcers

B. Non scarring alopecia

C. Synovitis involving >1 joint

D. Hemolytic anemia

Explanation:

Table: Systemic lupus international collaborating clinic criteria for classification of systemic lupus erythematosus	
Clinical Manifestations	**Immunologic Manifestations**
Skin • Acute, subacute cutaneous • LE (Photosensitive, malar, maculopapular, bullous) • Chronic cutaneous LE (discoid lupus, panniculitis, lichen planus-like, hypertrophic verrucous, chilblains) Oral or nasal ulcers Nonscarring alopecia Synovitis involving ≥ 2 joints Serositis (pleurisy, pericarditis)	ANA > reference negative value Anti-dsDNA > reference, if by ELISA 2x reference Anti-Sm Antiphospholipid (any of lupus anticoagulant, false-positive RPR, anti-cardiolipin, anti-β glycoprotein I Low serum complement (C3, C4 or CH50) Positive direct Coombs test in absence of hemolytic anemia
Renal • Prot/Cr ≥ 0.5 • RBC casts • Biopsy[a] Neurologic • Seizures, psychosis, mononeuritis, myelitis, peripheral or cranial neuropathies, acute confusional state Hemolytic anemia Leukopenia (< 4000/μl) or Lymphopenia (< 1000/Symboll) Thrombocytopenia (< 100,000/μl)	

Ans. C

72. In classification criteria for diagnosis of systemic sclerosis which feature carry 4 points?

A. Sclerodactyly
B. Mucocutaneous telangiectasia
C. Abnormal nails capillary pattern
D. PAH

Explanation:

Table: Classification criteria for diagnosis of systemic sclerosis		
Item	**Sub-Item**	**Weight/Score**
Skin thickening (bilateral)–fingers extending proximal to MCP joints		9
Skin thickening of fingers only	Puffy fingers Sclerodactyly (skin thickened distal to MCP joints)	2 4
Fingertip lesions	Digital tip ulcer or Pitting scar	2 3
Mucocutaneous telangiectasia		2
Abnormal nails capillary pattern		2
Lung involvement	PAH Interstitial lung disease	2 2
Raynaud's phenomenon		3
SSc-specific autoantibodies	ACA Scl-70 RNA polymerase III	3

Ans. A

73. Not a immunological manifestations in SLE for diagnosis is:

A. Anti Sm

B. Antiphospholipid

C. Low serum complement

D. Positive direct coombs test with hemolytic anemia

Explanation:

Table: Systemic lupus international collaborating clinic criteria for classification of systemic lupus erythematosus

Clinical Manifestations	Immunologic Manifestations
Skin • Acute, subacute cutaneous • LE (Photosensitive, malar, maculopapular, bullous) • Chronic cutaneous LE (discoid lupus, panniculitis, lichen planus-like, hypertrophic verrucous, chilblains) Oral or nasal ulcers Nonscarring alopecia Synovitis involving ≥ 2 joints Serositis (pleurisy, pericarditis) Renal • Prot/Cr ≥ 0.5 • RBC casts • Biopsy[a]	ANA > reference negative value Anti-dsDNA > reference, if by ELISA 2x reference Anti-Sm Antiphospholipid (any of lupus anticoagulant, false-positive RPR, anti-cardiolipin, anti-β glycoprotein I Low serum complement (C3, C4 or CH50) Positive direct Coombs test in absence of hemolytic anemia
Neurologic • Seizures, psychosis, mononeuritis, myelitis, peripheral or cranial neuropathies, acute confusional state Hemolytic anemia Leukopenia (< 4000/μl) or Lymphopenia (< 1000/μl) Thrombocytopenia (< 100,000/μl)	

Ans. D

74. Rhupus is likely is used for:

A. Fulfill criteria for both RA & SLE

B. Fulfill criteria for both RA & Polymyositis

C. Fulfill criteria for both APLA & SLE

D. Fulfill criteria for both MCTD

Explanation:

- Most people with SLE have intermittent polyarthritis, varying from mild to disabling, characterized by soft tissue swelling and tenderness in joints and/or tendons, most commonly in hands, wrists, and knees.
- Joint deformities (hands and feet) develop in only 10%.
- Erosions on joint X-rays are rare but can be identified by ultrasound in 10–50% of patients. Some individuals have rheumatoid-like arthritis with erosions and fulfill criteria for both RA and SLE ("rhupus").

Ans. A

75. Most common extra articular manifestation of ankylosing spondylitis is:

A. Acute anterior uveitis (U/L)
B. Acute anterior uveitis (B/L)
C. Aortic regurgitation
D. IBD

Explanation:

- Most common extra-articular manifestation is acute anterior uveitis, which occurs in up to 40% of patients and can antedate spondylitis.
- Attacks are typically unilateral, causing pain, photophobia, and increased lacrimation.
- These tend to recur, often in the opposite eye.
- Cataracts and secondary glaucoma may ensue. Up to 60% of patients with AS have inflammation in the colon or ileum.
- This is usually asymptomatic, but frank IBD occurs in 5–10% of patients with AS.

Ans. A

76. All autoantigen autoimmune disease combination correct except:

A. Amphiphysin in Neuropathy, small-cell lung cancer
B. Cyclin B1 in Hepatocellular carcinoma
C. DNA topoisomerase II in Paraneoplastic stiff-person syndrome
D. Desmoplakin in Paraneoplastic pemphigus

Explanation:

Autoantigen	Autoimmune Diseases
Aminoacyl-tRNA synthetase (several)	Polymyositis, dermatomyositis
Cardiolipin	Systemic lupus erythematosus, antiphospholipid syndrome
Carbonic anhydrase II	Systemic lupus erythematosus, Sjögren's syndrome, systemic sclerosis
Collagen (multiple types)	Rheumatoid arthritis, systemic lupus erythematosus, progressive systemic sclerosis
Centromere-associated proteins	Systemic sclerosis
DNA-dependent nucleoside-stimulated ATPase	Dermatomyositis
Fibrillarin	Scleroderma
Fibronectin	Systemic lupus erythematosus, rheumatoid arthritis, morphea
Glucose-6-phosphate isomerase	Rheumatoid arthritis
β2-Glycoprotein 1 (B2-GPI)	Primary antiphospholipid syndrome
Golgin (95, 97, 160, 180) Heat shock protein	Sjögren's syndrome, systemic lupus erythematosus, rheumatoid arthritis, Various immune-related disorders
Hemidesmosomal protein 180	Bullous pemphigoid, herpes gestationis, cicatricial pemphigoid
Histone H2A-H2B-DNA	Systemic lupus erythematosus
IgE receptor	Chronic idiopathic urticaria
Keratin	Rheumatoid arthritis

Contd.

Contd.

Ku-DNA-protein kinase	Systemic lupus erythematosus
Ku-nucleoprotein La phosphoprotein (La 55-B)	Connective tissue syndrome, Sjögren's sydrome
Myeloperoxidase	Necrotizing and crescentic glomerulonephritis (NCGN), systemic vasculitis
Proteinase 3 (PR3)	Granulomatosis with polyangiitis (Wegener's), Churg-Struss syndrome
RNA polymerase I-III (RNP)	Systemic sclerosis, systemic lupus erythematosus
Signal recognition protein (SRP54)	Polymyositis
Topoisomerase-1 (Scl-70)	Scleroderma, Raynaud's syndrome
Tublin	Chronic liver disease, visceral leishmaniasis
Vimentin	Systemic autoimmune disease

Ans. C

77. Causes of polyarticular a rthritis include all except:

A. Neisseria meningitides
B. Serum sickness
C. Osteoarthritis
D. HIV

Explanation:

Table: Differential diagnosis of arthritis syndromes

Acute Monarticular Arthritis	Chronic Monarticular Arthritis	Polyarticular Arthritis
Staphylococcus aureus	*Mycobacterium tuberculosis*	*Neisseria meningitidis*
Streptococcus pneumoniae	Nontuberculous mycobacteria	*N. gonorrhoeae*
β–Hemolytic streptococci	*Borrelia burgdorferi*	Nongonococcal bacterial arthritis
Gram-negative bacilli	*Treponema pallidum*	Bacterial endocarditis
Neisseria gonorrhoeae	*Candida spp.*	Candida spp.
Candida spp.	*Sporothrix schenckii*	Poncet's disease (tuberculous rheumatism)
Crystal-induced arthritis	*Coccidioides immitis*	Hepatitis B virus
Fracture	*Blastomyces dermatitidis*	Parvovirus B_{19}
Hemarthrosis	*Aspergilus spp.*	HIV
Foreign body	*Cryptococcus neoformans*	Human T-lymphotrophic virus type 1
Osteoarthritis	*Nocardia spp.*	Rubella virus
Ischemic necrosis	*Brucella spp.*	Arthropod-borne viruses
Monarticuar rheumatoid arthritis	Legg-Calvé-Perthes disease	Sickle cell disease flare
	Osteoarthritis	Reactive arthritis
		Serum sickness
		Acute rheumatic fever
		Inflammatory bowel disease
		Systemic lupus erythematosus
		Rheumatoid arthritis/Still's disease
		Other vasculitides
		Sarcoidosis

Ans. C

78. All are true about extraglandular (systemic) manifestations in Sjögren's syndrome except:

A. Extraglandular (systemic) manifestations are seen in one-third of patients with Sjögren's syndrome

B. Extraglandular (systemic) manifestations are very rare in patients whose Sjögren's syndrome is associated with rheumatoid arthritis

C. Arthritis in patients with primary Sjögren's syndrome is erosive

D. Myelitis associated with antibody to aquaporin 4 have been described

Explanation:

Table: Prevalence of extraglandular manifestations in primary Sjögren's syndrome

Clinical Manifestation	Percent	Remarks
Non-Specific		
Fatigability/Myalgias	25	Fibromyalgia
Arthralgias/Arthritis	60	Usually non-erosive, leading to Jaccoud's arthropathy
Raynaud's phenomenon	37	In one-third of patients, precedes sicca manifestations
Peri-Epithelial		
Lung involvement	14	Small airway disease/lymphocyte interstitial pneumonitis
Kidney involvement	9	Interstitial kidney disease is usually asymptomatic
Liver involvement	6	Primary biliary cirrhosis stage
Immune-Complex Mediated		
Small vessel vasculitis		Purpura, urticarial lesions
Peripheral neuropathy	2	Polyneuropathy, either sensory or sensorimotor
Glomerulonephritis		Membranoproliferative
Lymphoma		
Lymphoma	6	Glandular MALT[a] lymphoma is most common

Ans. C

79. Cardiac manifestation of polyarteritis nodosa are all except:

A. Myocarditis

B. Pericarditis

C. Myocardial infarction

D. Congestive heart failure

Explanation:

Table: Clinical manifestations related to organ system involvement in polyarteritis nodosa

Organ System	Percent Incidence	Clinical Manifestations
Renal	60	Renal failure, hypertension
Musculoskeletal	64	Arthritis, arthralgia, myalgia
Peripheral nervous system	51	Peripheral neuropathy, mononeuritis multiplex
Gastrointestinal tract	44	Abdominal pain, nausea and vomiting, bleeding, bowel infarction and perforation, cholecystitis, hepatic infarction, pancreatic infarction
Skin	43	Rash, purpura, nodules, cutaneous infarcts, livedo reticularis, Raynaud's phenomenon
Cardiac	36	Congestive heart failure, myocardial infarction, pericarditis
Genitourinary	25	Testicular, ovarian, or epididymal pain
Central nervous system	23	Cerebral vascular accident, altered mental status, seizure

Ans. A

80. Regarding RA all are correct except:

A. Subcutaneous nodules occur more commonly in those with low level of disease activity

B. Secondary sjögren syndrome seen in approximately 10%

C. Presence of ILD confers poor prognosis

D. ILD secondary to RA has good prognosis than Idiopathic ILD

Explanation:

- Subcutaneous nodules have been reported to occur in 30–40% of patients and more commonly in those with the highest levels of disease activity, the disease-related shared epitope (SE), a positive test for serum RF, and radiographic evidence of joint erosions.
- However, more recent cohort studies suggest a declining prevalence of subcutaneous nodules, perhaps, related to early and more aggressive disease-modifying therapy.
- When palpated, the nodules are generally firm; non tender; and adherent to periosteum, tendons, or bursae; developing in areas of the skeleton subject to repeated trauma or irritation such as the forearm, sacral prominences, and Achilles tendon.
- They may also occur in the lungs, pleura, pericardium, and peritoneum. Nodules are typically benign, although they can be associated with infection, ulceration and gangrene.

Ans. A

81. Which antibody high titres are SLE specific & in some patients correlate with disease activity?

A. ANA

B. Anti Sm

C. Anti ds DNA

D. Anti histone

Explanation:

Table: Autoantibodies in systemic lupus erythematosus (SLE)

Antibody	Prevalence, %	Antigen Recognised	Clinical Utility
Antinuclear antibodies	98	Multiple nuclear	Best screening test; repeated negative tests by immunofluorescence make SLE unlikely
Anti-dsDNA	70	DNA (double-stranded)	High titers are SLE-specific and in some patients correlate with disease activity, nephritis, vasculitis. Crithidia immunofluorescence is more specific for SLE than ELISA methods
Anti-Sm	25	Protein complexed to 6 species of nuclear U1 RNA	Specific for SLE; no definite clinical correlations; most patients also have anti-RNP; more common in blacks and Asians than whites
Anti-RNP	40	Protein complexed to U1 RNA	Not specific for SLE; high titers associated with syndromes that have overlap features of several rheumatic syndromes including SLE; more common in blacks than whites; correlates with high IFN-induced gene signature
Anti-Ro (SS-A)	30	Protein complexed to hY RNA, primarily 60 kDa and 52 kDa	Not specific for SLE; associated with sicca syndrome, predisposes to subacute cutaneous lupus, and to neonatal lupus with congenital heart block; associated with decreased risk for nephritis
Anti-La (SS-B)	10	47-kDa protein complexed to hY RNA	Usually associated with anti-Ro; associated with decreased risk for nephritis

Contd.

Contd.

Antithistone	70	Histones associated with DNA (in nucleosome, chromatin)	More frequent in drug-induced lupus than in SLE
Antiphospholipid	50	Phospholipids, β_2 glycoprotein 1 (β_2 G1) confactor, prothrombin	Three tests available–ELISAs for cardiolipin and β_2G1, sensitive prothrombin time (DRVVT) for lupus anticoagulant; predisposes to clotting, fetal loss, thrombocytopenia
Antierythrocyte	60	Erythrocyte membrane	Measured as direct Coombs test; a small proportion develops overt hemolysis
Antiplatelet	30	Surface and altered cytoplasmic antigens on platelets	Associated with thrombocytopenia, but sensitivity and specificity are not good; this is not a useful clinical test
Antineuronal (includes antiglutamate receptor 2)	60	Neuronal and lymphocyte surface antigens	In some series, a positive test in CSF correlates with active CNS lupus
Antiribosomal P	20	Protein in ribosomes	In some series, a positive test in serum correlates with depression or psychosis due to CNS lupus

Ans. C

82. Inflammatory myopathy having predilection for finger/wrist flexors & knee extensors is:

A. Dermatomyosistis

B. Polymyositis

C. IBM

D. Necrotizing myopathy

Explanation:

Table: Inflammatory myopathies: Clinical and laboratory features

Disorder	Sex	Age of Onset	Rash	Pattern of Weakness	Laboratory Features	Muscle Biopsy	Cellular Infiltrate	Response to IS Therapy	Common Associated Conditions
DM	F > M	Childhood and Adult	Yes	Proximal > distal	Normal or increased CK (up to 50 × normal or higher); Various MSAs (anti-MDA5, anti-TIF1, anti-Mi-2, anti-NXP2)	Perimysial and Perivascular Inflammation; IFN-1 regulated proteins (MHC-1, MxA), MAC deposition on capillaries	CD4+ Dendritic cells; B cells; macrophages	Yes	Myocarditis, ILD, Malignancy, Vasculitis, Other CTDs
PM	F > M	Adult	No	Proximal > distal	Increased CK (up to 50 × normal or higher)	Endomysial and perivascular inflammation; ubiquitous expression of MHC-1	CD8+ T-cells; Macrophages; plasma cells	Yes	Myocarditis, ILD, Other CTDs
NM	M = F	Children and adults	No	Proximal > distal	Elevated CK (> 10 × normal or higher); anti-HMGCR or anti-SRP antibodies	Necrotic muscle fibers; minimal inflammatory infiltrate	Macrophages in necrotic fibers undergoing phagocytosis	Yes	Malignancy, CTD, HMGCR antibody cases can be triggered by statin use

Contd.

Contd.

ASS	F > M	Children and adults	Some-times	Proximal > distal	Elevated CK (> 10 × normal or higher); antisynthetase antibodies	Perimysial and Perivascular Inflammation; perimysial fragmentation with alkaline phosphatase staining; perimysial muscle damage with necrosis	CD4+ Dendritic cells; B cells; macrophages	Yes	Non-erosive arthritis, ILD, Raynaud phenomenon, mechanic hands and fever
IBM	M > F	Older adults (> 50 years)	No	Proximal and distal; predilection for: finger/ wrist flexors, knee extensors	Normal or mildly increased CK (usually < 10 × normal); anti-cN-1A antibodies; large granular lymphocytes on flow cytometry and reduced CD4/ CD8 ratio with increased CD8 count	Endomysial and perivascular inflammation; ubiquitous expression of MHC-1; Rimmed Vacuoles; p62, LC3, TDP-43 aggregates; EM: 15-18 nm tubulofilaments; ragged red and COX negative fibers	CD8+ T cells; Macrophages; plasma cells; myeloid dendritic cells; large granular lymphocytes	None of Minimal	Granular lymphocytic leukemia/ lymphocytosis, sarcoidosis, SICCA or Sjögren syndrome

Ans. C

83. Preferred method of characterizing chest involvement in sarcoidosis is:

A. CECT
B. HRCT
C. Chest X-ray
D. MRI

Explanation:

- Lung involvement occurs in >90% of sarcoidosis patients. The most commonly used method for detecting lung disease is still the chest roentgenogram. Chest roentgenogram from a sarcoidosis patient shows bilateral hilar adenopathy.
- Although the computed tomography (CT) scan has changed the diagnostic approach to interstitial lung disease, the CT scan is not usually considered a monitoring tool for patients with sarcoidosis.
- Characteristic CT features, including peribronchial thickening and reticular nodular changes, which are predominantly subpleural.
- Peribronchial thickening seen on CT scan seems to explain the high yield of granulomas from bronchial biopsies performed for diagnosis.

Ans. C

84. Not true about Scleroderma is:

A. Describes group of localized skin disorders
B. Occurs more commonly in children than adults
C. Generally not complicated by Raynauds phenomenon
D. Significant internal organ involvement

Explanation:

- Term *scleroderma* describes a group of localized skin disorders. These occur more commonly in children than in adults, and in marked contrast to SSc, are generally not complicated by Raynaud's phenomenon or significant internal organ involvement.

- Morphea presents as solitary or multiple circular patches of thick skin or, rarely, as widespread induration (generalized or pansclerotic morphea); the fingers are generally spared. Linear scleroderma may affect subcutaneous tissues, leading to fibrosis and atrophy of supporting structures, tendons, muscle, and even bone. In children, the growth of affected long bones can be retarded. When linear scleroderma crosses large joints, significant contractures can develop.

Ans. D

85. Which of the following target enzyme produces p-ANCS associated vasculitis?

A. Myeloperoxidase
B. Cathepsin G
C. Lysozyme
D. Lactoferrin

Explanation:

- Terminology of *cytoplasmic ANCA* (cANCA) refers to the diffuse, granular cytoplasmic staining pattern observed by immunofluorescence microscopy when serum antibodies bind to indicator neutrophils.
- Proteinase-3, a 29-kDa neutral serine proteinase present in neutrophil azurophilic granules, is the major cANCA antigen.
- More than 90% of patients with typical active granulomatosis with polyangiitis (Wegener's) have detectable antibodies to proteinase-3.
- Terminology of *perinuclear ANCA* (pANCA) refers to the more localized perinuclear or nuclear staining pattern of the indicator neutrophils.
- Major target for pANCA is the enzyme myeloperoxidase; other targets that can produce a pANCA pattern of staining include elastase, cathepsin G, lactoferrin, lysozyme, and bactericidal/permeability-increasing protein.
- However, only antibodies to myeloperoxidase have been convincingly associated with vasculitis.

Ans. A

86. Antibody rarely associated against scleroderma renal crisis is:

A. DNA Topoisomerase 1
B. Centromere proteins
C. RNA Polymerase III
D. U3-RNP

Explanation:

Table: Major systemic sclerosis-specific autoantibodies and principal associated features

Target Antigen	SSc Subset	Prominent Characteristic Clinical Association
DNA Topoisomerase I (Scl-70) Speckled pattern	dcSSc	Tendon friction rubs, digital ischemic ulcers, scleroderma, extensive skin involvement, early ILD, cardiac involvement, scleroderma renal crisis
Centromere proteins Discreet speckled (centromere) pattern	lcSSc	Digital ischemic ulcers, calcinosis cutis, isolated PAH; renal crisis rare
RNA polymerase III Speckled pattern	dcSSc	Rapidly progressive skin, tendon friction rubs, joint contractures, GAVE, renal crisis, contemporaneous cancers; digital ulcers rare
U3-RNP (fibrillarin) Nucleolar pattern	dc/lcSSc	PAH, ILD, scleroderma renal crisis, GI tract involvement, myositis
Bacteria m/r_o Nucleolar pattern	lcSSc	ILD, PAH

Contd.

Contd.

PM/Scl Nucleolar pattern	lcSSc	Calcinosis cutis, ILD, myositis overlap
Ku Speckled pattern	Overlap	SLE, myositis overlap
U1-RNP Speckled pattern	MCTD	PAH, inflammatory arthritis, myositis overlap
U11/U12 RNP Speckled pattern	dc/lcSSc	ILD

Ans. B

87. All are true about reactive arthritis except:

A. First manifestation of HIV infection

B. HLA B27 significantly prolongs intracellular survival of Yersinia enterocolitica & Salmonella enteritidis in human

C. Upper extremities 1st involved

D. Arthritis typically persists for 3-5 months

Explanation:

- Clinical manifestations of ReA range from an isolated, transient monoarthritis or enthesitis to severe multisystem disease. A careful history will often elicit evidence of an antecedent infection 1–4 weeks before onset of symptoms of the reactive disease, particularly in postenteric ReA.
- However, in a sizable minority, no clinical or laboratory evidence of an antecedent infection can be found, particularly in case of postchlamydial ReA.
- In cases of presumed venereally acquired reactive disease, there is often a history of a recent new sexual partner, even without laboratory evidence of infection.
- Constitutional symptoms are common, including fatigue, malaise, fever, and weight loss. The musculoskeletal symptoms are usually acute in onset. Arthritis is usually asymmetric and additive, with involvement of new joints occurring over a few days to 1–2 weeks.
- Joints of the lower extremities, especially the knee, ankle, subtalar, metatarsophalangeal, and toe interphalangeal joints, are most commonly involved, but the wrist and fingers may be involved.
- Arthritis is usually quite painful, and tense joint effusions are not uncommon, especially in the knee. Dactylitis, or "sausage digit," a diffuse swelling of a solitary finger or toe, is a distinctive feature of ReA and other peripheral spondyloarthritides but can be seen in polyarticular gout and sarcoidosis.
- Tendinitis and fasciitis are particularly characteristic lesions, producing pain at multiple insertion sites (entheses), especially Achilles insertion, the plantar fascia, and sites along the axial skeleton.
- Back and buttock pain are quite common and may be caused by insertional inflammation, muscle spasm, acute sacroiliitis, or, presumably, arthritis in intervertebral joints.

Ans. C

88. True about cryoglobulinemic vasculitis is:

A. ANA almost always found

B. Hypercomplementemia occurs in 90% of patients

C. RF almost always found

D. Elevated ESR & Anemia occurs rarely

Explanation:

- Presence of circulating cryoprecipitates is the fundamental finding in cryoglobulinemic vasculitis.
- Rheumatoid factor is almost always found and may be a useful clue to the disease when cryoglobulins are not detected.
- Hypocomplementemia occurs in 90% of patients. An elevated ESR and anemia occur frequently. Evidence for hepatitis C infection must be sought in all patients by testing for hepatitis C antibodies and hepatitis C RNA.

Ans. C

89. Antibody found against which collagen type in Relapsing polychondritis?

A. Type 1

B. Type 2

C. Type 3

D. Type 4

Explanation:

- Immunoglobulin and complement deposits are found at sites of inflammation. In addition, antibodies to type II collagen and to matrilin-1 and immune complexes are detected in the sera of some patients.
- Possibility that an immune response to type II collagen may be important in the pathogenesis is supported experimentally by the occurrence of auricular chondritis in rats immunized with type II collagen.
- Antibodies to type II collagen are found in the sera of these animals, and immune deposits are detected at sites of ear inflammation.
- Humoral immune responses to type IX and type XI collagen, matrilin-1, and cartilage oligomeric matrix protein have been demonstrated in some patients. In a study, rats immunized with matrilin-1 were found to develop severe inspiratory stridor and swelling of nasal septum.
- Rats had severe inflammation with erosions of involved cartilage, which was characterized by increased numbers of CD4+ and CD8+ T cells in the lesions.
- Cartilage of the joints and ear pinna was not involved. All had IgG antibodies to matrilin-1.
- Matrilin-1 is a noncollagenous protein present in the extracellular matrix in cartilage. It is present in high concentrations in the trachea and is also present in the nasal septum but not in articular cartilage.
- A subsequent study demonstrated serum anti-matrilin-1 antibodies in ~13% of patients with relapsing polychondritis; ~70% of these patients had respiratory symptoms. Cell-mediated immunity may also be operative in causing tissue injury, since lymphocyte transformation can be demonstrated when lymphocytes of patients are exposed to cartilage extracts.
- T cells specific for type II collagen have been found in some patients, and CD4+ T cells have been observed at sites of cartilage inflammation.

Ans. B

90. Which of the following is not a single organ vasculitis?

A. Cutaneous leukocytoclastic angitis

B. Cutaneous arteritis

C. IgA Vasculitis

D. Primary CNS Vasculitis

Explanation:

Table: Vasculitis syndromes

Primary Vasculitis Syndromes	Secondary Vasculitis Syndromes
Granulomatosis with polyangiitis (Wegener's) Microscopic polyangiitis Eosinophilic granulomatosis with polyangiitis (Churg-Strauss) IgA vasculitis (Henoch-Schönlein) Cryoglobulinemic vasculitis Polyarteritis nodosa Kawasaki disease Giant cell arteritis Takayasu arteritis Behçet's disease Cogan's syndrome Single-organ vasculitis • Cutaneous leukocytoclastic angiitis • Cutaneous arteritis • Primary central nervous system vasculitis • Isolated aortitis	Vasculitis associated with probable etiology • Drug-induced vasculitis • Hepatitis C virus-associated cryoglobulinemic vasculitis • Hepatitis B virus-associated vasculitis • Cancer-associated vasculitis Vasculitis associated with systemic disease • Lupus vasculitis • Rheumatoid vasculitis • Sarcoid vasculitis

Ans. C

91. Not true about epidemiology of systemic sclerosis is:

A. Strong female predominance
B. Most pronounced in child bearing years
C. Increase after menopause
D. Less common in blacks

Explanation:

- SSc shows a strong female predominance (4.6:1), which is most pronounced in the childbearing years and declines after menopause. An additional risk factor is having an affected first-degree family member, which increases disease risk 13-fold. Although SSc can present at any age, the peak age of onset in women with both lcSSc and dcSSc is 65–74 years, although in blacks, disease onset occurs at an earlier age. Furthermore, blacks with SSc are more likely to have dcSSc, ILD, and a worse prognosis.

Ans. C

92. Risk factor for chronic disease in sarcoidosis include all except:

A. Bone cyst
B. Fibrosis on X-ray
C. 7th Nerve palsy
D. Renal calculi

Explanation:

- For the majority of patients, initial presentation occurs during granulomatous phase of the disease. It is clear that many patients resolve their disease within 2–5 years. These patients are felt to have acute, self-limiting sarcoidosis. However, there is a form of the disease that does not resolve within the first 2–5 years. These chronic patients can be identified at presentation by certain risk factors at presentation such as fibrosis on chest roentgenogram, presence of lupus pernio, bone cysts, cardiac or neurologic disease (except isolated seventh nerve paralysis), and presence of renal calculi due to hypercalciuria. In several studies, patients who required glucocorticoids for any manifestation of their disease in the first 6 months of presentation had a >50% chance of having chronic disease. In contrast, <10% of patients who require no systemic therapy in the first 6 months required chronic therapy.

Ans. C

93. For treatment of sarcoidosis which of the following is correct?

A. Steroid is drug of choice

B. Dosage of glucocorticoids is usually higher for neurosarcoidosis & cutaneous disease

C. Minocyclin steroid sparing agent

D. HCQ is less effective for skin than pulmonary disease

Explanation:

- For acute disease, no therapy remain stable option for patients with nor mild symptoms.
- For symptoms confined to only one organ, topical therapy is preferable.
- For multi-organ disease or disease too extensive for topical therapy, an approach to systemic therapy is outlined. Glucocorticoids remain the drugs of choice for this disease.
- However, the decision to continue to treat with glucocorticoids or to add steroid-sparing agents depends on the tolerability, duration, and dosage of glucocorticoids.
- According to available trials, evidence-based recommendations are made. Most of these recommendations are for pulmonary disease because most of trials were performed only in pulmonary disease.
- Treatment recommendations for extrapulmonary disease are usually similar with a few modifications. For example, the dosage of glucocorticoids is usually higher for neurosarcoidosis and lower for cutaneous disease.
- There was some suggestion that higher doses would be beneficial for cardiac sarcoidosis, but one study found that initial prednisone doses >40 mg/d were associated with a worse outcome because of toxicity.

Ans. A

94. True about lab investigation of scleroderma is:

A. ANA detected in almost all patients SSc

B. Topoisomerase 1 antibodies are not associated with increased risk of ILD & Poor outcomes

C. Nucleolar immunofluorescence pattern may indicate antibodies to RNA Polymerase III

D. Speckled immunoflourescence indicates antibodies to U3-RNP

Explanation:

- Antinuclear autoantibodies are detected in almost all patients with SSc.
- Anti-topoisomerase I (Scl-70) and anti-centromere antibodies are mutually exclusive and each is highly specific for SSc.
- Topoisomerase I antibodies are associated with increased risk of ILD and poor outcomes.
- Anticentromere antibodies are associated with PAH, but only infrequently with significant cardiac, pulmonary, or renal involvement. Nucleolar immunofluorescence pattern may indicate antibodies to U3-RNP (fibrillarin),
- Th/To, or PM/Scl, whereas speckled immunofluorescence indicates antibodies to RNA polymerase III.

Ans. A

95. Features highly consistent with sarcoidosis include all except:

A. Serum ACE Level >2 times upper limit normal

B. BAL Lymphocytes >2 times upper limit normal

C. 7th nerve palsy

D. Panda sign on gallium scan

Explanation:

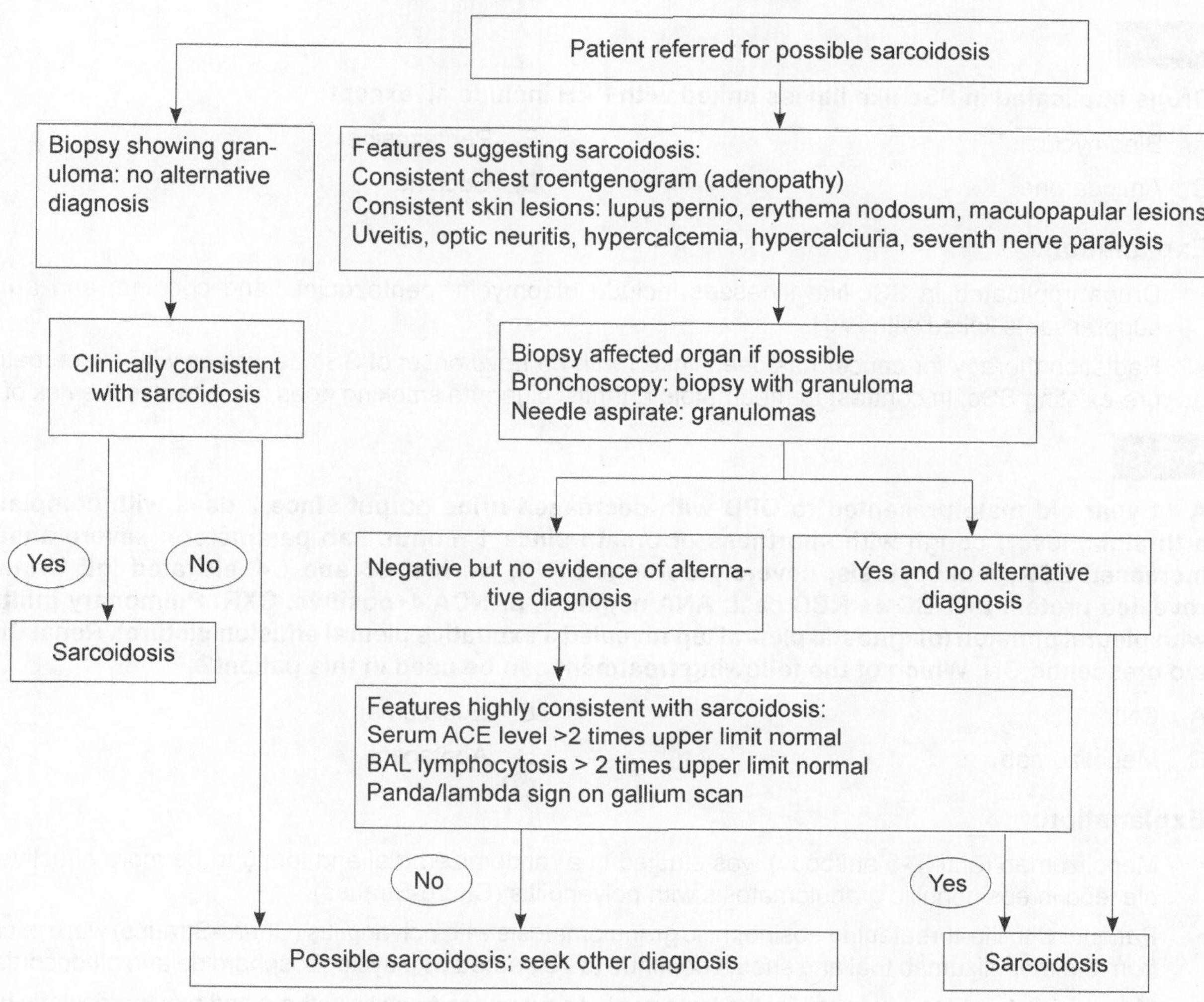

Ans. C

96. Drug having role in Ankylosing spondylitis:

A. Sulfasalazine
B. Methotrexate
C. Gold
D. Steroid

Explanation:

- Sulfasalazine, in doses of 2–3 g/d, has modest benefit, primarily for peripheral arthritis. Methotrexate, although widely used, has not been shown to be of benefit in AS, nor has any therapeutic role for gold or oral glucocorticoids been documented. Potential benefit in AS has been reported for thalidomide, 200 mg/d, perhaps acting through inhibition of TNF-α. The oral Jak inhibitor, tofacitinib, showed efficacy in AS, with reduction of inflammation evident on MRI, in a 16 week phase 2 study
- Most common indication for surgery in patients with AS is severe hip joint arthritis, the pain and stiffness of which are usually dramatically relieved by total hip arthroplasty. Rare patients may benefit from surgical correction of extreme flexion deformities of the spine or of atlantoaxial subluxation.
- Attacks of uveitis are usually managed effectively with local glucocorticoids and mydriatic agents, although systemic glucocorticoids, immunosuppressive drugs, or anti-TNF therapy may be required. TNF inhibitors reduce the frequency of attacks of uveitis in patients with ax-SpA, and adalimumab has recently been

approved by the FDA for treating uveitis. Cases of new or recurrent uveitis after use of a TNF inhibitor have been observed, especially with etanercept. Anti-IL-17 does not appear as effective for uveitis as anti-TNF therapy.

Ans. A

97. Drugs implicated in SSc like illness linked with PAH include all except:

A. Bleomycin
B. Pentazosine
C. Amiodarone
D. Cocaine

Explanation:

- Drugs implicated in SSc-like illnesses include bleomycin, pentazocine, and cocaine, and appetite suppressants linked with PAH.
- Radiation therapy for cancer has been linked with *de novo* onset of SSc as well as with exacerbation of pre-existing SSc. In contrast to rheumatoid arthritis, cigarette smoking does not increase the risk of SSc.

Ans. C

98. A 44 year old male presented to OPD with decreased urine output since 2 days with complaint of arthralgia, fever; cough with shortness of breath since 1 month. Lab parameters: severe anaemia; increased ESR; leukocytosis; severely deranged RFT; Normal C3 and C4, elevated IgE Urinalysis revealed protein 2+ RBC 4+ RBC cast; ANA negative, pANCA 4+positive. CXR: Pulmonary infiltrates with pleural effusion (diagnostic pleural tap revealed a exudative pleural effusion picture). Renal Biopsy s/o crescentic GN. Which of the following treatment can be used in this patient?

A. CNI
B. Eculizumab
C. Mepolizumab
D. Abatacept

Explanation:

- Mepolizumab (anti-IL-5 antibody) was studied in a randomized trial and found to be more effective than placebo in eosinophilic granulomatosis with polyangiitis (Churg-Strauss).
- Patients with life-threatening eosinophilic granulomatosis with polyangiitis (Churg-Strauss) were excluded from the mepolizumab trial and should continue to be treated with cyclophosphamide and glucocorticoids.
- Mepoluzimab is FDA approved for the treatment of severe eosinophilic asthma and may particularly have a role in the setting of relapsing or resistant asthma in eosinophilic granulomatosis with polyangiitis (Churg-Strauss).
- Rituximab has been examined only in small retrospective series, primarily in patients who have active disease despite conventional agents or who are intolerant of these medications.

Ans. C

99. A patient presented with angiokeratomas, peripheral neuropathy and Premature atherosclerosis. He was diagnosed as Fabrys disease. Which enzyme deficiency causes this?

A. Beta galactosidase
B. Beta glucosidase
C. Alpha glucosidase
D. Alpha galactosidase

Explanation:

- Fabry's disease (angiokeratoma corporis diffusum)- X-linked dominant disorder
- Burning or lancinating pain in the hands and feet often develops in males in late childhood or early adult life

- Associated premature atherosclerosis (e.g., hypertension, renal failure, cardiac disease, and stroke) that often lead to death by the fifth decade of life.
- Fabry's disease is caused by mutations in the alpha-galactosidase gene

Ans. D

100. A patient has mutation in PAHX gene which encodes for phytanoyl co A hydroxylase enzyme. Which of the following is not true about his disease?

A. Peripheral neuropathy
B. Retinitis pigmentosa
C. Cerebellar ataxia
D. Decreased CSF protein

Explanation:

- Refsums disease–Autosomal recessive
- Mutations in the gene that encodes for phytanoylCoA α-hydroxylase (PAHX)
- Accumulation of phytanic acid

Classic tetrad of:

- Peripheral neuropathy
- Elevated CSF protein concentration
- Retinitis pigmentosa
- Cerebellar ataxia

Ans. D

101. A 45 year-old male presents to his doctor with episodes of pre syncope; bilateral pedal oedema. He has family history of hypertrophic cardiomyopathy. An echocardiogram reveals a maximum left ventricular wall thickness of 18.6 mm. His 24 hour urine protein was: 3.1 gm. Renal biopsy reveals enlarged glomerular visceral epithelial cells packed with small clear vacuoles containing globotriaosylceramide. Which of the following treatment would you like to give to this patient?

A. RAAS inhibitors
B. Alpha-galactosidase enzyme
C. Renal transplant
D. All of the above

Explanation:

- Nephropathy of Fabry's disease typically presents in the third decade as mild to moderate proteinuria, sometimes with microscopic hematuria or nephrotic syndrome.
- Urinalysis may reveal oval fat bodies and birefringent glycolipid globules under polarized light (Maltese cross).
- Renal biopsy is necessary for definitive diagnosis. Progression to renal failure occurs by the fourth or fifth decade.
- Treatment with inhibitors of the renin-angiotensin system is recommended. Treatment with recombinant α-galactosidase A clears microvascular endothelial deposits of globotriaosylceramide from the kidneys, heart, and skin. In patients with advanced organ involvement including chronic kidney disease, progression of disease occurs despite enzyme replacement therapy.
- Variable responses to enzyme therapy may be due to the occurrence of neutralizing antibodies or differences in uptake of the enzyme. Graft and patient survival following renal transplantation in patients with Fabry's are similar to other causes of ESRD.

Ans. D

102. A 42 year-old male presents to his doctor with episodes of pre syncope; bilateral pedal oedema. He has family history of hypertrophic cardiomyopathy. An echocardiogram reveals a maximum left ventricular wall thickness of 18.6 mm. His 24 hour urine protein was: 3.1 gm. Full panel testing was ordered for hypertrophic cardiomyopathy (HCM). A hemizygous mutation was found in the GLA gene. Renal biopsy reveals enlarged glomerular visceral epithelial cells packed with small clear vacuoles containing globotriaosylceramide. Which of the following disease would you suspect?

A. Niemann Pick disease
B. Fabry's disease
C. Ataxia telangiectasia
D. Alport's syndrome

Explanation:

- Fabry's disease is an X-linked inborn error of globotriaosylceramide metabolism secondary to deficient lysosomal α-galactosidase. A activity, resulting in excessive intracellular storage of globotriaosylceramide.
- Affected organs include the vascular endothelium, heart, brain, and kidneys.
- Classically, Fabry's disease presents in childhood in males with acroparesthesias, angiokeratoma, and hypohidrosis.
- Over time male patients develop cardiomyopathy, cerebrovascular disease, and renal injury, with an average age of death around 50 years of age. Hemizygotes with hypomorphic mutations sometimes present in the fourth to sixth decade with single-organ involvement.
- Rarely, dominant-negative α-galactosidase A mutations or female heterozygotes with unfavourable X inactivation present with mild single-organ involvement.

Ans. B

103. A 68 year old obese women ,non-diabetic, euthyroid but hypertensive since 8 years presents to OPD with nephrotic range proteinuria. Urinalysis is negative for RBC/WBC. Which one of the following is least likely on renal biopsy?

A. Membranous nephropathy
B. Minimal change disease
C. Amyloidosis
D. Fibrillary GN

Explanation:

- Fibrillary-immunotactoid glomerulopathy is a rare (<1.0% of renal biopsies), morphologically defined disease characterized by glomerular accumulation of nonbranching randomly arranged fibrils.

Ans. D

104. Second most common clinical manifestation in SLE is related to:

A. Musculockeletal
B. Hematological
C. Cutaneous
D. Renal

Explanation:

Table: Clinical manifestations of SLE and prevalence over the entire course of disease[a]

Manifestation	Prevalence, %
Systemic: Fatigue, malaise, fever, anorexia, weight loss	95
Musculoskeletal	95
• Arthralgias/myalgias	95
• Nonerosive polyarthritis	60
• Hand deformities	10
• Myopathy/myositis	25/5
• Ischemic necrosis of bone	15

Contd.

Contd.

Cutaneous	80
• Photosensitivity	70
• Malar rash	50
• Oral ulcers	40
• Alopecia	40
• Discoid rash	20
• Vasculitis rash	20
• Other (e.g., urticaria, subacute cutaneous lupus)	15
Hematologic	85
• Anemia (chronic disease)	70
• Leukopenia (< 4000/μl)	65
• Lymphopenia (< 1500/μl)	50
• Thrombocytopenia (< 100,000/μl)	15
• Lymphadenopathy	15
• Splenomegaly	15
• Hemolytic anemia	10
Neurologic	60
• Cognitive disorder	50
• Mood disorder	40
• Depression	25
• Headache	25
• Seizures	20
• Mono-, polyneuropathy	15
• Stroke, TIA	10
• Acute confessional state or movement disorder	2-5
• Aseptic meningitis, myelopathy	< 1
Cardiopulmonary	60
• Pleurisy, pericarditis, effusions	30-50
• Myocarditis, endocarditis	10
• Lupus pneumonitis	10
• Coronary artery disease	10
• Interstitial fibrosis	5
• Pulmonary hypertension, ARDS, hemorrhage	< 5
• Shrinking lung syndrome	< 5
Renal	30-50
• Proteinuria ≥ 500 mg/24 h, cellular casts	30-60
• Nephrotic syndrome	25
• End-stage renal disease	5-10
Gastrointestinal	40
• Nonspecific (nausea, mild pain, diarrhea)	30
• Abnormal liver enzymes	40
• Vasculitis	5

Contd.

Contd.

Thrombosis • Venous • Arterial	15 10 5
Ocular • Sicca syndrome • Conjunctivitis, episcleritis • Vasculitis	15 15 10 5

Ans. B

105. A patient with muscular dystrophy has mutations in emerin gene. Which of following is false regarding this type of muscular dystrophy?

A. Can be autosomal dominant or X linked
B. Prominent contractures
C. Cardiomyopathy
D. Starts with hand muscle weakness

Explanation:

- Emerin mutations are the most common cause of X-linked EDMD
- Lamin A/C mutation are the most common cause of autosomal dominant EDMD Muscle
- Weakness affects humeral and peroneal muscles at first and later spreads to a limbgirdle
- Prominent contractures can be recognized in early childhood and teenage years, often preceding muscle weakness
- Cardiomyopathy is potentially life threatening and may result in sudden death

Ans. D

106. Muscle disease can be caused due to defects in various enzymes in glycogen metabolism. which is false combination?

A. Pompe's disease- α glucosidase
B. McArdles disease- myophosphorylase
C. Type 4 glycogenosis- branching enzyme deficiency
D. Type 5 glycogenosis- debranching enzyme deficiency

Ans. D

107. A patient with glycogen metabolism defect shows second wind phenomenon. He is likely to be suffering from:

A. Pompe's disease
B. McArdles disease
C. Andersons disease
D. Coris disease

Ans. B

108. Bilateral skin thickening is a characteristic feature of:

A. Scleroderma
B. Dermatomyositis
C. Peyronie's disease
D. Sticker Syndrome

Explanation:

- Bilateral symmetrical skin thickening is the hallmark of SSc that distinguishes it from other connective tissue diseases.

- Skin involvement starts in the fingers and characteristically advances from distal to proximal extremities in an ascending fashion.
- Some patients note diffuse taming in the absence of sun exposure as a very early manifestation. In dark skinned individuals, vitiligo like hypopigmentation may occur.
- Because pigment loss spares the perifollicular areas, the skin may have a "salt and pepper" appearance, most prominently on the scalp, upper back, and Chest.

Ans. A

109. Most common hematologic problem in sarcoidosis is:

A. Lymphocytosis
B. Lymphopenia
C. Anemia
D. Thrombocytopenia

Explanation:

- Most common hematologic problem is lymphopenia in patients with Sarcoidosis.
- This reflects sequestration of lymphocytes into areas of inflammation.

Ans. B

110. Most common ocular manifestation of Sarcoidosis is:

A. Retinitis
B. Pars planitis
C. Anterior uveitis
D. Optic neuritis

Explanation:

- Most common ocular manifestation in sarcoidosis is anterior uveitis.
- Retinitis and Pars planitis can also occur with sarcoidosis.

Ans. C

111. Not true about MCTD is:

A. lcSSc coexisting with features of SLE, polymyositis and rheumatoid arthritis
B. Generally associated with autoantibodies to U1-RNP
C. Often doesn't respond to glucocorticoids
D. Long term prognosis is better than that if SSc

Explanation:

- Patients who have lcSSc coexisting with features of SLE, polymyositis, and rheumatoid arthritis may have mixed connective tissue disease (MCTD).
- This overlap syndrome is generally associated with presence of high titers of autoantibodies to U1-RNP.
- Characteristic initial presentation is Raynaud's phenomenon associated with puffy fingers and myalgia. Over time, sclerodactyly, soft tissue calcinosis, and cutaneous telangiectasia may appear.
- Skin rash suggestive of SLE (malar erythema, photosensitivity) or dermatomyositis (heliotrope rash on the eyelids, erythematous rash on knuckles) occur.
- Arthralgia is common, and some patients develop erosive polyarthritis.
- Pulmonary fibrosis and isolated or secondary PAH may develop. Other manifestations include esophageal dysmotility, pericarditis, Sjögren's syndrome, and renal disease, especially membranous glomerulonephritis.
- Laboratory evaluation shows elevated ESR and hypergammaglobulinemia.
- While anti-U1RNP antibodies are detected in high titers, SSc-specific autoantibodies are absent. In contrast to SSc, MCTD often responds to glucocorticoids, and the long-term prognosis is better than that of SSc.
- Whether MCTD is truly a distinct entity or is a subset of SLE or SSc, remains controversial.

Ans. C

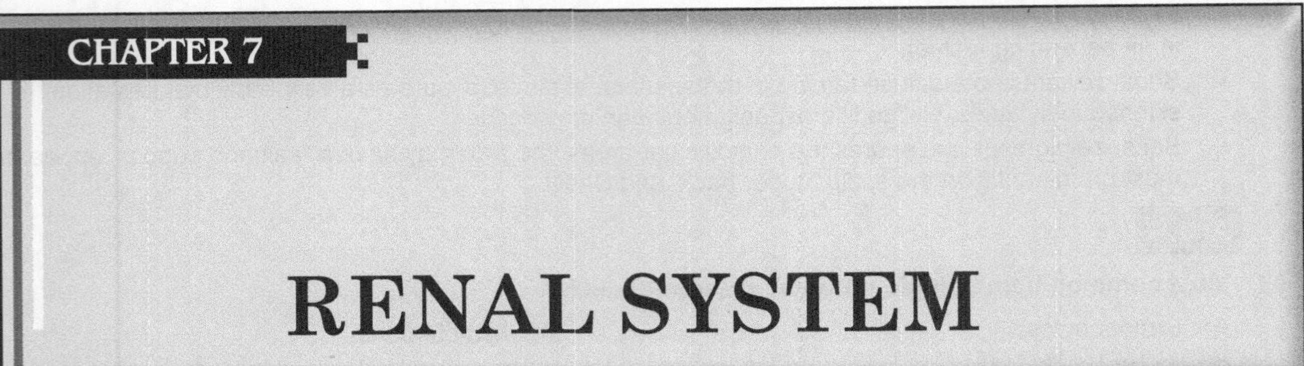

CHAPTER 7

RENAL SYSTEM

1. **Incorrect regarding Fabry's disease affecting kidney is:**

A. Zebra bodies are found in renal biopsy
B. Disease affects females in family
C. X linked disease
D. Renal biopsy picture is of FSGS

Explanation:

X-linked disease:

- Fabry's disease typically presents in childhood males
- Manifests with Angiokeratomas, hypohidrosis, corneal and lenticular opacities, acroparesthesias, progressive disease of kidney, heart and brain vasculature
- Angiokearatomas – most common between the umbilicus and knees(bathing suit area)
- Abdominal pain, recurrent diarrhoea and acroparesthesias- may appear in childhood
- Zebra bodies are seen on electron microscopy
- Kidney transplantation live saving in renal failure
- Renal biopsy picture is of FSGS

Ans. B

2. **Stage V Chronic kidney disease occurs when GFR falls below:**

A. 5ml/min/1.73 m2
B. 10ml/min/1.73 m2
C. 15ml/min/1.73 m2
D. 20ml/min/1.73 m2

Explanation:

- Stage V Chronic kidney disease occurs when GFR falls below 15ml/min/1.73m2

Ans. C

3. **All the following are seen in chronic kidney disease except:**

A. Hyperphosphatemia
B. Reduced ionized calcium in blood
C. Increased calcitriol
D. Increased PTH secretion

Explanation:

- In CKD there is reduced GFR that leads to reduced phosphate excretion- thus phosphate retention
- Retained phosphate causes increased FGF 23 & PTH Synthesis
- Decreased ionized levels occur due to suppression of calcitriol production by FGF 23

Ans. C

4. In healthy adults renal autoregulation usually falls once systolic blood pressure falls below?

A. 120mm Hg
B. 100mm Hg
C. 90mm Hg
D. 80mm Hg

Explanation:

- In healthy adults, renal autoregulation usually fails once the systolic blood pressure falls below 80 mmHg.

Ans. D

5. Renal cysts are seen in which type of MODY?

A. MODY 1
B. MODY 3
C. MODY 5
D. MODY 7

Explanation:

- Individuals with a HNF-1β mutation have progressive impairment of insulin secretion and hepatic insulin resistance, and require insulin treatment with minimal response to sulfonylureas.
- These individuals often have other abnormalities such as renal cysts, mild pancreatic exocrine insufficiency, and abnormal liver function tests.

Ans. C

6. All are phosphate binders used in CKD except:

A. Calcium carbonate
B. Calcium acetate
C. Calcium hydroxide
D. Lanthanum

Explanation:

- Hyperphosphatemia is common in CKDand can usually be treated by limiting intestinal absorption of phosphate using phosphate binders
- PHOSPHATE BINDERS

CALCIUM BASED

- Calcium carbonate
- Calcium acetate

NON-CALCIUM BASED

- Sevelamer
- Lanthanum
- Aluminium hydroxide

NEWER IRON BASED BINDERS

- Surcroferric oxyhydroxide
- Ferric citrate
- Tenapanor- newer phosphate lowering drug

Ans. C

7. A 12 years old male child presents with complaints of loose stools (10 episodes/day, watery) for the past 5 days. Child also gives history of decreased urine output for the past 2 days. On examination, the patient is dehydrated with decreased skin turgor. Which of the following would you expect to see in this patient?

A. Fractional excretion of sodium <1%
B. Urinary sodium >40
C. Urine/plasma creatinine <20
D. Urine osmolality <350

Explanation:

- The child is this scenario is presenting with ***pre renal acute kidney injury (AKI)*** due to several episodes of loose stools causing dehydration.
- Lab findings in pre renal acute kidney injury: BUN/Creatinine ratio >20:1, Urine sodium <20, Urine osmolality >500, Fractional excretion of sodium (FeNa) <1% and Urine/Plasma creatinine ratio >40

Ans. A

8. **Following is the immune-fluorescent staining for IgG stained kidney specimen. Suggestive of:**

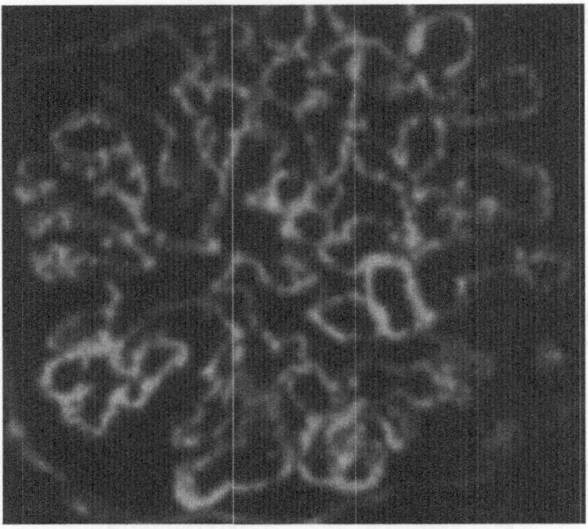

A. Systemic lupus erythematosus
B. Buerger's disease
C. Good pasture disease
D. Memberanous glomerulonephritis

Explanation:

- Image shows immunofluorescence of diffuse granular pattern characteristic of Membranous nephropathy.
- It is an immunologically mediated disease in which deposits of mainly IgG and complement collect in basement membrane as shown in figure.
- In systemic lupus erythematosus immunofluoroscence profile is full house meaning that IgG, IgA, IgM C3 and C1q are usually present.

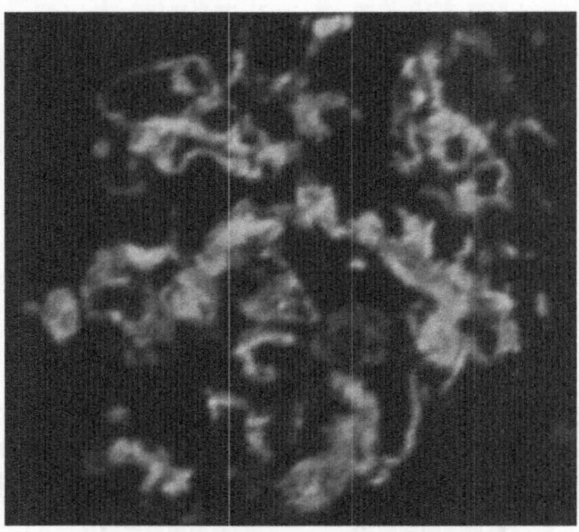

- Buerger's disease: ruled out as question clearly mentions IgG stained as in Buerger's IgA deposits are seen.

- In Good pasture syndrome smooth, diffuse linear pattern characteristic of glomerular basement membrane disease.

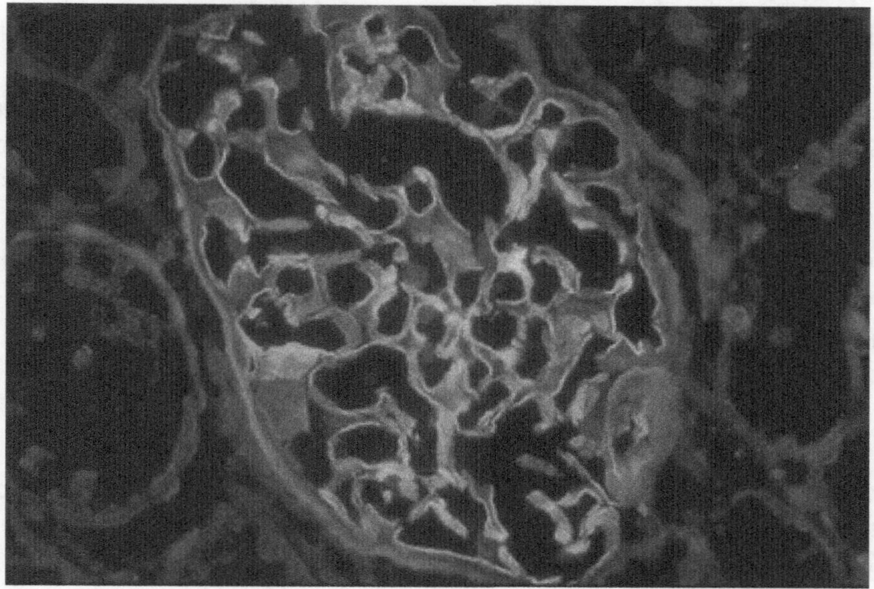

Ans. D

9. A 50 years old chronic kidney disease patient who is on thrice weekly hemodialysis presents with symptoms of non specific back pain & chest pain 1.5 hours into his dialysis session. His blood pressure is normal and he is afebrile. What is the complication of hemodialysis that patient has developed now?

A. Hemodialysis related hypotension
B. Type A reaction
C. Type B reaction
D. Dialysis disequilibrium syndrome

Explanation:

- Type B reaction consists of a symptom complex of non specific chest and back pain, which is due to complement activation and cytokine release. These symptoms typically occur several minutes into the dialysis run and typically resolve over time with continued dialysis.

Hemodialysis related complications:

- Hypotension (most common)
- Muscle cramps
- Dialysis disequilibrium syndrome
- Type A reaction
- Type B reaction
- Anaphylactoid reactions

Ans. C

10. A 60 years old chronic kidney disease patient who is currently on peritoneal dialysis, presents to the nephrology outpatient department with complaints of fever, severe abdominal pain with guarding a rigidity. Patient also reports that peritoneal dialysate has been cloudy for the past 3 days. What should be peritoneal fluid leucocyte count in this patient to diagnose peritoneal dialysis related peritonitis?

A. >250/mm^3
B. >150/mm^3
C. >100/mm^3
D. >50/mm^3

Explanation:

- This patient has developed ***peritoneal dialysis associated peritonitis.***
- Peritoneal dialysis related peritonitis typically develops when there has been a break in sterile technique during one or more of the exchange procedures.
- Peritonitis is usually defined by an ***elevated peritoneal fluid leukocyte count (100/mm3, of which at least 50% are polymorphonuclear neutrophils)***; these cut-offs are lower than in spontaneous bacterial peritonitis because of presence of dextrose in peritoneal dialysis solutions and rapid bacterial proliferation in this environment without antibiotic therapy.
- Clinical presentation typically consists of pain and cloudy dialysate, often with fever and other constitutional symptoms.
- Most common culprit organisms are gram-positive cocci, including Staphylococcus, reflecting the origin from the skin.

Ans. C

11. A 35 year old male patient who is a known case of chronic kidney disease is planned for regular hemodialysis. Which of the following vascular access for hemodialysis has the highest long-term patency rate?

A. Arteriovenous fistula
B. Arteriovenous grafts
C. Tunneled hemodialysis catheter
D. Central venous line

Explanation:

Types of vascular access for hemodialysis: (i) Arteriovenous fistula (ii) Arteriovenous graft (iii) Tunnelled hemodialysis catheter.

Fistulas have highest long-term patency rate of all hemodialysis access options.

- For patients in whom fistulas fail to mature, or in patients whose vasculature does not allow creation of a successful fistula (i.e., poor arterial inflow or recipient veins of inadequate caliber), patients undergo placement of an arteriovenous graft (i.e., the interposition of prosthetic material, usually polytetra-fluoroethylene, between an artery and a vein) or a tunnelled hemodialysis catheter.

Ans. A

12. A 40 years old patient who has been recently diagnosed with chronic kidney disease (patient not willing for dialysis) presents to the casualty with complaints of severe retrosternal chest pain. Patient says that his pain is partially relieved when he leans forward and worsens when he lies down. An ECG is immediately ordered and it reveals saddle shaped ST elevation and PR depression. What orders will you give the dialysis technician before starting hemodialysis in this particular scenario?

A. Sodium remodeling
B. 2.5 hours dialysis instead of 4 hours
C. Avoid heparin during hemodialysis
D. Low potassium in dialysate

Explanation:

- This patient has presented with classical signs and symptoms of pericarditis, and in this scenario the most likely cause is ***uremic pericarditis***.
- Because of the propensity to hemorrhage in pericardial fluid, hemodialysis should be performed without heparin. Chest pain with respiratory accentuation, accompanied by a friction rub, is diagnostic of pericarditis.
- Classic electrocardiographic abnormalities include PR-interval depression and diffuse ST-segment elevation.
- Pericarditis can be accompanied by pericardial effusion that is seen on echocardiography and can rarely lead to tamponade.

- Uremic pericarditis is an absolute indication for the urgent initiation of dialysis or for intensification of the dialysis prescription in those already receiving dialysis.
- Pericarditis is observed in advanced uremia, and with the advent of timely initiation of dialysis, is not as common as it once was. It is now more often observed in underdialyzed, non-adherent patients than in those starting dialysis.

Ans. C

13. A 45 years old chronic kidney disease patient presents to the nephrology clinic with history blackish ulcers over her abdomen. Patient was recently started on warfarin for atrial fibrillation that was detected on her previous visit. On examination there is livedo reticularis and skin necrosis and ulceration over anterior abdominal wall. What is the complication that has developed in this patient?

A. Scrub typhus
B. Atrial fibrillation related microthrombi
C. Calciphylaxis
D. Necrotizing fasciitis

Explanation:

- Calciphylaxis is a devastating condition seen almost exclusively in patients with advanced CKD. It is heralded by livedo reticularis and advances to patches of ischemic necrosis, especially on the legs, thighs, abdomen and breasts.
- Warfarin is commonly used in hemodialysis patients in whom most direct oral anticoagulants (DOACs) are contraindicated, and one of the effects of warfarin therapy is to decrease the vitamin K–dependent regeneration of matrix GLA protein. This latter protein is important in preventing vascular calcification.
- Thus, warfarin treatment is considered a risk factor for calciphylaxis, and if a patient develops this syndrome, this medication should be discontinued and replaced with another anticoagulant. Treatment is with hyperbaric oxygen, intravenous thiosulfate and discontinuation of warfarin.

Ans. C

14. A 25 year old male patient presents to the casualty with decreased urine output for the past 3 days. Patient gives history of bloody diarrhea (2-3 episodes/day) for the past one week. On examination the patient appears to be pale. Lab investigations reveal serum creatinine 3.5 mg/dL, raised LDH and schistocytes in peripheral smear. What is the organism that is commonly associated with this disease?

A. Enterohemorrhagic E.coli
B. Enteroaggregative E.coli
C. Enteroinvasive E.coli
D. Diffusely adherent E.coli

Explanation:

- This patient is presenting with Acute kidney injury, microangiopathic hemolytic anemia (since schistocytes are present in peripheral smear) following a history of dysentery.
- Presence of the constellation of these features strongly suggest a diagnosis of ***Hemolytic Uremic Syndrome.***
- HUS is loosely defined by the presence of MAHA and renal impairment. At least four variants are recognized. Most common is Shiga toxin–producing Escherichia coli (STEC) HUS, which is also known as D+ (diarrhea-associated) HUS or enterohemorrhagic E. coli (EHEC) HUS.
- Most cases involve children <5 years of age, but adults also are susceptible. Diarrhea, often bloody, precedes MAHA within 1 week in >80% of cases. Abdominal pain, cramping, and vomiting are frequent, whereas fever is typically absent. Most common STEC strain is O157:H7.

Ans. A

15. A 57 year old chronic kidney disease patient presents to the nephrology clinic with history of decreased sensation over both lower limbs (below his knees) for the past 3 months. On examination there is decreased sensation over both lower limbs from below the knees with diminished deep tendon reflexes. Plantar response is flexor. At what stage of chronic kidney disease does the complication seen in this patient start to appear?

A. Stage 1
B. Stage 2
C. Stage 3
D. Stage 4

Explanation:

- This patient is suffering from Uremic peripheral neuropathy that is usually seen after stage 4 chronic kidney disease.
- Peripheral neuropathy usually becomes clinically evident after the patient reaches stage 4 CKD, although electrophysiologic and histologic evidence occurs earlier. Initially, sensory nerves are involved more than motor, lower extremities more than upper, and distal part of the extremities more than proximal.
- Other CNS complications include mild disturbances in memory and concentration and sleep disturbance.
- Neuromuscular irritability, including hiccups, cramps, and twitching, becomes evident at later stages. In advanced untreated kidney failure, asterixis, myoclonus, seizures, and coma can be seen.

Ans. D

16. Assertion(A): Calcium Carbonate should not be used in achlorhydric patients.

Reason(R): Calcium Carbonate is a weekly dissociable supplement.

A. Both (A) and (R) are correct and (R) explains (A)
B. Both (A) and (R) are correct but (R) doesn't explain (A)
C. (R) is correct But (A) is false
D. (A) is correct But (R) is false

Explanation:

- Intestinal absorption of ingested calcium involves both active (transcellular) and passive (paracellular) mechanisms.
- Passive calcium absorption is nonsaturable and approximates 5% of daily calcium intake, whereas active absorption involves apical calcium entry via specific ion channels (TRPV5 and TRPV6), whose expression is controlled principally by 1,25(OH)2D, and normally ranges from 20 to 70%.
- Active calcium transport occurs mainly in the proximal small bowel (duodenum and proximal jejunum), although some active calcium absorption occurs in most segments of the small intestine.
- Optimal rates of calcium absorption require gastric acid. This is especially true for weakly dissociable calcium supplements such as calcium carbonate.
- In fact, large boluses of calcium carbonate are poorly absorbed because of their neutralizing effect on gastric acid.
- In achlorhydric subjects and for those taking drugs that inhibit gastric acid secretion, supplements should be taken with meals to optimize their absorption. Use of calcium citrate may be preferable in these circumstances. Calcium absorption may also be blunted in disease states such as pancreatic or biliary insufficiency, in which ingested calcium remains bound to unabsorbed fatty acids or other food constituents.

Ans. A

17. **Most common complication of Hemodialysis is:**

A. Hypotension
B. Muscle cramps
C. Chest pain
D. Anaphylaxis

Explanation:

- Hypotension is the most common acute complication of hemodialysis, particularly among patients with diabetes mellitus.
- Numerous factors appear to increase the risk of hypotension, including excessive ultrafiltration with inadequate compensatory vascular filling, impaired vasoactive or autonomic responses, osmolar shifts, overzealous use of antihypertensive agents, and reduced cardiac reserve.
- Muscle cramps during dialysis are also a common complication.
- Anaphylactoid reactions to the dialyzer, particularly on its first use, have been reported most frequently with the bioincompatible cellulosic containing membranes.

Ans. A

18. **A 30 year old male presents to the OPD with complaints of chronic cough and new onset hematuria. He is being evaluated as a case of pulmonary renal syndrome. Differential diagnosis include:**

A. Granulomatosis with polyangiitis
B. Hanta virus
C. Paraquat poisoning
D. All of the above

Explanation:

Pulmo-renal syndromes are uncommon conditions but are often rapidly progressive and fatal if untreated. Causes include:

(a) Autoimmune

- Goodpasture's syndrome
- ANCA associated vasculitis (microscopic polyangitis, granulomatosis with poly angiitis, eosinophilic granulomatosis with polyangiitis)
- SLE

(b) Medications and Toxins

- Paraquat poisoning
- Chemotherapy agents (e.g., Gemcitabine)

(c) Infections

- Leptospirosis
- Hanta virus
- HIV

(d) Congenital Diseases

- AV malformation
- Hereditary haemorrhagic telangiectasia.

Ans. D

19. **Commonly accepted criteria for initiating patients on maintainance dialysis include all except:**

A. Presence of uremic symptoms
B. Persistent extracellular volume expansion despite diuretic therapy

C. Bleeding diathesis

D. Creatinine clearance or estimated GFR <20ml/min per 1.73 m2

Explanation:

- Commonly accepted criteria for initiating patients on maintenance dialysis include the presence of uremic symptoms, presence of hyperkalemia unresponsive to conservative measures, persistent extracellular volume expansion despite diuretic therapy, acidosis refractory to medical therapy, a bleeding diathesis, and a creatinine clearance or estimated glomerular filtration rate (GFR) <10 mL/min per 1.73 m2.

Ans. D

20. Baby born with a renal condition is died within one month of birth. What is the most possible diagnosis?

A. Autosomal dominant PKD
B. Autosomal recessive PKD
C. Von Hippel Lindau syndrome
D. Medullary cystic disease

Explanation:

- Classic ARPKD is generally diagnosed in utero or within the neonatal period, and characterized by greatly enlarged echogenic kidneys in diseased fetuses.
- Reduced fetal urine production may contribute to oligohydroaminos and pulmonary hypoplasia.
- About 30% of affected neonates die shortly after birth due to respiratory insufficiency.
- Close to 60% of mortality occurs within the first month of life. In the classic group, most patients are born with renal insufficiency and ESRD.
- However, infants often have a transient improvement in their GFR; death from renal insufficiency at this stage is rare.
- Some patients are diagnosed after neonatal stage, which form older group.
- Morbidity and mortality in this group often involve systemic hypertension, progressive renal insufficiency, and liver manifestations.

Ans. B

21. Most common type of stone in adult polycystic kidney disease is:

A. Uric acid
B. Calcium oxalate
C. Struvite
D. Calcium phosphate

Explanation:

- Kidney stones occur in ~20% of patients with ADPKD. Different from the general population, more than half of the stones in patients with ADPKD are composed of uric acid, with the remainder due to calcium oxalate.

Ans. A

22. All of the following medications may be useful in the treatment of benign prostatic hypertrophy except:

A. Alfuzosin
B. Bosentan
C. Dutasteride
D. Finasteride

Explanation:

- Benign prostatic hypertrophy (BPH) is a pathologic process that contributes to the development of lower urinary tract symptoms in men.

- Such symptoms, arising from lower urinary tract dysfunction, are further subdivided into obstructive symptoms (urinary hesitancy, straining, weak stream, terminal dribbling, prolonged voiding, incomplete emptying) and irritative symptoms (urinary frequency, urgency, nocturia, urge incontinence, small voided volumes).
- Lower urinary tract symptoms and other sequelae of BPH are not just due to a mass effect, but are also likely due to a combination of the prostatic enlargement and age-related detrusor dysfunction.
- Asymptomatic patients do not require treatment regardless of the size of the prostate gland.
- Symptomatic relief is the most common reason men seek treatment for BPH, and therefore, the goal of therapy for BPH is usually relief of these symptoms.
- Selective α-adrenergic receptor antagonists, such as alfuzosin, are thought to treat the dynamic aspect of BPH by reducing sympathetic tone of the bladder outlet, thereby decreasing resistance and improving urinary flow.
- 5α-Reductase inhibitors, like dutasteride and finasteride, are thought to treat static aspect of BPH by reducing prostate volume and having a similar, albeit delayed effect.
- They have also proven to be beneficial in the prevention of BPH progression, as measured by prostate volume, the risk of developing acute urinary retention, and the risk of having BPH-related surgery.
- Use of an α-adrenergic receptor antagonist and a 5α-reductase inhibitor as combination therapy seeks to provide symptomatic relief while preventing progression of BPH.
- Another class of medications that has shown improvement in lower urinary tract symptoms secondary to BPH is phosphodiesterase-5 (PDE5) inhibitors, used currently in the treatment of erectile dysfunction.
- All three of the PDE5 inhibitors available in the United States, sildenafil, vardenafil, and tadalafil, appear to be effective in the treatment of symptoms secondary to BPH.
- Use of PDE5 inhibitors is not without controversy, however, given the fact that short-acting PDE5 inhibitors such as sildenafil need to be dosed separately from α-blockers because of potential hypotensive effects. Bosentan is a nonselective endothelin receptor antagonist used in the treatment of pulmonary arterial hypertension.

Ans. B

23. Identify the image:

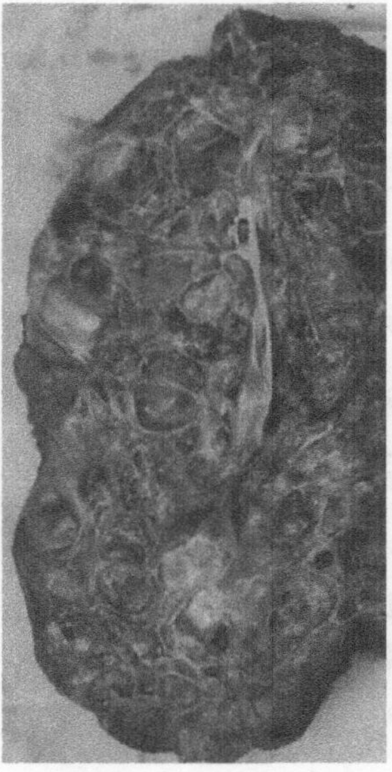

A. Autosomal dominant Polycystic kidney
B. Autosomal recessive polycystic kidney
C. Medullary sponge kidney
D. Renal cystic dysplasia

Explanation:

- Image shows enlarged kidney with complete loss of demarcation between cortex and medulla and replacement of renal parenchyma by variauable sizes cysts diagnostic of autosomal dominant polycystic kidney.
- In autosomal recessive tiny fusion cysts are seen.

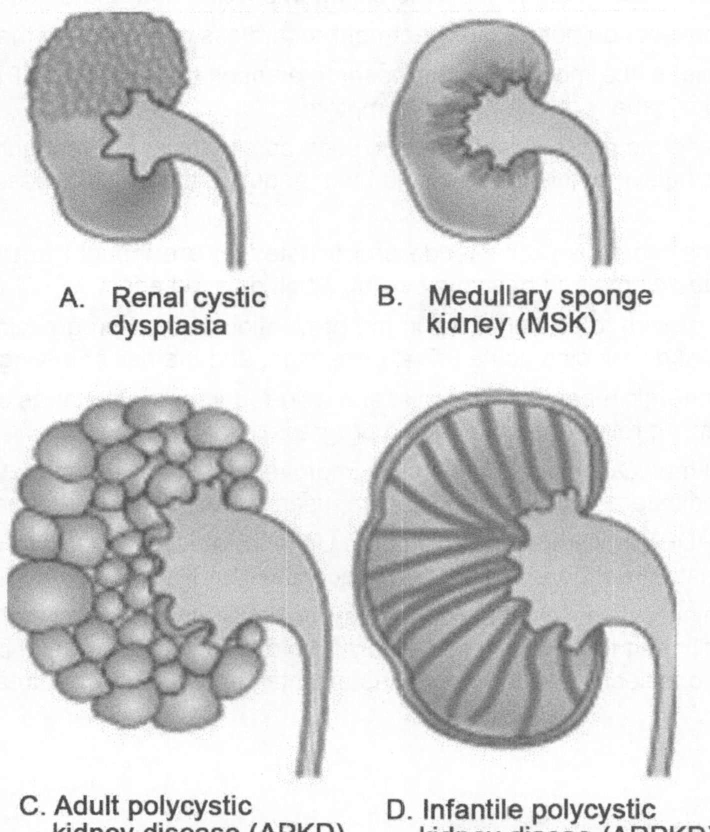

Ans. A

24. Which of the following is not true about ADPKD?

A. Cardiovascular complications are most common cause of death.

B. Mitral valve prolapse is seen in 80% of cases

C. Aortic and tricuspid valves may also involved

D. Risk of Colonic diverticula is increased.

Explanation:

- In autosomal dominant polycystic kidney there are numerous cysts are seen in parenchyma with loss of demarcation between cortex and medulla.
- Mitral valve prolapse is seen in 30% cases not 80% cases.
- Rest options are true regarding autosomal dominant polycystic kidney.

Ans. B

25. All are true about response of kidney to different situations except:

A. Under conditions of acidemia the kidney preferentially uses type A intercalated cells to secrete excess H+ and generate more HCO3−

B. Renal natriuretic peptide is secreted by renal afferent arteriole

C. Aquaporin 1 is constitutively active in all water-permeable segments

D. Aquaporin 2, 3, and 4 in the collecting duct promote vasopressin-regulated water permeability

Explanation:

- Inner medullary collecting duct cells share many similarities with principal cells of the cortical collecting duct. They have apical Na+ and K+ channels that mediate Na+ reabsorption and K+ secretion, respectively. Sodium reabsorption by inner medullary collecting duct cells is also inhibited by the natriuretic peptides called *atrial natriuretic peptide* or *renal natriuretic peptide* (urodilatin); the same gene encodes both peptides but uses different posttranslational processing of a common preprohormone to generate different proteins.
- Atrial natriuretic peptides are secreted by atrial myocytes in response to volume expansion, whereas urodilatin is secreted by renal tubular epithelia. Natriuretic peptides interact with either apical (urodilatin) or basolateral (atrial natriuretic peptides) receptors on inner medullary collecting duct cells to stimulate guanylyl cyclase and increase levels of cytoplasmic cGMP. This effect in turn reduces the activity of apical Na+ channel in these cells and attenuates net Na+ reabsorption, producing natriuresis.

Ans. B

26. Acute fibrinoid necrosis of afferent arterioles, followed by intimal proliferation (onion-skin pattern) in kidney is seen in all below conditions except:

A. Scleroderma renal crisis

B. TTP

C. ITP

D. HUS

Explanation:

- In the kidneys, vascular lesions affecting the interlobular and arcuate arteries predominate.
- Chronic renal ischemia is associated with shrunken glomeruli.
- Patients with scleroderma renal crisis show acute fibrinoid necrosis of afferent arterioles, followed by intimal proliferation (onion-skin pattern), and ischemic collapse of glomeruli.
- These changes are reminiscent of thrombotic microangiopathies such as atypical hemolytic-uremic syndrome and are accompanied by complement deposition, thrombosis, thrombocytopenia due to platelet consumption, and intravascular hemolysis.
- Extensive vascular thrombosis, glomerular collapse and sclerosis, and peritubular capillary deposits in renal biopsy are associated with irreversible renal failure.

Ans. C

27. Basement membrane syndrome can present in all way except:

A. Mild to heavy proteinuria

B. Gross hematuria

C. Hypertension

D. Raised creatinine

Explanation:

- Patients with a *basement membrane syndrome* either have genetically abnormal basement membranes (Alport's syndrome) or an autoimmune response to basement membrane collagen IV (Goodpasture's syndrome) associated with microscopic hematuria, mild to heavy proteinuria, and hypertension with variable elevations in serum creatinine.

Ans. B

28. All stains and the structures they are used to see are correct except:

A. Periodic acid Schiff (PAS) to stain carbohydrate

B. Jones methenamine silver to assess cellularity and architecture

C. Congo red for amyloid deposits

D. Masson's trichrome to identify collagen deposition

Explanation:

- A renal biopsy in the setting of glomerulonephritis quickly identifies type of glomerular injury and often suggests a course of treatment.
- The biopsy is processed for light microscopy using stains for *hematoxylin and eosin* (*H&E*) to assess cellularity and architecture, *periodic acid–Schiff* (*PAS*) to stain carbohydrate moieties in the membranes of the glomerular tuft and tubules, *Jones-methenamine silver* to enhance basement membrane structure, *Congo red* for amyloid deposits, and *Masson's trichrome* to identify collagen deposition and assess the degree of glomerulosclerosis and interstitial fibrosis.

Ans. B

29. Not true about endocrine abnormalities in women with CKD is:

A. Estrogen levels are low

B. Menstrual abnormalities

C. Infertility

D. When GFR has declined to 50ml/min, pregnancy is associated with high rate of spontaneous abortion

Explanation:

- In women with CKD, estrogen levels are low, and menstrual abnormalities, infertility, and inability to carry pregnancies to term are common.
- When the GFR has declined to ~40 mL/min, pregnancy is associated with a high rate of spontaneous abortion, with only ~20% of pregnancies leading to live births, and pregnancy may hasten progression of the kidney disease itself.
- Women with CKD who are contemplating pregnancy should consult first with a nephrologist in conjunction with an obstetrician specializing in high-risk pregnancy.
- Men with CKD have reduced plasma testosterone levels, and sexual dysfunction and oligospermia may supervene.
- Sexual maturation may be delayed or impaired in adolescent children with CKD, even among those treated with dialysis.
- Many of these abnormalities improve or reverse with intensive dialysis or with successful renal transplantation.

Ans. D

30. Hyaline cast is commonly seen in all except:

A. Malignant hypertension
B. Pre renal azotemia
C. Post renal azotemia
D. Scleroderma renal crisis

Explanation:

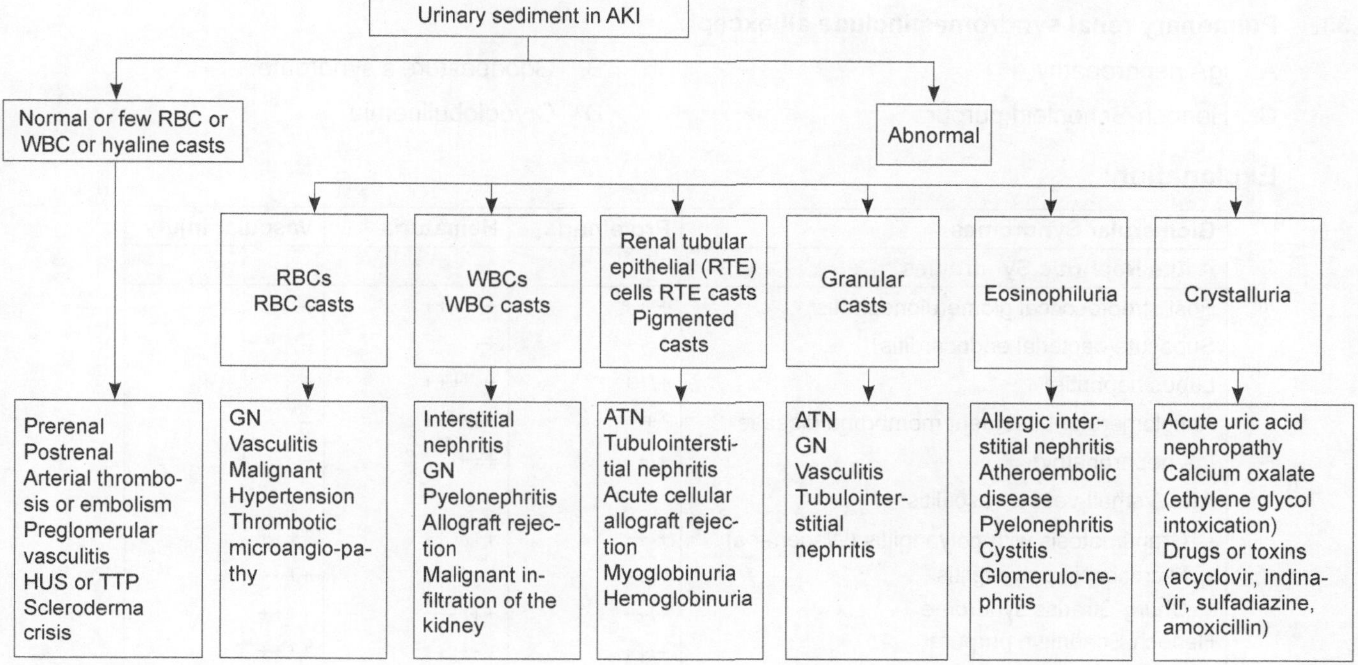

Ans. A

31. Prolonged period of pre-renal azotemia may lead to:

A. Acute glomerulonephritis
B. Acute tubular necrosis
C. Hemolytic uremic syndrome
D. Chronic glomerulonephritis

Explanation:

- Prolonged periods of pre-renal azotemia may lead to ischemic injury, often termed acute tubular necrosis (ATN).
- By definition, pre-renal azotemia involves no parenchymal damage to kidney and is rapidly reversible once parenchymal blood flow and intra-glomerular hemodynamics are restored.

Ans. B

32. All are true about diabetic nephropathy except:

A. More than 90% of patients with type 1 diabetes and nephropathy have diabetic retinopathy
B. Almost 100% of patients with type 2 diabetes and nephropathy have diabetic retinopathy
C. Absence of retinopathy in type 1 patients with proteinuria should prompt consideration of a diagnosis other than diabetic nephropathy
D. There is a significant correlation between the presence of retinopathy and the presence of Kimmelstiel-Wilson nodules

Explanation:

- More than 90% of patients with type 1 diabetes and nephropathy have diabetic retinopathy, so the absence of retinopathy in type 1 patients with proteinuria should prompt consideration of a diagnosis other than diabetic nephropathy; only 60% of patients with type 2 diabetes with nephropathy have diabetic retinopathy.

- There is a significant correlation between the presence of retinopathy and the presence of Kimmelstiel-Wilson nodules.
- Also, characteristically, patients with advanced diabetic nephropathy have normal to enlarged kidneys, in contrast to many other glomerular diseases where kidney size is usually decreased.

Ans. B

33. Pulmonary renal syndromes include all except:

A. IgA nephropathy
B. Goodpasture's syndrome
C. Henoch-Schönlein purpura
D. Cryoglobulinemia

Explanation:

Glomerular Syndromes	Proteinuria	Hematuria	Vascular Injury
Acute Nephritic Syndromes			
Post streptococcal glomerulonephritis[a]	+/++	++/+++	–
Subacute bacterial endocarditis[a]	+/++	++	–
Lupus nephritis[a]	+/++	++/+++	+
Antiglomerular basement membrane disease[a]	++	++/+++	–
IgA nephropathy[a]	+/++	+++[c]	–
ANCA small-vessel vasculitis[a]			
• Granumatosis with polyangiitis (Wegener's)	+/++	++/+++	++++
• Microscopic polyangiitis	+/++	++/+++	++++
• Churg-Strauss syndrome	+/++	++/+++	++++
Henoch-Schönlein purpura[a]	+/++	++/+++	++++
Cryoglobulinemia[a]	+/++	++/+++	++++
Membranoproliferative glomerulonephritis[a]	++	++/+++	–
C_3 Glomerulopathies	++	++/+++	–
Mesangioproliferative glomerulonephritis	+	+/++	–
Pulmonary-Renal Syndromes			
Goodpasture's syndrome[a]	++	++/+++	–
ANCA small-vessel vasculitis[a]			
• Granulomatosis with polyangiitis (Wegener's)	+/++	++/+++	++++
• Microscopic polyangliitis	+/++	++/+++	++++
• Churg-Strauss syndrome	+/++	++/+++	++++
Henoch-Schönlein purpura[a]	+/++	++/+++	++++
Cryoglobulinemia[a]	+/++	++/+++	++++

Ans. A

34. Commonly used urine determinations include all except:

A. Metanephrine
B. Free cortisol
C. Calcium
D. Thyroxine

Explanation:

- A 24-h urine-free cortisol measurement largely reflects the amount of unbound cortisol, thus providing a reasonable index of biologically available hormone.

- Other commonly used urine determinations include 17-hydroxycorticosteroids, 17-ketosteroids, vanillylmandelic acid, metanephrine, catecholamines, 5-hydroxyindoleacetic acid, and calcium.

Ans. D

35. All are true about toxin induced AKI except:

A. Metabolite of Aristolochic acid by name 2-hydroxyethoxyacetic acid (HEAA) is responsible for tubular injury

B. Melamine contamination of foodstuffs has led to nephrolithiasis and AKI

C. Uromodulin is the most common protein in normal urine

D. Proton pump inhibitors and NSAIDS are commonly used drugs that have been associated with acute tubulointerstitial nephritis

Explanation:

- Ethylene glycol, present in automobile antifreeze, is metabolized to oxalic acid, glycolaldehyde, and glyoxylate, which may cause AKI through direct tubular injury and tubular obstruction.
- Diethylene glycol is an industrial agent that has caused outbreaks of severe AKI around the world due to adulteration of pharmaceutical preparations.
- Metabolite 2-hydroxyethoxyacetic acid (HEAA) is thought to be responsible for tubular injury.
- Melamine contamination of foodstuffs has led to nephrolithiasis and AKI, either through intratubular obstruction or possibly direct tubular toxicity.
- Aristolochic acid was found to be the cause of "Chinese herb nephropathy" and "Balkan nephropathy" due to contamination of medicinal herbs or farming.
- List of environmental toxins is likely to grow and contribute to a better understanding of previously catalogued "idiopathic" chronic tubular interstitial disease, a common diagnosis in both the developed and developing world.

Ans. A

36. A 45 year old male was prescribed Sildenafil for his erectile dysfunction. What is the mechanism of action of sildenafil?

A. PDE4 inhibition

B. PDE5 inhibition

C. Guanyl cyclase agonist

D. Prostaglandin E agonist

Explanation:

- Sildenafil is potent and selective inhibition of PDE5. Onset of action is 30-120mins. Contraindications include hypotension, drugs like nitrates.

Ans. B

37. Adenosine is a potent vasoconstrictor of:

A. Afferent arteriole

B. Vasa recta

C. Efferent arteriole

D. Renal vein

Explanation:

- TGF changes the rate of filtration and tubular flow by reflex vasoconstriction or dilatation of the afferent arteriole. TGF is mediated by specialized cells in thick ascending limb of the loop of Henle called the *macula densa* that act as sensors of solute concentration and tubular fluid flow rate.
- With high tubular flow rates, a proxy for an inappropriately high filtration rate, there is increased solute delivery to the macula densa that evokes vasoconstriction of the afferent arteriole causing GFR to return toward normal.

- One component of the soluble signal from the macula densa is adenosine triphosphate (ATP) released by the cells during increased NaCl reabsorption. ATP is metabolized in the extracellular space to generate adenosine, a potent vasoconstrictor of the afferent arteriole.
- During conditions associated with a fall in filtration rate, reduced solute delivery to the macula densa attenuates TGF, allowing afferent arteriolar dilatation and restoring GFR to normal levels.
- Angiotensin II and reactive oxygen species enhance, while nitric oxide (NO) blunts TGF.

Ans. A

38. Chronic TIN all are true except:

A. Polyuria
B. Fanconi syndrome
C. Hyperkalemia
D. Proteinuria (always >2g/d)

Explanation:

Table: Chronic tubulointerstitial disorders
• Vesicoureteral reflux/reflux nephropathy • Sickle cell disease • Chronic exposure to toxins or therapeutic agents • Analgesics, especially those containing phenacetin • Lithium • Heavy metals (lead, cadmium) • Aristolochic acid (Chinese herbal and Balkan endemic nephropathies) • Calcineurin inhibitors (cyclosporine, tacrolimus)

Ans. D

39. All are true about C3 glomerulopathy except:

A. C3GN is defined morphologically with dense deposits forming ribbons in GBM
B. DDD is primarily a disease of children and young adults
C. Partial lipodystrophy and Drusen bodies in the retina may also be present in DDD
D. Increasing evidence suggests a benefit of therapy with eculizumab, a monoclonal antibody directed at C5 which is activated by C3

Explanation:

- C3 glomerulopathy is a recent disease classification that is defined by the glomerular accumulation of C3 with little or no immunoglobulin and encompasses dense deposit disease (DDD), formerly MPGN type II (see below), and C3 glomerulonephritis (C3GN).
- DDD is defined morphologically with dense deposits forming ribbons in the GBM. In the absence of this specific morphology the entity is categorized as C3GN. Both are associated with the presence of a complement mutation believed to cause the renal pathology, including mutations in the complement factor H regulatory proteins (CFHR's) genes.
- DDD is primarily a disease of children and young adults while the other C3 glomerulopathies are reported to present in an older age group (mean age 30). By definition kidneys with C3 glomerulopathy show sole or dominant staining for C3 but can have variable light microscopy with mesangial proliferative or membranoproliferative patterns seen most commonly.
- Morphologically, many cases are not distinguishable from recovering post-infections GN.
- Patients with DDD present with proteinuria and/or hematuria with nephrotic range proteinuria in up to 2/3 of patients.

- Partial lipodystrophy and Drusen bodies in the retina may also be present.
- Prognosis is poor with 50% of patients progressing to ESRD. C3GN patients are clinically less well defined but ~2/3 have hematuria and 1/3 proteinuria.
- In addition to renal biopsy serological and genetic evaluation may be indicated including measurement of C3 levels which are typically low with normal C4 levels, C3 nephritic factor, Factor H, paraprotein detection and specific CFHR genetic mutations.
- Optimal therapies remain undefined but include inhibition of the renin-angiotensin system, anticoagulants, steroids and other immunosuppressants.
- Increasing evidence suggests a benefit of therapy with eculizumab, a monoclonal antibody directed at C5 which is activated by C3.

Ans. A

40. Selective proteinuria is due to:

A. Albumin
B. Globulin
C. Labda chain
D. Kappa chain

Explanation:

- Proteinuria only seen with upright posture is called *orthostatic proteinuria* and has a benign prognosis. Isolated proteinuria sustained over multiple clinic visits is found in many glomerular lesions.
- Proteinuria in most adults with glomerular disease is *nonselective*, containing albumin and a mixture of other serum proteins, whereas in children with *minimal change disease* (MCD), proteinuria is *selective* and composed largely of albumin

Ans. A

41. All are possible contraindications for renal biopsy except:

A. Bilaterally small kidneys
B. Active urinary tract infection
C. Worsening GFR
D. Severe obesity

Explanation:

- In the patient with bilaterally small kidneys, renal biopsy is not advised because (1) it is technically difficult and has a greater likelihood of causing bleeding and other adverse consequences, (2) there is usually so much scarring that the underlying disease may not be apparent, and (3) the window of opportunity to render disease-specific therapy has passed.
- Other contraindications to renal biopsy include uncontrolled hypertension, active urinary tract infection, bleeding diathesis (including ongoing anticoagulation), and severe obesity.
- Ultrasound-guided percutaneous biopsy is the favored approach, but a surgical or laparoscopic approach can be considered, especially in the patient with a single kidney where direct visualization and control of bleeding are crucial. In the CKD patient in whom a kidney biopsy is indicated (e.g., suspicion of a concomitant or superimposed active process such as interstitial nephritis or in the face of accelerated loss of GFR), the bleeding time should be measured, and if increased, desmopressin should be administered immediately prior to the procedure.

Ans. C

42. All are true about peritoneal dialysis except:

A. Most common additives to peritoneal dialysis solutions are antibiotics

B. Icodextrin is a non-absorbable carbohydrate that can be used in place of dextrose

C. Most common culprit organisms for peritonitis are gram-positive cocci

D. Non-peritonitis catheter associated infections are often termed tunnel infections

Explanation:

- Most common additives to peritoneal dialysis solutions are heparin to prevent obstruction of the dialysis catheter lumen with fibrin and antibiotics during an episode of acute peritonitis.
- Insulin may also be added in patients with diabetes mellitus.

Ans. A

43. Acute papillary necrosis may be seen with all except:

A. Sickle cell disease
B. Analgesic nephropathy
C. Diabetes
D. Amyloidosis

Explanation:

- Patients with diabetes may present with obstructive uropathy associated with acute papillary necrosis when sloughed papillae obstruct the ureter.
- Papillary necrosis may also be evident in some cases of pyelonephritis complicated by obstruction, sickle cell disease, analgesic nephropathy, or combinations of these conditions.
- In the rare cases of bilateral papillary necrosis, a rapid rise in the serum creatinine level may be the first indication of the condition.

Ans. D

44. A 30 year old woman presents with polyuria, investigations revealed diabetes insipidus. She had met with road traffic accident and head injury. Which part of the nephron is most affected?

A. Cortical and medullary collecting tubules
B. Distal convoluted tubule
C. Thin ascending loop of Henle
D. Glomerular efferent arterioles

Explanation:

- ADH plays a central role in urinary concentration by increasing the water permeability of the normally impermeable cortical and medullary collecting tubules. In the absence of ADH, little water is reabsorbed in the collecting tubules and dilute urine is excreted.

Ans. A

45. All are true about antihypertensive in CKD except:

A. Reduction in proteinuria is a surrogate for improved renal outcome
B. In the absence of an anti proteinuric response with either agent alone, combined treatment with both ACE inhibitors and ARBs has been considered
C. Combination of ACE and ARB is associated with a greater reduction in proteinuria compared to either agent alone
D. ACE inhibitor plus ARB therapy should be advised in patients with CKD

Explanation:

- Increased intraglomerular filtration pressures and glomerular hypertrophy develop as a response to loss of nephron number. This response is maladaptive, as it promotes the ongoing decline of kidney function even if the inciting process has been treated or spontaneously resolved.
- Control of glomerular hypertension is important in slowing the progression of CKD.
- Moreover, elevated blood pressure increases proteinuria by increasing its flux across glomerular capillaries.
- Conversely, renoprotective effect of antihypertensive medications is gauged through consequent reduction of proteinuria.

- Thus, the more effective a given treatment is in lowering protein excretion, the greater the subsequent impact on protection from decline in GFR. This observation is the basis for the treatment guideline establishing 130/80 mmHg as a target blood pressure in proteinuric CKD patients.
- Several controlled studies have shown that ACE inhibitors and ARBs are effective in slowing the progression of renal failure in patients with advanced stages of both diabetic and nondiabetic CKD, in large part through effects on efferent vasodilatation and subsequent decline in glomerular hypertension.
- In the absence of an anti-proteinuric response with either agent alone, combined treatment with both ACE inhibitors and ARBs has been considered.
- Combination is associated with a greater reduction in proteinuria compared to either agent alone. Insofar as reduction in proteinuria is a surrogate for improved renal outcome, the combination would appear to be advantageous.
- However, there is a greater incidence of acute kidney injury and adverse cardiac events from such combination therapy. On balance, therefore, ACE inhibitor plus ARB therapy should be avoided.
- Progressive increase in serum creatinine concentration with these agents may suggest presence of renovascular disease within the large or small arteries.
- Development of side effects may mandate the use of second-line antihypertensive agents instead of ACE inhibitors/ARBs.
- Among the calcium channel blockers, diltiazem and verapamil may exhibit superior antiproteinuric and renoprotective effects compared to dihydropyridines.
- At least 2 different categories of response can be considered: one in which progression is strongly associated with systemic and intraglomerular hypertension and proteinuria (e.g. diabetic nephropathy, glomerular diseases) and in which ACE inhibitors and ARBs are likely to be first choice; and another in which proteinuria is mild or absent initially (e.g., adult polycystic kidney disease and other tubulointerstitial diseases), where contribution of intraglomerular hypertension is less prominent and other antihypertensive agents can be useful for control of systemic hypertension.

Ans. D

46. All are true about donor kidney evaluation except:

A. The 5 year survival rates still favor a partially matched (3/6 HLA mismatched) family donor over a randomly selected cadaver donor

B. For both living and deceased donors the 5 year outcomes are somewhat poorer if there is a complete (6/6) HLA mismatch

C. Selective renal arteriography need not be performed on donors

D. Living donors provide the advantage of immediate availability

Explanation:

- Selective renal arteriography should be performed on donors to rule out the presence of multiple or abnormal renal arteries, because the surgical procedure is difficult, and ischemic time of the transplanted kidney is long when there are vascular abnormalities.
- Transplant surgeons commonly use a laparoscopic approach to isolate and remove the living donor's kidney.
- This operation has the advantage of less evident surgical scars, and, as there is less tissue trauma, laparoscopic donors have a substantially shorter hospital stay and less discomfort than those who undergo an open nephrectomy.

Ans. C

47. Basement membrane syndromes include:

A. Alport's syndrome
B. Goodpasture's syndrome
C. Both of the above
D. None of the above

Explanation:

- Patients with a *basement membrane syndrome* either have genetically abnormal basement membranes (Alport's syndrome) or an autoimmune response to basement membrane collagen IV (Goodpasture's syndrome) associated with microscopic hematuria, mild to heavy proteinuria, and hypertension with variable elevations in serum creatinine.

Ans. C

48. Most common cause of peritonitis in patients undergoing continuous ambulatory peritoneal dialysis is:

A. Bacteroides fragilis
B. Staphylococcus aureus
C. Streptococcus
D. E.coli

Explanation:

- Most common organisms are *Staphylococcus* species, which accounted for ~45% of cases in one series.
- Historically, coagulase negative staphylococcal species were identified most commonly in these infections, but these isolates have more recently been decreasing in frequency.
- *Staphylococcus aureus* is more often involved among patients who are nasal carriers of the organism than among those who are not, and this organism is the most common pathogen in overt exit-site infections.
- Gram-negative bacilli and fungi such as *Candida* species are also found. Vancomycin-resistant enterococci and vancomycin-intermediate *S. Aureus* have been reported to produce peritonitis in CAPD patients.
- Finding of more than one organism in dialysate culture should prompt evaluation for secondary peritonitis.
- As with PBP, culture of dialysate fluid in blood culture bottles improves the yield.
- To facilitate diagnosis, several hundred milliliters of removed dialysis fluid should be concentrated by centrifugation before culture.

Ans. B

49. A 36 year old female presents to GN clinic with complaints of generalised body swelling with decreased urine output. Her 24 hour urine protein is 4.4 gm. Urine dipstick revealed protein 3+, RBC 2+. Renal biopsy was done. LM: doubling of GBM with mesangial and endocapillary hypercellularity. What diagnosis would you like to keep in this patient?

A. Mesangiocapillary GN
B. Mesangioproliferative GN
C. MCD
D. Membranous nephropathy

Explanation:

Type I MPGN, the most proliferative of the three types, shows mesangial proliferation with lobular segmentation on renal biopsy and mesangial interposition between the capillary basement membrane and endothelial cells, producing a double contour sometimes called *tram-tracking.* Subendothelial deposits with low serum levels of C3 are typical, although 50% of patients have normal levels of C3 and occasional intramesangial deposits. Low serum C3 and a dense thickening of the GBM containing ribbons of dense deposits and C3 characterize type II MPGN, *dense deposit disease.* Classically, the glomerular tuft has a lobular appearance; intramesangial deposits are rarely present and subendothelial deposits are generally absent. Proliferation in type III MPGN is less common than the other two types and is often focal; mesangial interposition is rare, and subepithelial deposits can occur along widened segments of the GBM that appear laminated and disrupted.

Ans. A

50. A 23 year old male, heavy smoker presented to ER with bouts of hemoptysis. His lab parameters indicated severe anaemia, urinalysis: protein 3+, RBC: 3+, severely deranged RFT. Renal biopsy was done. IF: linear staining for IgG. What is the differential diagnosis for this linear staining of IgG in IF apart from the obvious diagnosis of antiGBM disease?

A. Amyloidosis
B. Diabetic Glomerulosclerosis
C. MCD
D. MPGN

Explanation:

Within 1–2 years after the onset of clinical diabetes, morphologic changes appear in the kidney. Thickening of the GBM is a sensitive indicator for the presence of diabetes but correlates poorly with the presence or absence of clinically significant nephropathy. The composition of the GBM is altered notably with a loss of heparan sulfate moieties that form the negatively charged filtration barrier. This change results in increased filtration of serum proteins into the urine, predominately negatively charged albumin. The expansion of the mesangium due to the accumulation of extracellular matrix correlates with the clinical manifestations of diabetic nephropathy. This expansion in mesangial matrix is associated with the development of *mesangial sclerosis.* Some patients also develop eosinophilic, PAS+ nodules called *nodular glomerulosclerosis* or *Kimmelstiel-Wilson nodules.* Immunofluorescence microscopy often reveals the nonspecific deposition of IgG (at times in a linear pattern) or complement staining without immune deposits on electron microscopy.

Ans. B

51. A 18 year old male presented to OPD with complaint of hematuria. Urine dipstick was done in OPD which did not show any evidence of proteinuria. What differential pathologic diagnosis of glomerular hematuria without proteinuria, RBC cast or renal insufficiency should come to your mind?

A. IgA nephropathy
B. TBM nephropathy
C. Hereditary nephritis
D. All of the above

Explanation:

Table: Patterns of clinical glomerulonephritis

Glomerular Syndromes	Proteinuria	Hematuria	Vascular Injury
Acute Nephritic Syndromes			
Poststreptococcal glomerulonephritis[a]	+/++	+/+++	–
Subacute bacterial endocarditis[a]	+/++	++	–
Lupus nephritis[a]	+/++	++/+++	+
Antiglomerular basement membrane disease[a]	++	++/+++	–
IgA nephropathy[a]	+/++	+++[a]	–
ANCA small-vessel vasculitis[a]			
• Granulomatosis with polyangiitis (Wegener's)	+/++	++/+++	++++
• Microscopic polyangiitis	+/++	++/+++	++++
• Churg-Strauss syndrome	+/++	++/+++	++++
Henoch-Schönlein purpura[a]	+/++	++/+++	++++
Cryoglobulinemia[a]	+/++	++/+++	++++
Membranoproliferative glomerulonephritis[a]	++	++/+++	–
C_3 Glomerulopathies	++	++/+++	–
Mesangioproliferative glomerulonephritis	+	+/++	–

Contd.

Contd.

Pulmonary-Renal Syndromes			
Goodpasture's syndrome[a]	++	++/+++	–
ANCA small-vessel vasculitis[a]			
• Granulomatosis with polyangiitis (Wegener's)	+/++	++/+++	++++
• Microscopic polyangiitis	+/++	++/+++	++++
• Churg-Strauss syndrome	+/++	++/+++	++++
Henoch-Schölein purpura[a]	+/++	++/+++	++++
Cryoglobulinemia[a]	+/++	++/+++	++++
Nephrotic Syndromes			
Minimal change disease	++++	–	–
Focal segmental glomerulosclerosis	+++/++++	+	–
Membranous glomerulonephritis	++++	+	–
Diabetic nephropathy	++/++++	–/+	–
AL and AA amyloidosis	+++/++++	+	+/++
Light-chain deposition disease	+++	+	–
Fibrillary-immunotactoid disease	+++/++++	+	+
Fabry's disease	+	+	–
Basement Membrane Syndromes			
Anti-GBM disease[a]	++	++/+++	–
Alport's syndrome	++	++	–
Thin basement membrane disease	+	++	–
Nail-patella syndrome	++/+++	++	–
Glomerular Vascular Syndromes			
Atherosclerotic nephropathy	+	+	+++
Hypertensive nephropathy[b]	+/++	+/++	++
Cholesterol emboli	+/++	++	+++
Sickle cell disease	+/++	+++[c]	+++
Thrombotic microangiopathies	++	++	+++
Antiphospholipid syndrome	++	++	+++
ANCA small-vessel vasculitis[a]			
• Granulomatosis with polyangiitis (Wegener's)	+/++	++/+++	++++
• Microscopic polyangiitis	+/++	++/+++	++++
• Churg-Strauss syndrome	+++	++/+++	++++
Henoch-Schönlein purpura[b]	+/++	++/+++	++++
Cryoglobulinemia[a]	+/++	++/+++	++++
AL and AA amyloidosis	+++/++++	+	+/++
Infectious Disease-Associated Syndromes			
Poststreptococcal glomerulonephiritis[a]	+/++	++/+++	–
Subacute bacterial endocarditis[a]	+/++	++	–
HIV	+++	+/++	–
Hepatitis B and C	+++	+/++	–
Syphilis	+++	+	–
Leprosy	+++	+	–
Malaria	+++	+/++	–
Schistosomiasis	+++	+/++	–

Ans. D

52. A 45 year old male known case of type 2 DM presented with complaint of generalised body swelling; hypertension; oliguria. Urine R/M did not reveal any abnormalities. Which of the following anti diabetic drug may be associated with this sort of picture of nephritic syndrome?

A. Tolbutamide
B. Linagliptin
C. Saxagliptin
D. Dapagliflozin

Explanation:

There is an *acute nephritic syndrome* producing 1–2 g/24 h of proteinuria, hematuria with red blood cell casts, pyuria, hypertension, fluid retention, and a rise in serum creatinine associated with a reduction in glomerular filtration. If glomerular inflammation develops slowly, the serum creatinine will rise gradually over many weeks, but if the serum creatinine rises quickly, particularly over a few days, acute nephritis is sometimes called *rapidly progressive glomerulonephritis* (RPGN); the histopathologic term *crescentic glomerulonephritis* is the pathologic equivalent of the clinical presentation of RPGN. When patients with RPGN present with lung hemorrhage from Goodpasture's syndrome, antineutrophil cytoplasmic antibodies (ANCA)-associated small-vessel vasculitis, lupus erythematosus, or cryoglobulinemia, they are often diagnosed as having a *pulmonary-renal syndrome.*

Ans. A

53. A 26 year old male; athlete by profession had his routine tests done. Urine R/M revealed Urine protein:2+. Which of the following statement regarding orthostatic proteinuria is correct?

A. Most common in elderly
B Proteinuria in recumbent position
C. Maximum have damaged glomeruli in LM
D. Maximum with proteinuria of <1gm/day

Explanation:

Sustained proteinuria >1–2 g/24 h is also commonly associated with glomerular disease. Patients often will not know they have proteinuria unless they become edematous or notice foaming urine on voiding. *Sustained proteinuria* has to be distinguished from lesser amounts of so-called *benign proteinuria* in the normal population. This latter class of proteinuria is nonsustained, generally <1 g/24 h, and is sometimes called *functional* or *transient proteinuria.* Fever, exercise, obesity, sleep apnea, emotional stress, and congestive heart failure can explain transient proteinuria. Proteinuria only seen with upright posture is called *orthostatic proteinuria* and has a benign prognosis. Isolated proteinuria sustained over multiple clinic visits is found in many glomerular lesions. Proteinuria in most adults with glomerular disease is *nonselective*, containing albumin and a mixture of other serum proteins, whereas in children with *minimal change disease* (MCD), the proteinuria is *selective* and composed largely of albumin.

Ans. D

54. A 8 year old female presented with complaints of generalised body swelling. Urine dipstick revealed Protein: 4+; RBC:2+. Renal biopsy was planned. Which of the following is the most common IF finding in MCD?

A. Low level mesangial staining for IgM
B. Mesangial electron dense deposits
C. Well defined irregular focal/segmental stain for IgM
D. All of the above

Explanation:

MCD on renal biopsy shows no obvious glomerular lesion by light microscopy and is negative for deposits by immunofluorescent microscopy, or occasionally shows small amounts of IgM in the mesangium Electron microscopy, however, consistently demonstrates an effacement of the foot processes supporting the epithelial podocytes with weakening of slit-pore membranes.

Ans. A

55. A 18 year old athletic man with no significant past medical history is found to have isolated asymptomatic microscopic hematuria on routine examination. Which of the following observations suggests hematuria of glomerular origin?

A. >40% dysmorphic RBC or 5% acanthocytes
B. >20% dysmorphic RBC or 2% acanthocytes
C. >10% dysmorphic RBC or 10% acanthocytes
D. >50% dysmorphic RBC or 3% acanthocytes

Explanation:

As few as 3–5 red blood cells in the spun sediment from first-voided morning urine is suspicious. The diagnosis of glomerular injury can be delayed because patients will not realize they have *microscopic hematuria*, and only rarely with the exception of IgA nephropathy and sickle cell disease is *gross hematuria* present.

Ans. A

56. A 28 year old female is referred by a physician for complete evaluation of isolated proteinuria (Urine R/M: Protein: 2+). Her 24 hour protein is 1.4gm/day. Her RFT are normal. What would be the future status of her renal function in coming 10 years?

A. No relationship between proteinuria and renal disease
B. Detrimental with progressive renal disease
C. Require renal biopsy
D. Impossible to predict at this time

Explanation:

Table: Urine assays for albuminuria/Proteinuria				
	24-h Albumin[a] (mg/24 h)	Albumin[a]/ Creatinine Ratio (mg/g)	Dipstick Proteinuria	24-h Urine Protein[b] (mg/24 h)
Normal	8–10	< 30	–	< 150
Microalbuminuria	30–300	30–300	–/Trace/1+	–
Proteinuria	> 300	> 300	Trace–3+	> 150

Ans. B

57. A 8 year old male presented to OPD for the first time with generalised body swelling with slightly decreased urine output. His Urine R/M revealed protein: 4+. His RFT, C3, C4 were normal. Keeping the clinical diagnosis as MCD he was started on full dose steroids. Which of the following is true with respect to MCD?

A. First described by Munk
B. Also known as lipoid nephrosis
C. Maximum in less then 10 yrs of age
D. All of the above

Explanation:

MCD, sometimes known as *nil lesion,* causes 70–90% of nephrotic syndrome in childhood but only 10–15% of nephrotic syndrome in adults. MCD usually presents as a primary renal disease but can be associated with several other conditions, including Hodgkin's disease, allergies, or use of nonsteroidal anti-inflammatory agents; significant interstitial nephritis often accompanies cases associated with nonsteroidal drug use.

Ans. D

58. A child was referred to endocrinologist from pediatric surgeon with history of penoscrotal hypospadias. And was diagnosed to have Reifenstein syndrome which is:

A. Complete testosterone resistance
B. Partial testosterone resistance
C. Complete oestrogen resistance
D. Partial oestrogen resistance

Explanation:

- **Paritial AIS (Reifenstein's syndrome) results from androgen receptor mutations that maintain residual function. Patients often present in infancy with penoscrotal hypospadias and undescended testes and with gynecomastia at the time of puberty.**

Ans. B.

59. A 10 year old male with diagnosis of MCD was started on oral steroids. Which of the following classifies this patient as a primary responder?

A. Complete remission with 1 course of steroids
B. Complete remission within 1 year of treatment
C. Complete remission within 6 months of treatment
D. Complete remission with 2 course of steroids

Explanation:

- Although up to 30% of children have a spontaneous remission, all children today are treated with steroids; only children who are nonresponders are biopsied in this setting.
- Primary responders are patients who have a complete remission (<0.2 mg/24 h of proteinuria) after a single course of prednisone; steroid-dependent patients relapse as their steroid dose is tapered. Frequent relapsers have two or more relapses in the 6 months following taper, and steroid-resistant patients fail to respond to steroid therapy. Adults are not considered steroid-resistant until after 4 months of therapy.
- Ninety to 95% of children will develop a complete remission after 8 weeks of steroid therapy, and 80–85% of adults will achieve complete remission, but only after a longer course of 20–24 weeks.
- Patients with steroid resistance may have FSGS on repeat biopsy.
- Some hypothesize that if the first renal biopsy does not have a sample of deeper corticomedullary glomeruli, then the correct diagnosis of FSGS may be missed.

Ans. A

60. All are true about albuminuria except:

A. Mean of 8 to 10 mg/24 h of albumin appears in the urine in the absence of kidney disease
B. Sustained proteinuria >1 to 2 g/24 h is also commonly associated with glomerular disease
C. Proteinuria only seen with upright posture is called orthostatic proteinuria and has worse prognosis
D. Greater than 300 mg/24 h of albuminuria represents frank proteinuria and more advanced renal disease

Explanation:

- Sustained proteinuria >1–2 g/24 h is also commonly associated with glomerular disease. Patients often will not know they have proteinuria unless they become edematous or notice foaming urine on voiding.
- Sustained proteinuria has to be distinguished from lesser amounts of so-called benign proteinuria in the normal population. This latter class of proteinuria is nonsustained, generally <1 g/24 h, and is sometimes called functional or transient proteinuria. Fever, exercise, obesity, sleep apnea, emotional stress, and congestive heart failure can explain transient proteinuria.
- **Proteinuria only seen with upright posture is called orthostatic proteinuria and has a benign prognosis.** Isolated proteinuria sustained over multiple clinic visits is found in many glomerular lesions.
- Proteinuria in most adults with glomerular disease is nonselective, containing albumin and a mixture of other serum proteins, selective and composed largely of albumin.

Ans. C

61. Both PLCO and ERSPC trials are done for:

A. Lung cancer screening
B. Prostate cancer screening
C. Ovarian cancer screening
D. Cervical cancer screening

Explanation:

- European Randomized Study of Screening for Prostate Cancer (ERSPC) was a multinational study that randomized ~182,000 men between age 50 and 74 years (with a predefined "core" screening group of men age 55–69 years) to receive PSA testing or no screening.
- Recruitment and randomization procedures, as well as actual frequency of PSA testing, varied by country.
- After a median follow-up of 13 years, a 21% relative reduction in the risk of prostate cancer death in screened arm was noted in the "core" screening group.
- Trial found that 781 (95% CI 490–1,929) men would need to be invited to screening, and 27 (95% CI 17–66) cases of prostate cancer detected, to avert 1 death from prostate cancer. Of the seven countries included in the mortality analysis, two demonstrated statistically significant reductions in prostate cancer deaths, whereas five did not.
- There was also an imbalance in treatment between the two study arms, with a higher proportion of men with clinically localized cancer receiving radical prostatectomy in screening arm and receiving it at experienced referral centers.

Ans. B

62. Disorders involving proximal tubule include all except:

A. Cystinuria
B. Bartters syndrome
C. Dent disease
D. Hartnup syndrome

Explanation:

Table: Disorders involving the proximal tubule

Disease or syndrome	Gene
Proximal renal tubular acidosis	Sodium bicarbonate cotransporter (*SLC4A4,* 4q21)
Fanconi-Bickel syndrome	Glucose transporter, GLUT2 (*SLC2A2,* 3q26.2)
Isolated renal glycosuria	Sodium glucose cotransporter (*SLC5A2,* 16p11.2)
Cystinuria	
• Type I	Cystine, dibasic and neutral amino acid transporter (*SLC3A1,* 2p16.3)
• Non-type I	Amino acid transporter, light subunit (*SLC7A9,* 19q13.1)
Lysinuric protein intolerance	Amino acid transporter (*SLC7A7,* 4q11.2)
Hartnup disorder	Neutral amino acid transporter (*SLC6A19,* 5p15.33)
Hereditary hypophosphatemic rickets with hypercalcemia	Sodium phosphate cotransporter (*SLC34A,* 9q34)
Renal hypouricemia	
• Type 1	Urate-anion exchanger (*SLC22A12,* 11q13)
• Type 2	Urate transporter, GLUT9 (*SLC2A9,* 4p16.1)
Dent disease	Chloride channel, CIC-5 (*CLCN5,* Xp11.22)
X-linked recessive nephrolithiasis with renal failure	Chloride channel, CIC-5 (*CLCN5,* Xp11.22)
X-linked recessive hypophosphatemic rickets	Chloride channel, CIC-5 (*CLCN5,* Xp11.22)

Ans. B

63. All are true statements except:

A. Apical membrane face the tubular lumen & basolateral membrane face interstitium
B. Renal epithelial cells are polarized
C. Proximal tubule contains leaky epithelia, collecting duct contain tight epithelia
D. Leaky epithelia are allow for more refined control and regulation of transport, whereas tight epithelia most well suited for bulk fluid reabsorption

Explanation:

- There are two types of epithelial transport. Movement of fluid and solutes sequentially across the apical and basolateral cell membranes (or vice versa) mediated by transporters, channels, or pumps is called cellular transport.
- By contrast, movement of fluid and solutes through the narrow passageway between adjacent cells is called paracellular transport.
- Paracellular transport occurs through tight junctions, indicating that they are not completely "tight" or occlusive.
- Indeed, some epithelial cell layers allow rather robust paracellular transport to occur (leaky epithelia), whereas other epithelia have more restrictive tight junctions (tight epithelia).
- In addition, because the ability of ions to flow through the paracellular pathway determines the electrical resistance across the epithelial monolayer, leaky and tight epithelia are also referred to as low- or high-resistance epithelia, respectively.
- Proximal tubule contains leaky epithelia, whereas distal nephron segments, such as the collecting duct, contain tight epithelia.
- Leaky epithelia are most well suited for bulk fluid reabsorption, whereas tight epithelia allow for more refined control and regulation of transport.

Ans. D

64. Type of RTA seen in Multiple myeloma is:

A. Type 1
B. Type 2
C. Type 3
D. Type 4

Explanation:

- Earliest manifestation of this tubular damage is the adult Fanconi's syndrome (a type 2 proximal renal tubular acidosis), with loss of glucose & amino acids, as well as defects in ability of the kidney to acidify and concentrate urine.
- Proteinuria is not accompanied by hypertension & protein is nearly all light chains.

Ans. B

65. Accepted threshold for bacteriuria to meet definition of catheter associated UTI is:

A. >/= 10^3 CFU/ml of urine
B. >/= 10^4 CFU/ml of urine
C. >/= 10^5 CFU/ml of urine
D. >/= 10^6 CFU/ml of urine

Explanation:

- Multiple institutions have released guidelines for the treatment of CAUTI, which is defined by bacteriuria and symptoms in a catheterized patient. The signs and symptoms either are localized to urinary tract or can include otherwise unexplained systemic manifestations, such as fever.
- Accepted threshold for bacteriuria to meet the definition of CAUTI is $\geq 10^3$ CFU/mL of urine, while the threshold for bacteriuria to meet the definition of ASB is $\geq 10^5$ CFU/mL.

Ans. A

66. Conditions predispose to stone formation are all except:

A. Primary hyperparathyroidism
B. Obesity
C. Type 1 DM
D. Distal RTA

Explanation:

- Several conditions predispose to stone formation, including gastrointestinal malabsorption (e.g., Crohn's disease, gastric bypass surgery), primary hyperparathyroidism, obesity, type 2 diabetes mellitus, and distal renal tubular acidosis.

- A number of other medical conditions are more likely to be present in individuals with a history of nephrolithiasis, including hypertension, gout, cardiovascular disease, cholelithiasis, reduced bone mineral density, and chronic kidney disease.

Ans. C

67. Dipeptidyl peptidase 4 inhibitors safe in renal disease is:

A. Alogliptin B. Linagliptin

C. Saxagliptin D. Sitagliptin

Explanation:

Table: Agents used for treatment of type 1 or type 2 diabetes

	Mechanism of Action	Examples[a]	HBA_{1C} Reduction (%)[b]	Agent-Specific Advantages	Agent-Specific Disadvantages	Contraindi-ca-tions
Oral						
Biguanides[C+]	↓ Hepatic glucose production	Metformin	1-2	Weight neutral, do not cause hypoglycemia, inexpensive, extensive experience, ↓CV events	Diarrhea, nausea, lactic acidosis, vitamin B_{12} deficiency	Renal insufficiency (see text for GFR < 45 ml/min), CHF, radiographic contrast studies, hospitalized patients, acidosis
α-Glucosidase inhibitors[c++]	↓ GI glucose absorption	Acarbose, miglitol, voglibose	0.5-0.8	Reduce postprandial glycemia	GI flatulence, liver function tests	Renal/liver disease
Dipeptidyl peptidase IV inhibitors[c+++]	Prolong endogenous GLP-1 action; ↑Insulin ↓glucagon	Alogliptin, linagliptin, saxagliptin, sitagliptin, vildagliptin	0.5-0.8	Well tolerated, do not cause hypoglycemia	Angioedema/ urticarial and immune-mediated dermatologic effects	Reduced dose with renal disease
Insulin secretagogues: Sulfonylureas[c+]	↑ Insulin secretion	Glibomuride, gliclazide, glimepiride, glipizide, gliquidone, glyburide, glyclopyramide	1-2	Short onset of action, lower postprandial glucose, inexpensive	Hypoglycemia, weight gain	Renal/liver disease
Insulin secretagogues: Non-sulfonylureas[c+++]	↑ Insulin secretion	Mitiglinide nateglinide, repaglinide	0.5-1.0	Short onset of action, lower postprandial glucose	Hypoglycemia	Renal/liver disease
Sodium-glucose contransporter 2 inhibitors***	↑ Renal glucose excretion	Canagliflazin, dapagliflazin, empagliflozin, ertugliflozin	0.5-1.0	Do not cause hypoglycemia, ↓ weight and BP; see text for CVD effect	Urinary and genital infections, polyuria, dehydration, exacerbate tendency to hyperkalemia and DKA; see text	Moderate renal insufficiency, insulin-deficient DM
Thiazolidinediones[c+++]	↓ Insulin resistance, ↑ glucose utilization	Pioglitazone, rosiglitazone	0.5-1.4	Lower insulin requirements	Peripheral edema, CHF, weight gain, fractures, macular edema	CHF, liver disease

Ans. B

68. True about treatment & prognosis of HSP is:

A. No spontaneous recovery
B. Renal biopsy used for diagnosis
C. Treatment different for children & adults
D. Steroid not useful in skin & renal disease

Explanation:

- Prognosis of IgA vasculitis (Henoch-Schönlein) is excellent. Mortality is exceedingly rare, and 1–5% of children progress to end-stage renal disease.
- Most patients recover completely, and some do not require therapy. Treatment is similar for adults and children.
- When glucocorticoid therapy is required, prednisone, in doses of 1 mg/kg/d and tapered according to clinical response, has been shown to be useful in decreasing tissue edema, arthralgias, and abdominal discomfort; however, it has not proved beneficial in the treatment of skin or renal disease and does not appear to shorten the duration of active disease or lessen the chance of recurrence.
- Patients with rapidly progressive glomerulonephritis have been anecdotally reported to benefit from intensive plasma exchange combined with cytotoxic drugs.
- Disease recurrences have been reported in 10–40% of patients.

Ans. D

69. Grossly kidney has subcapsular hemorrhage with flea bitten appearance in which acute nephritis syndrome?

A. Lupus nephritis
B. Post streptococcal nephritis
C. Subacute bacterial endocarditis
D. All of the above

Explanation:

- Endocarditis-associated glomerulonephritis is typically a complication of SBE, particularly in patients who remain untreated for a long time, have negative blood cultures, or have right-sided endocarditis.
- Common comorbidities are valvular heart disease, intravenous drug use, hepatitis C, and diabetes mellitus.
- Glomerulonephritis is unusual in acute bacterial endocarditis because it takes 10–14 days to develop immune complex–mediated injury, by which time the patient has been treated, often with emergent surgery.
- Grossly, the kidneys in SBE have subcapsular hemorrhages with a "flea-bitten" appearance, and microscopy on renal biopsy reveals focal proliferation around foci of necrosis associated with abundant mesangial, subendothelial, and subepithelial immune deposits of IgG, IgM, and C3.
- Commonly patients present with a clinical picture of RPGN and have crescents on biopsy.
- Embolic infarcts or septic abscesses may also be present.

Ans. C

70. Which class of Lupus nephritis is having high titer of dsDNA Antibody?

A. Class II
B. Class III
C. Class IV
D. Class V

Explanation:

- Class IV describes *global, diffuse proliferative lesions* involving the vast majority of glomeruli. Patients with class IV lesions commonly have high antiDNA antibody titers, low serum complement, hematuria, red blood cell casts, proteinuria, hypertension, and decreased renal function; 50% of patients have nephrotic-range proteinuria. Patients with crescents on biopsy often have a rapidly progressive decline in renal function.

Ans. C

71. Not true about Nephrotic syndrome is:

A. Higher the 24 hr urine protein excretion, more rapid is decline in GFR

B. All patients with hypercholesterolemia are treated with lipid lowering agents

C. Venous complications treated with anticoagulants

D. Proteinuria treated with CCB

Explanation:

- Therapies for various causes of nephrotic syndrome are noted under individual disease headings below. In general, all patients with hypercholesterolemia secondary to nephrotic syndrome should be treated with lipid-lowering agents because they are at increased risk for cardiovascular disease. Edema secondary to salt and water retention can be controlled with the judicious use of diuretics, avoiding intravascular volume depletion. Venous complications secondary to the hypercoagulable state associated with nephrotic syndrome can be treated with anticoagulants.
- Losses of various serum binding proteins, such as thyroid-binding globulin, lead to alterations in functional tests. Lastly, proteinuria itself is hypothesized to be nephrotoxic, and treatment of proteinuria with inhibitors of the renin-angiotensin system can lower urinary protein excretion.

Ans. D

72. True about drug induced lupus is:

A. Syndrome of +ve ANA associated with symptoms such as fever, malaise, arthritis or intense arthralgia/myalgia, serositis &/or rash

B. Predominant in blacks, has less female predilicton than SLE

C. Commonly associated with anti ds DNA & anti histone antibodies

D. ANA usually appears after symptoms develop

Explanation:

- This is a syndrome of positive ANA associated with symptoms such as fever, malaise, arthritis or intense arthralgias/myalgias, serositis, and/or rash.
- Syndrome appears during therapy with certain medications and biologic agents, is predominant in whites, has less female predilection than SLE, rarely involves kidneys or brain, is rarely associated with anti-dsDNA, is commonly associated with antibodies to histones, and usually resolves over several weeks after discontinuation of offending medication.
- List of substances that can induce lupus like disease is long. Among the most frequent are the antiarrhythmics procainamide, disopyramide, and propafenone; the anti-hypertensive hydralazine; several angiotensin-converting enzyme inhibitors and beta blockers; the antithyroid propylthiouracil; the antipsychotics chlorpromazine and lithium; the anticonvulsants carbamazepine and phenytoin; the antibiotics isoniazid, minocycline, and nitrofurantoin (Macrodantin); the antirheumatic sulfasalazine; the diuretic hydrochlorothiazide; the antihyperlipidemics lovastatin and simvastatin.
- Biologics that can cause drug-induced lupus (DIL) include inhibitors of IFNs and TNF. In DIL, ANA usually appears before symptoms; however, many of the medications mentioned above induce ANA in patients who never develop symptoms of drug-induced lupus. It is appropriate to test for ANA at the first hint of relevant symptoms and to use test results to help decide whether to withdraw the suspect agent.

Ans. A

73. Clinical features of Amphotericin B nephrotoxicity include all except:

A. Polyuria
B. Hypomagnesemia
C. Hypophosphatemia
D. Hypocalcemia

Explanation:

- Amphotericin B causes renal vasoconstriction from an increase in tubuloglomerular feedback as well as direct tubular toxicity mediated by reactive oxygen species.
- Nephrotoxicity from amphotericin B is dose and duration dependent. This drug binds to tubular membrane cholesterol and introduces pores.
- Clinical features of amphotericin B nephrotoxicity include polyuria, hypomagnesemia, hypocalcemia, and nongap metabolic acidosis.

Ans. C

74. Uromodulin most common protein in urine produced in which part:

A. PCT
B. Thick ascending limb of loop of henle
C. DCT
D. CD

Explanation:

- Pathogenic factors for AKI due to endogenous toxins include intrarenal vasoconstriction, direct proximal tubular toxicity, and mechanical obstruction of the distal nephron lumen when myoglobin or hemoglobin precipitates with Tamm-Horsfall protein (uromodulin, the most common protein in urine and produced in the thick ascending limb of the loop of Henle), a process favored by acidic urine.
- Tumor lysis syndrome may follow initiation of cytotoxic therapy in patients with high-grade lymphomas and acute lymphoblastic leukemia; massive release of uric acid (with serum levels often exceeding 15 mg/dL) leads to precipitation of uric acid in the renal tubules and AKI.

Ans. B

75. In chronic renal failure which is seen?

A. Normal anion gap
B. Increased anion gap
C. Decreased anion gap
D. Metabolic alkalosis

Explanation:

- In CKD, Anion gap increased
- Other conditions associated with increased anion gap- Milk alkali syndrome, Uremia, DKA, Lactic acidosis, Salicylates & Isoniazid toxicity

Ans. B

76. A 28 year old male presented to OPD with anuria since 2 days with c/o arthralgia, fever since 1 month. Lab parameters: severe anaemia; severely deranged RFT; Normal C3 and C4,Urinalysis revealed protein 2+ RBC 4+ RBC cast; ANA negative, cANCA 4+positive.CXR :cavity lesions. Which of the following patterns in renal biopsy is expected?

A. MCD
B. MPGN
C. FSGS
D. Crescentic GN

Explanation:

- In its earliest form, renal involvement is characterized by a focal and segmental glomeruli is that may evolve into a rapidly progressive crescentic glomerulonephritis.
- Granuloma formation is only rarely seen on renal biopsy. In contrast to other forms of glomerulonephritis, evidence of immune complex deposition is not found in the renal lesion of granulomatosis with polyangiitis

(Wegener's). In addition to the classic triad of disease of the upper and lower respiratory tracts and kidney, virtually any organ can be involved with vasculitis, granuloma, or both.

- Immunopathogenesis of this disease is unclear, although the involvement of upper airways and lungs with granulomatous vasculitis suggests an aberrant cell-mediated immune response to an exogenous or even endogenous antigen that enters through or resides in the upper airway.
- Chronic nasal carriage of *Staphylococcus aureus* has been reported to be associated with a higher relapse rate of granulomatosis with polyangiitis (Wegener's); however, there is no evidence for a role of this organism in the pathogenesis of the disease.

Ans. D

77. A 32 year old female presents to GN clinic with complaints of generalised body swelling with decreased urine output. Her 24 hour urine protein is 4.2 gm. Urine dipstick revealed protein 3+, RBC 2+. Renal biopsy was done. IF revealed intense capillary wall band like staining for C3 without Ig/C4/C1q. Fundoscopy shows Drusen bodies in the retina. Which of the following treatment has been tried for this disease?

A. Eculizumab B. Mepolizumab

C. Bevacizumab D. Anakinra

Explanation:

- C3GN patients are clinically less well defined but ~2/3 have hematuria and 1/3 proteinuria. In addition to renal biopsy serological and genetic evaluation may be indicated including measurement of C3 levels which are typically low with normal C4 levels, C3 nephritic factor, Factor H, paraprotein detection and specific CFHR genetic mutations.
- Optimal therapies remain undefined but include inhibition of the renin-angiotensin system, anticoagulants, steroids and other immunosuppressant. Increasing evidence suggests benefit of therapy with eculizumab, monoclonal antibody directed at C5 which is activated by C3.

Ans. A

78. A 22 year old male presented to OPD with generalised body swelling with nocturia. His urine dipstick: Protein: 3+; RBC: 2+. His USG KUB was suggestive of HDUN. Cystoscopy revealed "sandy patches". Which helminth may be associated with this picture?

A. Instestinal flukes B. Lung flukes

C. Schistosomiasis D. All of the above

Explanation:

- Signs and symptoms of *S. haematobium* infection relate to the worms' predilection for the veins of the urogenital tract.
- Two stages of infection are recognized.
- An active stage occurring mainly in children, adolescents, and younger adults is characterized by egg excretion in urine, with proteinuria and macroscopic or microscopic hematuria and deposition of eggs in the urinary tract.
- Chronic stage in older individuals is characterized by sparse or no urinary egg excretion despite urogenital tract pathology.
- A characteristic sign in the active stage is painless, terminal hematuria. Dysuria and suprapubic discomfort or pain are associated with active urogenital schistosomiasis and may persist throughout the course of active infection.
- Eggs deposited in the bladder mucosa may give rise to an intense inflammatory response of the bladder wall, which may cause ureteric obstruction and lead to hydroureter and hydronephrosis. These early inflammatory lesions, including obstructive uropathy, can be visualized by ultrasonography.
- As the infection progresses, the inflammatory component decreases and fibrosis becomes more prominent. The symptoms at this stage are nocturia, urine retention, dribbling, and incontinence. Cystoscopy reveals "sandy patches" composed of large numbers of calcified eggs surrounded by fibrous tissue and an atrophic

mucosal surface. The ureters are less commonly involved, but ureteral fibrosis can cause irreversible obstructive uropathy that can progress to uremia.

Ans. C

79. A 26 year old female presents to GN clinic with complaints of generalised body swelling with decreased urine output. Her 24 hour urine protein is 4.4 gm. Urine dipstick revealed protein 3+, RBC 2+. Low C3 and normal C4. Renal biopsy was done. LM: doubling of GBM with mesangial and endocapillary hyper-cellularity. Which of the following MPGN subtypes is the "most proliferative"?

A. Type 1
B. Type 2
C. Type 3
D. Type 4

Explanation:

- Type I MPGN, the most proliferative of the three types, shows mesangial proliferation with lobular segmentation on renal biopsy and mesangial interposition between the capillary basement membrane and endothelial cells, producing a double contour sometimes called *tram-tracking*

Ans. A

80. A 28 year old female presents to GN clinic with complaints of generalised body swelling with decreased urine output. Her 24 hour urine protein is 4.4 gm. Urine dipstick revealed protein 3+, RBC 2+. Low C3 and low C4. Renal biopsy was done. LM: doubling of GBM with mesangial and endocapillary hypercellularity. Which of the following complement pathway is activated?

A. Classic
B. Alternative
C. Lectin
D. None of the above

Explanation:

- Minority of cases of MPGN type I have C3 but not immunoglobulin deposits on biopsy and are best considered as in the category of a C3 glomerulopathy.
- *Types II and III MPGN* can be idiopathic, and immunoglobulin-mediated disease (driven by the classical complement pathway) but the majority of cases formerly defined as MPGN type II and III are non-immunoglobulin-mediated and driven by the alternate complement pathway.

Ans. A

81. Following schematic figure represents which of the following glomerulonephritis?

Glomerular schematic 3

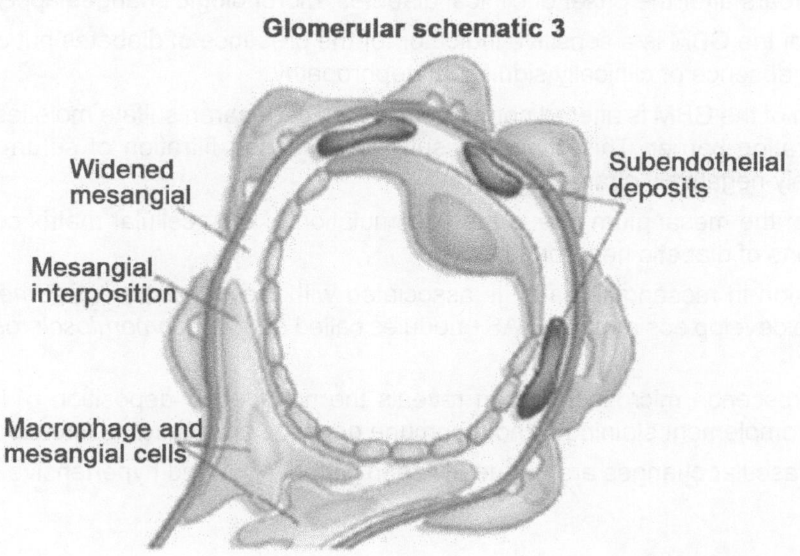

A. Membranoproliferative GN type 1
B. Mesangioproliferative GN
C. Diabetic glomerulosclerosis
D. FSGS

Explanation:

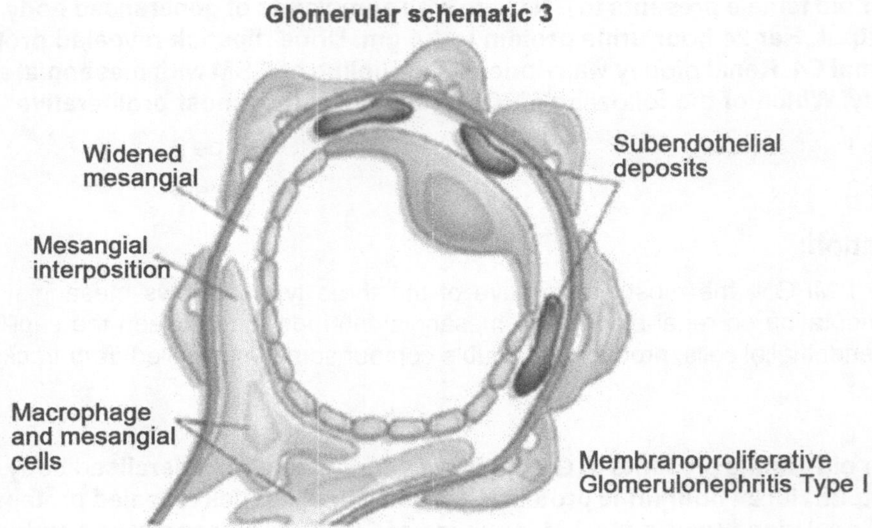

Ans. A

82. A type 2 DM patient is referred from CHC to your hospital. His 24 hour urine protein is 2.2 gm. His BP is 150/80mm Hg. His HbAIC is 7.2%. Which one of the following statements is false with respect to Diabetic Nephropathy?

A. Natural history of diabetic nephropathy in patients with types 1 and 2 diabetes is similar
B. Expansion of the mesangium due to the accumulation of extracellular matrix correlates with the clinical manifestations of diabetic nephropathy
C. Thickening of the GBM is a sensitive indicator for the presence of diabetes only
D. Thickening of the GBM is sensitive indicator for the presence of diabetic nephropathy

Explanation:

- Within 1–2 years after the onset of clinical diabetes, morphologic changes appear in the kidney.
- Thickening of the GBM is a sensitive indicator for the presence of diabetes but correlates poorly with the presence or absence of clinically significant nephropathy.
- Composition of the GBM is altered notably with a loss of heparan sulfate moieties that form the negatively charged filtration barrier. This change results in increased filtration of serum proteins into the urine, predominately negatively charged albumin.
- Expansion of the mesangium due to the accumulation of extracellular matrix correlates with the clinical manifestations of diabetic nephropathy.
- This expansion in mesangial matrix is associated with the development of *mesangial sclerosis.* Some patients also develop eosinophilic, PAS+ nodules called *nodular glomerulosclerosis* or *Kimmelstiel-Wilson nodules*.
- Immunofluorescence microscopy often reveals the nonspecific deposition of IgG (at times in a linear pattern) or complement staining without immune deposits on electron microscopy.
- Prominent vascular changes are frequently seen with hyaline and hypertensive arteriosclerosis.

Ans. D

83. A 18 year old male presents to nephrology OPD with mild body swelling. Urine dipstick revealed Protein: 3+; RBC: 2+. Slit lamp examination: Anterior lenticonus. Renal biopsy: EM revealed following picture. Most likely diagnosis is:

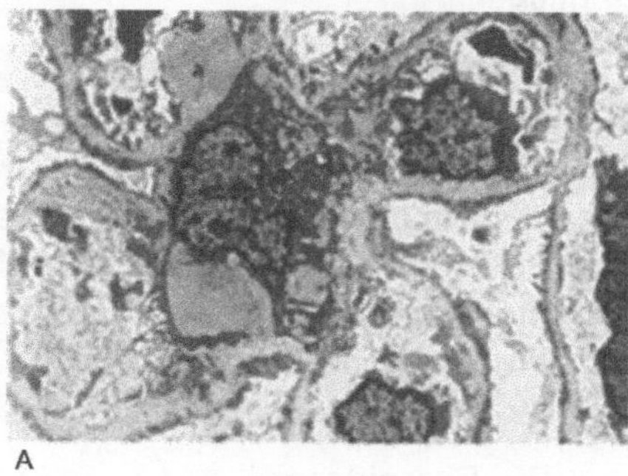
A

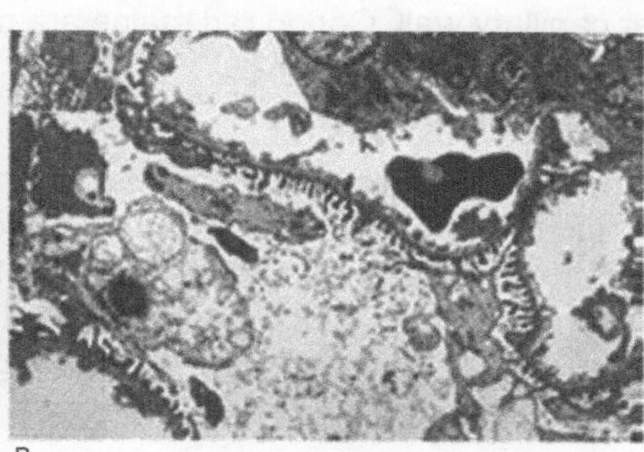
B

A. Fabry's disease
B. Nail-patella syndrome
C. TBM disease
D. Alport syndrome

Explanation:

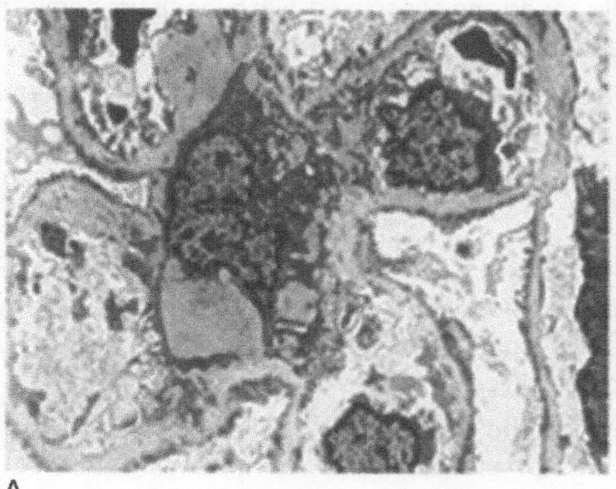
A

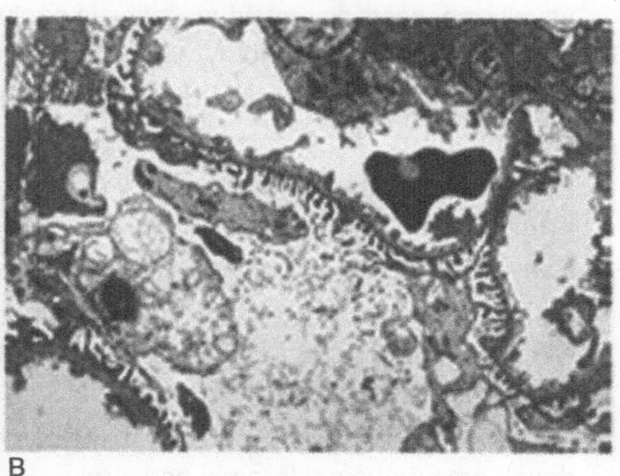
B

Figure: Alport's syndrome and thin glomerular basement membrane lesion. In Alport's syndrome, there is irregular thinning alternating with thickened so-called basket-weaving abnormal organization of the glomerular basement membrane **(A)** In benign familial hematuria, or in early cases of Alport's syndrome or female carriers, only extensive thinning of the glomerular basement membrane is seen by electron microscopy **(B)** (ABN Nanderbilt Collection)

Ans. D

84. Match the following disease states with EM findings of the glomeruli:

1. Amyloidosis	**A. Randomly arranged fibrils with 12-24 nm in diameter**
2. Fibrillary GN	**B. Randomly arranged fibrils with 8-12 nm in diameter**
3. Immunotactoid GN	**C. Microtubular structures with diameter of >30 nm in diameter**

A. 1A,2B,3C
B. 1B,2A,3C
C. 2A,1C,3B
D. 3A,1C,2B

Explanation:

- Some classify amyloid and nonamyloid fibril-associated renal diseases all as fibrillary glomerulopathies with immunotactoid glomerulopathy reserved for nonamyloid fibrillary disease not associated with a systemic illness.

- Others define fibrillary glomerulonephritis as a nonamyloid fibrillary disease with fibrils 12–24 nm and immunotactoid glomerulonephritis with fibrils >30 nm. In either case, fibrillar/microtubular deposits of oligoclonal or oligotypic immunoglobulins and complement appear in the mesangium and along the glomerular capillary wall. Congo red stains are negative.

Ans. B

85. A 60 year old male presented to OPD with generalised body swelling, decreased urine output, severe backache. On examination he was found to have macroglossia. Lab parameters: anaemia; reversed albumin globulin ratio; deranged renal function tests. ECG shows low voltage in the limb leads with a pseudo-infarct pattern; ECHO: concentrically thickened ventricles and diastolic dysfunction. Urine dipstick: protein 4+; 24 hour urine protein: 6.2gm. Which of the following is the most appropriate diagnosis?

A. Lupus Nephritis
B. Sarcoidosis
C. Amyloidosis
D. Scleroderma

Explanation:

- Kidneys are the most frequently involved organ and are affected in 70–80% of patients. Renal amyloidosis usually manifests as proteinuria, often in nephrotic range and associated with hypoalbuminemia, secondary hypercholesterolemia and hypertriglyceridemia, and edema or anasarca.
- In some patients, interstitial rather than glomerular amyloid deposition can produce azotemia without proteinuria.
- Heart is the second most commonly affected organ (50–60% of patients), and cardiac involvement is the leading cause of death from AL amyloidosis.
- Early on, the electrocardiogram may show low voltage in the limb leads with a pseudo-infarct pattern.
- Echocardiographic features of disease include concentrically thickened ventricles and diastolic dysfunction with an abnormal global longitudinal strain pattern; a "sparkly" appearance has been described but is often not seen with modern high-resolution echocardiographic techniques.
- Poor atrial contractility occurs even in sinus rhythm, and patients with cardiac amyloidosis are at risk for development of atrial thrombi and stroke.
- Cardiac MRI can show increased wall thickness, and characteristic delayed enhancement of the subendocardium has been described following injection of gadolinium contrast.

Ans. C

86. A 50 year old woman presented to medicine OPD with complaints of generalised body swelling. Urinalysis revealed nephrotic range proteinuria and microhematuria. Her serum creatinine is 2.8mg/dL. She is referred to nephrologist for evaluation. Renal biopsy was planned which revealed following in Congo red stain. What would be your diagnosis?

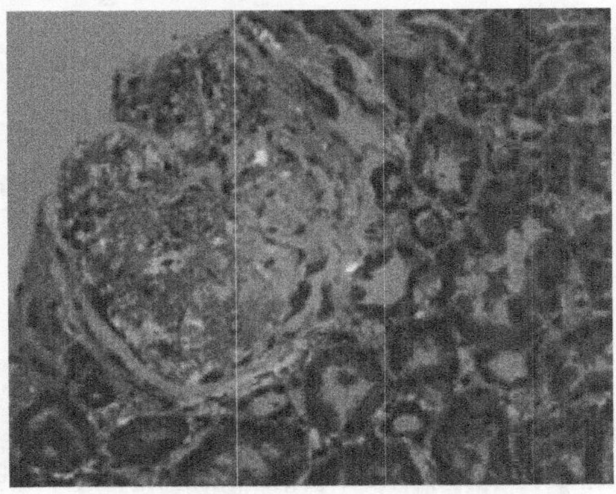

A. Light chain deposition disease
B. Fibrillary GN
C. Immunotactoid GN
D. Amyloidosis

Explanation:

- Biopsy of involved liver or kidney is diagnostic 90% of the time when the pretest probability is high; abdominal fat pad aspirates are positive about 70% of the time, but apparently less so when looking for AA amyloid.
- Amyloid deposits are distributed along blood vessels and in the mesangial regions of the kidney.
- Treatment for primary amyloidosis, melphalan, and autologous hematopoietic stem cell transplantation can delay course of disease in about 30% of patients.
- Secondary amyloidosis is also relentless unless the primary disease can be controlled.
- Some new drugs in development that disrupt the formation of fibrils may be available in the future.

Ans. D

87. A 60 year old woman presented to nephrology OPD with complaints of generalised body swelling. Her BP was 160/100mmHg.Urinalysis revealed nephrotic range proteinuria and microhematuria. Her serum creatinine is 3.8mg/dL. She is referred to a nephrologist for evaluation. Renal biopsy was planned which revealed: Nodular glomerulosclerosis with mesangial material of acellular eosinophilic material. Congo red negative. EM showed following picture.

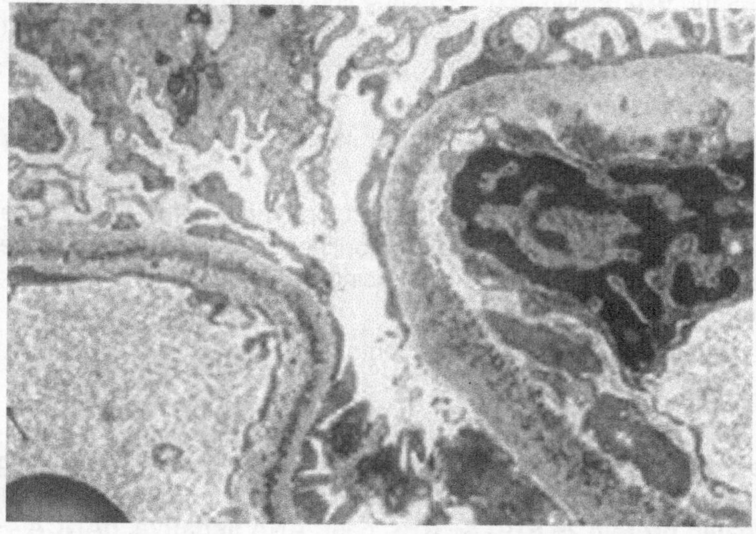

A. Light chain deposition disease
B. Amyloidosis
C. Membranous nephropathy
D. FSGS

Explanation:

- Biochemical characteristics of nephrotoxic light chains produced in patients with light chain malignancies often confer a specific pattern of renal injury; that of either *cast nephropathy* which causes renal failure but not heavy proteinuria or amyloidosis, or light chain deposition disease, which produces nephrotic syndrome with renal failure.
- These latter patients produce kappa light chains that do not have the biochemical features necessary to form amyloid fibrils. Instead, they self-aggregate and form granular deposits along the glomerular capillary and mesangium, tubular basement membrane, and Bowman's capsule.
- When predominant in glomeruli, nephrotic syndrome develops, and about 70% of patients progress to dialysis. Light-chain deposits are not fibrillar and do not stain with Congo red, but they are easily detected with anti–light chain antibody using immunofluorescence or as granular deposits on electron microscopy.
- Combination of the light chain rearrangement, self-aggregating properties at neutral pH, and abnormal metabolism probably contribute to the deposition.

- Treatment for light chain deposition disease is treatment of the primary disease and, if possible, autologous stem cell transplantation.

Ans. A

88. A 32 year old female presents with nephrotic range proteinuria; microhematuria; SCr=3.1 mg/dl. She has a family history of glaucoma and proteinuria, but none on dialysis. Her serum ANA is negative. Her serum complement levels are normal. A 24-h urine collection reveals 3.6 g of proteinuria. The renal biopsy findings are as follows: EM: thickened BMs with irregular lucent areas and moth-eaten appearance. Which of the following would be your diagnosis?

A. Fabry's disease
B. Nail patella syndrome
C. MCD
D. Pierson syndrome

Explanation:

- Patients with nail-patella syndrome develop iliac horns on the pelvis and dysplasia of the dorsal limbs involving the patella, elbows, and nails, variably associatec with neural-sensory hearing impairment, glaucoma, and abnormalities of the GBM and podocytes, leading to hematuria, proteinuria and FSGS.
- Syndrome is autosomal dominant, with haploinsufficiency for the *LIM* homeodomain transcription factor LMX1B; pedigrees are extremely variable in the penetrance for all features of the disease.
- LMX1B regulates the expression of genes encoding α3 and α4 chains of collagen IV, interstitial type III collagen, podocin, and CD2AP that help form the slit-pore membranes connecting podocytes.
- Mutations in the LIM domain region of *LMX1B* associate with glomerulopathy, and renal failure appears in as many as 30% of patients.
- Proteinuria or isolated hematuria is discovered throughout life, but usually by the third decade, and is inexplicably more common in females.
- On renal biopsy there is focal sclerosing glomerulonephritis with specific lucent damage to the lamina densa of the GBM, an increase in collagen III fibrils along glomerular capillaries and in the mesangium, and damage to the slit-pore membrane, producing heavy proteinuria not unlike that seen in congenital nephrotic syndrome.
- Patients with renal failure do well with transplantation.

Ans. B

89. A 57 year old male presented to OPD with anuria since 2 days with c/o arthralgia, fever since 1 month. Lab parameters: severe anaemia; increased ESR; leukocytosis; severely deranged RFT; Normal C3 and C4. Urinalysis revealed protein 2+ RBC 4+ RBC cast; ANA negative, pANCA 4+positive. CXR: Normal. Renal Biopsy suggestive of crescentic GN. Which of the following treatment would you consider giving in this patient?

A. Etanercept
B. Cyclophosphamide
C. Steroids
D. Rituximab

Explanation:

- 5-year survival rate for patients with treated microscopic polyangiitis is 74%, with disease-related mortality occurring from alveolar hemorrhage or gastrointestinal, cardiac, or renal disease.
- Studies on treatment have come from trials that have included patients with granulomatosis with polyangiitis (Wegener's) or microscopic polyangiitis.
- Currently, the treatment approach for microscopic polyangiitis is the same as is used for granulomatosis with polyangiitis.

Ans. B

90. A 42 year-old male presents to his doctor with episodes of pre syncope; bilateral pedal oedema, angiokeratoma. He has a family history of hypertrophic cardiomyopathy. An echocardiogram reveals a maximum left ventricular wall thickness of 18.6 mm. His 24 hour urine protein was: 3.1 gm. Full panel testing was ordered for hypertrophic cardiomyopathy (HCM). Hemizygous mutation was found in the GLA gene. Renal biopsy will reveal which of the following?

A. MCD
B. MPGN
C. FSGS
D. IgAN

Explanation:

- Renal biopsy reveals enlarged glomerular visceral epithelial cells packed with small clear vacuoles containing globotriaosylceramide; vacuoles may also be found in parietal and tubular epithelia.
- These vacuoles of electron-dense materials in parallel arrays (zebra bodies) are easily seen on electron microscopy. Ultimately, renal biopsies reveal FSGS.
- Nephropathy of Fabry's disease typically presents in the third decade as mild to moderate proteinuria, sometimes with microscopic hematuria or nephrotic syndrome.

Ans. C

91. A 35 year-old male presents to his doctor with episodes of pre syncope; bilateral pedal oedema, angiokeratoma, hypohydrosis. He has a family history of hypertrophic cardiomyopathy. His 24 hour urine protein was: 3.1 gm. Renal biopsy reveals enlarged glomerular visceral epithelial cells packed with small clear vacuoles containing globotriaosylceramide. Renal biopsy reveals:

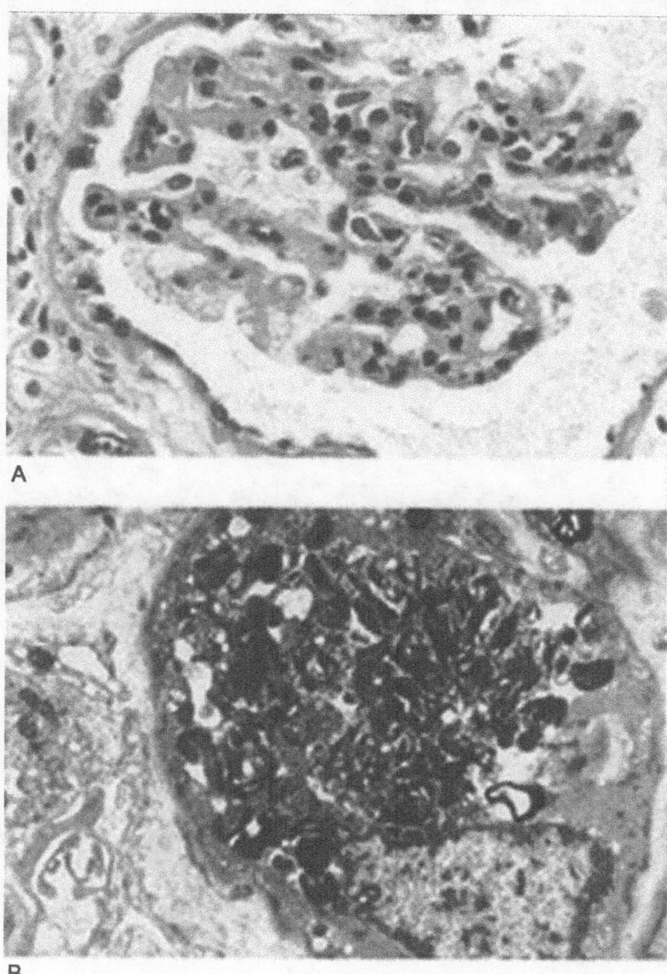

What would be your diagnosis?

A. Fabry's disease
B. Beta mannosidosis
C. Fucosidosis
D. Any of the above

Explanation:

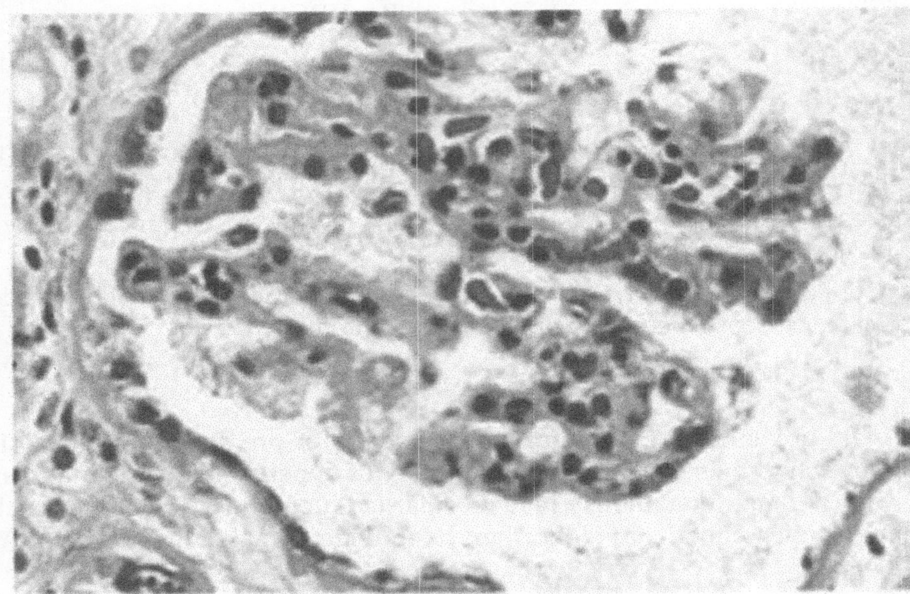

A

B

Figure: Fabry's disease. Due to deficiency of α-galactosidase, there is abnormal accumulation of glycolipids, resulting in foamy podocytes by light microscopy (A). These deposits can be directly visualized by electron microscopy (B), where the glycosphingolipid appears as whorled so-called myeloid bodies, particularly in the podocytes *(ABF/Vanderbilt Collection)*

Ans. A

92. A 16-year-old male student is diagnosed with Alport syndrome. Which one of the following statements is false regarding this syndrome?

A. Usually females from X-linked pedigrees have only microhematuria, but up to 25% of carrier females have been reported to have more severe renal manifestations

B. Female carriers have variable penetrance depending on the type of mutation or the degree of mosaicism created by X inactivation

C. Fifteen percent of patients have autosomal recessive disease of the α3(IV) or α4(IV) chains on chromosome 2q35–37

D. All of the above

Explanation:

- Approximately 85% of patients with Alport's syndrome have an X-linked inheritance of mutations in α5(IV) collagen chain on chromosome Xq22–24.
- Female carriers have variable penetrance depending on the type of mutation or the degree of mosaicism created by X inactivation.
- Fifteen percent of patients have autosomal recessive disease of the α3(IV) or α4(IV) chains on chromosome 2q35–37.
- Rarely, some kindred have an autosomal dominant inheritance of dominant-negative mutations in α3(IV) or α4(IV) chains.

Ans. D

93. A 21 year old female; known case of sick cell disease presents to OPD with deranged renal function tests. Renal biopsy revealed FSGS pattern. Which of the following is true with respect to sick cell nephropathy?

A. Renal function can be overestimated due to the increased tubular secretion of creatinine seen in many patients with SS-sickle cell

B. By second/third decade of life, persistent vasoocclusive disease in kidney leads to varying degrees of renal failure, and some patients end up on dialysis

C. Patients with homozygous SS-sickle cell disease and less commonly SC-sickle cell disease develop chronic vasoocclusive disease in many organs. Polymers of deoxygenated SS-hemoglobin distort shape of red

D. All of the above

Explanation:

- Renal function can be overestimated due to the increased tubular secretion of creatinine seen in many patients with SS-sickle cell.
- By second or third decade of life, persistent vasoocclusive disease in kidney leads to varying degrees of renal failure, and some patients end up on dialysis.
- Their prognosis on dialysis is poor and anemia management with erythropoiesis-stimulating agents complicated.

Ans. D

94. A 16 year old male presents to nephrology OPD with mild body swelling. Urine dipstick revealed protein: 3+; RBC:2+. Slit lamp examination: anterior lenticonus. Renal biopsy revealed splitting of basement membrane. What treatment would you like to initiate in this patient?

A. ACE inhibitors

B. Cyclophosphamide

C. Cyclosporine

D. Bevacizumab

Explanation:

- All affected members of a family with X-linked Alport's syndrome should be identified and followed, including mothers of affected males.
- Primary treatment is control of systemic hypertension and use of ACE inhibitors to slow renal progression.
- Although patients who receive renal allografts usually develop anti- GBM antibodies directed toward the collagen epitopes absent in their native kidney, overt Goodpasture's syndrome is rare and graft survival is good.

Ans. A

95. A 48 year old male with years of uncontrolled hypertension presents to OPD with features of renal failure. Provisional diagnosis of hypertensive nephrosclerosis was kept. Which of the following statements is true with respect to hypertensive nephrosclerosis?

A. *Hypertensive nephrosclerosis* is five-fold more frequent in African Americans than whites

B. Risk alleles associated with *APOL1*

C. Kidney biopsies in patients with hypertension, microhematuria, and moderate proteinuria demonstrate arteriolosclerosis, chronic nephrosclerosis, and interstitial fibrosis in the absence of immune deposits

D. All of the above

Explanation:

- Systemic hypertension causes permanent damage to the kidneys in about 6% of patients with elevated blood pressure.
- As many as 27% of patients with end-stage kidney disease have hypertension as a primary cause.
- Although there is not a clear correlation between the extent or duration of hypertension and the risk of end-organ damage, *hypertensive nephrosclerosis* is fivefold more frequent in African Americans than whites.
- Risk alleles associated with *APOL1*, a functional gene for apolipoprotein L1 expressed in podocytes, substantially explains the increased burden of ESRD among African Americans.
- Associated risk factors for progression to end-stage kidney disease include increased age, male gender, race, smoking, hypercholesterolemia, duration of hypertension, low birth weight, and preexisting renal injury.
- Kidney biopsies in patients with hypertension, microhematuria, and moderate proteinuria demonstrate arteriolosclerosis, chronic nephrosclerosis, and interstitial fibrosis in the absence of immune deposits.

Ans. D

96. All of the following medications may be useful in the treatment of benign prostatic hypertrophy except:

A. Alfuzosin

B. Bosentan

C. Dutasteride

D. Finasteride

Explanation:

- Benign prostatic hypertrophy (BPH) is a pathologic process that contributes to the development of lower urinary tract symptoms in men.
- Such symptoms, arising from lower urinary tract dysfunction, are further subdivided into obstructive symptoms (urinary hesitancy, straining, weak stream, terminal dribbling, prolonged voiding, incomplete emptying) and irritative symptoms (urinary frequency, urgency, nocturia, urge incontinence, small voided volumes).
- Lower urinary tract symptoms and other sequelae of BPH are not just due to a mass effect, but are also likely due to a combination of the prostatic enlargement and age-related detrusor dysfunction.
- Asymptomatic patients do not require treatment regardless of the size of the prostate gland.

- Symptomatic relief is the most common reason men seek treatment for BPH, and therefore, the goal of therapy for BPH is usually relief of these symptoms.
- Selective α-adrenergic receptor antagonists, such as alfuzosin, are thought to treat the dynamic aspect of BPH by reducing sympathetic tone of the bladder outlet, thereby decreasing resistance and improving urinary flow.
- 5α-Reductase inhibitors, like dutasteride and finasteride, are thought to treat static aspect of BPH by reducing prostate volume and having a similar, albeit delayed effect.
- They have also proven to be beneficial in the prevention of BPH progression, as measured by prostate volume, the risk of developing acute urinary retention, and the risk of having BPH-related surgery.
- Use of an α-adrenergic receptor antagonist and a 5α-reductase inhibitor as combination therapy seeks to provide symptomatic relief while preventing progression of BPH.
- Another class of medications that has shown improvement in lower urinary tract symptoms secondary to BPH is phosphodiesterase-5 (PDE5) inhibitors, used currently in the treatment of erectile dysfunction.
- All three of the PDE5 inhibitors available in the United States, sildenafil, vardenafil, and tadalafil, appear to be effective in the treatment of symptoms secondary to BPH.
- Use of PDE5 inhibitors is not without controversy, however, given the fact that short-acting PDE5 inhibitors such as sildenafil need to be dosed separately from α-blockers because of potential hypotensive effects. Bosentan is a nonselective endothelin receptor antagonist used in the treatment of pulmonary arterial hypertension.

Ans. B

97. Most common acute complication of Hemodialysis is:

A. Hypotension
B. Muscle cramps
C. Chest pain
D. Anaphylaxis

Explanation:

- Hypotension is the most common acute complication of hemodialysis, particularly among patients with diabetes mellitus.
- Numerous factors appear to increase the risk of hypotension, including excessive ultrafiltration with inadequate compensatory vascular filling, impaired vasoactive or autonomic responses, osmolar shifts, overzealous use of antihypertensive agents, and reduced cardiac reserve.
- Muscle cramps during dialysis are also a common complication.
- Anaphylactoid reactions to the dialyzer, particularly on its first use, have been reported most frequently with the bioincompatible cellulosic-containing membranes.

Ans. A

98. Generally patients do not develop symptomatic uremia until GFR reduces to:

A. 40 ml/min
B. 20 ml/min
C. 15 ml/min
D. 10 ml/min

Explanation:

- Generally, patients do not develop symptomatic uremia until renal insufficiency is severe (GFR <15 mL/min).

Ans. C

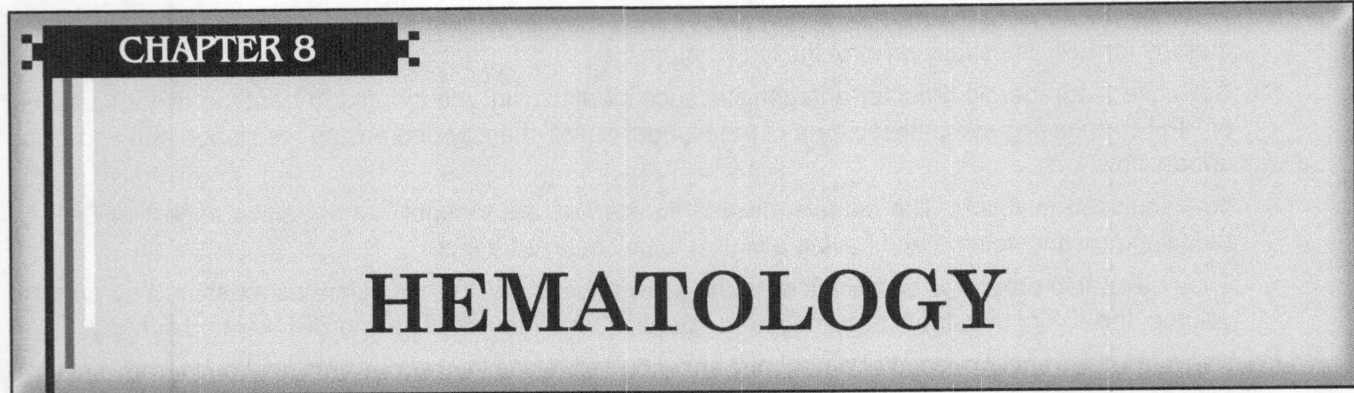

CHAPTER 8

HEMATOLOGY

1. **Assessment of red cell mass by using hematocrit may underestimate degree of erythrocytosis in which of the following conditions?**

A. Polycythemia vera
B. Smokers
C. COPD
D. High altitude

Explanation:

- In polycythemia vera, there is expansion of plasma volume which can mask elevated red cell mass.

Ans. A

2. **In Hemochromatosis timely phlebotomy is advised to keep serum ferritin level below:**

A. 100 μg/L
B. 50 μg/L
C. 30 μg/L
D. 200 μg/L

Explanation:

- Treatment of choice* for Hemochromatosis is timely *phlebotomy* to remove the excess iron from the body .
- Therefore, in patients with advanced disease, weekly phlebotomy may be required for 1–2 years, and it should be continued until the serum ferritin level is ≤100 μg/L.
- Thereafter, phlebotomies are performed at appropriate intervals to *maintain ferritin levels at ≤100 μg/L.*

Ans. A

3. **Factor VIII (F8) present in one bag of cryoprecipitate:**

A. 80 IU
B. 50 IU
C. 120 IU
D. 250 IU

Explanation:

- Cryoprecipitate is enriched with FVIII protein (each bag contains ~80 IU of FVIII).

Ans. A

4. **What is the Absolute lymphocyte count needed to make a diagnosis of CLL?**

A. >3500 cells
B. >5000 cells
C. >4000 cells
D. >1500 cells

Explanation:

- Chronic lymphocytic leukemia (CLL) is a monoclonal proliferation of mature B lymphocytes defined by an absolute number of malignant cells in the blood (>5000 cells).

Ans. B

5. Most common inherited bleeding disorder is:

A. Hemophilia A
B. Vitamin K deficiency
C. Von Willebrand's Disease
D. Glanzmann's thrombasthenia

Explanation:

- VWD is the most common inherited bleeding disorder.
- VWD has been classified into three major types, with four subtypes of type 2.
- The most common type is VWD type 1.
- Mild type 1 VWD first manifests with dental extractions, particularly wisdom tooth extraction, or tonsillectomy.
- Treatment of choice - DDAVP.

Ans. C

6. Extramedullary Plasmacytoma treatment of choice:

A. Local radiotherapy
B. High dose Melphalan
C. Surgical resection
D. Lenalidomide + Dexamethasone

Explanation:

There are two important variants of myeloma

1. Solitary bone plasmacytoma
2. Solitary extramedullary plasmacytoma.
   - These lesions are associated with an M component in <30% of the cases, ***without marrow plasmacytosis***. They may affect younger individuals.

Solitary bone plasmacytoma

1. Single lytic bone lesion
2. Most common site vertebra.
3. May recur in other bony sites or evolve into myeloma.

Extramedullary plasmacytoma

1. Usually involve submucosal lymphoid tissue of nasopharynx or paranasal sinuses.
2. Rarely recur or progress.
   - **Both tumors are highly responsive to local radiation therapy.**

Ans. A

7. A 68-year-old man with stage IV renal failure is receiving erythropoietin with a target hemoglobin of 14 g/dL. Which is the most directly increased risk as a result of this therapy?

A. Peripheral neuropathy
B. Ischemic stroke
C. Seizures
D. Dementia

Explanation:

- Administration of erythropoiesis-stimulating agents (ESA) to patients with renal impairment has come under scrutiny in recent years.
- Whereas historical treatment goals were to obtain normal hemoglobin levels, recent evidence from large randomized trials has demonstrated an increased cardiovascular and stroke risk in patients treated to normal hemoglobin values.
- Peripheral neuropathy risk is increased with chronic uremia, but not by ESA administration. Seizure risk may be increased with electrolyte disarray or severe uremia, but is generally not increased with ESA administration.
- Dementia risk is increased by both chronic renal failure and cerebrovascular events, but not directly from ESA. Headaches may relate to polycythemia, but are otherwise not directly related to ESA administration.

Ans. B

8. **Statement not true about Hepcidin is:**

A. Made by Liver
B. Increased by IL 1 mediated pathway
C. Acts to suppress iron absorption
D. Inhibits iron release from storage sites

Explanation:

- Hepcidin, made by the liver, is increased in inflammation via an IL-6 ediated pathway, and acts to suppress iron absorption and iron release from storage sites.
- Overall result is a chronic hypoproliferative anemia with classic changes in iron metabolism.
- Anemia is further compounded by a mild to moderate shortening in red cell survival.

Ans. B

9. **Mc Leod phenotype is:**

A. Kell
B. Weak Kell antigen
C. Duffy
D. Kidd

Explanation:

- *Kell* protein is very large (720 amino acids), and its secondary structure contains many different antigenic epitopes. The immunogenicity of Kell is third behind the ABO and Rh systems.
- Kell protein is linked to another blood group protein termed Kx.
- Rare absence of this protein (controlled by a gene on X) is associated with weak KEL antigen, acanthocytosis, shortened RBC survival, and progressive form of muscular dystrophy that includes cardiac defects. This rare condition is called *McLeod phenotype*.
- Duffy antigens are codominant alleles, Fya and Fyb, that also serve as receptors for Plasmodium vivax.

Ans. B

10. **True about Anemia of chronic disease is:**

A. Red cells are typically normocytic & hypochromic
B. In acute renal failure, correlation between anemia and renal function is weaker
C. Anemia of chronic kidney disease patients usually present with decreased serum iron, TIBC & Ferritin levels
D. Reticulocytes are reduced

Explanation:

- Progressive CKD is usually associated with a moderate to severe hypoproliferative anemia; level of anemia correlates with the stage of CKD.
- Red cells are typically normocytic and normochromic, and reticulocytes are decreased.
- Anemia is primarily due to a failure of EPO production by diseased kidney and a reduction in red cell survival.
- In certain forms of acute renal failure, the correlation between anemia and renal function is weaker.
- Patients with the hemolytic-uremic syndrome increase erythropoiesis in response to hemolysis, despite renal failure.
- Polycystic kidney disease also shows a smaller degree of EPO deficiency for a given level of renal failure.
- By contrast, patients with diabetes or myeloma have more severe EPO deficiency for a given level of renal failure.
- Assessment of iron status provides information to distinguish the anemia of CKD from the other forms of hypoproliferative anemia and to guide management.
- Patients with the anemia of CKD usually present with normal serum iron, TIBC, and ferritin levels.
- However, those maintained on chronic hemodialysis may develop iron deficiency from blood loss through the dialysis procedure. Iron must be replenished in these patients to ensure an adequate response to EPO therapy.

Ans. D

11. Imerslund Grasbeck syndrome is related to which of the following:

A. Cobalamine deficiency
B. Iron deficiency
C. Folate deficiency
D. Thalasemmia

Explanation:

Selective Malabsorption of Cobalamin with Proteinuria (Imerslund's Syndrome; Imerslund-Gräsbeck Syndrome; Congenital Cobalamin Malabsorption; Autosomal Recessive Megaloblastic Anemia; MGA1)

- This autosomally recessive disease is the most common cause of megaloblastic anemia due to cobalamin deficiency in infancy in Western countries.
- More than 200 cases have been reported with familial clusters in Finland, Norway, the Middle East, and North Africa.
- Patients secrete normal amounts of IF and gastric acid but are unable to absorb cobalamin.
- In Finland, impaired synthesis, processing, or ligand binding of cubilin due to inherited mutations is found.
- In Norway, mutation of gene for *AMN* has been reported. Other tests of intestinal absorption are normal. Over 90% of these patients show nonspecific proteinuria, but renal function is otherwise normal, and renal biopsy has not shown any consistent renal defect.
- Few have shown aminoaciduria and congenital renal abnormalities, such as duplication of the renal pelvis.

Ans. A

12. Cause of rebound thrombocytosis is:

A. Folate deficiency
B. Vitamin B1 deficiency
C. Malignancy
D. Iron deficiency anemia

Explanation:

Table: Causes of thrombocytosis	
Tissue inflammation: Collagen vascular disease, inflammatory bowel disease	Hemorrhage
Malignancy	Iron-deficiency anemia
Infection	Surgery
Myeloproliferative disorders: Polycythemia vera, primary myelofibrosis, essential thrombocytosis, chronic myelogenous leukemia	**Rebound:** Correction of vitamin B_{12} or folate deficiency, post-ethanol abuse
Myelodysplastic disorders: 5 q-syndrome, idiopathic refractory sideroblastic anemia	Hemolysis
Postsplenectomy or hyposplenism	**Familial:** Thrombopoietin overproduction, *JAK2* or *MPL* mutations

Ans. A

13. **Intermediate grade Non Hodgkin's lymphoma is:**
   A. CLL/SCL
   B. DLBCL
   C. Mantle cell lymphoma
   D. Follicular lymphoma

Explanation:

- Among the aggressive diseases, the most common are NHL and DLBCL; and the most rapidly prolific are NHL and BL.
- FL is the second most common NHL and the most common indolent NHL.
- Other indolent NHLs include MZL, lymphoplasmacytic lymphoma (LPL), and hairy cell leukemia (HCL).
- MCL is an intermediate grade lymphoma that shares some characteristics with the aggressive lymphomas (fairly urgent need for treatment and aggressive upfront combination chemotherapy regimens), but like the indolent lymphomas, it is not readily curable with conventional dose therapies.

Ans. C

14. **Agammaglobulinemia is charcaterized by:**
   A. Caused by mutation in BTK gene that is located on Y chromosome
   B. Not a manifestation of Myelodysplastic syndrome
   C. No role of Immunoglobulin replacement
   D. Profound hypo-gammaglobulinemia is also observed in adults in association with thymoma

Explanation:

- Agammaglobulinemia is characterized by a profound defect in B cell development (<1% of the normal B cell blood count).
- In most patients, very low residual Ig isotypes can be detected in serum.
- In 85% of cases, agammaglobulinemia is caused by a mutation in the BTK gene that is located on the X chromosome.
- BTK gene product is a kinase that participates in (pre) B cell receptor signaling.
- When the kinase is defective, there is a block (albeit a leaky one) at pre-B to B cell stage.
- Detection of BTK by intracellular immunofluorescence of monocytes, and lack thereof in patients with X-linked agammaglobulinemia (XLA), is a useful diagnostic test.

- Not all of the mutations in BTK result in agammaglobulinemia, since some patients have a milder form of hypogammaglobulinemia and low but detectable B cell counts.
- These cases should not be confused with common variable immunodeficiency .
- About 10% of agammaglobulinemia cases are caused by alterations in genes encoding elements of the pre-B cell receptor, i.e., the μ heavy chain, λ5 surrogate light chain, Igα or Igβ, the scaffold protein BLNK, and p85 α subunit of phosphatidylinositol 3 phosphate kinase (P13K) and the Ikaros transcription factor.
- In 5% of cases, the defect is unknown.
- It is noteworthy that agammaglobulinemia can be observed in patients with ICF syndrome, despite the presence of normal peripheral B cell counts.
- Lastly, agammaglobulinemia can be a manifestation of a myelodysplastic syndrome (associated or not with neutropenia).
- Treatment of agammaglobulinemic patients is based on immunoglobulin replacement.
- Profound hypogammaglobulinemia is also observed in adults, in association with thymoma.

Ans. D

15. **Best predictor of outcome in NHL is:**

A. Rai & Binnet score
B. Ann Arbor staging
C. IPI (International Prognostic index)
D. Kadish staging

Explanation:

- International Prognostic Index (IPI) is perhaps the best predictor of outcome.
- IPI was developed based on the analysis of over 2000 patients with aggressive NHLs treated with an anthracycline containing regimen.
- Age (≤60 vs >60); serum LDH (≤normal vs >normal); performance status (0 or 1 vs 2–4); stage (I or II vs III or IV); and extranodal involvement (<1 site vs >1 site) were identified as independently prognostic for overall survival (OS).
- A point is awarded for each risk factor and then summed, defining four risk groups: low-risk (0 or 1); low-intermediate (2); high-intermediate (3); and high (4–5). The 5-year OS rates for patients with scores of 0 to 1, 2, 3, and 4–5 were 73, 51, 43 and 26%, respectively.

Table: International prognostic index for NHL

Five Clinical Risk Factors	
Age ≥ 60 years Serum lactate dehydrogenase levels elevated Performance status ≥2 (ECOG) or ≤ 70 (Karnofsky) Ann Arbor stage III or IV > 1 site of extranodal involvement	
For Diffuse Large B-cell Lymphoma	
0,1 factor=low risk	35% of cases; 5-year survival, 73%
2 factors = low-intermediate risk	27% of cases; 5-year survival, 51%
3 factors=high-intermediate risk	22% of cases; 5-year survival, 43%
4, 5 factor=high risk	16% of cases; 5-year survival, 26%
For Diffuse Large B-cell Lymphoma Treated with R-CHOP	
0 factor = good	10% of cases; 4-year survival, 94%
1, 2 factors = intermediate	45% of cases; 4-year survival, 80%
3,4,5 factors = poor	45% of cases; 4-year survival, 53%

Ans. C

16. At what wavelengths oxyhemoglobin reflects light more effectively than does deoxyhemoglobin?

A. 660 nm
B. 740 nm
C. 860 nm
D. 940 nm

Explanation:

- At wavelengths of 660 nm, oxyhemoglobin reflects light more effectively than does deoxyhemoglobin, whereas the reverse is true in the infrared spectrum (940 nm).

Ans. A

17. Which of the following endocrine abnormality does not cause Anemia?

A. Hypothyroidism
B. Hyperthyroidism
C. Hyperparathyroidism
D. Hypopituitarism

Explanation:

- Patients who are hypothyroid or have deficits in pituitary hormones also may develop a mild anemia.
- Pathogenesis may be complicated by other nutritional deficiencies because iron and folic acid absorption can be affected by these disorders. Usually, correction of the hormone deficiency reverses anemia.
- Anemia may be more severe in Addison's disease, depending on level of thyroid and androgen hormone dysfunction; however, anemia may be masked by decreases in plasma volume. Once such patients are given cortisol and volume replacement, hemoglobin level may fall rapidly.
- Mild anemia complicating hyperparathyroidism may be due to decreased EPO production as a consequence of the renal effects of hypercalcemia or to impaired proliferation of erythroid progenitors.

Ans. B

18. Plasmapheresis is used in the treatment of:

A. Autoimmune haemolytic anemia
B. Disseminated intravascular coagulation
C. Thrombotic thrombocytopenic purpura
D. Hemolytic uremic syndrome

Explanation:

- Main stay of treatment in TTP is plasmapheresis. Best response is seen in idiopathic TTP. The treatment must be continued till the platelet count becomes normal and Hemolytic signs were resolved.

Ans. C

19. All of the following are typically increased in a patient with hemolytic anemia except:

A. Aspartate aminotransferase
B. Haptoglobin
C. LDH
D. MCV

Explanation:

- Differentiates hemolytic anemias (HAs) from other anemias is that the patient has signs and symptoms arising directly from hemolysis.
- At the clinical level, the main sign is jaundice; in addition, the patient may report discoloration of the urine. In many cases of HA, the spleen is enlarged, because it is a preferential site of hemolysis; and in some cases, the liver may be enlarged as well.
- Laboratory features of HA are related to hemolysis per se and the erythropoietic response of the bone marrow. Hemolysis regularly produces an increase in unconjugated bilirubin and aspartate aminotransferase (AST) in serum; urobilinogen will be increased in both urine and stool. If hemolysis is mainly intravascular,

telltale sign is hemoglobinuria (often associated with hemosiderinuria); in the serum, there is hemoglobin, LDH is increased, and haptoglobin is reduced. In contrast, the bilirubin level may be normal or only mildly elevated.

- Main sign of the erythropoietic response by the bone marrow is an increase in reticulocytes (a test all too often neglected in initial workup of a patient with anemia).
- Usually the increase will be reflected in both the percentage of reticulocytes (the more commonly quoted figure) & absolute reticulocyte count (more definitive parameter).
- Increased number of reticulocytes is associated with an increased mean corpuscular volume (MCV) in the blood count. On blood smear, this is reflected in the presence of macrocytes; there is also polychromasia, and sometimes, one sees nucleated red cells.

Ans. B

20. Drug that cause thrombocytopenia within 24 hours of its initial exposure is:

A. Abciximab
B. Ibuprofen
C. Acetaminophen
D. Ampicillin

Explanation:

- Abciximab is a Gp 2b-3a inhibitor and it causes production of antibodies against platelet surface antigen resulting in thrombocytopenia.
- Usually it will occur after 7 days of exposure to drugs and resolve within 7-10 days after withdrawal of drug except for Gp 2b-3a inhibitor which causes thrombocytopenia within 24 hours of exposure to the drug.

Ans. A

21. Most common chronic Myeloproliferative disorder is:

A. Chronic myeloid leukemia
B. Essential thrombocytosis
C. Primary myelofibrosis
D. Polycythemia vera

Explanation:

It is the most common Myeloproliferative disorder and it most commonly affect females.

Ans. D

22. Most common cytogenetic abnormality in Polycythemia vera is:

A. CAL mutation
B. MPL mutation
C. JAK 6 mutation
D. JAK 2 mutation

Explanation:

- JAK 2 mutation will cause constitutional activation of erythropoietic and thrombopoietic receptors leading to Polycythemia vera.

Ans. D

23. Pancytopenia with hypercellular marrow is seen in all except:

A. Paroxysmal nocturnal hemoglobinuria
B. Fanconi anemia
C. Megaloblastic anemia
D. Myelodysplastic syndromes

Explanation:

- Fanconi anemia shows pancytopenia with hypocellular bone marrow. It is an Autosomal recessive disorder.
- Other features of Fanconi anemia include short stature, hypogonadism, esophageal atresia.

Ans. B

24. Janus associated kinase receptor inhibitor used in Polycythemia vera is:

A. Dabrafenib
B. Nilotinib
C. Eculizumab
D. Ruxolitinib

Explanation:

- Ruxolitinib is used in the treatment of Polycythemia vera. Dabrafenib used for treating melanoma. Nilotinib used for treating chronic myeloid leukemia. Eculizumab used in the treatment of paroxysmal nocturnal hehemoglobinuria

Ans. D

25. Which of the following is not a cause of acquired aplastic anemia?

A. Eosinophilic fascitis
B. Thymoma
C. Hepatitis A
D. Carbamazepine

Explanation:

- Hepatitis A won't cause acquired aplastic anemia
- Causes of acquired aplastic anemia include
- Carbamazepine, chloramphenicol
- HIV and Epstein Barr virus infection
- Thymoma, Eosinophilic fascitis
- Paroxysmal nocturnal hemoglobinuria
- Pregnancy

Ans. C

26. Which of the following conditions predisposes to acute myeloid leukemia?

A. Down's syndrome
B. Alkylating agents
C. Ataxia telangiectasia
D. All of the above

Explanation:

- Down's syndrome is associated with AML
- Inherited disorders associated with AML include Fanconi anemia and ataxia telangiectasia.
- **Drugs causing AML includes** Cyclophosphamide, Dacarbazine & Etoposide.

Ans. D

27. All are frontline therapies in CML except:

A. Imatinib
B. Dasatinib
C. Ponatinib
D. Nilotinib

Explanation:

Chronic Myeloid Leukemia

- With TKI therapy, the estimated 10-year survival in CML is 85%.
- Six agents have been approved by the U.S. FDA for the treatment of CML. These include five oral TKIs: (Tyrosine kinase inhibitors)
- First generation - Imatinib
- Second generation- Nilotinib, Dasatinib & Bosutinib
- Third generation- Ponatinib
- Sixth approved agent is omacetaxine, a protein synthesis inhibitor with presumed more selective inhibition of the synthesis of the BCR-ABL1 oncoprotein.
- In that Imatinib, nilotinib, and dasatinib are all acceptable frontline therapies in CML.

Ans. C

28. Which of the following is not seen in Polycythemia vera?

A. Leucocytosis
B. Hepatic vein thrombosis
C. Digital ischemia
D. Triphosphate stones in kidney

Explanation:

- Isolated thrombocytosis, leukocytosis, or splenomegaly may be the initial presenting manifestation of PV. Uncontrolled erythrocytosis causes hyperviscosity, leading to neurologic symptoms such as vertigo, tinnitus, headache, visual disturbances, and transient ischemic attacks (TIA).
- Hepatic venous thrombosis (Budd-Chiari syndrome) is particularly common in young women and may be catastrophic if sudden and complete obstruction of the hepatic vein occurs.
- Indeed, PV should be suspected in any patient who develops hepatic vein thrombosis.
- Digital ischemia, easy bruising, epistaxis, acid-peptic disease, or gastrointestinal hemorrhage may occur due to vascular stasis or thrombocytosis.
- Given large turnover of hematopoietic cells, hyperuricemia with secondary gout, uric acid stones, and symptoms due to hypermetabolism can also complicate the disorder.

Ans. D

29. A 24-year-old man returns to the acute care clinic complaining of 1 day of worsening malaise, weakness, abdominal pain, and discoloured dark urine. He was at the clinic yesterday where he was diagnosed with a possible staphylococcal skin carbuncle and treated with empiric trimethoprim/sulfamethoxazole. His physical examination is notable for mild jaundice, normal vital signs, and no focal findings other than the carbuncle in his left axilla. His CBC shows that his hemoglobin has fallen from 13 g/dL to 8 g/dL and his bilirubin has gone from normal to 3.0 mg/dL. His urine dipstick is positive for bilirubin. Which of the following is the most likely cause of his new anemia?

A. Glucose 6-phosphate dehydrogenase (G6PD) deficiency
B. Hemolytic-uremic syndrome
C. Hereditary spherocytosis
D. Iron deficiency anemia

Explanation:

- Peripheral blood smear shows bite cells anisocytosis, and spherocytes.
- Combination of the smear, jaundice, and hyperbilirubinemia 1 day after receiving sulfamethoxazole makes glucose 6-phosphate dehydrogenase (G6PD) deficiency most likely.
- G6PD deficiency is widely distributed in tropical and subtropical parts of the world (Africa, Southern Europe, Middle East, Southeast Asia, and Oceania) and wherever people from those areas have migrated.
- Conservative estimate is that at least 400 million people have a G6PD deficiency gene. In several of these areas, frequency of a G6PD deficiency gene may be as high as 20% or more.
- G6PD gene is X-linked; thus, males have only one G6PD gene (i.e., they are hemizygous for this gene); therefore, they must be either normal or G6PD deficient.
- Hemolytic anemia in patients with G6PD deficiency can develop as a result of fava beans, infections and drugs.
- Common drugs include primaquine, dapsone, sulfamethoxazole, and nitrofurantoin.
- Typically, a hemolytic attack starts with malaise, weakness, and abdominal or lumbar pain.
- After an interval of several hours to 2–3 days, patient develops jaundice and often dark urine.
- Onset can be extremely abrupt, especially with favism in children.
- There may be hemoglobinemia, hemoglobinuria, high LDH, and low or absent plasma haptoglobin. G6PD deficiency may be diagnosed by semiquantitative or quantitative RBC tests or by DNA testing.
- Hemolytic-uremic syndrome and thrombotic thrombocytopenic purpura cause microangiopathic hemolytic anemia with prominent schistocytes.
- Iron deficiency causes a microcytic and hypochromic anemia.

Ans. A

30. **A 19-year-old collegiate rower who has been in excellent health and takes no chronic medications, for new-onset severe fatigue and left upper abdominal pain. She was treated 2 days ago in the health center for presumed gonorrhea with ceftriaxone and azithromycin. Her past medical history is only notable for one prior episode of presumed gonorrhea when she was 17 years old. Her physical examination is notable for a heart rate of 100 bpm and a palpable spleen. Stool is negative for heme. Laboratory examination is notable for a hemoglobin of 5 g/dL with normal WBC and platelets. Peripheral blood smear shows an excess of spherocytes. Which of the following tests will most likely confirm the diagnosis?**

A. ADAMTS-13 activity assay
B. Direct antiglobulin (Coombs) test
C. Flow cytometry
D. G6PD deficiency assay

Explanation:

- Patient has autoimmune hemolytic anemia (AIHA) with development of warm immunoglobulin G (IgG) antibodies due to ceftriaxone exposure.

Classification of Acquired Immune Hemolytic Anemia:

- AIHA is a serious condition; without appropriate treatment, it may have a mortality of approximately 10%. The onset is often abrupt and can be dramatic.
- Hemoglobin level can drop within days to as low as 4 g/dL; the massive red cell removal will produce jaundice; and sometimes the spleen is enlarged. When this triad is present, the suspicion of AIHA must be high.

Clinical Setting	Type of Antibody	
	Cold, Mostly IgM, Optimal Temperature 4-30°C	**Warm, Mostly IgG, Optimal Temperature 37°C, or Mixed**
Primary	CAD	AIHA (idiopathic)
Secondary to viral infection	EBV CMV Other	HIV Viral vaccines
Secondary to other infection	Mycoplasma infection: Paroxysmal cold hemoglobinuria	
Secondary to/associated with other disease	CAD in: Waldenstrom disease Lymphoma	AIHA inc SLE CLL Other malignancy Chronic inflammatory disorders (e.g., IBD) After allogeneic HSCT
Secondary to drugs: Drug induced immune hemolytic anemia	Small minority (e.g., with lenalidomide)	Majority: currently most common culprit drugs are cefotetan, ceftriaxone, piperacillin
	Drug-dependent: Antibody destroys red cells only when drug present (e.g., rarely penicillin) **Drug-independent:** Antibody can destroy red cells even when drug no longer present (e.g., methyldopa)	

- Diagnostic test for AIHA is the direct antiglobulin (Coombs) test, which detects the presence of antibody on the red cells. When the test is positive, it clinches the diagnosis; when it is negative, the diagnosis is unlikely.
- Immediate treatment almost invariably includes transfusion of red cells. This may pose a special problem because, if the antibody involved is nonspecific, all of the blood units cross-matched will be incompatible.
- Whenever the anemia is not immediately life threatening, blood transfusion should be withheld (because compatibility problems may increase with each unit of blood transfused), and medical treatment started immediately with prednisone (1 mg/kg/d), which will produce a remission promptly in at least one-half of patients.
- Rituximab (anti-CD20) was regarded as second-line treatment, but it is increasingly likely that a relatively low dose (100 mg/wk × 4) of rituximab together with prednisone will become a first-line standard.
- It is especially encouraging that this approach seems to reduce the rate of relapse, a common occurrence in AIHA. G6PD deficiency is unlikely in this previously healthy female only exposed to ceftriaxone.
- ADAMTS-13 activity assay is used to diagnose thrombotic thrombocytopenic purpura. Flow cytometry may be used to diagnose paroxysmal nocturnal hemoglobinuria. Hemoglobin electrophoresis is used to diagnose congenital hemoglobinopathies.

Ans. B

31. A 73-year-old man comes to primary care clinic complaining of 4–6 weeks of increasing malaise, fatigue, dyspnea on exertion, and occasional night sweats. His past medical history is notable for hypertension and hyperlipidemia. Medications include lisinopril and atorvastatin. He had a screening colonoscopy 6 months ago, at which time his laboratory studies were normal. His physical examination today is only notable for a heart rate of 105 bpm and pale mucous membranes. Lungs are clear, and there are

no new cardiac findings. Electrocardiogram (ECG) shows sinus tachycardia but no acute changes. Laboratory studies show normal electrolytes, but his WBC is 1300/μL, platelet count is 35,000/μL, and hemoglobin is 7.5 g/dL. Examination of his peripheral smear confirms the pancytopenia and notes the red blood cells are macrocytic, and there are 3% blasts present. All of the following statements regarding his condition are true except:

A. Azacitidine may improve his blood counts and prolong survival.

B. Children with Down syndrome are also at risk.

C. He is at high risk of developing acute myeloid leukemia.

D. Hematopoietic stem cell transplantation is contraindicated.

Explanation:

- This patient likely has idiopathic myelodysplastic syndrome.
- Myelodysplastic syndromes (MDS) are a heterogeneous group of hematologic disorders broadly characterized by both (1) cytopenias due to bone marrow failure and (2) a high risk of development of acute myeloid leukemia.
- Anemia, often with thrombocytopenia and neutropenia, occurs with dysmorphic (abnormal-appearing) and usually cellular bone marrow, which is evidence of ineffective blood cell production. In patients with "low-risk" MDS, marrow failure dominates the clinical course. In other patients, myeloblasts are present at diagnosis, chromosomes are abnormal, and the "high risk" is due to leukemic progression.
- MDS may be fatal due to complications of pancytopenia or incurability of leukemia, but large proportion of patients will die of concurrent disease, comorbidities typical in an elderly.
- **Idiopathic MDS is a disease of the elderly; mean age at onset is older than 70 years.**
- There is a slight male predominance. MDS is a relatively common form of bone marrow failure, with reported incidence rates of 35 to >100 per million persons in general population and 120 to >500 per million persons in older adults.
- MDS is rare in children but is increased in children with Down syndrome. MDS is associated with environmental exposures such as radiation and benzene.
- Secondary MDS occurs as a late toxicity of cancer treatment, usually combination of radiation & radiomimetic alkylating agents such as busulfan, nitrosourea, or procarbazine (with a latent period of 5–7 years) or DNA topoisomerase inhibitors (2-year latency).
- Anemia dominates the early course of MDS.
- Most symptomatic patients complain of the gradual onset of fatigue and weakness, dyspnea, and pallor, but at least one-half of patients are asymptomatic, and their MDS is discovered only incidentally on routine blood counts.
- Physical examination is typical for signs of anemia, with approximately 20% of patients having splenomegaly. Some unusual skin lesions, including Sweet syndrome (febrile neutrophilic dermatosis), occur with MDS.
- Median survival times of patients with MDS vary widely, but prognosis worsens with increasing percent blasts in bone marrow, cytogenetic abnormalities, and lineages affected by cytopenia. Only hematopoietic stem cell transplantation offers cure of MDS.
- Current survival rate in selected patient cohorts is approximately 50% at 3 years and is improving. New epigenetic modulator drugs are believed to act through a demethylating mechanism to alter gene regulation and allow differentiation to mature blood cells from the abnormal MDS stem cell.
- Azacitidine and decitabine are two epigenetic modifiers frequently used in bone marrow failure clinics.
- Azacitidine improves blood counts and survival in MDS, compared to best supportive care.

WHO Classification of Myelodysplastic Syndromes (MDS)/Neoplasms

Name	WHO Estimated Proportion of Patients with MDS	Peripheral Blood: Key Features	Bone Marrow: Key Features
Refractory cytopenias with unilineage dysplasia (RCUD):			
• Refractory anemia (RA)	10%-20%	Anemia < 1% of blasts	Unilineage erythroid dysplasia (in ≥ 10% of cells) < 5% blasts
• Refractory neutropenia (RN)	<1%	Neutropenia <1% blasts	Unilineage granulocytic dysplasia < 5% blasts
• Refractory thrombocytopenia (RT)	<1%	Thrombocytopenia <1% blasts	Unilineage megakaryocytic dysplasia < 5% blasts
Refractory anemia with ringed sideroblasts (RARS)	3%-11%	Anemia No blasts	Unilineage erythroid dysplasia ≥ 15% of erythroid precursors are ringed sideroblasts < 5% blasts
Refractory cytopenias with multilineage dysplasia (RCMD)	30%	Cytopenia(s) < 1% blasts No Auer rods	Multilineage dysplasia ± ringed sideroblasts < 5% blasts No Auer rods
Refractory anemia with excess blasts, type 1 (RAEB-1)	40%	Cytopenia(s) <5% blasts No Auer rods	Unilineage or multilineage dysplasia
Refractory anemia with excess blasts, type 2 (RAEB-2)		Cytopenia(s) 5%-19% blasts ± Auer rods	Unilineage or multilineage dysplasia 10%-19% blasts ± Auer rods
MDS associated with isolated del (5q) [del(5q)]	Uncommon	Anemia Normal or high platelet count <1% blasts	Isolated 5q31 chromosome deletion Anemia; hypolobated megakaryocytes < 5% blasts
Childhood MDS, including refractory cytopenia of childhood *(provisional)* (RCC)	<1%	Pancytopenia	<5% marrow blasts for RCC Marrow usually hypocellular
MDS, unclassifiable (MDS-U)	?	Cytopenia ≤ 1% blasts	Does not fit other categories Dysplasia < 5% blasts If no dysplasia, MDS associated karyotype

Ans. D

32. A 53-year-old man was sent to you for evaluation of an elevated hematocrit found incidentally on lab testing. He was removing dry wall in a house and cut his upper arm. A CBC before his arm was stitched revealed a hematocrit of 59% with hemoglobin of 20 g/dL, WBC count of 15.4/μL with a normal differential, and platelet count of 445,000/μL. His physical examination is notable for a room air oxygen saturation of 95%, blood pressure of 145/85 mmHg, and a palpable spleen. He has no past medical history, is a non-smoker, drinks rarely on social occasions, and is taking no medications. The patient

reports his last contact with a physician was 2–3 years ago, and he recalls no abnormalities reported on blood testing. Which of the following is the next diagnostic step?

A. Arterial blood gas
B. Erythropoietin (EPO) level
C. Red blood cell (RBC) mass
D. Pulmonary function tests

Explanation:

- This patient has polycythemia, likely due to PV, with the elevation of hemoglobin, WBC count, and platelets. The next step in his evaluation is measurement of RBC mass. After finding an elevated RBC mass, measurement of erythropoietin levels will distinguish between PV and other causes of polycythemia such as renal cell carcinoma, lung disease, hypoxemic states, or chronic carbon monoxide poisoning.

An Approach to Diagnosing Patients with Polycythemia

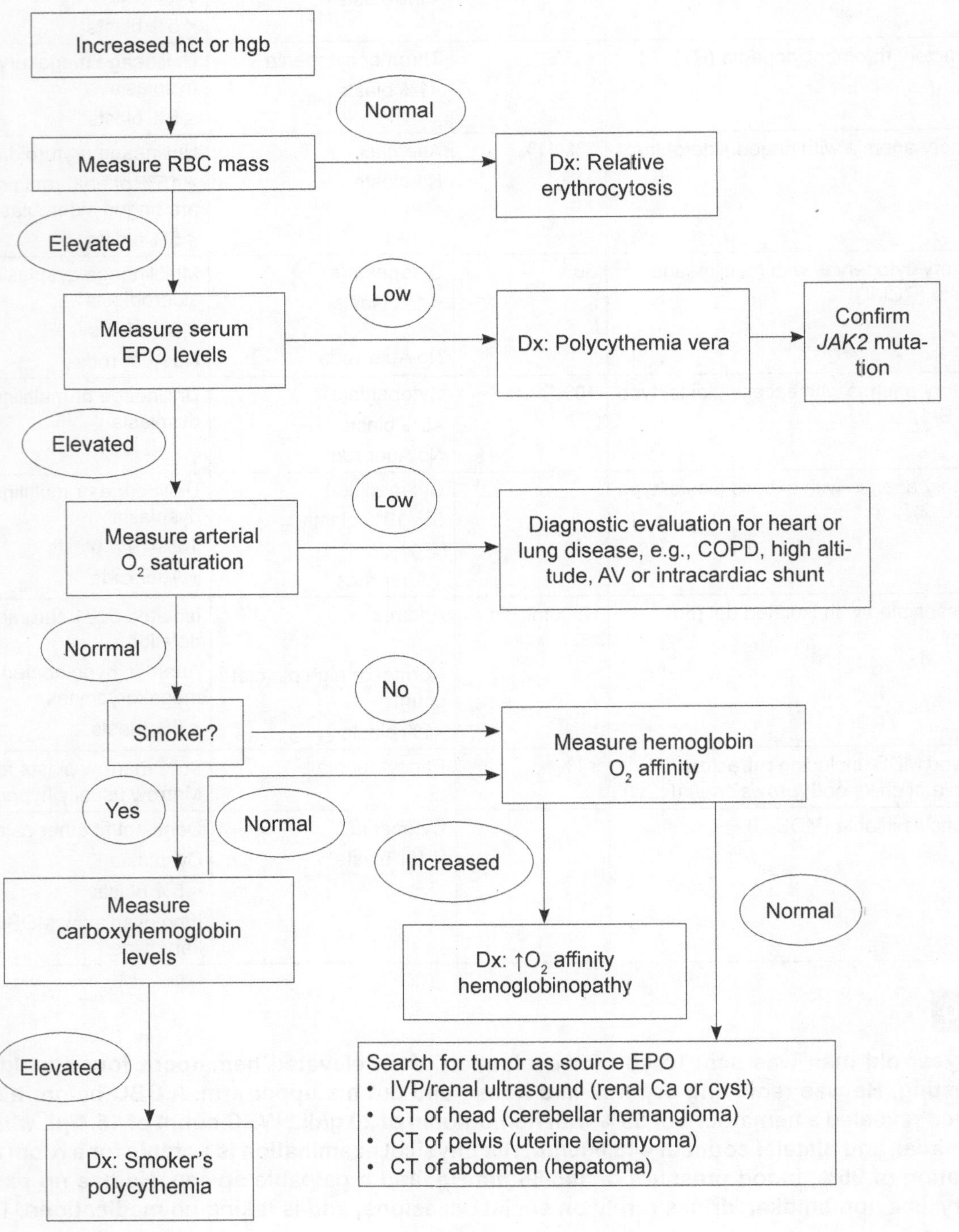

- PV is a clonal disorder involving a multipotent hematopoietic progenitor cell in which phenotypically normal red cells, granulocytes, and platelets accumulate in the absence of a recognizable physiologic stimulus.
- Etiology of PV is unknown. A mutation in the autoinhibitory pseudokinase domain of the tyrosine kinase JAK2, that replaces valine with phenylalanine (V617F) causing constitutive kinase activation, appears to have a central role in the pathogenesis of PV.

Ans. C

33. Which of the following is the most likely finding in a patient with a "dry" bone marrow aspiration?

A. Chronic myeloid leukemia
B. Hairy cell leukemia
C. Metastatic carcinoma infiltration
D. Normal marrow

Explanation:

- A "dry tap" is defined as the inability to aspirate bone marrow and is reported in approximately 4% of attempts. It is rare in the case of normal bone marrow.
- Differential diagnosis includes metastatic carcinoma infiltration (17%), chronic myeloid leukemia (15%), myelofibrosis (14%), hairy cell leukemia (10%), acute leukemia (10%), and lymphomas including Hodgkin disease (9%)

Table: Differential diagnosis of "Dry tap"–Inability to aspirate bone marrow	
Dry taps occur in about 4% of attempts and are associated with:	
• Metastatic carcinoma infiltration	17%
• Chronic myeloid leukemia	15%
• Myelofibrosis	14%
• Hairy cell leukemia	10%
• Acute leukemia	10%
• Lymphomas, Hodgkin disease	9%
• Normal marrow	Rare

Ans. D

34. In patients with multiple myeloma, which of the following results is the most powerful predictor of survival?

A. Bone involvement on radiograph
B. Renal function
C. Serum albumin
D. Serum β2-microglobulin

Explanation:

- Serum β2-microglobulin is the single most powerful predictor of survival and can substitute for staging. Patients with β2-microglobulin levels <0.004 g/L have a median survival of 43 months, and those with levels >0.004 g/L have a survival of only 12 months.
- Combination of serum β2-microglobulin and albumin levels forms the basis for a three-stage International Staging System (ISS) that predicts survival.
- Other factors that may influence prognosis are the presence of cytogenetic abnormalities and hypodiploidy by karyotype, fluorescent in situ hybridization (FISH)–identified chromosome 17p deletion, and translocations t(4;14), (14;16), and t(14;20).
- Chromosome 13q deletion, previously thought to predict poor outcome, is not a predictor following the use of newer agents.
- Microarray profiling and comparative genomic hybridization have formed basis for RNA- and DNA-based prognostic staging systems, respectively.
- ISS system, along with cytogenetic changes, is the most widely used method for assessing prognosis.

Risk Stratification in Myeloma

Table: Chromosomal abnormalities		
Method	**Standard Risk (80%) (expected survival 6-7 + years)**	**High Risk (20%) (expected survival 2-3 years)**
Karyotype	No chromosomal aberration	Any abnormality on conventional karyotype
FISH	t(11:14) t(6:14) del(13)	Del(17p) t(4:14) t(14:16) t(14:20)
International Staging System		
	Stage	**Median Survival, Months**
β_2M <3.5, alb >3.5	I (28%)*	62
β_2M <3.5, alb <3.5 or β_2M = 3.5-5.5	II (39%)	44
β_2M > 5.5	III (33%)	29
Other features suggesting high-risk disease: • De novo plasma cell leukemia • Extramedullary disease • Elevated lactate dehydrogenate (LDH) • High-risk gene expression profile		

Ans. D

35. All of the following disorders are considered by World Health Organization classification as chronic myeloproliferative neoplasms except:

A. Chronic myeloid leukemia (Bcr-Abl positive)
B. Essential thrombocytosis
C. Polycythemia vera
D. All are chronic myeloproliferative neoplasms

Explanation:

- World Health Organization (WHO) classification of the chronic myeloproliferative neoplasms (MPNs) includes eight disorders, some of which are rare or poorly characterized but all of which share an origin in a multipotent hematopoietic progenitor cell; overproduction of one or more of the formed elements of the blood without significant dysplasia; and a predilection to extramedullary hematopoiesis, myelofibrosis, and transformation at varying rates to acute leukemia.

World Health Organization Classification of Chronic Myeloproliferative Neoplasms

Chronic myeloid leukemia, Bcr-Abl positive
Chronic neutrophilic leukemia
Chronic eosinophilic leukemia, not otherwise specified
Polycythemia vera
Primary myelofibrosis
Essential thrombocytosis
Mastocytosis
Myeloproliferative neoplasms, unclassifiable

- Within this broad classification, however, significant phenotypic heterogeneity exists.
- Some diseases such as chronic myelogenous leukemia (CML), chronic neutrophilic leukemia (CNL), and chronic eosinophilic leukemia (CEL) express primarily a myeloid phenotype, whereas in other diseases,

such as polycythemia vera (PV), primary myelofibrosis (PMF), and essential thrombocytosis (ET), erythroid or megakaryocytic hyperplasia predominates.

- Latter three disorders, in contrast to the former three, also appear capable of transforming into each other.
- Such phenotypic heterogeneity has a genetic basis; CML is the consequence of the balanced translocation between chromosomes 9 and 22 [t(9;22)(q34;11)]; CNL has been associated with t(15;19) translocation; and CEL occurs with deletion or balanced translocations involving PDGFRα gene.
- By contrast, to a greater or lesser extent, PV, PMF, and ET are characterized by a mutation, V617F, that causes constitutive activation of JAK2, a tyrosine kinase essential for the function of the erythropoietin and thrombopoietin receptors but not granulocyte colony-stimulating factor receptor.
- This important distinction is also reflected in the natural histories of CML, CNL, and CEL, which are usually measured in years, and their high rate of leukemic transformation.
- By contrast, the natural history of PV, PMF, and ET is usually measured in decades, and transformation to acute leukemia is uncommon in PV and ET in the absence of exposure to mutagenic drugs.

Ans. D

36. All are frontline therapies in CML except:

A. Imatinib B. Dasatinib

C. Ponatinib D. Nilotinib

Explanation:

Chronic Myeloid Leukemia

- With TKI therapy, the estimated 10-year survival in CML is 85%.
- Six agents have been approved by the U.S. FDA for the treatment of CML. These include five oral TKIs: (Tyrosine kinase inhibitors)
- First generation - Imatinib
- Second generation- Nilotinib, Dasatinib & Bosutinib
- Third generation- Ponatinib
- Sixth approved agent is omacetaxine, a protein synthesis inhibitor with presumed more selective inhibition of the synthesis of the BCR-ABL1 oncoprotein.
- In that Imatinib, nilotinib, and dasatinib are all acceptable frontline therapies in CML

Ans. C

37. All of the following are typically increased in a patient with hemolytic anemia except:

A. Aspartate aminotransferase (AST) B. Haptoglobin

C. LDH D. MCV

Explanation:

- Differentiates hemolytic anemias (HAs) from other anemias is that the patient has signs and symptoms arising directly from hemolysis.
- At the clinical level, the main sign is jaundice; in addition, the patient may report discoloration of the urine.
- In many cases of HA, the spleen is enlarged, because it is a preferential site of hemolysis; and in some cases, the liver may be enlarged as well.
- Laboratory features of HA are related to hemolysis per se & erythropoietic response of the bone marrow.
- Hemolysis regularly produces an increase in unconjugated bilirubin and aspartate aminotransferase (AST) in serum; urobilinogen will be increased in both urine and stool.

- If hemolysis is mainly intravascular, telltale sign is hemoglobinuria (often associated with hemosiderinuria); in serum, there is hemoglobin, LDH is increased & haptoglobin is reduced.
- In contrast, the bilirubin level may be normal or only mildly elevated.
- Main sign of the erythropoietic response by the bone marrow is an increase in reticulocytes (a test all too often neglected in the initial workup of a patient with anemia).
- Usually the increase will be reflected in both percentage of reticulocytes (the more commonly quoted figure) & absolute reticulocyte count (the more definitive parameter).
- Increased number of reticulocytes is associated with an increased mean corpuscular volume (MCV) in the blood count.
- On the blood smear, this is reflected in presence of macrocytes; there is also polychromasia, and sometimes, one sees nucleated red cells.

Ans. B

38. Time taken for hematopoietic progenitors to become mature cells is:

A. 2-5 days
B. 5-8 days
C. 10-14 days
D. 15-20 days

Explanation:

- The time it takes for hematopoietic progenitors to become mature cells is ~10–14 days in humans, evident clinically by the interval between cytotoxic chemotherapy and blood count recovery in patients.

Ans. C

39. Splenectomy is an effective secondary or tertiary treatment for below lymphomas except:

A. Hairy cell leukemia
B. Prolymphocytic leukemia
C. Marginal zone lymphoma
D. Nodular sclerosis

Explanation:

- Splenectomy is an effective secondary or tertiary treatment for two chronic B cell leukemias, hairy cell leukemia and prolymphocytic leukemia, and for the very rare splenic mantle cell or marginal zone lymphoma. Splenectomy in these diseases may be associated with significant tumor regression in bone marrow and other sites of disease. Similar regressions of systemic disease have been noted after splenic irradiation in some types of lymphoid tumors, especially chronic lymphocytic leukemia and prolymphocytic leukemia. This has been termed the *abscopal effect*.

Ans. D

40. Unstable hemoglobin presenting as polycythemia is:

A. Hb Yakima
B. Hb Kansas
C. HbM Iwata
D. Hb Koln

Explanation:

Table: Representative abnormal hemoglobins with altered synthesis or function

Designation	Mutation	Population	Main Clinical Effects[a]
Sickle or S	$\beta^{6Glu \to Val}$	African	Anemia, ischemic infarcts
C	$\beta^{6Glu \to Lys}$	African	Mild anemia; interacts with Hbs
E	$\beta^{26Glu \to Lys}$	Southeast Asian	Microcytic anemia, splenomegaly, thalassemic phenotype

Contd.

Contd.

Köln	$\beta^{98Val \rightarrow Met}$	Sporadic	Hemolytic anemia, Heinz bodies when splenectomized
Yakima	$\beta^{99Asp \rightarrow His}$	Sporadic	Polycythemia
Kansas	$\beta^{102Asn \rightarrow Lys}$	Sporadic	Mild anemia
M Iwata	$\alpha^{87His \rightarrow Tyr}$	Sporadic	Methemoglobinemia

Ans. A

41. All are true about diagnosis of Essential thrombocytosis except:

A. Hyperkalemia in these patients is usually associated with electrocardiographic abnormalities
B. Arterial oxygen measurements can be inaccurate unless thrombocythemic blood is collected on ice
C. The prothrombin and partial thromboplastin times are normal
D. Abnormalities of platelet function such as a prolonged bleeding time and impaired platelet aggregation can be present

Explanation:

- Anemia is unusual, but a mild neutrophilic leukocytosis is not.
- Blood smear is most remarkable for the number of platelets present, some of which may be very large.
- Large mass of circulating platelets may prevent the accurate measurement of serum potassium due to release of platelet potassium upon blood clotting.
- This type of hyperkalemia is a test tube artifact and not associated with electrocardiographic abnormalities.
- Similarly, arterial oxygen measurements can be inaccurate unless thrombocythemic blood is collected on ice.
- Prothrombin and partial thromboplastin times are normal, whereas abnormalities of platelet function such as a prolonged bleeding time and impaired platelet aggregation can be present.
- However, despite much study, no platelet function abnormality is characteristic of ET, and no platelet function test predicts the risk of clinically significant bleeding or thrombosis.
- Elevated platelet count may hinder marrow aspiration, but marrow biopsy usually reveals megakaryocyte hypertrophy and hyperplasia, as well as an overall increase in marrow cellularity.
- If marrow reticulin is increased, another diagnosis should be considered.
- Absence of stainable iron demands an explanation because iron deficiency alone can cause thrombocytosis, and absent marrow iron in presence of marrow hypercellularity is a feature of PV.

Ans. A

42. Antithrombotic which need not be stopped for EGD or colonoscopy with dilation includes:

A. Aspirin
B Clopidogrel
C. Dabigatran
D. Edoxaban

Explanation:

Table: Management of antithrombotic drugs prior to endoscopic procedures

Drug	Bleeding Risk of Procedure	Management	Interval Between Last Dose and Procedure	Comments
Warfarin	Low[a]	Continue	N/A	Ensure that INR is not supratherapeutic
	High[b]	Discontinue	3-7 days (usually 5), INR should be ≤1.5 for procedure	Consider bridging therapy with heparin;[c] usually safe to resume warfarin on the same or next day

Contd.

Contd.

Dabigatran, rivaroxaban, apixaban, edoxaban	Low[a]	Continue or hold morning dose on day of procedure	N/A	
Dabigatran	High[b]	Discontinue	2-3 days if GFR is ≥ 50 ml/min, 3-4 days if GFR is 30-49 ml/min	Bridging therapy not recommended; resume drug when bleeding risk is low
Rivaroxaban, apixaban, edoxaban	High[a]	Discontinue	2 days if GFR is ≥60 ml/min, 3 days if GFR is 30-59 ml/min 4 days if GFR is < 30 ml/min	Bridging therapy not recommended; resume drug when bleeding risk is low
Heparin	Low[a] High[b]	Continue Discontinue	N/A 4–6 h for unfractionated heparin	 Skip one dose if using low-molecular-weight heparin
Aspirin	Any	Continue	N/A	Low-dose aspirin does not substantially increase the risk of endoscopic procedures
Aspirin with dipyridamole	Low[a] High[b]	Continue Discontinue	N/A 2-7 days	 Consider continuing aspirin monotherapy
P2Y12 receptor antagonists (clopidogrel, prasugrel, ticlopidine, ticagrelor, cangrelor)	Low[a] High[b]	Continue Coronary stent in place: discuss with cardiologist No coronary stent: Discontinue, consider substituting to aspirin	N/A 5 days (clopidogrel or ticagrelor), 7 days (prasugrel), 10-4 days (ticlopidine)	 Risk of stent thrombosis for 12 months after insertion of drug-eluting coronary stent or 1 month after insertion of bare metal coronary stent

Ans. A

43. All can be seen in hemolytic anemia except:

A. Increased reticulocytes

B. Increased unconjugated bilirubin

C. Haptoglobin elevated in intravascular hemolysis

D. Upto 10 times elevated LDH in intravascular hemolysis

Explanation:

Table: Features common to most patients with a hemolytic disorder	
General examination	Jaundice, pallor
Other physical findings	Spleen may be enlarged; bossing of skull in severe congenital cases
Hemoglobin level	From normal to severely reduced
MCV, MCH	Usually increased
Reticulocytes	Usually increased
Bilirubin	Almost always increased (mostly unconjugated)
LDH	Increased (up to 10 × normal with intravascular hemolysis)
Haptoglobin	Reduced to absent if hemolysis is at least in part intravascular

Ans. C

44. All are true about AML presentation except:

A. Hemorrhagic complications are most commonly and, classically, found in APL
B. APL patients often present with DIC-associated minor hemorrhage
C. Bleeding associated with coagulopathy may also occur in monocytic AML
D. Retinal hemorrhages are detected in 30% of patients

Explanation:

- Fever, infection, and hemorrhage are often found at time of diagnosis; splenomegaly, hepatomegaly, lymphadenopathy, and "bone pain" may also be present less commonly.
- Hemorrhagic complications are most commonly and, classically, found in APL. APL patients often present with DIC-associated minor hemorrhage but may have significant gastrointestinal bleeding, intrapulmonary hemorrhage, or intracranial hemorrhage.
- Likewise, thrombosis is another less frequent but well recognized clinical feature of DIC in APL.
- Bleeding associated with coagulopathy may also occur in monocytic AML and with extreme degrees of leukocytosis or thrombocytopenia in other morphologic subtypes.
- Retinal hemorrhages are detected in 15% of patients.
- Infiltration of the gingiva, skin, soft tissues, or meninges with leukemic blasts at diagnosis is characteristic of the monocytic subtypes and those with 11q23 chromosomal abnormalities.

Ans. D

45. B-cell markers for Mantle cell lymphoma include all except:

A. CD19
B. CD5
C. CD10
D. CD20

Explanation:

- Pathognomonic cytogenetic finding in MCL is t(11;14), which brings the gene for the cell cycle control protein cyclin D1 under control of the immunoglobulin heavy chain gene promoter on chromosome.
- This translocation is present in >90% of cases.
- The remaining cases usually overexpress cyclin D2, cyclin D3, or cyclin E.
- Tumor cells also are positive for B-cell markers CD19 and CD20, as well as CD5.
- **Usually lack CD10 and CD23.**

Ans. C

46. **Congenital neutropenia with increased risk of AML is termed as:**

A. Kostmann disease
B. Bloom syndrome
C. Fanconi anemia
D. Hemolytic uremic syndrome

Explanation:

- Congenital neutropenia with increased risk of AML is termed as Kostmann disease
- It is due to mutation in G- colony stimulating factor and neutrophil elastase which eventually leads to AML.

Ans. A

47. **Which of the following is a feature of myeloblast?**

A. Prominent nucleoli
B. Phi bodies
C. Auer rods
D. All the above

Explanation:

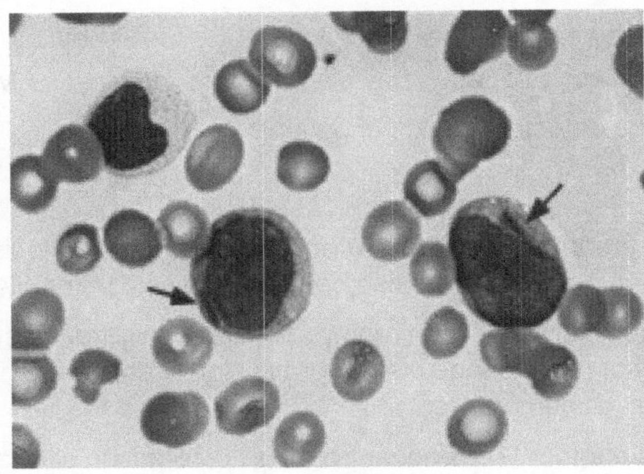

- ***Auer rods:** Needle shaped intracytoplasmic inclusion bodies, azurophilic in nature formed by fusion of lysosomes. Those black arrows pointing Auer rods.
- ***Phi bodies:** Spindle shaped rods similar to Auer rods which requires staining with hydroperoxidases.

Ans. D

48. **Which of the following predisposes to Chronic myeloid leukemia?**

A. Family history
B. Polycythemia vera
C. Exposure to ionising Radiation
D. Both B and C

Explanation:

- There is no familial association for CML.
- Exposure to ionising Radiation predisposes to CML. High dose ionising Radiation may develop into CML after 5-10 years EXAMPLE Treatment for ankylosing spondylitis.
- Hematological association: Essential thrombocytosis and primary myelofibrosis.

Ans. D

49. **Treatment of choice in chronic myeloid leukemia is:**

A. Monoclonal antibodies
B. Tyrosine kinase inhibitors
C. Janus kinase inhibitors
D. Allogenic hematopoietic stem cell transplantation

Explanation:

- Allogenic hematopoietic stem cell transplantation is the treatment of choice before the introduction of tyrosine kinase inhibitors but AHSCT is the treatment modality with curative potential.

Tyrosine kinase inhibitors

- **1st Generation-** Imatinib
- **2nd generation-** Dasatinib, Nilotinib
- **3rd generation-** Ponatinib.

Ans. B

50. An old aged patient presented with fatigue and early satiety. Philadelphia chromosome is found to be positive. What is the characteristic finding in clinical examination?

A. Pallor
B. Lymphadenopathy
C. Hepatomegaly
D. Splenomegaly

Explanation:

- **Splenomegaly is the most common finding in CML**
- Other features include Hepatomegaly, Lymphadenopathy and extramedullary disease like skin lesions

***Phases in CML**

- Chronic phase
- Accelerated phase
- Blastic phase

Ans. D

51. Most common symptom in multiple myeloma is:

A. Easy fatiguability
B. Bone pain
C. Renal failure
D. Fever

Explanation:

- Bone pain most commonly seen in 70-75 percent of the patient. It is due to the imbalance between osteoclastic and osteoblastic activity. That is osteoclast is activated more and osteoblast have got suppressed.
- Renal injury is mostly due to hypercalcaemia.
- Other causes of renal injury include: Hyperurcemia, Amyloid deposits and Infiltration of kidney by myeloma cells

Ans. B

52. Treatment of choice in multiple myeloma is:

A. Lenalidomide + Borteozomib + Dexamethasone
B. Thalidomide + Dexamethasone
C. Rituximab + Cyclophosphamide
D. Rituximab + Borteozomib

Explanation:

- Combination of Lenalidomide, Borteozomib and Dexamethasone achieves close to 100 percentage response which makes the patient condition suitable for further treatment.

- Autologous stem cell transplantation will improve the chance of survival.

Ans. A

53. Most common bleeding manifestation in Severe hemophilia is:

A. Recurrent hematoma
B. Recurrent hemarthrosis
C. Hematuria
D. Intracranial hemorrhage

Explanation:

- Most common bleeding manifestation in severe hemophilia is Recurrent Hemarthrosis and the most commonly affect joint is knee joint.
- Acute manifestation of the disease is characterized by local pain, erythema and swelling, muscle contracture due to fixed positioning.
- Chronic manifestation of the disease is characterized by synovial thickening and synovitis due to intra articular blood collection.

Ans. B

54. Bethesda assay is used for the detection of inhibitors against:

A. Factor VIII
B. Factor II
C. Factor VII
D. Factor X

Explanation:

- Formation of alloantibodies against factor VIII is one of the significant complication of hemophilia treatment. After this the patient won't respond to factor replacement at ordinary doses.
- Usually in a patient suffering from hemophilia prolonged aPTT is corrected by 1:1 mixture of patient plasma and normal plasma.
- In inhibitor presence it will be prolonged even after the administration of 1:1 mixture (due to the consumption of normal factors by inhibitors).

Ans. A

55. Most sensitive test for diagnosing Disseminated intravascular coagulation is:

A. Fibrin degradation products (FDP) level.
B. D-Dimer assay
C. Fibrinogen level
D. Activated Partial thromboplastin time.

Explanation:

- It shows 100 percent sensitivity and 86 percent diagnostic efficiency better than any other tests.

Ans. A

56. An isolated prolongation of prothrombin time suggests:

A. Factor VII deficiency
B. Factor V deficiency
C. Factor XI deficiency
D. Factor II deficiency

Explanation:

- Prothrombin time is time taken for plasma to clot when exposed to tissue factor.
- Normal prothrombin time is 12-16 seconds.

- Extrinsic pathway of coagulation can be assessed using prothrombin time.

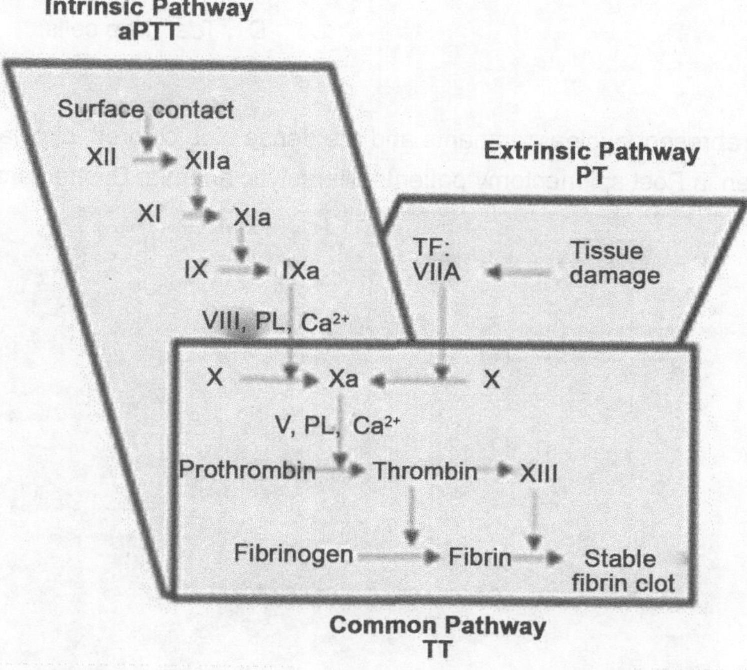

Ans. A

57. Below shown haematological picture is seen in which of the following disorder:

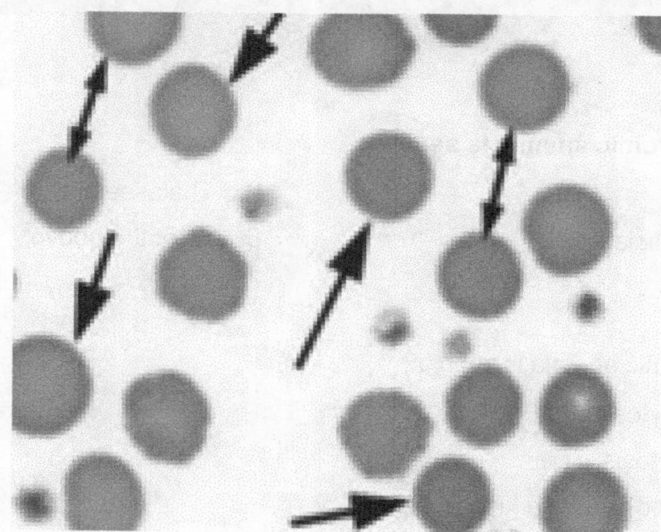

A. Thalassemia
B. Iron deficiency anemia
C. Autoimmune haemolysis
D. Sickle cell anemia

Explanation:

- Spherocytes are small red cells with compact appearance and absent central pallor. Macrophages in spleen remove membranes coated by antibodies leading to spherocytes formation resulting in autoimmune hemolysis.

Ans. C

58. **Which of the following cells is seen in patient suffering from hyposplenism?**

A. Howell-Jolly bodies
B. Spherocytes
C. Elliptocytes
D. Tear drop cells

Explanation:

- These cells represent nuclear remnants and are dense blue colored, circular in shape.
- They are seen in Post splenectomy patients, Hemolytic anemia, Dyshematopoiesis, Hyposplenism.

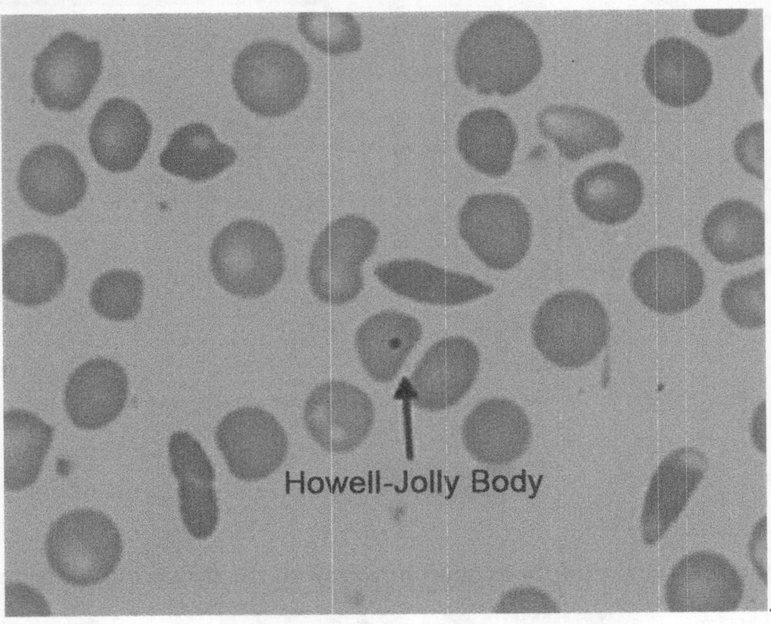

Ans. A

59. **Normocytic normochromic anemia is seen in:**

A. Sickle cell anemia
B. Thalassemia
C. Pyruvate kinase deficiency
D. All of the above

Explanation:

Normocytic normochromic anemia is seen in:

- Hereditary spherocytosis
- Hereditary Elliptocytosis
- G6PD deficiency and pyruvate kinase deficiency
- Parvovirus B19 infection.
- Chronic kidney disease.

Ans. C

60. **Iron absorption takes place in:**

A. Stomach
B. Proximal small intestine
C. Distal small intestine
D. Large intestine

Explanation:

- Iron absorption mainly takes place in proximal small intestine under acidic conditions.
- Acidity favors conversion of ferric iron to ferrous form which is then easily absorbed.

Ans. B

61. Transport of iron across brush border cells is facilitated by:

A. DMT-1
B. Nramp 2
C. Ferroportin
D. Both A and B

Explanation:

- Transport of iron across brush border cells is facilitated by DMT-1 (Divalent metal Transporter-1). It is also called as Natural resistance associated macrophage protein type 2(Nramp2).

Ans. D

62. Life span of platelet is:

A. 48 hours
B. 4 days
C. 7 days
D. 3 weeks

Explanation:

- Average life span of platelet is 7-10 days.
- Thrombopoietin is the hormone that stimulates platelet production.

Ans. C

63. Thrombocytopenia is not seen in:

A. Thrombotic thrombocytopenic purpura
B. Henoch-Schönlein purpura
C. Hemolytic uremic syndrome
D. Disseminated intravascular coagulation

Explanation:

- *Plateletcount <1,50,000/microlitre is termed as thrombocytopenia but in henoch-schönlein purpura platelet count and coagulation profile were normal.
- *Henoch-schönlein purpura is characterized by vasculitis which is IgA mediated usually affects children and young adults.

Ans. B

64. Condition in which immune mediated destruction of platelet is seen in:

A. Chronic lymphocytic leukemia
B. HIV infection
C. Systemic lupus erythematosus
D. All of the above

Explanation:

- Immune mediated platelet destruction is seen in * Chronic and acute idiopathic thrombocytopenic purpura, *Systemic lupus erythematosus,*Following blood transfusion.

- HIV Infection and *Dengue fever.

Ans. D

65. Combination of autoimmune Hemolytic anemia and idiopathic thrombocytopenic purpura together called as:

A. Rosenthal syndrome
B. Fechtner syndrome
C. Evans syndrome
D. All of the above

Explanation:

- *Evans syndrome is the combination of autoimmune Hemolytic anemia and ITP.
- *Rosenthal syndrome is factor eleven deficiency.
- *Fechtner syndrome is an Autosomal Dominant disorder characterized by sensory neural hearing loss, bleeding, glomerulonephritis and eye abnormalities.

Ans. C

66. IPSS score for Primary myelofibrosis include all except:

A. Platelet count
B. Age
C. Anemia
D. Leukocytosis

Explanation:

Table: Three current scoring systems for estimating prognosis in PMG patients

Risk Factor	IPSS (2009)[a]	DIPSS (2010)[b]	DIPSS Plus (2011)[c]
Anemia (<10 g/dl)	X	X	X
Leukocytosis (>25,000/μl)	X	X	X
Peripheral blood blasts (≥1%)	X	X	X
Constitutional symptoms	X	X	X
Age (> 65 years)	X	X	X
Unfavorable karyotype			X
Platelet count (<100,000/μl)			X
Transfusion dependence			X

Ans. A

67. In aplastic anemia, severe disease is defined by all except:

A. Absolute neutrophil count <500/μL
B. Platelet count <30,000/μL
C. Corrected reticulocyte count <1%
D. Absolute reticulocyte count <60,000/μL

Explanation:

- Severe disease historically has been defined by the presence of two of three parameters: absolute neutrophil count <500/μL, platelet count <20,000/μL, and corrected reticulocyte count <1% (or absolute reticulocyte count <60,000/μL).
- In the era of effective immunosuppressive therapies, absolute numbers of reticulocytes (>25,000/μL) and lymphocytes (>1000/μL) may be better predictors of response to treatment and long-term outcome.

Ans. B

68. Most common physical finding in CML is:

A. Splenomegaly
B. Hepatomegaly
C. Lymphadenopathy
D. Skin/Subcutaneous lesions

Explanation:

- Splenomegaly is the most common physical finding, occurring in 20–70% of patients depending on health care screening frequency.
- Other less common findings include hepatomegaly (5–10%), lymphadenopathy (5–10%), and extramedullary disease (skin or subcutaneous lesions).
- Latter indicates CML transformation if a biopsy confirms predominance of blasts. Other physical findings are manifestations of complications of high tumor burden (e.g., cardiovascular, cerebrovascular, bleeding).
- High basophil counts may be associated with histamine overproduction causing pruritus, diarrhea, flushing, and even gastrointestinal ulcers.

Ans. A

69. Intravascular hemolysis is differentiated from extravascular type by which of the following feature?

A. Normal LDH
B. Normal Haptoglobin
C. No splenomegaly
D. Presence of hemoglobinuria

Explanation:

- In most cases hemolysis is largely extravascular, and it produces an increase in unconjugated bilirubin and aspartate aminotransferase (AST) in serum; urobilinogen will be increased in both urine and stool.
- If hemolysis is mainly intravascular, the telltale sign is hemoglobinuria (often associated with hemosiderinuria); in the serum there is free hemoglobin, lactate dehydrogenase (LDH) is increased, and haptoglobin is reduced. In contrast, the serum bilirubin level may be normal or only mildly elevated. The main sign of the erythropoietic response by the bone marrow is an increase in reticulocytes (a test all too often neglected in the initial workup of a patient with anemia). Usually increase will be reflected in both the percentage of reticulocytes (more commonly quoted figure) and in the absolute reticulocyte count (more definitive parameter).

Ans. D

70. Not a part of International prognostic score in Classical HL:

A. Female sex
B. Stage 4 disease
C. Serum albumin <4g/dL
D. WBC >15,000/μL

Explanation:

- Prognosis in advanced stage disease is best predicted by the International Prognostic Score (IPS), which ascribes a point for male sex, older age (>45 years), stage IV disease, serum albumin <4 g/dL, hemoglobin <10.5 g/dL, white blood cell count ≥15,000/μL, and a lymphocyte count <600/μL and/or <8% of white blood cell count.
- Five-year progression-free survival ranges from 88% for patients with no risk factors, to 62% for patients with four or more factors, but very few patients have multiple risk factors.

Ans. A

71. All are components of PNH except:

A. Intravascular hemolysis
B. Pancytopenia
C. Venous thrombosis
D. Arterial thrombosis

Explanation:

- PNH is an acquired chronic HA characterized by persistent intravascular hemolysis with occasional or frequent recurrent exacerbations. In addition to (i) hemolysis, there may be (ii) pancytopenia and (iii) a distinct tendency to venous thrombosis.
- This triad makes PNH a truly unique clinical condition; however, when not all of these three features are manifest on presentation, the diagnosis is often delayed, although it can always be made by appropriate laboratory investigations.

Ans. D

72. Ring sideroblasts are formed due to accumulation of iron in:

A. Endoplasmic reticulum
B. Lysosomes
C. Mitochondria
D. Nucleus

Explanation:

- Normally, when the marrow smear is stained for iron, 20–40% of developing erythroblasts—called *sideroblasts*—will have visible ferritin granules in their cytoplasm.
- This represents iron in excess of that needed for hemoglobin synthesis.
- In states in which release of iron from storage sites is blocked, RE iron will be detectable, and there will be few or no sideroblasts.
- In the myelodysplastic syndromes, mitochondrial dysfunction can occur, and accumulation of iron in mitochondria appears in a necklace fashion around the nucleus of the erythroblast. Such cells are referred to as *ring sideroblasts*.

Ans. C

73. Spur cells are due to:

A. Excess of iron
B. Excess of folate
C. Excess of Cholesterol
D. Excess of glucose

Explanation:

- Mild hypoproliferative anemia may develop in patients with chronic liver disease from nearly any cause.
- Peripheral blood smear may show spur cells and stomatocytes from the accumulation of excess cholesterol in membrane from a deficiency of lecithin-cholesterol acyltransferase.
- Red cell survival is shortened, and the production of EPO is inadequate to compensate.
- In alcoholic liver disease, nutritional deficiencies are common and complicate the management.
- Folate deficiency from inadequate intake, as well as iron deficiency from blood loss and inadequate intake, can alter the red cell indices

Ans. C

74. Myeloproliferative Hypereosinophilic syndrome may include all except:

A. Decreased serum vitamin B12
B. Increased tryptase
C. Anemia
D. Splenomegaly

Explanation:

- Clinical and laboratory findings in myeloproliferative HES may include dysplastic peripheral eosinophils, increased serum vitamin B12, increased tryptase, anemia, thrombocytopenia, splenomegaly, bone marrow cellularity >80%, spindle-shaped mast cells, and myelofibrosis.

- Evaluation for lymphocytic HES includes searching for abnormal T cell clonal populations.

Ans. A

75. Tear drop cells are seen in:

A. Hereditary spherocytois
B. Myelofibrosis
C. Sickle cell anemia
D. Parasitic infection

Explanation:

Tear drop cells also called Dacrocytes. Seen in:

- Thalassemia
- Myelofibrosis
- Myelodysplastic syndromes
- Severe iron deficiency.

Ans. B

76. MCHC >34:

A. Hereditary spherocytosis
B. Hereditary elliptocytosis
C. Hereditary stomatocytosis
D. Thalessemia major

Explanation:

- Anemia is usually normocytic, with the characteristic morphology that gives the disease its name. An increased mean corpuscular hemoglobin concentration (MCHC >34) on an ordinary blood count report should raise the suspicion of HS, because HS is almost the only condition in which this abnormality occurs.

Ans. A

77. Frequent first symptom among AML patients is:

A. Fatigue
B. Anorexia
C. Weight loss
D. Bone pain

Explanation:

- Patients with AML usually present with nonspecific symptoms that begin gradually, or abruptly, and are the consequence of anemia, leukocytosis, leukopenia/leukocyte dysfunction, or thrombocytopenia.
- Nearly half have symptoms for ≤3 months before leukemia is diagnosed.
- Fatigue is a frequent first symptom among AML patients.
- Anorexia and weight loss are common. Fever with or without an identifiable infection is the initial symptom in ~10% of patients.
- Signs of abnormal hemostasis (bleeding, easy bruising) are common.
- Bone pain, lymphadenopathy, nonspecific cough, headache, or diaphoresis may also occur

Ans. A

78. Complete remission in ALL:

A. <1% blast cells in bone marrow
B. <5% blast cells in bone marrow
C. <10 % blast cells in bone marrow
D. <15% blast cells in bone marrow

Explanation:

Table: Response parameters according to MRD	
Terminology	**Definition**
Complete (hematologic) remission	Leukemic cells not detectable by light microscopy (<5% blast cells in bone marrow)
Complete molecular remission MRD-negativity	Patient in complete remission, MRD not detectable, ≤ 0.01% = ≤1 leukemia blast cell in 10,000
Molecular failure/MRD-positivity	Patient in complete hematologic remission but not in molecular complete remission >0.01%
Molecular relapse/MRD-positivity	Patient still in complete remission had prior molecular complete remission Leukemic blast cells detectable in bone marrow not detectable (<5%)
Hematologic relapse	>5% ALL cells in bone marrow/blood

Ans. B

79. AML is associated with:

A. Kostmann syndrome
B. Fanconi anemia
C. Bloom syndrome
D. All of the above

Explanation:

- Several genetic syndromes with somatic cell chromosome aneuploidy, such as Down syndrome with trisomy 21, are associated with an increased incidence of AML.
- Down syndrome–associated AML in young children (<4 years) is typically of the acute megakaryocytic subtype and is associated with mutation in the *GATA1* gene.
- Such patients have excellent clinical outcomes but require dose modification of chemotherapy due to high treatment-related toxicities.
- Inherited diseases with defective DNA repair (e.g., Fanconi anemia, Bloom syndrome, and ataxia-telangiectasia) are also associated with AML.
- Each syndrome is associated with unique clinical features and atypical toxicities with chemotherapy, requiring expert care.
- Congenital neutropenia (Kostmann syndrome), due to mutations in genes encoding granulocyte colony-stimulating factor receptor and neutrophil elastase is another disorder that may evolve into AML.

Ans. D

80. Which type of von willebrand disease is called as autosomal haemophilia?

A. 2A
B. 2B
C. 2M
D. 2N

Explanation:

- Type 2N VWD is due to variants in the *VWF* gene that affect binding of FVIII.
- As FVIII is stabilized by binding to VWF, the FVIII in patients with type 2N VWD has a very short half-life, and the FVIII level is markedly decreased. This is sometimes termed *autosomal hemophilia*.
- Type 3 VWD, or severe VWD, describes patients with virtually no VWF protein and FVIII levels <10%. Patients experience mucosal and joint bleeding, surgery-related bleeding, and other bleeding symptoms.
- Some patients with type 3 VWD, particularly those with large VWF gene deletions, are at risk of developing antibodies to infused VWF.

Ans. D

81. All are causes of hypocellular bone marrow with or without pancytopenia except:

A. Hairy cell leukemia
B. Q fever
C. Leigionnaires disease
D. Anorexia nervosa

Explanation:

Table: Differential diagnosis of pancytopenia	
Pancytopenia with Hypocellular Bone Marrow	
Acquired aplastic anemia	
Constitutional aplastic anemia (Fanconi anemia, dyskeratosis congenita and others)	
Hypocellular myelodysplastic syndrome	
Rare aleukemic leukemia	
Some acute lymphoid leukemia	
Rare lymphomas of bone marrow	
Copper deficiency	
Pancytopenia with Cellular Bone Marrow	
Primary bone marrow diseases	Secondary to systemic disease
• Myelodysplastic syndromes	• Systemic lupus erythematosus
• Paroxysmal nocturnal hemoglobinuria (PNH)	• Hypersplenism
	• B_{12}, folate deficiency
	• Copper deficiency
• Mylofibrosis	• Alcohol
• Aleukemic leukemia	• HIV infection
• Myelophthisis	• Brucellosis
Bone marrow lymphoma	• Sarcoidosis
Hairy cell leukemia	• Tuberculosis
	• Leishmaniasis
	• Sepsis
Hypocellular Bone Marrow ± Pancytopenia	
Q fever	
Legionnaires' disease	
Anorexia nervosa, starvation	
Mycobacterium	

Ans. A

82. Condition causing microcytic erythrocytosis are all except:

A. Beta thalassemia trait
B. Hypoxic erythrocytosis
C. PNH
D. PV

Explanation:

- When PV presents with erythrocytosis in combination with leukocytosis, thrombocytosis, or splenomegaly or any combination of these, the diagnosis is apparent.
- However, when patients present with an elevated hemoglobin, hematocrit, or red cell count alone, the diagnostic evaluation is more complex because of the many diagnostic possibilities.

Table: Causes of erythrocytosis	
Relative Erythrocytosis	
Hemoconcentration secondary to dehydration, diuretics, ethanol abuse, androgens or tobacco abuse	
Absolute Erythrocytosis	
Hypoxia	**Tumors**
Carbon monoxide intoxication	Hypernephroma
High-oxygen-affinity hemoglobins	Hepatoma
High altitude	Cerebellar hemangioblastoma
Pulmonary disease	Uterine myoma
Right-to-left cardiac or vascular shunts	Adrenal tumors
Sleep apnea syndrome	Meningioma
Hepatopulmonary syndrome	Pheochromocytoma
Renal Disease	**Drugs**
Renal artery stenosis	Androgens
Focal sclerosing or membranous glomerulonephritis	Recombinant erythropoietin
Postrenal transplantation	**Familial (with normal hemoglobin function)**
Renal cysts	Erythropoietin receptor mutations
Bartter's syndrome	*VHL* mutations (Chuvash polycythemia)
	2, 3-BPG mutation
	PHD2 and HIF2α mutations
	Polycythemia vera

Ans. C

83. Which drug doesn't cause TTP?

A. Quinine
B. Ticlopidine
C. Ticagrelor
D. Clopidogrel

Explanation:

- ADAMTS13 deficiency is found in fewer than half of patients with clopidogrel-associated TTP.
- Quinine appears to induce autoantibodies to granulocytes, lymphocytes, endothelial cells, and platelet glycoprotein Ib/IX or IIb/IIIa complexes, but not to ADAMTS13. Quinine-associated TTP is more common among women.
- TMA has also been reported with drugs that inhibit vascular endothelial growth factor, such as bevacizumab; the mechanism is not completely understood

Ans. C

84. Most common cause of renal failure in multiple myeloma is:

A. Hypercalcemia
B. Amyloid deposits
C. Hyperuricemia
D. Frequent use of NSAID's

Explanation:

- Renal failure occurs in nearly 25% of myeloma patients, and some renal pathology is noted in >50%.
- Of many contributing factors, hypercalcemia is the most common cause of renal failure.
- Glomerular deposits of amyloid, hyperuricemia, recurrent infections, frequent use of NSAID's for pain control, use of iodinated contrast dye for imaging, bisphosphonate use, and occasional infiltration of the kidney by myeloma cells all may contribute to renal dysfunction.
- However, tubular damage associated with the excretion of light chains is almost always present.

- Normally, light chains are filtered, reabsorbed in the tubules, and catabolized.
- With the increase in the amount of light chains presented to the tubule, the tubular cells become overloaded with these proteins, and tubular damage results either directly from light chain toxic effects or indirectly from release of intracellular lysosomal enzymes.
- Earliest manifestation of this tubular damage is the adult Fanconi's syndrome (a type 2 proximal renal tubular acidosis), with loss of glucose and amino acids, as well as defects in the ability of the kidney to acidify and concentrate the urine.

Ans. A

85. All are possible treatment options for CML in pregnancy except:

A. Leukapheresis B. Hydroxyurea

C. Imatinib D. Interferon alpha

Explanation:

- Interferon α is considered in combination with TKIs (an investigational approach), sometimes after CML failure on TKIs, occasionally in patients during pregnancy, or as part of investigational strategies with TKIs to eradicate residual molecular disease.
- Women with CML who become pregnant should discontinue TKI therapy immediately.
- Babies delivered to women with CML who discontinued imatinib therapy as soon as the pregnancy was known, three babies were born with neurologic, skeletal, and renal malformations, suggesting teratogenicity of imatinib known from animal studies.
- A similar experience has been reported with dasatinib, the incidence of malformations was reported to be higher, 10–12%.

Ans. C

86. All are possible surrogate markers for CLL diagnosis except:

A. IGHV sequencing B. ZAP-70 methylation

C. CD 34 expression D. CD 38 expression

Explanation:

- Because IGHV sequencing was initially cumbersome to perform, a number of surrogate factors have been identified; however, none yet have been shown to be equal or superior to IGVH sequencing.
- Most prevalent of these surrogate markers are Zap-70 expression, *ZAP-70* methylation, and surface CD38 expression.
- Zap-70 protein is a normal intracellular T-cell signaling protein that is aberrantly expressed in most IGHV unmutated CLL cells.
- CD38 is a marker that is also more highly expressed on the surface of IGHV unmutated CLL cells. Both these prognostic factors are widely used but limited in their applicability. Zap-70 protein status is difficult to measure by flow cytometry, and it has low reproducibility.
- Measurement of methylation status of *ZAP-70* promoter is much more precise but not widely available.
- CD38 expression is easier to measure by flow cytometry but not as highly predictive of outcomes and can change during the course of disease.

Ans. C

87. All are causes of pancytopenia with hypocellular bone marrow except:

A. Copper deficiency B. Fanconi anemia

C. PNH D. Acquired aplastic anemia

Explanation:

<table>
<tr><th colspan="2">Pancytopenia with Hypocellular Bone Marrow</th></tr>
<tr><td colspan="2">• Acquired aplastic anemia
• Constitutional aplastic anemia (Fanconi anemia, dyskeratosis congenita and others)
• Hypocellular myelodysplastic syndrome
• Rare aleukemic leukemia
• Some acute lymphoid leukemia
• Rare lymphomas of bone marrow
• Copper deficiency</td></tr>
<tr><th colspan="2">Pancytopenia with Cellular Bone Marrow</th></tr>
<tr><td>• Primary bone marrow diseases
– Myelodysplastic syndromes
– Paroxysmal nocturnal hemoglobinuria (PNH)
– Mylofibrosis
– Aleukemic leukemia
– Myelophthisis
• Bone marrow lymphoma
• Hairy cell leukemia</td><td>• Secondary to systemic diseases
– Systemic lupus erythematosus
– Hypersplenism
– B_{12}, folate deficiency
– Copper deficiency
– Alcohol
– HIV infection
– Brucellosis
– Sarcoidosis
– Tuberculosis
– Leishmaniasis
– Sepsis</td></tr>
<tr><th colspan="2">Hypocellular Bone Marrow ± Pancytopenia</th></tr>
<tr><td colspan="2">• Q fever
• Legionnaires' disease
• Anorexia nervosa, starvation
• Mycobacterium</td></tr>
</table>

Ans. C

88. All are true about associations of aplastic anemia except:

A. Hepatitis which is associated with aplastic anemia is seronegative (non-A, non- B, non-C)

B. Aplastic anemia can rarely follow infectious mononucleosis

C. Aplastic anemia is strongly associated with the parvovirus B19 infection

D. Pancytopenia with marrow hypoplasia can also occur in systemic lupus erythematosus

Explanation:

- Posthepatitis marrow failure accounts for ~5% of etiologies in most series.
- Patients are usually young men who have recovered from a bout of liver inflammation 1–2 months earlier; the subsequent pancytopenia is very severe.
- Hepatitis is seronegative (non-A, non-B, non-C); intensive laboratory efforts including deep sequencing have not disclosed an infectious agent.
- Fulminant liver failure in childhood also follows seronegative hepatitis, and marrow failure occurs at a high rate in these patients.
- Aplastic anemia can rarely follow infectious mononucleosis.
- Parvovirus B19 does not usually cause generalized bone marrow failure.
- Transient, mild blood count depression is frequent in the course of many viral and bacterial infections.

Ans. C

89. If the fever occurs during every 21st day of its cycle is seen in:

A. Hodgkin lymphoma
B. Brucellosis
C. Cyclic neutropenia
D. Familial Mediterranean fever

Explanation:

- In Cyclic Neutropenia fever occurs during every 21 days and it is accompanied by neutropenia.

Ans. C

90. Sweet syndrome is most often in association with:

A. AML
B. ALL
C. CLL
D. CML

Explanation:

- *Sweet syndrome*, or *febrile neutrophilic dermatosis*, was originally described in women with elevated white blood cell (WBC) counts.
- Disease is characterized by the presence of leukocytes in the lower dermis, with edema of the papillary body.
- Ironically, this disease now is usually seen in neutropenic patients with cancer, most often in association with acute myeloid leukemia (AML) but also in association with a variety of other malignancies.
- Sweet syndrome usually presents as red or bluish-red papules or nodules that may coalesce and form sharply bordered plaques.
- Edema may suggest vesicles, but on palpation the lesions are solid, and vesicles probably never arise in this disease.
- Lesions are most common on the face, neck, and arms.
- On the legs, they may be confused with erythema nodosum.
- Development of lesions is often accompanied by high fevers and an elevated erythrocyte sedimentation rate.
- Both the lesions and the temperature elevation respond dramatically to glucocorticoid administration.
- Treatment begins with high doses of glucocorticoids (prednisone, 60 mg/d) followed by tapered doses over the next 2–3 weeks.

Ans. A

91. Thrombocytosis seen in all except:

A. Wagener's granulomatosis
B. Kawasaki disease
C. RA
D. APLA

Explanation:

- Thrombocytosis may be seen as an acutephase reactant. Approximately 90% of patients with active granulomatosis with polyangiitis (Wegener's) have a positive antiproteinase-3 ANCA. However, in the absence of active disease, the sensitivity drops to ~60–70%. A small percentage of patients with granulomatosis with polyangiitis (Wegener's) may have antimyeloperoxidase rather than antiproteinase-3 antibodies, and up to 20% may lack ANCA.
- APLA Syndrome is associated with Thrombocytopenia.

Ans. D

92. Pneumoniae/H.Influenzae/N.Meningitidis common in all except:

A. Hodgkin lymphoma
B. CLL
C. Multiple myeloma
D. Post splenectomy

Explanation:

Table: Disruption of normal barriers in patients with cancer that may predispose them to infections					
Type of Defense	**Specific Lesion**	**Cells Involved**	**Organism**	**Cancer Association**	**Disease**
Physical barrier	Breaks in skin	Skin epithelial cells	Staphylococci, streptococci	Head and neck, squamous cell carcinoma	Cellulitis, extensive skin infection
Emptying of fluid collections	Occlusion of orifices; ureters, bile duct, colon	Luminal epithelial cells	Gram-negative bacilli	Renal, ovarian biliary tree, metastatic diseases of many cancers	Rapid, overwhelming bacteremia; urinary tract infection
Lymphatic function	Node dissection	Lymph nodes	Staphylococci, streptococci	Breast cancer surgery	Cellulitis
Splenic clearance of microorganisms	Splenectomy	Splenic reticuloendothelial cells	*Streptococcus pneumoniae, Haemophilus influenzae, Neisseria meningitidis, Babesia, Capnocytophaga canimorsus*	Hodgkin's disease, leukemia	Rapid, overwhelming sepsis
Phagocytosis	Lack of granulocytes	Granulocytes (neutrophils)	Staphylococci, streptococci, enteric organisms, fungi	Acute myeloid and acute lymphocytic leukemias, hairy cell leukemia	Bacteremia
Humoral immunity	Lack of antibody	B cells	*S. pneumoniae, H. influenzae, N. meningitidis*	Chronic lymphocytic leukemia, multiple myeloma	Infections with encapsulated organisms, sinusitis, pneumonia
Cellular immunity	Lack of T cells	T cells and macrophages	*Mycobacterium tuberculosis, Listeria, herpersviruses, fungi, intracellular* parasites	Hodgkin's disease, leukemia, T cell lymphoma	Infections with intracellular bacteria, fungi, parasites; virus reactivation

Ans. A

93. **Single most powerful predictor of survival and can substitute for staging in multiple myeloma is:**

A. Serum beta 2 microglobulin
B. Extramedullary disease
C. Lactate dehydrogenase (LDH)
D. High risk gene expression profile

Explanation:

- Serum β2-microglobulin is the single most powerful predictor of survival and can substitute for staging. β2-Microglobulin is the light chain of the class I major histocompatibility antigens (HLA-A, -B, -C) on the surface of every cell. Combination of serum β2-microglobulin and albumin levels forms the basis for a three-stage International Staging System (ISS) that predicts survival.
- With the use of high dose therapy and the newer agents, the Durie-Salmon staging system is unable to predict outcome and thus is no longer used.

Ans. A

94. Which of the following is not T cell lymphoid malignancy?

A. Anaplastic large cell lymphoma ALK+
B. Anaplastic large cell lymphoma ALK-
C. Mycosis fungoides
D. Hairy cell leukemia

Explanation:

Table: WHO classification of lymphoid malignancies	
B Cell	**T Cell**
Mature (peripheral) B-cell neoplasms • Lymphoplasmacytic lymphoma (Waldenstrom's macroglobulinemia) • Hairy cell leukemia • Splenic marginal zone B-cell lymphoma • Extranodal marginal zone B-cell lymphoma of MALT type • Nodal marginal zone B-cell lymphoma • Follicular lymphoma • Mantle cell lymphoma • Diffuse large B-cell lymphoma (including subtypes) • High grade B-cell lymphoma with MYC and BCL2 and/or BCL6 rearrangements • High grade B-cell lymphoma NOS • Burkitt's lymphoma/Burkitt's cell leukemia • Primary mediastinal large B-cell lymphoma • Plasmablastic lymphoma • Primary effusion lymphoma • HHV8+ DLBCL NOS • Intravascular large B-cell lymphoma • ALK+ large B-cell lymphoma	**Mature (peripheral) T-cell neoplasms** • T-cell granular lymphocytic leukemia • Adult T-cell leukemia/lymphoma (HTLV-1+) • Extranodal NK/T-cell lymphoma, nasal type • Enteropathy-associated T-cell lymphoma • Hepatosplenic T-cell lymphoma • Subcutaneous panniculitis-like T-cell lymphoma • Mycosis fungoides • Sezary syndrome • Peripheral T-cell lymphoma, NOS • Angioimmunoblastic T-cell lymphoma • Anaplastic large cell lymphoma, ALK+ • Anaplastic large cell lymphoma ALK–

Ans. D

95. Treatment of choice for MGUS is:

A. Bortezomib
B. Nilotinib
C. Thalidomide
D. No specific treatment required

Explanation:

- No specific intervention is indicated for patients with MGUS.
- Follow-up once a year or less frequently is adequate except in higher risk MGUS, where serum protein electrophoresis, complete blood count, creatinine, and calcium should be repeated every 6 months.
- A patient with MGUS and severe polyneuropathy is considered for therapeutic intervention if a causal relationship can be assumed, especially in the absence of any other potential causes for neuropathy. Therapy can include plasmapheresis and occasionally rituximab in patients with IgM MGUS or myeloma-like therapy in those with IgG or IgA disease. About 10% of patients have smoldering MM (SMM) and will have an indolent course demonstrating only slow progression of disease over many years. For patients with SMM, no specific therapeutic intervention is indicated, although early intervention with lenalidomide and dexamethasone may prevent progression from high-risk SMM to active MM.

Ans. D

96. Not true about Microvascular thrombotic crisis is:

A. Occurs most commonly in young patients with lupus nephritis

B. Most useful lab tests are identification of schistocytes on peripheral blood smears, elevated serum LDH and antibodies to ADAMS 13

C. Plasma exchange or extensive plasmapheresis is usually life saving

D. Cytotoxic drugs are effective

Explanation:

Microvascular Thrombotic Crisis (Thrombotic Thrombocytopenic Purpura, Hemolytic-Uremic Syndrome)

- This syndrome of hemolysis, thrombocytopenia, and microvascular thrombosis in kidneys, brain, and other tissues carries a high mortality rate and occurs most commonly in young individuals with lupus nephritis.
- Most useful laboratory tests are identification of schistocytes on peripheral blood smears, elevated serum levels of lactate dehydrogenase, and antibodies to ADAMS13.
- Plasma exchange or extensive plasmapheresis is usually life-saving; most authorities recommend concomitant glucocorticoid therapy; there is no evidence that cytotoxic drugs are effective.

Ans. D

97. Megaloblastic anemia not due to cobalamin or folate deficiency or altered metabolism is seen in all except:

A. Fanconi anemia

B. Antimetabolite drug

C. HAART

D. Thiamine responsive

Explanation:

Megaloblastic Anemia not Due to Cobalamin or Folate Deficiency or Altered Metabolism

- This may occur with many antimetabolic drugs (e.g., hydroxyurea, cytosine arabinoside, 6-mercaptopurine) that inhibit DNA replication.
- Antiviral nucleoside analogues used in treatment of HIV infection may also cause macrocytosis and megaloblastic marrow changes.
- In the rare disease orotic aciduria, two consecutive enzymes in purine synthesis are defective.
- Condition responds to therapy with uridine, which bypasses the block. In thiamine-responsive megaloblastic anemia, there is a genetic defect in the high-affinity thiamine transport (*SLC19A2*) gene.
- This causes defective RNA ribose synthesis through impaired activity of transketolase, a thiamine-dependent enzyme in the pentose cycle. This leads to reduced nucleic acid production.
- It may be associated with diabetes mellitus and deafness and the presence of many ringed sideroblasts in the marrow.
- Explanation is unclear for megaloblastic changes in the marrow in some patients with acute myeloid leukemia and myelodysplasia.

Ans. A

98. Not true about hematological findings in CML:

A. Thrombocytosis common

B. Blast <5%

C. Low LAP

D. Thrombocytopenia associated with good prognosis

Explanation:

- In untreated CML, leukocytosis ranging from 10–500 × 109/L is common. The peripheral blood differential shows left-shifted hematopoiesis with predominance of neutrophils and the presence of bands, myelocytes, metamyelocytes, promyelocytes, and blasts (usually ≤5%). Basophils and/or eosinophils are frequently increased.
- Thrombocytosis is common, but thrombocytopenia is rare and, when present, suggests a worse prognosis, disease acceleration, or an unrelated etiology.
- Anemia is present in 1/3rd of patients. Cyclic oscillations of counts are noted in 10–20% of patients without treatment.
- Biochemical abnormalities include a low leukocyte alkaline phosphatase score and high levels of vitamin B12, uric acid, lactic dehydrogenase, and lysozyme.
- Presence of unexplained and sustained leukocytosis, with or without splenomegaly, should lead to a marrow examination and cytogenetic analysis.

Ans. D

99. All are poor prognostic factors in early of advanced HL:

A. Lymphocyte count <600/μL
B. ESR>30
C. Serum albumin <4gm/dL
D. Hb <10.5 gm/dL

Explanation:

- Patients with early stage disease have a better prognosis overall but are further classified as favorable or unfavorable based on a variety of factors.
- These factors vary from study to study but include bulky disease, number of lymph node areas involved, an elevated ESR (>30 if B symptoms are present; >50 if B symptoms are absent), and age.
- Prognosis in advanced stage disease is best predicted by the International Prognostic Score (IPS), which ascribes a point for male sex, older age (>45 years), stage IV disease, serum albumin <4 g/dL, hemoglobin <10.5 g/dL, white blood cell count ≥15,000/μL, and a lymphocyte count <600/μL and/or <8% of white blood cell count.
- Five-year progression-free survival ranges from 88% for patients with no risk factors, to 62% for patients with four or more factors, but very few patients have multiple risk factors.

Ans. B

100. Not true about Waldenstrom's macroglobulinemia is:

A. Disease similar to myeloma in being slightly more common in men & increased incidence with increased age
B. Associated with bone lesions or hypercalcemia
C. Bone marrow shows >10% infiltration with lymphoplasmacytic cells
D. M component is present in serum in excess of 30gm/dL

Explanation:

- Disease is similar to myeloma in being slightly more common in men and occurring with increased incidence with increasing age (median 64 years).
- IgM in some patients with macroglobulinemia may have specificity for myelin-associated glycoprotein (MAG), a protein that has been associated with demyelinating disease of the peripheral nervous system and may be lost earlier and to a greater extent than the better known myelin basic protein in patients with multiple sclerosis.
- Sometimes patients with macroglobulinemia develop a peripheral neuropathy, and half of these patients are positive for anti-MAG antibody. The neuropathy may precede the appearance of the neoplasm.

- The whole process may begin with a viral infection that may elicit an antibody response that cross-reacts with a normal tissue component.
- Like myeloma, the disease involves the bone marrow, but unlike myeloma, it does not cause bone lesions or hypercalcemia.
- Bone marrow shows >10% infiltration with lymphoplasmacytic cells (surface IgM+, CD19+, CD20+, and CD22+, rarely CD5+, but CD10− and CD23−) with an increase in number of mast cells.
- Like myeloma, an M component is present in the serum in excess of 30 g/L (3 g/dL), but unlike myeloma, the size of the IgM paraprotein results in little renal excretion, and only ~20% of patients excrete light chains.
- Therefore, renal disease is not common. The light chain isotype is kappa in 80% of the cases. Patients present with weakness, fatigue, and recurrent infections similar to myeloma patients, but epistaxis, visual disturbances, and neurologic symptoms such as peripheral neuropathy, dizziness, headache, and transient paresis are much more common in macroglobulinemia. Presence of *MYD88* and *CXCR4* mutations also affects disease presentation.
- Presence of *CXCR4* mutations is associated with higher bone marrow disease burden and higher incidence of hyperviscosity. Patients with wild-type *MYD88* show lower bone marrow disease burden.

Ans. B

101. Dry tap is most commonly seen in:

A. CML

B. Myelofibrosis

C. Hairy cell leukemia

D. Metastatic carcinoma infiltration

Explanation:

Table: Differential diagnosis of "Dry tap"–Inability to aspirate bone marrow	
Dry taps occur in about 4% of attempts and are associated with:	
• Metastatic carcinoma infiltration	17%
• Chronic myeloid leukemia	15%
• Myelofibrosis	14%
• Hairy cell leukemia	10%
• Acute leukemia	10%
• Lymphomas, Hodgkin's disease	9%
• Normal marrow	Rare

Ans. D

102. True about etiology of CML is:

A. No familial association

B. Risk increased in monozygotic twins

C. Associations exist with exposures to benzene or other toxins

D. Frequent secondary leukemia following alkylating agents and/or radiation

Explanation:

- There are no familial associations in CML. The risk of developing CML is not increased in monozygotic twins or in relatives of patients.
- No etiologic agents are incriminated, and no associations exist with exposures to benzene or other toxins, fertilizers, insecticides, or viruses.
- CML is not a frequent secondary leukemia following therapy of other cancers with alkylating agents and/ or radiation.

- Exposure to ionizing radiation (e.g., nuclear accidents, radiation treatment for ankylosing spondylitis or cervical cancer) has increased the risk of CML, which peaks at 5–10 years after exposure and is dose-related.
- Median time to development of CML among atomic bomb survivors was 6.3 years.
- Following the Chernobyl accident, the incidence of CML did not increase, suggesting that larger dose exposures of radiation are required to cause CML.
- Because of adequate protection, the risk of CML is not increased in individuals working in the nuclear industry or among radiologists in recent times.

Ans. A

103. Not true regarding lab investigation in PNH is:

A. Normocytic anemia
B. Reduced MCV
C. Increased Reticulocyte count
D. Bone marrow cellular initially but later stage aplastic

Explanation:

- Most consistent blood finding is anemia, which may range from mild to moderate to very severe. The anemia is usually normo-macrocytic, with unremarkable red cell morphology. If the MCV is high, it is usually largely accounted for by reticulocytosis, which may be quite marked (up to 20%, or up to 400,000/μL). The anemia may become microcytic if patient is allowed to become iron-deficient as a result of chronic iron loss through hemoglobinuria. Unconjugated bilirubin is mildly or moderately elevated; LDH is typically markedly elevated (values in thousands are common); & haptoglobin is usually undetectable. All of these findings make diagnosis of HA compelling. Hemoglobinuria may be overt in a random urine sample; if it is not, it may be helpful to obtain serial urine samples because hemoglobinuria can vary dramatically from day to day and even from hour to hour.
- Bone marrow is usually cellular, with marked to massive erythroid hyperplasia, often with mild to moderate dyserythropoietic features (these overlap with those seen in myelodysplastic syndromes, but PNH remains a separate entity). At some stage of the disease, marrow may become hypocellular or even frankly aplastic.

Ans. B

104. Major diagnostic criteria for systemic mastocytosis is:

A. Multifocal dense infiltrates of mast cells (>15 mast cells per aggregate) in bone marrow
B. Abnormal mast cell morphology
C. Detection of codon 816 mutation
D. Total serum tryptase >20ng/ml

Explanation:

Table: Diagnostic criteria for systemic mastocytosis[a]
Major:
• Multifocal dense infiltrates of mast cells (>15 mast cells per aggregate) in bone marrow or other extracutaneous tissues
Minor:
• Abnormal mast cell morphology (spindle shape, bi- or multi-lobed or eccentric nucleus, hypogranulated cytoplasm
• Aberrant mast cell surface phenotype with expression of CD25 (IL-2 receptor alpha chain) and/or CD2
• Detection of codon 816 mutation in peripheral blood cells, bone marrow cells, or an extracutaneous lesional tissue
• Total serum tryptase > 20 ng/ml

Ans. A

105. Causes of Thrombocytosis include all except:

A. Hemorrhage
B. Malignancy
C. Vitamin B6 Deficiency
D. Iron deficiency anemia

Explanation:

Table: Causes of thrombocytosis	
Tissue inflammation: Collagen vascular disease, inflammatory bowel disease	Hemorrhage
Malignancy	Iron-deficiency anemia
Infection	Surgery
Myeloproliferative disorders: Polycythemia vera, primary myelofibrosis, essential thrombocytosis, chronic myelogenous leukemia	Rebound: Correction of vitamin B_{12} or folate deficiency, post-ethanol abuse
Myelodysplastic disorders: 5q–syndrome, idiopathic refractory sideroblastic anemia	Hemolysis
Postsplenectomy or hyposplenism	Familial: Thrombopoietin overproduction, *JAK2* or *MPL* mutations

Ans. C

106. Peripheral blood smear showing leukemia cells with typical "flower shaped" nucleus in:

A. Angioimmunoblastic T cell lymphoma
B. Anaplastic Large cell lymphoma
C. Adult T cell leukemia/lymphoma
D. Extranodal NK/T cell lymphoma- Nasal type

Explanation:

- Adult T-cell leukemia/ lymphoma (ATLL) is a disease that is most prevalent in Japan and Caribbean basin. It is a neoplasm that is driven by HTLV-1, often contracted through the breast milk of infected mothers.
- Average age at diagnosis is 60, so there is a long latency between viral infection and viral transformation, and only 4% of infected patients will develop disease.
- This suggests that HTLV-1 may not be sufficient to cause malignant phenotype. There are four disease variants: acute (60% of patients), lymphomatous (20% of patients), chronic (15% of patients), and smoldering (5% of patients).
- Prognosis varies across these groups with median survivals of 6 months, 10 months, 24 months, and not yet reached, respectively.
- Presentation depends on the subtype, but most commonly patients present with circulating disease and bone marrow involvement, hypercalcemia, lytic bone lesions, lymphadenopathy, heptosplenomegaly, skin lesions, and opportunistic infections.
- Pathognomonic finding is the malignant "flower cell" that is positive for CD4 and CD25, as well as CD2, CD3, and CD5 but lacking CD7.

Ans. C

107. Overexpression of which predicts favourable outcome both in CN-AML & Cytogenetically abnormal AML?

A. miR-181a
B. miR- 155
C. miR- 3151
D. All of the above

Explanation:

- Overexpression of *miR-155* and *miR-3151* predicts unfavorable outcome in CN-AML, whereas overexpression of *miR-181a* predicts favorable outcome both in CN-AML and cytogenetically abnormal AML.

Ans. A

108. Exception of hereditary intracorpuscular defect is:

A. Hemoglobinopathies
B. Enzymopathies
C. Membrane cytoskeletal defects
D. PNH

Explanation:

Table: Classification of hemolytic anemias[a]		
	Intracorpuscular Defects	**Extracorpuscular Factors**
Inherited	Hemoglobinopathies Enzymopathies Membrane-cytoskeletal defects	Familial (atypical) hemolytic-uremic syndrome
Acquired	Paroxysmal nocturnal hemoglobinuria (PNH)	Mechanical destruction (microangiopathic) Toxic agents Drugs Infectious Autoimmune

Ans. D

109. Erythropoetin level in zidovudine associated anemia is:

A. Increased
B. Decreased
C. No effect
D. First decreased then increased

Explanation:

- Erythropoietin levels in patients with HIV infection and anemia are generally lower than expected given the degree of anemia.
- Treatment with erythropoietin may result in an increase in hemoglobin levels.
- An exception to this is a subset of patients with zidovudine-associated anemia in whom erythropoietin levels may be quite high.

Ans. A

110. A 71 year old male presented to OPD with generalised body swelling, decreased urine output, severe backache and sternal tenderness. On examination he was found to have macroglossia. Lab parameters: anaemia; reversed albumin globulin ratio; deranged renal function tests. ECG: show low voltage in the limb leads with a pseudo-infarct pattern; ECHO: concentrically thickened ventricles and diastolic dysfunction. Urine dipstick: protein 4+; 24-hour urine protein: 6.2gm. Which of the following is the most appropriate investigation to substantiate your diagnosis?

A. Serum fibrinogen
B. FLC assay
C. Serum electrophoresis
D. All of the above

Explanation:

- Identification of an underlying clonal plasma cell or B lymphoproliferative process and a clonal LC are key to the diagnosis of AL amyloidosis.
- Serum protein electrophoresis and urine protein electrophoresis, although of value in multiple myeloma, are *not* useful screening tests if AL amyloidosis is suspected because the clonal LC or whole immunoglobulin often is not present in sufficient amounts to produce a monoclonal "M-spike" in serum or LC (Bence Jones) protein in urine.
- However, more than 90% of patients with AL amyloidosis have serum or urine monoclonal LC or whole immunoglobulin detectable by immunofixation electrophoresis of serum (SIFE) or urine (UIFE) or by nephelometric measurement of serum "free" LCs (i.e., LCs circulating in monomeric form rather than in an immunoglobulin tetramer with heavy chain).

- Examining the ratio as well as the absolute amount of serum-free LCs is essential, as renal insufficiency reduces LC clearance, nonspecifically elevating both isotypes.
- In addition, an increased percentage of plasma cells in the bone marrow— typically 5–30% of nucleated cells—is found in ~90% of patients.
- Kappa or lambda clonality should be demonstrated by flow cytometry, immunohistochemistry, or in situ hybridization for LC mRNA.

Ans. B

111. A 62 year old woman presented to medicine OPD with complaints of generalised body swelling. Urinalysis revealed nephrotic range proteinuria and microhematuria. Her serum creatinine is 2.8mg/dL. She is referred to a nephrologist for evaluation. Renal biopsy was planned which revealed amorphous, acellular expansion of mesangium, with material often also infiltrating glomerular basement membranes, vessels, and the interstitium, with apple-green birefringence by polarized Congo red stain. What would be your line of management?

A. CNI
B. Rituximab
C. Bortezomib
D. Carboplatin

Explanation:

- Novel anti–plasma cell agents have been investigated for treatment of plasma cell diseases.
- Immunomodulators thalidomide, lenalidomide, and pomalidomide display activity; dosing may need to be adjusted compared to their usage for myeloma.
- Proteasome inhibitor bortezomib has also been found to be effective in single-center and multicenter trials.
- Anti-fibril small molecules and humanized monoclonal antibodies are also being tested. Clinical trials are essential in improving therapy for this rare disease.

Ans. C

112. Not a marker for Hairy cell leukemia is:

A. CD22
B. CD25
C. CD20
D. CD103

Explanation:

- Hairy cell leukemia is a tumor of small lymphocytes with oval nuclei, abundant cytoplasm, and distinctive membrane projections (hairy cells).
- Patients have splenomegaly and diffuse BM involvement.
- While some circulating cells are noted, clinical picture is dominated by symptoms from the enlarged spleen and pancytopenia.
- Mechanism of the pancytopenia is not completely clear and may be mediated by both inhibitory cytokines and marrow replacement.
- Marrow has an increased level of reticulin fibers; indeed, hairy cell leukemia is a common cause of inability to aspirate BM or so-called "dry tap"
- Monocytopenia is profound and may explain a predisposition to atypical mycobacterial infection that is observed clinically.
- Tumor cells have strong expression of CD22, CD25, and CD103; soluble CD25 level in serum is an excellent tumor marker for disease activity. The cells also express tartrate-resistant acid phosphatase.
- Immunoglobulin genes are rearranged and mutated, indicating the influence of a germinal center.
- No specific cytogenetic abnormality has been found, but most cases contain the activating *BRAF* mutation V600E.

Ans. C

113. A 24-year-old man returns to the acute care clinic complaining of 1 day of worsening malaise, weakness, abdominal pain, and discolored dark urine. He was at the clinic yesterday where he was diagnosed with a possible staphylococcal skin carbuncle and treated with empiric trimethoprim/sulfamethoxazole. His physical examination is notable for mild jaundice, normal vital signs, and no focal findings other than the carbuncle in his left axilla. His CBC shows that his hemoglobin has fallen from 13 g/dL to 8 g/dL and his bilirubin has gone from normal to 3.0 mg/dL. His urine dipstick is positive for bilirubin. Which of the following is the most likely cause of his new anemia?

A. Glucose 6-phosphate dehydrogenase (G6PD) deficiency

B. Hemolytic-uremic syndrome

C. Hereditary spherocytosis

D. Iron deficiency anemia

Explanation:

- Peripheral blood smear shows bite cells, anisocytosis, and spherocytes.
- Combination of the smear, jaundice, and hyperbilirubinemia 1 day after receiving sulfamethoxazole makes glucose 6-phosphate dehydrogenase (G6PD) deficiency most likely.
- G6PD deficiency is widely distributed in tropical and subtropical parts of the world (Africa, southern Europe, Middle East, Southeast Asia, and Oceania) and wherever people from those areas have migrated.
- Conservative estimate is that at least 400 million people have a G6PD deficiency gene. In several of these areas, frequency of a G6PD deficiency gene may be as high as 20% or more.
- G6PD gene is X-linked; thus, males have only one G6PD gene (i.e., they are hemizygous for this gene); therefore, they must be either normal or G6PD deficient.
- Hemolytic anemia in patients with G6PD deficiency can develop as a result of fava beans, infections, and drugs.
- Common drugs include primaquine, dapsone, sulfamethoxazole, and nitrofurantoin.
- Typically, a hemolytic attack starts with malaise, weakness, and abdominal or lumbar pain.
- After an interval of several hours to 2–3 days, patient develops jaundice and often dark urine.
- Onset can be extremely abrupt, especially with favism in children.
- There may be hemoglobinemia, hemoglobinuria, high LDH, and low or absent plasma haptoglobin. G6PD deficiency may be diagnosed by semiquantitative or quantitative RBC tests or by DNA testing.
- Hemolytic-uremic syndrome and thrombotic thrombocytopenic purpura cause microangiopathic hemolytic anemia with prominent schistocytes.
- Iron deficiency causes a microcytic and hypochromic anemia.

Ans. A

114. A 19-year-old collegiate rower who has been in excellent health and takes no chronic medications, for new-onset severe fatigue and left upper abdominal pain. She was treated 2 days ago in the health center for presumed gonorrhea with ceftriaxone and azithromycin. Her past medical history is only notable for one prior episode of presumed gonorrhea when she was 17 years old. Her physical examination is notable for a heart rate of 100 bpm and a palpable spleen. Stool is negative for heme. Laboratory examination is notable for a hemoglobin of 5 g/dL with normal WBC and platelets. Peripheral blood smear shows an excess of spherocytes. Which of the following tests will most likely confirm the diagnosis?

A. ADAMTS-13 activity assay

B. Direct antiglobulin (Coombs) test

C. Flow cytometry

D. G6PD deficiency assay

Explanation:

- Patient has autoimmune hemolytic anemia (AIHA) with development of warm immunoglobulin G (IgG) antibodies due to ceftriaxone exposure.

Classification of Acquired Immune Hemolytic Anemia:

Clinical Setting	Type of Antibody	
	Cold, Mostly IgM, Optimal Temperature 4-30°C	**Warm, Mostly IgG, Optimal Temperature 37°C; or Mixed**
Primary	CAD	AIHA (idiopathic)
Secondary to viral infection	EBV CMV Other	HIV Viral vaccines
Secondary to other infection	*Mycoplasma* infection: Paroxysmal cold hemoglobinuria	
Secondary to/associated with other disease	CAD in: Waldenström disease Lymphoma	AIHA in: SLE CLL Other malignancy Chronic inflammatory disorders (e.g., IBD) After allogeneic HSCT
Secondary to drugs: Drug induced immune hemolytic anemia	Small minority (e.g., with lenalidomide)	**Majority:** Currently most common culprit drugs are cefotetan, ceftriaxone, piperacillin
	Drug-dependent: Antibody destroys red cells only when drug present (e.g., rarely penicillin) **Drug-independent:** Antibody can destroy red cells even when drug no longer present (e.g., methyldopa)	

- AIHA is a serious condition; without appropriate treatment, it may have a mortality of approximately 10%. The onset is often abrupt and can be dramatic.
- Hemoglobin level can drop within days to as low as 4 g/dL; the massive red cell removal will produce jaundice; and sometimes the spleen is enlarged. When this triad is present, the suspicion of AIHA must be high.
- Diagnostic test for AIHA is the direct antiglobulin (Coombs) test, which detects the presence of antibody on the red cells. When the test is positive, it clinches the diagnosis; when it is negative, the diagnosis is unlikely.
- Immediate treatment almost invariably includes transfusion of red cells. This may pose a special problem because, if the antibody involved is nonspecific, all of the blood units cross-matched will be incompatible.
- Whenever the anemia is not immediately life threatening, blood transfusion should be withheld (because compatibility problems may increase with each unit of blood transfused), and medical treatment started immediately with prednisone (1 mg/kg/d), which will produce a remission promptly in at least one-half of patients.
- Rituximab (anti-CD20) was regarded as second-line treatment, but it is increasingly likely that a relatively low dose (100 mg/wk × 4) of rituximab together with prednisone will become a first-line standard.
- It is especially encouraging that this approach seems to reduce the rate of relapse, a common occurrence in AIHA. G6PD deficiency is unlikely in this previously healthy female only exposed to ceftriaxone.
- ADAMTS-13 activity assay is used to diagnose thrombotic thrombocytopenic purpura. Flow cytometry may be used to diagnose paroxysmal nocturnal hemoglobinuria. Hemoglobin electrophoresis is used to diagnose congenital hemoglobinopathies.

Ans. B

115. Which of the following is the most likely finding in a patient with a "dry" bone marrow aspiration?

A. Chronic myeloid leukemia
B. Hairy cell leukemia
C. Metastatic carcinoma infiltration
D. Normal marrow

Explanation:

- A "dry tap" is defined as the inability to aspirate bone marrow and is reported in approximately 4% of attempts. It is rare in the case of normal bone marrow.
- Differential diagnosis includes metastatic carcinoma infiltration (17%), chronic myeloid leukemia (15%), myelofibrosis (14%), hairy cell leukemia (10%), acute leukemia (10%), and lymphomas including Hodgkin's disease (9%).

Differential Diagnosis of "Dry Tap"—Inability to Aspirate Bone Marrow

Dry taps occur in about 4% of attempts and are associated with:	
• Metastatic carcinoma infiltration	17%
• Chronic myeloid leukemia	15%
• Myelofibrosis	14%
• Hairy cell leukemia	10%
• Acute leukemia	10%
• Lymphomas, Hodgkin disease	9%
• Normal marrow	Rare

Ans. D

116. In patients with multiple myeloma, which of the following results is the most powerful predictor of survival?

A. Bone involvement on radiograph
B. Renal function
C. Serum albumin
D. Serum β2-microglobulin

Explanation:

- Serum β2-microglobulin is the single most powerful predictor of survival and can substitute for staging. Patients with β2-microglobulin levels <0.004 g/L have a median survival of 43 months, and those with levels >0.004 g/L have a survival of only 12 months.
- Combination of serum β2-microglobulin and albumin levels forms the basis for a three-stage International Staging System (ISS) that predicts survival.
- Other factors that may influence prognosis are the presence of cytogenetic abnormalities and hypodiploidy by karyotype, fluorescent in situ hybridization (FISH)–identified chromosome 17p deletion, and translocations t(4;14), (14;16), and t(14;20).
- Chromosome 13q deletion, previously thought to predict poor outcome, is not a predictor following the use of newer agents.
- Microarray profiling and comparative genomic hybridization have formed the basis for RNA- and DNA-based prognostic staging systems, respectively.
- ISS system, along with cytogenetic changes, is the most widely used method for assessing prognosis.

Risk Stratification in Myeloma:

Table: Chromosomal abnormalities		
Method	**Standard Risk (80%) (expected survival 6-7 + years)**	**High Risk (20%) (expected survival 2-3 years)**
Karyotype	No chromosomal aberration	Any abnormality on conventional karyotype
FISH	t(11:14) t(6:14) del(13)	Del(17p) t(4:14) t(14:16) t(14:20)
International Staging System		
	Stage	**Median Survival, Months**
$\beta_2M < 3.5$, alb ≥ 3.5 $\beta_2M < 3.5$, alb < 3.5 or $\beta_2M = 3.5\text{-}5.5$ $\beta_2M > 5.5$	I (28%)[a] II (39%) III (33%)	62 44 29
Other features suggesting high-risk disease: • De novo plasma cell leukemia • Extramedullary disease • Elevated lactate dehydrogenate (LDH) • High-risk gene expression profile		

Ans. D

117. All of the following infectious agents are associated with the development of a lymphoid malignancy except:

A. Epstein-Barr virus
B. H.pylori
C. HIV
D. JC virus

Explanation:

- A number of infectious agents are associated with the development of lymphoid malignancies. JC virus is associated with progressive multifocal leukoencephalopathy (PML) in immunodeficient individuals .

Infectious Agents Associated with the Development of Lymphoid Malignancies

Table: Infectious agents associated with the development of lymphoid malignancies	
Infectious Agent	**Lymphoid Malignancy**
Epstein-Barr virus	Burkitt lymphoma Post-organ transplant lymphoma Primary CNS diffuse large B-cell lymphoma Hodgkin lymphoma Extranodal NK/T-cell lymphoma, nasal type
HTLV-1	Adult T-cell leukemia/lymphoma
HIV	Diffuse large B-cell lymphoma Burkitt lymphoma
Hepatitis C virus	Lymphoplasmacytic lymphoma
Helicobacter pylori	Gastric MALT lymphoma
Human herpesvirus 8	Primary effusion lymphoma Multicentric Castleman disease

Ans. D

118. All of the following disorders are considered by World Health Organization classification as chronic myeloproliferative neoplasms except:

A. Chronic myeloid leukemia (Bcr-Abl positive)
B. Essential thrombocytosis
C. Polycythemia vera
D. All are chronic myeloproliferative neoplasms

Explanation:

- World Health Organization (WHO) classification of the chronic myeloproliferative neoplasms (MPNs) includes eight disorders, some of which are rare or poorly characterized but all of which share an origin in a multipotent hematopoietic progenitor cell; overproduction of one or more of the formed elements of the blood without significant dysplasia; and a predilection to extramedullary hematopoiesis, myelofibrosis, and transformation at varying rates to acute leukemia.

World Health Organization Classification of Chronic Myeloproliferative Neoplasms:

- Chronic myeloid leukemia, Bcr-Abl positive
- Chronic neutrophilic leukemia
- Chronic eosinophilic leukemia, not otherwise specified
- Polycythemia vera
- Primary myelofibrosis
- Essential thrombocytosis
- Mastocytosis
- Myeloproliferative neoplasms, unclassifiable

- Within this broad classification, however, significant phenotypic heterogeneity exists.
- Some diseases such as chronic myelogenous leukemia (CML), chronic neutrophilic leukemia (CNL), and chronic eosinophilic leukemia (CEL) express primarily a myeloid phenotype, whereas in other diseases, such as polycythemia vera (PV), primary myelofibrosis (PMF), and essential thrombocytosis (ET), erythroid or megakaryocytic hyperplasia predominates.
- Latter three disorders, in contrast to the former three, also appear capable of transforming into each other.
- Such phenotypic heterogeneity has a genetic basis; CML is the consequence of the balanced translocation between chromosomes 9 and 22 [t(9;22)(q34;11)]; CNL has been associated with a t(15;19) translocation; and CEL occurs with deletion or balanced translocations involving PDGFRα gene.
- By contrast, to a greater or lesser extent, PV, PMF, and ET are characterized by a mutation, V617F, that causes constitutive activation of JAK2, a tyrosine kinase essential for the function of the erythropoietin and thrombopoietin receptors but not granulocyte colony-stimulating factor receptor.
- This important distinction is also reflected in the natural histories of CML, CNL, and CEL, which are usually measured in years, and their high rate of leukemic transformation.
- By contrast, the natural history of PV, PMF, and ET is usually measured in decades, and transformation to acute leukemia is uncommon in PV and ET in the absence of exposure to mutagenic drugs.

Ans. D

119. Most common histologic subtype of non-Hodgkin's Lymphoma?

A. Diffuse Large B cell lymphoma
B. Burkitt's Lymphoma
C. Follicular lymphoma
D. Mature B cell Lymphoma

Explanation:

- Diffuse large B-cell lymphoma (DLBCL) is the most common histologic subtype of NHL diagnosed, representing about one-third of all cases.
- Previously felt to be "one disease" it is now recognized as a heterogeneous collection of multiple entities. It is slightly more common in Caucasians and men, and the median age at diagnosis is 64.
- Relative risk of DLBCL is higher amongst people with affected first-degree relatives (RR 3.5-fold), and patients with congenital or acquired immunodeficiency, patients on immunosuppression, and patients with autoimmune disorders also have a higher risk of developing DLBCL, often EBV-related.

Ans. A

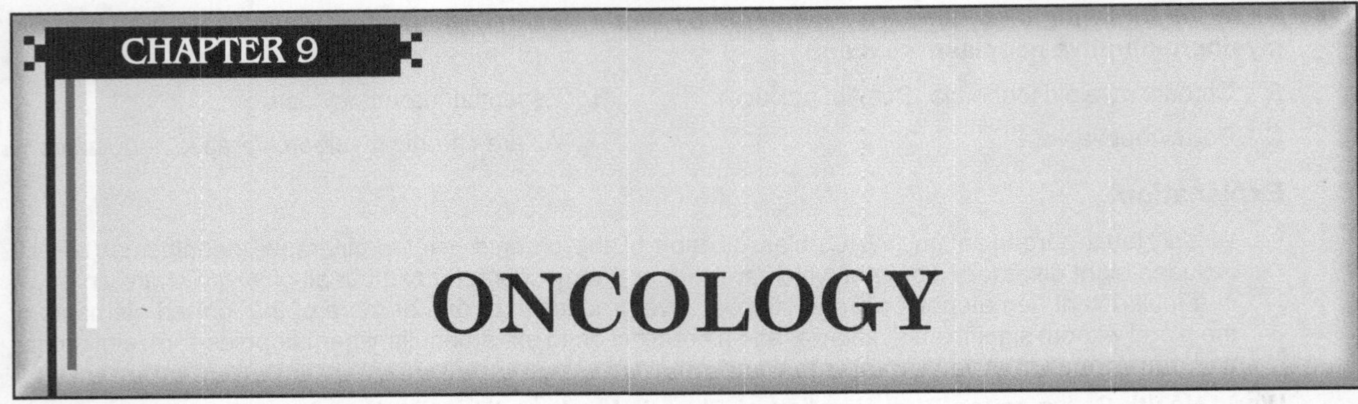

CHAPTER 9

ONCOLOGY

1. Most common cause for Pituitary secondary is:

A. CA Breast
B. CA Lung
C. CA Ovary
D. All of the above

Explanation:

- Pituitary metastases occur in ~3% of cancer patients. Blood borne metastatic deposits are found almost exclusively in the posterior pituitary.
- Accordingly, diabetes insipidus can be a presenting feature of lung, gastrointestinal, breast, and other pituitary metastases. About half of pituitary metastases originate from breast cancer.
- MRI diagnosis of a metastatic lesion may be difficult to distinguish from an aggressive pituitary adenoma; the diagnosis may require histologic examination of excised tumor tissue.
- Primary or metastatic lymphoma, leukemias, and plasmacytomas also occur within the sella.
- Most common cause of secondary in brain is CA Lung (small cell carcinoma of lung).

Ans. A

2. Which of the following sarcoma metastasize to the lung?

A. GIST
B. Myxoid liposarcoma
C. Clear cell sarcoma
D. Leiomyosarcoma

Explanation:

- Lymph node metastases occur in 5%, except in synovial and epithelioid sarcomas, clear-cell sarcoma (melanoma of the soft parts), angiosarcoma, and rhabdomyosarcoma, where nodal spread may be seen in 17%.
- Pulmonary parenchyma is the most common site of metastases.
- Exceptions are GISTs, which metastasize to the liver; myxoid liposarcomas, which seek fatty tissue; and clear-cell sarcomas, which may metastasize to bones.
- Central nervous system metastases are rare, except in alveolar soft part sarcoma.

Ans. D

3. Which organism causes pelvic infection that mimic's the malignancy of endometrium?

A. Actinomycosis
B. Gardenella vaginalis
C. Chlamydia
D. Niesseria gonorrhea

Explanation:

- Actinomycotic involvement of the pelvis occurs most commonly in association with an IUCD but can also be associated with other foreign bodies, such as surgical mesh.
- When an IUCD is in place or has been used but removed, pelvic symptoms should prompt consideration of actinomycosis. The risk, although not quantified, appears small.
- Disease rarely develops when the IUCD has been in place for <1 year, but the risk increases with time.
- Symptoms are typically indolent; fever, weight loss, abdominal pain, and abnormal vaginal bleeding or discharge are the most common.
- Earliest stage of disease—often endometritis—commonly progresses to pelvic masses or a tuboovarian abscess.
- Unfortunately, because the diagnosis is often delayed, a “frozen pelvis” mimicking malignancy or endometriosis can develop by the time of recognition, which may lead to unnecessary surgery.
- Cancer antigen 125 levels may be elevated, further contributing to misdiagnosis.

Ans. A

4. **A 50 year old male presents with right shoulder pain, ptosis, myosis and anhidrosis. Which of the following is the most likely diagnosis?**

A. Mesothelioma
B. Pancoast tumour
C. Carcinoid
D. Hodgkin’s lymphoma

Explanation:

- Pancoast tumour or superior sulcus tumour are characterized by a distinct constellation of presenting signs and symptoms due to their location. Most of the tumours are non-small cell lung cancer. Lesions in the superior sulcus of the lung may result in shoulder and arm pain due to the involvement of C8, T1 and T2 dermatomes.
- Horner’s syndrome consists of ipsilateral ptosis, myosis, enophthalmos and anhidrosis. It’s caused by the involvement of paravertebral sympathetic chain and the inferior cervical ganglion.

Ans. B

5. **Multicentric Castleman’s disease is caused by:**

A. EBV
B. HTLV1
C. HIV
D. HHV 8

Table: Infectious agents associated with the development of lymphoid malignancies

Infectious Agent	Lymphoid Malignancy
Epstein-Barr virus	Burkitt’s lymphoma Post-organ transplant lymphoma Primary CNS diffuse large B-cell lymphoma Hodgkin’s lymphoma Extranodal NK/T-cell lymphoma, nasal type
HTLV-1	Adult T-cell leukemia/lymphoma
HIV	Diffuse large B-cell lymphoma Burkitt’s lymphoma
Hepatitis C virus	Lymphoplasmacytic lymphoma
Helicobacter pylori	Gastric MALT lymphoma
Human herpesvirus 8	Primary effusion lymphoma Multicentric Castleman’s disease

Ans. D

6. Which of the following is at more risk for seminoma?

A. Undescended testis

B. History of Father with Seminoma

C. Descended testes without another

D. Seminoma on one testis earlier

Explanation:

- Although most patients with GCTs do not have a family history of this disease, there are rare familial cases.
- Strongest risk factors for testicular GCT include a prior history of disease, cryptorchidism, and a history of testicular intratubular germ cell neoplasia (ITGCN). Patients with a prior history of testicular GCT have 2% risk of developing a contralateral GCT.
- These are more commonly metachronous than synchronous.
- Men with cryptorchidism have approximately a four- to sixfold increased risk of developing testicular GCT.
- Orchidopexy before puberty decreases but does not eliminate this risk.
- Interestingly, contralateral descended testis is also at risk for this disease.
- Men undergoing infertility evaluation in which a testicular biopsy demonstrates ITGCN have a 50% risk of developing GCT.

Ans. A

7. All of the following infectious agents are associated with development of a lymphoid malignancy except:

A. Epstein-Barr virus

B. H.pylori

C. HIV

D. JC virus

Explanation:

- A number of infectious agents are associated with the development of lymphoid malignancies. JC virus is associated with progressive multifocal leukoencephalopathy (PML) in immunodeficient individuals.

Table: Infectious agents associated with the development of lymphoid malignancies

Infectious Agent	Lymphoid Malignancy
Epstein-Barr virus	Burkitt lymphoma Post-organ transplant lymphoma Primary CNS diffuse large B-cell lymphoma Hodgkin lymphoma Extranodal NK/T-cell Lymphoma, nasal type
HTLV-1	Adult T-cell leukemia/lymphoma
HIV	Diffuse large B-cell lymphoma Burkitt lymphoma
Hepattis C virus	Lymphoplasmacytic lymphoma
Helicobacter pylori	Gastric MALT lymphoma
Human herpesvirus B	Primary effusion lymphoma Multicentric Castleman disease

Ans. D

8. A 26-year-old man presents with pain and swelling of his right testicle that has persisted after an empiric treatment for epididymitis. Ultrasound confirms a 1.5 × 2 cm solid mass, suspicious for testicular cancer. Radical inguinal orchiectomy confirms the mass as a seminoma with disease limited to testis (tumor stage pT1). Chest, abdomen, and pelvis CT shows no evidence of metastatic disease

or lymphadenopathy. Results of serum tumor markers demonstrate the following (normal values in parentheses): α-fetoprotein (AFP) 5 ng/mL (<10 ng/mL), β-human chorionic gonadotropin (β-hCG) 182 U/L (0.2–0.8 U/L), and lactate dehydrogenase (LDH) 432 U/L (100–190 U/L). Following resection, all tumor markers become undetectable after an appropriate interval. Which is the next best step in this patient's treatment?

A. Immediate retroperitoneal radiation therapy

B. Nerve-sparing retroperitoneal lymph node dissection

C. Surveillance alone with treatment only if relapse detected

D. Either A or C, because both are associated with a near 100% cure rate

Explanation:

- Seminomas have the best survival of all forms of testicular cancer and represent approximately 50% of all germ cell tumors.
- Median age of presentation is the fourth decade of life, and approximately 80% of individuals present with stage I disease, indicating any disease limited to the testis no matter the size at initial presentation.
- All men presenting with a testicular mass should be referred for radical inguinal orchiectomy as this approach mirrors the embryonic development of the testis and does not breach anatomic barriers to allow for other pathways of spread.
- In the staging workup of testicular cancers, men should undergo CT imaging of the chest, abdomen, and pelvis as well as measurement of the serum tumor markers AFP and β-human chorionic gonadotropin (β-hCG), in addition to lactate dehydrogenase (LDH) levels.
- These tumor markers assist with both diagnosis and prognosis in testicular cancer and help with determining the appropriate postorchiectomy treatment. In pure seminomas,
- AFP levels should not be elevated. If the AFP level is elevated, this indicates an occult nonseminomatous component, which may require more aggressive initial treatment with either retroperitoneal lymph node dissection or adjuvant chemotherapy depending on local surgical expertise and preference of the patient and treating physician.
- β-hCG levels may be elevated in pure seminomas, although this too is infrequent in men without advanced disease. LDH levels are less specific, but are increased in up to 80% of patients with advanced seminoma.
- After resection, the tumor markers should return to normal values within their expected half-lives following first-order kinetics.
- Half-life of β-hCG is 24–36 hours, and that of AFP is 5–7 days. In stage I seminoma, survival is near 100% with either immediate postorchiectomy radiation or with surveillance alone (option E).
- Given the concern about secondary malignancy due to radiation exposure, many providers chose watchful waiting with surveillance alone in men who are compliant with follow-up.
- However, approximately 15% of patients will experience relapse, and 5% of relapses occur after 5 years. Thus, extended follow-up is required.
- Single dose of carboplatin has been investigated as an alternative to radiation therapy, but long-term outcomes are as yet unknown.

Ans. D

9. **Most significant risk factor for cancer overall is:**

A. Smoking
B. Alcohol
C. Sex
D. Age

Explanation:

- The most significant risk factor for cancer overall is age; two-thirds of all cases were in those aged >65 years. Cancer incidence increases as the third, fourth, or fifth power of age in different sites. For the interval between birth and age 49 years, 1 in 29 men and 1 in 19 women will develop cancer; for the interval between ages 50 and 59 years, 1 in 15 men and 1 in 17 women will develop cancer; for the interval between ages 60 and 69 years, 1 in 6 men and 1 in 10 women will develop cancer and for people aged ≥70, 1 in 3 men and 1 in 4 women will develop cancer. Overall, men have a 44% risk of developing cancer at some time during their lives; women have a 38% lifetime risk.

Ans. D

10. A 60 year old male is advised lung cancer screening since he is chronic smoker. Which among the following statements is false regarding lung cancer screening?

A. Screening is done in people > 55 years
B. Done in individuals with minimum 30 pack year history
C. Done in people who have smoked in the past 15 years
D. Done using conventional CT chest

Explanation:

- Low dose chest CT is recommended for lung cancer screening among pts aged 55–80 with at least a 30 pack-year smoking history, who have smoked in the past 15 years. With appropriate data reanalysis, chest CT scans can provide a three-dimensional reconstruction of the airways down to at least the sixth generation, providing a virtual bronchoscopy. Virtual bronchoscopies may be helpful in assessing stenotic airways and in planning therapeutic bronchoscopy procedures.
- Refinements of CT scanning techniques have led to the evaluation of low-dose helical computed tomography (LDCT) for lung cancer screening. New multidetector CT scanners generate high-resolution imaging with significantly less radiation exposure than diagnostic chest CT scanning.

Ans. D

11. Pain is unrelated to cancer in:

A. 10%
B. 20%
C. 30%
D. 40%

Explanation:

- In ~20% of cases, pain is related to a surgical or invasive medical procedure, to radiation injury (mucositis, enteritis, or plexus, or spinal cord injury), or to chemotherapy injury (mucositis, peripheral neuropathy, phlebitis, steroid-induced aseptic necrosis of the femoral head).
- **In 10% of cases, pain is unrelated to cancer or its treatment.**

Ans. A

12. Forced diuresis with mannitol to prevent kidney damage is given with hydration in treatment with:

A. Cisplatin
B. Doxorubicin
C. Bleomycin
D. Mitoxantrone

Explanation:

- Cisplatin was discovered fortuitously by observing that bacteria present in electrolysis solutions with platinum electrodes could not divide.

- Only the *cis* diamine configuration is active as an antitumor agent.
- In the intracellular environment, a chloride is lost from each position, being replaced by a water molecule.
- Resulting positively charged species is an efficient bifunctional interactor with DNA, forming Pt-based cross-links.
- Cisplatin requires administration with adequate hydration, including forced diuresis with mannitol to prevent kidney damage; even with the use of hydration, gradual decrease in kidney function is common, along with noteworthy anemia.
- Hypomagnesemia frequently attends cisplatin use and can lead to hypocalcemia and tetany.
- Other common toxicities include neurotoxocity with stocking-and-glove sensorimotor neuropathy.
- Hearing loss occurs in 50% of patients treated with conventional doses.
- Cisplatin is intensely emetogenic, requiring prophylactic antiemetics.
- Myelosuppression is less evident than with other alkylating agents.
- Chronic vascular toxicity (Raynaud's phenomenon, coronary artery disease) is a more unusual toxicity.
- Carboplatin displays less nephro-, oto-, and neurotoxicity.
- However, myelosuppression is more frequent, and because drug is exclusively cleared through the kidney, adjustment of dose for creatinine clearance must be accomplished through use of various dosing nomograms. Oxaliplatin is a platinum analogue with noteworthy activity in colon cancers refractory to other treatments. It is prominently neurotoxic.

Ans. A

13. All are given orally except:

A. Everolimus
B. Ribociclib
C. Pertuzumab
D. Neratinib

Explanation:

Table: Common agents added to endocrine therapies for metastatic breast cancer			
Class	**How Administered**	**Agents**	**Common Toxicities**
Anti-mTOR	Oral	Everolimus	Mucositis, diarrhea, rash
CDK4/6 inhibitors	Oral	Palbociclib, ribociclib, abemaciclib (not FDA approved)	Neutropenia; uncommon leukopenia, fatigue and nausea

Table: Common anti-HER2 agents for breast cancer			
Class	**How Administered**	**Agents**	**Common Toxicities**
Humanized monoclonal antibodies	IV	Trastuzumab, pertuzumab	Cardiac dysfunction GI (diarrhea)
Tyrosine kinase inhibitors	Oral	Lapatinib neratinib (not FDA approved)	Diarrhea, mucositis, rash
Antibody-drug conjugate	IV	Ado-trastuzumab emtansine	Peripheral neuropathy, thrombocytopenia

Ans. C

14. Predictors of poor outcome following total surgical resection of colorectal cancer are all except:

A. Perforation
B. Venous invasion
C. Preoperative CEA titre (<5 ng/ml)
D. Right sided location of primary tumor

Explanation:

Table: Predictors of poorer outcomes following total surgical resection of colorectal cancer
• Tumor spread to regional lymph nodes
• Number of regional lymph nodes involved
• Tumor penetration through the bowel wall
• Poorly differentiated histology
• Perforation
• Tumor adherence to adjacent organs
• Venous invasion
• Preoperative elevation of CEA titer (>5 ng/ml)
• Specific chromosomal deletion (e.g., mutation in the *b-raf* gene)
• Right-sided location of primary tumor

Ans. C

15. All autoantigen autoimmune disease combination correct except:

A. Ri protein in Paraneoplastic cerebellar degeneration

B. βIV spectrin in Lower motor neuron syndrome

C. Synaptotagmin in Lambert-Eaton myasthenic syndrome

D. Voltage-gated calcium channels in Lambert-Eaton myasthenic syndrome

Explanation:

Table: Recombinant or purified autoantigens recognized by autoantibodies associated with human autoimmune disorders (Continued)	
Autoantigen	**Autoimmune Disease**
Cancer and Paraneoplastic Autoimmunity (Continued)	
Hu proteins	Paraneoplastic encephalomyelitis
Neuronal nicotinic acetylcholine receptor	Subacute autonomic neuropathy, cancer
P53	Cancer, systemic lupus erythematosus
P62 (IGF-II mRNA-binding protein)	Hepatocellular carcinoma (China)
Recoverin	Cancer-associated retinopathy
Ri protein	Paraneoplastic opsoclonus myoclonus ataxia
βIV spectrin	Lower motor neuron syndrome
Synaptotagmin	Lambert-Eaton myasthenic syndrome
Voltage-gated calcium channels	Lambert-Eaton myasthenic syndrome
Yo protein	Paraneoplastic cerebellar degeneration

Ans. A

16. All are second line therapy for advanced stage HCC except:

A. Regorafenib
B. Cabozantinib
C. Ramucirumab
D. Lenvatinib

Explanation:

- Patients at very early stages (stage 0) can be considered first for ablation in case they have contraindications for liver transplantation.
- Patients in Child-Pugh class C should be first considered for liver transplantation.
- Treatment stage migration: Consider the next efficacious treatment in algorithm when previous therapies fail.
- Sorafenib and lenvatinib in first line; and regorafenib, cabozantinib, and ramucirumab in second line.

Ans. D

17. Lung cancer more common in nonsmokers and woman:

A. Small cell
B. Adenocarcinoma
C. Squamous cell
D. Large cell

Explanation:

- EGFR mutations are associated with younger age, light (<10 pack-year) and nonsmokers, and adenocarcinoma histology.
- Approximately 90% of these mutations are exon 19 deletions or exon 21 L858R point mutations within EGFR TK domain, resulting in hyperactivation of both EGFR kinase activity and downstream signaling.
- Lung tumors that harbor activating mutations within the EGFR kinase domain display high sensitivity to small-molecule EGFR TKIs.
- Erlotinib, gefitinib, and afatinib are FDA-approved oral small-molecule TKIs that inhibit EGFR.
- Several large, international, phase III studies have demonstrated improved response rates, progression-free survival, and overall survival in patients with EGFR mutation–positive NSCLC patients treated with an EGFR TKI as compared with standard first-line chemotherapy regimens.

Ans. B

18. All can precipitate flushes in carcinoid syndrome except:

A. Alcohol
B. Smoking
C. Pentagatrin
D. Cheese

Explanation:

- Flushing and diarrhea are the two most common symptoms, occurring in a mean of 69–70% of patients initially and in up to 78% of patients during the course of the disease.
- Characteristic flush is of sudden onset; it is deep red or violaceous erythema of upper body, especially neck and face, often associated with a feeling of warmth and occasionally associated with pruritus, lacrimation, diarrhea, or facial edema.
- Flushes may be precipitated by stress; alcohol; exercise; certain foods, such as cheese; or certain agents, such as catecholamines, pentagastrin; and serotonin reuptake inhibitors.
- Flushing episodes may be brief, lasting 2–5 min, especially initially, or may last hours, especially later in the disease course.
- Flushing usually is associated with metastatic midgut NETs (carcinoids) but can also occur with foregut NETs (carcinoids).
- With bronchial NETs (carcinoids), flushes frequently are prolonged for hours to days, reddish in color, and associated with salivation, lacrimation, diaphoresis, diarrhea, and hypotension.

- Flush associated with gastric NETs (carcinoids) can also be reddish in color, but with a patchy distribution over the face and neck, although the classic flush seen with midgut NETs (carcinoids) can also be seen with gastric NETs (carcinoids). It may be provoked by food and have accompanying pruritus.

Ans. B

19. Cells which mediate Warburg effect include:

A. Astrocytes
B. Endothelial cells
C. Stem cells
D. Cancer cells

Explanation:

- Many cancer cells utilize aerobic glycolysis (the Warburg effect) to metabolize glucose leading to increased lactic acid production whereas normal cells utilize oxidative phosphorylation in mitochondria under aerobic conditions, a much more efficient process for generating ATP for energy utilization but one that does not produce the same level of building blocks needed for new cells.
- One consequence is increased glucose uptake by cancer cells, a fact utilized in fluorodeoxyglucose (FDG)-positron emission tomography (PET) scanning to detect tumors.

Ans. D

20. A patient of breast cancer being treated with chemotherapy referred to you from oncologist as patient developed exertional intolerance and dyspnea of new onset. CXR was done which was normal. PFT done which was normal. ECG was done suggestive of left ventricular hypertrophy changes. You advised 2 D ECHO which was suggestive of dilated cardiomyopathy. Which of the following drug must be responsible for patients condition?

A. Bleomycin
B. Doxorubicin
C. Carboplatin
D. Dacarbazine

Explanation:

- Anthracyclines (doxorubicin) used in cancer treatment can caused cardiomyopathy.
- Patient in above question has developed cardiomyopathy due to treatment of breast cancer with doxorubicin causing her symptoms. When taken for long time cardiomyopathy occurs with anthracyclines but can be seen within 1 year of exposure.
- Risk factors include higher doses, preexisting cardiac condition, women, chest irradiation, extreme age.
- Anthracyclines characteristically causes vacuolar degeneration and myofibrillar loss on histology examination.
- Other drugs causing cardiomyopathy are transtuzumab, pertuzumab used in breast cancer.
- Cyclophosphamide, ifosfamide carfilozomib, bortezomib are cardiotoxic.

Ans. B

21. All are second line therapy for advanced stage HCC except:

A. Regorafenib
B. Cabozantinib
C. Ramucirumab
D. Lenvatinib

Explanation:

- BCLC staging system has been externally validated by numerous studies. It is an evolving system that allows incorporation of new therapies and treatment-dependent variables as new evidence emerges.
- Six treatments have been demonstrated to improve survival in HCC, five are adopted by guidelines and BCLC classification: surgical resection, liver transplantation, radiofrequency (RF) ablation, chemoembolization, and systemic therapies (sorafenib, regorafenib, lenvatinib, cabozantinib, ramucirumab).

- BCLC system will also incorporate lenvatinib in first line and regorafenib as standard of care in patients with advanced HCC progressing on sorafenib as a consequence of a positive randomized controlled trial (RCT).
- BCLC assigns each patient with a given treatment allocation. Treatment stage migration is also applied by this scheme, meaning that if patients are not candidates for the selected therapy, the next effective therapy at more advanced stages can be given.

Ans. D

22. Screening test for colorectal cancer between age 50-75 yrs by sigmoidoscopy every:

A. 1 year
B. 3 year
C. 5 year
D. 7 year

Explanation:

Table: Screening tests recommended by the U.S. preventive services task force for average-risk adults

Disease	Test	Population	Frequency
Abdominal aortic aneurysm	Ultrasound	Men 65-75 who have ever smoked	Once
Alcohol misuse	Alcohol use disorders identification test	All adults	Unknown
Breast cancer	Mammography with or without clinical breast examination	Women 50-75	Every 2 years
Cervical cancer	Pap smear Pap smear and HPV testing	Women 21-65 Women 30-65	Every 3 years Every 5 years if HPV negative
Chlamydia/ gonorrhea	Nucleic acid amplification test on urine or cervical swab	Sexually active women < 25	Unknown
Colorectal cancer	Fecal occult blood testing Sigmoidoscopy Colonoscopy (or occult blood testing combined with sigmoidoscopy)	50-75 50-75 50-75	Every year Every 5 years Every 10 years
Depression	Screening questions	All adults	Periodically
Diabetes	Fasting blood glucose of HgbA1c	Adults overweight, obese or with hypertension	Every 3 years
Hepatitis C	Anti-HCV antibody followed by confirmatory PCR	Adults born between 1945 and 1965	Once
HIV	Reactive immunoassay or rapid HIV followed by confirmatory test	15-65	At least once
Hyperlipidemia	Cholesterol	40-75	Unknown
Hypertension	Blood pressure	All adults	Periodically
Intimate partner violence	Screening questions	Women of childbearing age	Unknown
Obesity	Body mass index	All adults	Unknown
Osteoporosis	DEXA	Women > 65 or >60 with risk factors	Unknown

Ans. C

23. All are true statements except:

A. Ramucirumab, Gastric cancer

B. Sorafenib, Prostate cancer

C. Ziv aflibercept, Colorectal cancer

D. Sunitinib, GIST

Explanation:

- Sorafenib, originally developed as a Raf kinase inhibitor but with potent activity against VEGFR and PDGFR, has activity against RCC, differentiated thyroid and hepatocellular cancers as well as desmoid tumors.
- A closely related molecule to sorafenib, regorafenib, has activity against colorectal cancer, GIST, and hepatocellular cancer.
- Other inhibitors of the VEGF pathway approved for the treatment of various cancers include axitinib, pazopanib, lenvatinib, and cabozantinib

Ans. B

24. Hypercalcemia in lung cancer is primarily related to:

A. Adenocarcinoma

B. Large cell carcinoma

C. Squamous carcinoma

D. Small cell carcinoma

Explanation:

- Endocrine syndromes are seen in 12% of patients; hypercalcemia resulting from ectopic production of parathyroid hormone (PTH), or more commonly, PTH-related peptide, is the most common life-threatening metabolic complication of malignancy, primarily occurring with squamous cell carcinomas of the lung.

Ans. C

25. Partial response of cancer is:

A. At least 25% tumor reduction

B. At least 50% tumor reduction

C. At least 75%tumor reduction

D. 100% reduction

Explanation:

- Partial response (PR) is defined conventionally as a decrease by at least 50% in a tumor's bidimensional area; a complete response (CR) connotes disappearance of all tumor; progression of disease signifies an increase in size of existing lesions by >25% from baseline or best response or development of new lesions; and stable disease fits into none of the above categories.

Ans. B

26. All the following act on RAF except:

A. Vemurafenib

B. Dabrafenib

C. Sorafenib

D. Trametinib

Explanation:

- Trametinib, acting downstream of *BRAF* V600E by directly inhibiting MEK serine kinase by a non-ATP binding site mechanism, also displayed noteworthy responses in *BRAF* V600E–mutated melanomas, and the combination of trametinib and dabrafenib is even more active, by targeting *BRAF* V600E–driven pathway at two points in the pathway leading to gene activation.
- Vemurafenib and dabrafenib, with selective capacity to inhibit the *BRAF* V600E serine kinase activity, were each shown to cause noteworthy responses in patients with *BRAF* V600E– mutated melanomas, although early relapse occurred in many patients treated with the drugs as single agents.

Ans. D

27. Most common mutations in oncogenes in cancers is:

A. RAS
B. HER
C. MET
D. BRAF

Explanation:

- Major effort is underway to develop targeted therapies for mutations in the *ras* family of genes which are the most common mutations in oncogenes in cancers (especially *kras*) but have proved to be very difficult targets for a number of reasons related to the structure of RAS proteins as well as mechanisms of activation and inactivation.
- Targeted therapies against a subset of proteins downstream of RAS in the signaling pathway (including BRAF and mitogen-activated protein [MAP] kinase) have proven to have significant antitumor activity against V600E BRAF mutant melanoma, with improved efficacy when they are used in combination.

Ans. A

28. Rate-limiting step for metastasis is:

A. Ability to adhere to foreign endothelium of the metastatic site
B. Ability for tumor cells to survive and expand in novel microenvironment of metastatic site
C. Ability to multiply at the metastatic site
D. Ability to divide at the rate more than normal cells at the metastatic site

Explanation:

- Rate-limiting step for metastasis is the ability for tumor cells to survive and expand in the novel microenvironment of the metastatic site, and multiple host-tumor interactions determine the ultimate outcome.

Ans. B

29. All are true statements except:

A. Aortopulmonary lymph nodes (levels 5, 6) are commonly sampled by doing the Chamberlain procedure
B. EUS-FNA is performed via the esophagus and is ideally suited for sampling lymph nodes in the posterior mediastinum (levels 7, 8, 9)
C. Area directly posterior to the trachea cannot accurately be assessed and is a "blind spot" for EUS-FNA
D. EBUS-FNA can visualize the anterior lymph nodes and can complement EUS-FNA

Explanation:

- As an alternative to surgery, a bronchoscope can be used to perform TBNA to obtain tissue from the mediastinum, and, when combined with EBUS, can allow access to the same lymph node stations associated with mediastinoscopy, but also extend access out to the hilar lymph nodes (levels 10, 11).
- Finally, endoscopic ultrasound (EUS)– fine-needle aspiration (FNA) is a second procedure that complements EBUS-FNA in the staging of lung cancer.
- EUS-FNA is performed via esophagus and is ideally suited for sampling lymph nodes in posterior mediastinum (levels 7, 8, 9). Because US imaging cannot penetrate air-filled spaces, the area directly anterior to the trachea cannot accurately be assessed and is a "blind spot" for EUS-FNA.
- However, EBUS-FNA can visualize the anterior lymph nodes and can complement EUS-FNA. The combination of EUS-FNA and EBUS-FNA with the use of radial probes has made these techniques a clear non operative alternative for staging the mediastinum in thoracic malignancies.

Ans. C

30. Physical activity is associated with decreased risk of:

A. Colon cancer
B. Breast cancer
C. Both of the above
D. None of the above

Explanation:

- Physical activity is associated with a decreased risk of colon and breast cancer.
- A variety of mechanisms have been proposed. However, such studies are prone to confounding factors such as recall bias, association of exercise with other health-related practices, and effects of preclinical cancers on exercise habits (reverse causality).

Ans. C

31. Trastuzumab targets:

A. HIF-1
B. HER2
C. cMET
D. VEGFR

Explanation:

Table: Monoclonal antibodies alone

Drug	Molecular Target	Disease	Mechanism Of Action
Trastuzumab	HER2/neu (ERBB2)	Breast cancer	Binds HER2 on tumor cell surface and induces receptor internalization
Pertuzumab	HER2/neu (ERBB2)	Breast cancer	Binds HER2 on tumor cell surface at distinct site from Trastuzumab and prevents binding to other receptors
Cetuximab	EGFR	Colon cancer, squamous cell carcinoma of the head and neck	Binds extracellular domain of EGFR and blocks binding of EGF and TGF-α; induces receptor internalization. Potentiates the efficacy of chemotherapy and radiotherapy
Panitumumab	EGFR	Colon cancer	Similar to Cetuximab but fully humanized rather than chimeric
Necitumumab	EGFR	Squamous NSCLC	Binds EGFR
Rituximab	CD20	B-cell lymphomas and leukemias that express CD20	Multiple potential mechanisms, including direct induction of tumor cell apoptosis and immune mechanisms
Alemtuzumab	CD52	Chronic lymphocytic leukemia and CD52-expressing lymphoid tumors	Immune mechanisms
Bevacizumab	VEGF	Colorectal, lung cancers, RCC, glioblastoma	Inhibits angiogenesis by high-affinity binding to VEGF
Ziv-Aflibercept	VEGFA, VEGFB, PLGF	Colorectal cancers	Inhibits angiogenesis by high-affinity binding to VEGFA, B and PLGF
Ramucirumab	VEGFR	Gastric, colorectal, lung cancers	Inhibits angiogenesis by binding to VEGFR

Ans. B

32. All can cause cancer except:

A. Silica
B. Asbestos
C. Coal dust
D. Beryllium

Explanation:

Table: Categories of occupational exposure and associated respiratory conditions		
Occupational Exposures	**Nature of Respiratory Responses**	**Comment**
Inorganic Dusts		
Asbestos: Mining, processing, construction, ship repair	Fibrosis (asbestosis), pleural disease, cancer, mesothelioma	Virtually all new mining and construction with asbestos done in developing countries
Silica: Mining, stone cutting, sandblasting, quarrying	Fibrosis (silicosis), progressive massive fibrosis (PMF), cancer, tuberculosis, chronic obstructive pulmonary disease (COPD)	Improved protection in United States; persistent risk in developing countries
Coal dust: Mining	Fibrosis (coal worker's pneumoconiosis), PMF, COPD	Risk persists in certain areas of United States, increasing in countries where new mines open
Beryllium: Processing alloys for high-tech industries	Acute pneumonitis (rare), chronic granulomatous disease, lung cancer (high suspect)	Risk in high-tech industries persists
Other metals: Aluminum, chromium, cobalt, nickel, titanium, tungsten carbide or 'hard metal' (contains cobalt)	Wide variety of conditions from acute pneumonitis to lung cancer and asthma	New diseases appear with new process development
Organic Dusts		
Cotton dust: Milling, processing	Byssinosis (an asthma-like syndrome), chronic bronchitis, COPD	Increasing risk in developing countries with drop in United States as jobs shift overseas
Grain dust: Elevator agents, dock workers milling bakers	Asthma, chronic bronchitis, COPD	Risk shifting more to migrant labor pool
Other agricultural dusts: Fungal spores, vegetable products, insect fragments, animal dander, bird and rodent feces, endotoxins, micoorganisms, pollens	Hypersensitivity pneumonitis (farmer's lung), asthma, chronic bronchitis	Important in migrant labor pool but also resulting from in-home exposures
Toxic chemicals: Wide variety of industries; see Table 283-2	Asthma, chronic bronchitis, COPD, hypersensitivity pneumonitis, pneumoconiosis and cancer	Reduced risk with recognized hazards; increasing risk for developing countries where controlled labor practices are less stringent
Other Environmental Agents		
Uranium and radon daughters, secondhand tobacco smoke, polycyclic aromatic hydrocarbons (PAHs), biomass smoke, diesel exhaust, welding fumes, wood finishing	Occupational exposures estimated to contribute to up to 10% of all lung cancers; chronic bronchitis, COPD and fibrosis	In-home exposures important; in developing countries, biomass smoke is a major risk factor for COPD among women in these countries

Ans. C

33. Third generation TKI among the following is:

A. Dasatinib B. Nilotinib

C. Bosutinib D. Ponatinib

Explanation:

- Among patients developing resistance to TKIs, several resistance mechanisms have been observed. The most clinically relevant one is development of different *ABL1* kinase domain mutations that may prevent the binding of TKIs to the catalytic site (ATP-binding site) of the kinase or maintain the kinase activity despite the presence of a TKI.
- More than 100 *BCR-ABL1* mutations have now been described, many of which confer relative or absolute resistance to imatinib. This has resulted in the development of second-generation TKIs (i.e., dasatinib, nilotinib, bosutinib) and of a **third-generation TKI (ponatinib)** with significant efficacy against T315I, a "gatekeeper" mutation that prevents binding of and causes resistance to all other TKIs.

Ans. D

34. Cancers which have a particularly high incidence of intracranial bleeding include all except:

A. Melanoma
B. Germ cell tumors
C. Lung cancer
D. Renal cell cancer

Explanation:

- Melanoma, germ cell tumors, and renal cell cancers have a particularly high incidence of intracranial bleeding.
- Tumor mass and surrounding edema may cause obstruction of the circulation of CSF, with resulting hydrocephalus.

Ans. C

35. Which of the following is not caused by EBV?

A. Burkitt lymphoma
B. Primary CNS diffuse large B cell lymphoma
C. Primary effusion lymphoma
D. Extranodal NK/T cell lymphoma- Nasal type

Explanation:

Table: Infectious agents associated with the development of lymphoid malignancies

Infectious Agent	Lymphoid Malignancy
Epstein-Barr virus	Burkitt's lymphoma Post-organ transplant lymphoma Primary CNS diffuse large B-cell lymphoma Hodgkin's lymphoma Extranodal NK/T-cell lymphoma, nasal type
HTLV-1	Adult T-cell leukemia/lymphoma
HIV	Diffuse large B-cell lymphoma Burkitt's lymphoma
Hepatitis C virus	Lymphoplasmacytic lymphoma
Helicobacter pylori	Gastric MALT lymphoma
Human herpesvirus 8	Primary effusion lymphoma Multicentric Castleman's disease

Ans. C

36. A 41-year-old male with features of Cushing's syndrome was referred to endocrinology OPD for further evaluation. 24 hr urinary cortisol and ONDST confirmed the Cushing's syndrome. To differentiate Cushing's disease from adrenal Cushing's ACTH was ordered. Sample for ACTH should be collected in:

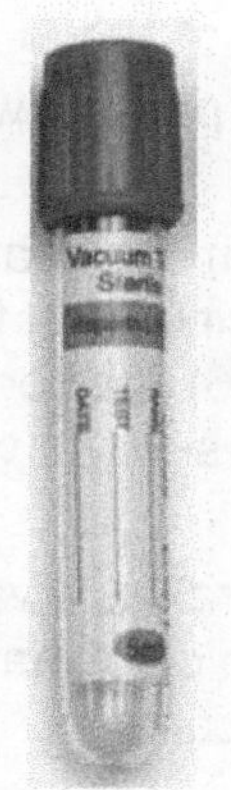
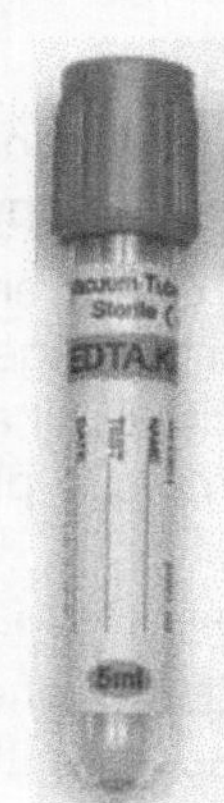
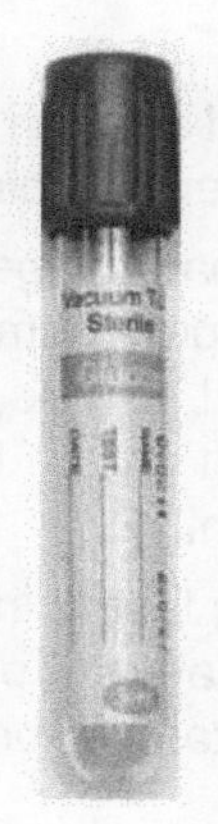
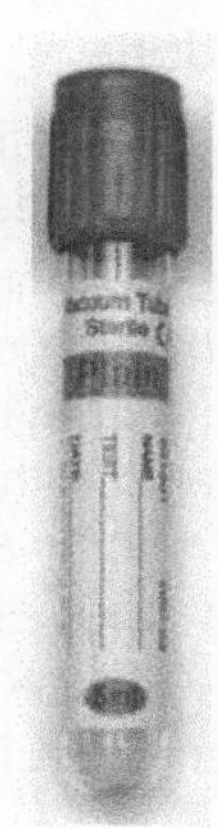

A. Green vacutainer
B. Purple vacutainer
C. Grey vacutainer
D. Red vacutainer

Explanation:

Secreted by lung tumors. Ideally, nonstressed resting subjects should have venous blood withdrawn between 6 AM and 9 AM. As ACTH is relatively unstable at room temperature and has a propensity to adhere to glass, plasma samples should immediately be separated in iced siliconized glass tubes containing ethylenediaminetetra-acetic acid (EDTA) and stored below –20°C for transport. Morning (8 AM) plasma ACTH levels range from 8 to 25 ng/l. Episodic secretion and short plasma half-life result in wide and rapid fluctuation of plasma measurements.

Ans. B

37. A 60 year old male who is a known smoker presented to the OPD with gradual onset cough, breathlessness, hoarseness of voice and dysphagia. He gives history of working in shipbuilding industry with exposure to asbestos fibres. Which among the following statements regarding mesothelioma is false?

A. Immunohistochemistry is used to confirm the diagnosis
B. Thoracoscopy is the standard procedure
C. Relatively brief asbestos exposure can lead to mesothelioma
D. Related to smoking

Explanation:

- Lung cancer is clearly associated with asbestos exposure but does not typically present for at least 15 years after initial exposure. The lung cancer risk increases multiplicatively with cigarette smoking.
- In addition, mesotheliomas (both pleural and peritoneal) are strongly associated with asbestos exposure, but they are not related to smoking.
- Relatively brief asbestos exposures may lead to mesotheliomas, which typically do not develop for decades after the initial exposure.
- Biopsy of pleural tissue, typically by thoracoscopic surgery, is required for diagnosing mesothelioma.

Ans. D

38. All the below agents are CDK4/6 inhibitors except:

A. Palbociclib
B. Ribociclib
C. Lapatinib
D. Abemaciclib

Explanation:

- At least two different targeted agents have been shown to enhance outcomes of patients with ER-positive metastatic breast cancer when combined with endocrine therapy.
- Addition of an inhibitor of mammalian target of rapamycin (mTOR), everolimus, to the hormonal treatment can lead to AIs, tamoxifen, or fulvestrant improves time to progression, and this agent is now being explored as front-line therapy and in the adjuvant setting. Likewise, inhibitors of cyclin D kinase 4/6 (CDK4/6) (palbociclib, ribociclib, abemaciclib) have also been shown to substantially improve progression-free survival when combined either with an AI or fulvestrant.
- These agents are also being tested in the adjuvant setting. Data regarding overall survival benefits from mTOR or CDK4/6 inhibitors are still pending, but addition of one or the other in combination with ET for women with ER-positive metastatic breast cancer is becoming the standard of care.

Ans. C

39. Hormone secreting tumors most commonly secrete:

A. GH
B. FSH
C. LH
D. Prolactin

Explanation:

- Hormone secreting tumors most commonly secrete prolactin.
- Hyperprolactinemia is the most common pituitary hormone hypersecretion syndrome in both men and women.
- PRL-secreting pituitary adenomas (prolactinomas) are the most common cause of PRL levels >200 μg/L.

Ans. D

40. 89 year old male presented to OPD for routine health checkup. Found to have marginally high PSA. On local examination found to have prostatomegaly. With advanced aging, size of testis will:

A. Increase
B. Decrease
C. No change
D. Any of the above

Explanation:

Testicular volume is best assessed by using a Prader orchidometer. Testes range from 3.5 to 5.5 cm in length, which corresponds to a volume of 12-25 ml. **Advanced age does not influence testicular size, although the consistency becomes less firm.** Asian men generally have smaller testes than western Europeans, independent of differences in body size.

Ans. C

41. Gompertzian growth curve is regarding:

A. Tumor growth
B. Skin growth
C. Puberty
D. None of the above

Explanation:

- Tumors follow a Gompertzian growth curve with the apparent growth fraction of a neoplasm being high with small tumor burdens and declining until, at time of diagnosis, with a tumor burden of 1–5 × 10^9 tumor cells, growth fraction is usually 1–4% for many solid tumors.
- By this view, the most rapid growth rate occurs before the tumor is detectable.
- An alternative explanation for such growth properties may also emerge from the ability of tumors at metastatic sites to recruit circulating tumor cells from the primary tumor or other metastases.

- An additional key feature of successful tumor is ability to stimulate development of a new supporting stroma through angiogenesis and production of proteases to allow invasion through basement membranes and normal tissue barriers.

Ans. A

42. Most common primary cardiac tumor of heart is:

A. Metastasis from CA breast
B. Lymphoma
C. Myxoma
D. Sarcoma

Explanation:

- Myxoma is an most common primary heart tumor.
- Most common site is interatrial septum in viscinity of fossa ovalis particularly in left atrium.
- Most commonly in 3rd to 6th decade with female > male
- Most of them 90 % are sporadic, 10 % familial with autosomal dominant inheritance.
- Most commonly clinically mimics mitral valve disease (mitral stenosis or mitral regurgitation). Fever, weight loss, cachexia, rash digital clubbing, arthralgias, raynauds phenomenon seen.
- Tumor plop is heard over mitral are in early or mid diastole

Familial variety occur as part of some syndromes like

- A.carney complex : myxomas, lentigines, pigmented nevi and endocrinopathies like primary adrenal cortical disease with or without Cushing's syndrome, testicular tumours, gigantism, acromegaly.
- B. NAME syndrome: **N**evi, **A**trial myxoma, **M**yxoid neurofibroma and **E**phelides
- C.LAMB syndrome : **l**entigines , **a**trial myoma , **b**lue nevi.

Ans. C

43. A 21-year-old man is treated with induction chemotherapy for acute lymphoblastic leukemia. His initial white blood cell count prior to treatment was 156,000/µL. All of the following are expected complications during his treatment except:

A. Acute kidney injury
B. Hypercalcemia
C. Hyperkalemia
D. Hyperphosphatemia

Explanation:

- Tumor lysis syndrome occurs most commonly in individuals undergoing chemotherapy for rapidly proliferating malignancies, including acute leukemias and Burkitt lymphoma. In rare instances, it can be seen in chronic lymphoma or solid tumors.
- As the chemotherapeutic agents act on these cells, there is massive tumor lysis that results in release of intracellular ions and nucleic acids. This leads to a characteristic metabolic syndrome of hyperuricemia, hyperphosphatemia, hyperkalemia, and hypocalcemia.
- Acute kidney injury is frequent and can lead to renal failure requiring hemodialysis if uric acid crystallizes within the renal tubules.
- Lactic acidosis and dehydration increase the risk of acute kidney injury.
- Hyperphosphatemia occurs due to the release of intracellular phosphate ions and causes a reciprocal reduction in serum calcium.
- This hypocalcemia can be profound, leading to neuromuscular irritability and tetany.
- Hyperkalemia can become rapidly life-threatening and cause ventricular arrhythmia. Knowing characteristics of tumor lysis syndrome, one can attempt to prevent the known complications from occurring. It is important to monitor serum electrolytes frequently during treatment.

- Laboratory studies should be obtained no less than three times daily, but more frequent monitoring is often needed.
- Allopurinol should be administered prophylactically at high doses.
- If allopurinol fails to control uric acid to less than 8 mg/dL, rasburicase, a recombinant urate oxidase, can be added at a dose of 0.2 mg/kg. Throughout this period, the patient should be well hydrated with alkalinization of the urine to a pH of greater than 7.0.
- This is accomplished by administration of intravenous normal or half-normal saline at a dose of 3000 mL/m2 daily with sodium bicarbonate. Prophylactic hemodialysis is not performed unless there is underlying renal failure prior to starting chemotherapy.

Ans. B

44. Which of the following statements describes the relationship between testicular tumors and serum markers?

A. β-hCG and AFP should be measured when following the progress of a tumor
B. β-hCG is limited in its usefulness as a marker because it is identical to human luteinizing hormone
C. Measurement of tumor markers the day after surgery for localized disease is useful in determining completeness of the resection
D. More than 40% of nonseminomatous germ cell tumors produce no cell markers

Explanation:

- 90 percent of persons with nonseminomatous germ cell tumors produce either AFP or β-hCG; in contrast, persons with pure seminomas usually produce neither.
- These tumor markers are present for some time after surgery; if the presurgical levels are high, 30 days or more may be required before meaningful postsurgical levels can be obtained.
- Half-lives of AFP and β-hCG are 6 days and 1 day, respectively.
- After treatment, unequal reduction of β-hCG and AFP may occur, suggesting that the two markers are synthesized by heterogeneous clones of cells within the tumor; thus, both markers should be followed. β-hCG is similar to luteinizing hormone except for its distinctive β subunit.

Ans. A

45. A 47-year-old woman with known HIV/AIDS (CD4+ lymphocyte = 106/ μL and viral load = 35,000/mL) presents with painful growths on the side of her tongue as shown in Figure. What is the most likely diagnosis?

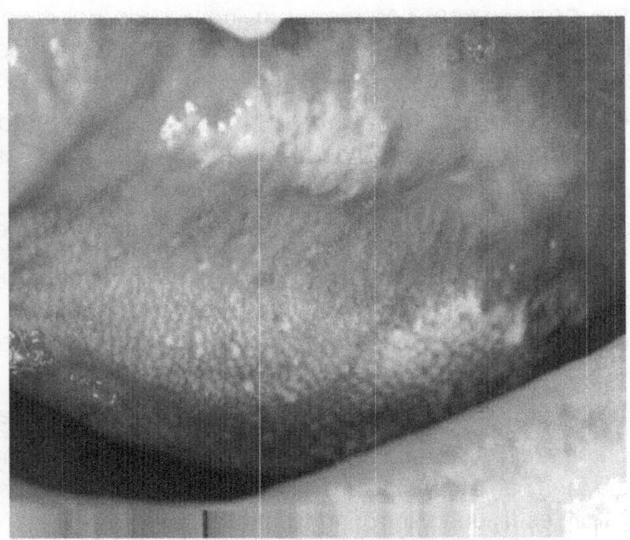

A. Aphthous ulcers
B. Hairy leukoplakia
C. Herpes stomatitis
D. Oral candidiasis

Explanation:

- Oral hairy leukoplakia is caused by a severe overgrowth of Epstein-Barr virus infection in T-cell–deficient patients.
- It is not premalignant and is often unrecognized by the patient but is sometimes a cosmetic, symptomatic, and therapeutic nuisance.
- White, thickened folds on the side of the tongue can be pruritic or painful and sometimes resolve with acyclovir derivatives or topical podophyllin resin.
- Ultimate resolution occurs after immune reconstitution with antiretroviral therapy.
- Oral candidiasis or thrush is a very common, relatively easy-to-treat condition in HIV patients and takes on an appearance of white plaques on the tongue, palate, and buccal mucosa that bleed with blunt removal.
- Herpes simplex virus (HSV) recurrences or aphthous ulcers present as painful ulcerating lesions.
- Latter should be considered when oral ulcers persist, do not respond to acyclovir, and do not culture HSV.
- Kaposi's sarcoma is uncommon in the oropharynx and takes on a violet hue, suggesting its highly vascularized content.

Ans. B

46. Regarding Chromosomal translocations all are true except:

A. 9;22 – CML
B. 11;14 – Prostate
C. 11;22 – Ewing's sarcoma
D. 2;3 – Thyroid

Explanation:

Table: Representative oncogenes at chromosomal translocations

Gene (Chromosome)	Translocation	Malignancy
BCR-ABL	(9;22) (q34;q11)	Chronic myeloid leukemia
BCL1 (11q13.3)–*IgH* (14q32)	(11;14) (q13;q32)	Mantle cell lymphoma
BCL2 (18q21.3)–*IgH* (14q32)	(14;18) (q32;q21)	Follicular lymphoma
FLI-EWSR1	(11;22) (q24;q12)	Ewing's sarcoma
LCK-TCRB	(1;7) (p34; q35)	T-cell acute lymphocytic leukemia
PAX3–FOXO1	(2;13) (q35;q14)	Rhabdomyosarcoma
PAX8–PPARG	(2;3) (q13;p25)	Thyroid
IL21R–BCL6	(3;16) (q27;p11)	Non-Hodgkin's lymphoma
TAL1–TCTA	(1;3) (p34;p21)	Acute T cell leukemia
TMPRSS2-ERG	Rearrangement on Chr21q22	Prostate

Ans. B

47. All act on RAF except:

A. Vemurafenib
B. Dabrafenib
C. Sorafenib
D. Trametinib

Explanation:

- BRAF V600E mutation has been detected in a notable fraction of melanomas, thyroid tumors, and hairy cell leukemia, and preclinical models supported the concept that BRAF V600E drives oncogenic signaling in these tumors.

- Vemurafenib and dabrafenib, with selective capacity to inhibit the BRAF V600E serine kinase activity, were each shown to cause noteworthy responses in patients with BRAF V600E–mutated melanomas, although early relapse occurred in many patients treated with the drugs as single agents.
- Trametinib, acting downstream of BRAF V600E by directly inhibiting the MEK serine kinase by a non-ATP binding site mechanism, also displayed noteworthy responses in BRAF V600E–mutated melanomas, and the combination of trametinib and dabrafenib is even more active, by targeting BRAF V600E–driven pathway at two points in the pathway leading to gene activation.

Ans. D

48. Excellent hydration must be maintained while using:

A. Cyclophosphamide
B. Bleomycin
C. Procarbazine
D. Melphalan

Explanation:

- Cyclophosphamide is inactive unless metabolized by the liver to 4-hydroxy-cyclophosphamide, which decomposes into an alkylating species, as well as to chloroacetaldehyde and acrolein.
- Latter causes chemical cystitis; therefore, excellent hydration must be maintained while using cyclophosphamide.
- If severe, cystitis may be attenuated or prevented altogether (if expected from dose of cyclophosphamide to be used) by mesna (2 *m*ercaptoethane*s*ulfo*na*te).
- Liver disease impairs cyclophosphamide activation. Sporadic interstitial pneumonitis leading to pulmonary fibrosis can accompany the use of cyclophosphamide, and high doses used in conditioning regimens for bone marrow transplant can cause cardiac dysfunction.
- Ifosfamide is a cyclophosphamide analogue also activated in liver, but more slowly, and it requires coadministration of mesna to prevent bladder injury.
- CNS effects, including somnolence, confusion, and psychosis, can follow ifosfamide use; the incidence appears related to low body surface area or decreased creatinine clearance.

Ans. A

49. Autoantigen related to liver cancer is:

A. Amphiphysin
B. DNA Topoisomerase II
C. Desmoplakin
D. Gephyrin

Explanation:

Table: Cancer and paraneoplastic autoimmunity	
Amphiphysin	Neuropathy, small-cell lung cancer
Cyclin B1	Hepatocellular carcinoma
DNA topoisomerase II	Liver cancer
Desmoplakin	Paraneoplastic pemphigus
Gephyrin	Paraneoplastic stiff-person syndrome

Ans. B

50. Autoantigen associated with paraneoplastic opsoclous-myoclonus ataxia is:

A. Ri protein
B. B-IV Spectrin
C. Synaptotagmin
D. Yo protein

Explanation:

Autoantigen	Autoimmune Diseases
Ri protein	Paraneoplastic opsoclonus myoclonus ataxia
βIV spectrin	Lower motor neuron syndrome
Synaptotagmin	Lambert-Eaton myasthenic syndrome
Voltage-gated calcium channels	Lambert-Eaton myasthenic syndrome
Yo protein	Paraneoplastic cerebellar degeneration

Ans. A

51. Breast & Lung carcinoma tend to occur in close temporal association with onset of SSc particularly who have antibodies against:

A. RNA Polymerase III
B. DNA Topoisomerase I
C. Centromere proteins
D. U3-RNP

Explanation:

- Lung cancer & esophageal adenocarcinoma typically occur in setting of long-standing ILD or GERD and may be caused by chronic inflammation and repair.
- In contrast, breast, lung, and ovarian carcinomas and lymphomas tend to occur in close temporal association with the onset of SSc, particularly in patients who have autoantibodies to RNA polymerase III.
- In this scenario, SSc may represent a paraneoplastic syndrome triggered by the anti-tumor immune response.

Ans. A

52. A person with larynx carcinoma has undergone radiation therapy. Which is false regarding radiation induced brachial plexopathy?

A. Occurs after months to years after radiation
B. Usually painless
C. Involves lower trunk
D. Associated with microvascular abnormalities

Explanation:

- Radiation can be associated with microvascular abnormalities and fibrosis of surrounding tissues, which can damage the axons and the Schwann cells.
- Radiation-induced plexopathy can develop months or years following therapy and is dose dependent.
- Tumor invasion is usually painful and more commonly affects the lower trunk, whereas radiation injury is often painless and affects the upper trunk.

Ans. C

53. A 50 year old smoker, recently diagnosed with lung mass on routine examination. Recently developed symptoms of confusion, weakness and tiredness. Which of the following types of cancer is most commonly associated with SIADH?

A. Small cell lung cancer
B. Non-small cell lung cancer
C. Mesothelioma
D. Thymoma

Explanation:

- Most commonly discovered in a symptomatic individuals as a result of serum electrolyte measurements, hyponatremia is usually due to tumor secretion of arginine vasopressin, a condition called syndrome of inappropriate antidiuretic hormone secretion (SIADH).
- Atrial natriuretic hormone also may produce hyponatremia. SIADH occurs most commonly in small cell lung cancer (15%) and head and neck cancer (3%).

Ans. A

54. What stage of non-small cell lung cancer is most appropriate for a patient who has a 3-cm mass in the right upper lobe, mediastinal adenopathy, and a 2-cm nodule in the right lobe of the liver?

A. Stage IIB
B. Stage IIIA
C. Stage IIIB
D. Stage IV

Explanation:

<table>
<tr><th colspan="8">Table: Distant metastasis (M)</th></tr>
<tr><td>M0</td><td colspan="3">No distant metastasis</td><td colspan="4">M0 No distant metastasis</td></tr>
<tr><td>M1</td><td colspan="3">Distant metastasis</td><td colspan="4">Distant metastasis</td></tr>
<tr><td>• M1a</td><td colspan="3">Separate tumor nodule(s) in a contralateral lobe; tumor with pleural nodules or malignant pleural or pericardial effusion</td><td colspan="4">M1a separate nodule(s) in a contralateral tumor with pleural nodules or malignant pleural or pericardial effusion</td></tr>
<tr><td>• M1b</td><td colspan="3">Distant metastasis (in extrathoracic organs)</td><td colspan="4">Single metastasis in a single organ</td></tr>
<tr><td>• M1c</td><td colspan="3"></td><td colspan="4">Multiple metastases in a single organ or in several organs</td></tr>
<tr><td>Stage IV</td><td>Any T</td><td>Any N</td><td>M1a or M1b</td><td>Stage IVA</td><td>Any T</td><td>Any N</td><td>M1a/M1b</td></tr>
<tr><td></td><td></td><td></td><td></td><td>Stage IVB</td><td>Any T</td><td>Any N</td><td>M1c</td></tr>
</table>

Ans. D

55. A 65-year-old man who has smoked two packs of cigarettes per day for the past 40 years has had drooping of the left eyelid for the past 3 weeks. A chest radiograph reveals a mass in the apex of the left lung. What is the cause for drooping of left eyelid?

A. Horner's syndrome
B. Glaucoma
C. Facial palsy
D. Paraneoplastic syndrome

Explanation:

- Lung tumors involving the apex of the lung (superior sulcus tumors) are also known as Pancoast tumors.
- If they involve the cervical sympathetic nerves in the neck, these tumors result in Horner syndrome.
- This syndrome is characterized by ptosis (drooping of the eyelid), anhidrosis (absence of sweating), and miosis (constricted pupil) on the same side as the tumor.
- Other manifestations of Pancoast tumor include pain and weakness in the upper extremity (owing to involvement of the brachial plexus), rib destruction, and destruction of vertebral bodies. Treatment depends on local and distant spread of the tumor.

Ans. A

56. A 50 year old female was diagnosed with right upper lobe mass lesion. Which among the following is the non ionizing imaging modality that will aid in taking a biopsy from the mass?

A. Chest X-ray
B. Computed tomography scan
C. PET CT
D. Ultrasound

Explanation:

- Diagnostic ultrasound is a non ionizing imaging approach which is safe to perform on pregnant women and children. It can detect and localize pleural abnormalities and guide thoracentesis of a pleural effusion.

Ans. D

CHAPTER 10

GIT – GASTROINTESTINAL SYSTEM

1. Most common CNS manifestation of Whipple's disease is:

A. Seizure

B. Ataxia

C. Ophthalmoplegia

D. Dementia

Explanation:

- Whipple's disease is a chronic multisystemic disease associated with diarrhea, steatorrhea, weight loss, arthralgia, and central nervous system (CNS) and cardiac problems; it is caused by the bacterium Tropheryma whipplei.
- Most common CNS manifestation is Dementia (cognitive dysfunction).
- Dementia generally a late manifestation with extremely poor prognostic sign.
- Recurrence of disease activity, especially with dementia, is an *extremely poor prognostic sign* and requires an antibiotic that crosses the blood brain barrier.

Ans. D

2. Not protective for Inflammatory bowel disease is:

A. Vitamin D

B. ↑ω-6 fatty acids

C. ↑ω-3 fatty acids

D. All of the above

Explanation:

- In Caucasian populations, smoking is an important risk factor in IBD with opposite effects on UC and CD, whereas in other ethnic groups with different genetic susceptibility, smoking may play a lesser role.
- There is a protective effect of previous appendectomy with confirmed appendicitis (risk reduction of 13–26%), particularly at a young age, on the development of UC across different geographical regions and populations.
- There is a modest association with the development of CD but this may be due to diagnostic bias.
- Oral contraceptive use is associated with the risk of CD with a reported hazard ratio as high as 2.82 among current users and 1.39 among past users. Association between oral contraceptive use and UC is limited to women with a history of smoking.
- There is an association between antibiotic use and the development of childhood IBD with children who received one or more dispensations of antibiotics during the first year of life having a 2.9-fold increase in the risk of developing IBD during childhood.

- Breastfeeding may also protect against the development of IBD.
- Infectious gastroenteritis with pathogens (e.g., *Salmonella*, *Shigella*, *Campylobacter* spp., *Clostridium difficile*) increases IBD risk by two- to threefold.
- **Diets high in animal protein, sugars, sweets, oils, fish and shellfish, and dietary fat, especially ω-6 fatty acids, and low in ω-3 fatty acids have been implicated in increasing the risk of IBD.**
- A protective effect of vitamin D on the risk of CD has been reported

Ans. B

3. Which of the following is not true about risk factor for Alcoholic liver disease?

A. Two drinks per day is probably safe

B. Patatin-like phospholipase domain-containing protein 3 (PNPLA3) has been associated with alcoholic cirrhosis.

C. HCV infection concurrent with alcoholic liver disease is associated with older age for severity, more advanced histology, and decreased survival

D. Alcohol injury does not require malnutrition, but obesity and nonalcoholic fatty liver are risk factors.

Explanation:

Table: Risk factors for alcoholic liver disease

Risk Factor	Comment
Quantity	In men, 40-80 g/d of ethanol produces fatty liver; 160 g/d for 10-20 years causes hepatitis or cirrhosis. Only 15% of alcoholics develop alcoholic liver disease
Gender	Women exhibit increased susceptibility to alcoholic liver disease at amounts > 20 g/d; two drinks per day is probably safe
Hepatitis C	HCV infection concurrent with alcoholic liver disease is associated with younger age for severity, more advanced histology and decreased survival
Genetics	Patatin-like phospholipase domain-containing protein 3 (PNPLA3) has been associated with alcoholic cirrhosis
Fatty liver	Alcohol injury does not require malnutrition, but obesity and non-alcoholic fatty liver are risk factors. Patients should receive vigorous attention to nutritional support

Ans. C

4. Hy law is related to:

A. Small intestinal obstruction

B. Acute pancreatitis

C. Drug induced liver injury

D. GERD

Explanation:

- More valid as a predictor of severe hepatotoxicity is the occurrence of jaundice in patients enrolled in a clinical drug trial, so-called "Hy's Law," named after Hyman Zimmerman, one of the pioneers of the field of drug hepatotoxicity.
- He recognized that, if jaundice occurred during a phase III trial, more serious liver injury was likely, with a 10:1 ratio between cases of jaundice and liver failure—10 patients with jaundice to 1 patient with acute liver failure.
- Thus, finding of such Hy's Law cases during drug development often portends failure of approval, particularly if any of the subjects sustains a bad outcome.

Ans. C

5. A 36-year-old male with a history of gastric bypass surgery developed numbness in his legs over the last 2 months. Three weeks ago he started having falls. He presented to the emergency department because he could no longer void on his own. His neurological examination shows prominent loss of sensation to vibration and proprioception in his lower extremities along with mild weakness in his legs. He seems to have maintained strength and sensation in his arms. He has brisk reflexes at the knees, but his reflexes at his ankles are absent. Which of the following is the most likely diagnosis?

A. Vitamin E deficiency
B. Vitamin D deficiency
C. Vitamin B6 toxicity
D. Vitamin B12 deficiency

Explanation:

- This patient presents with signs and symptoms of subacute combined degeneration of the spinal cord, which is a severe consequence of vitamin B12 deficiency, which affects the posterior columns and lateral columns of the spinal cord. This causes a loss of sensation to vibration and proprioception and can result in weakness in severe cases. Vitamin B12 deficiency is common in patients who have pernicious anemia, are vegan, or have had gastric bypass surgery. Vitamin E deficiency leads to a clinical picture of a spinocerebellar ataxia. Vitamin B6 toxicity, usually doses of more than 200 mg/day, can cause a predominantly sensory polyneuropathy and, in severe cases, sensory ganglionopathy. Vitamin A toxicity is associated with dry pruritic skin, joint pain, and pseudotumor cerebri. The most common neurological presentation of vitamin D deficiency is a mild myopathy with proximal leg weakness. It is also associated with diffuse bone pain and muscle pain.

Ans. D

6. Drugs that cause cholestatic hepatitis include all except:

A. OC Pills
B. Erythromycin
C. Chlorpromazine
D. Both B & C

Explanation:

Cholestatic conditions that can cause Jaundice

I. Intrahepatic
- A. Viral hepatitis
  1. Fibrosing cholestatic hepatitis–hepatitis B and C
  2. Hepatitis A, Epstein-Barr virus infection, cytomegalovirus infection
- B. Alcoholic hepatitis
- C. Drug toxicity
  1. Pure cholestasis–anabolic and contraceptive steroids
  2. Cholestatic hepatitis–chlorpromazine, erythromycin estolate
  3. Chronic cholestasis–chlorpromazine and prochlorperazine
- D. Primary biliary cholangitis
- E. Primary sclerosing cholangitis
- F. Vanishing bile duct syndrome
  1. Chronic rejection of liver transplants
  2. Sarcoidosis
  3. Drugs
- G. Congestive hepatopathy and ischemic hepatitis
- H. Inherited conditions
  1. Progressive familial intrahepatic cholestasis
  2. Benign recurrent intrahepatic cholestasis

Contd.

Contd.

- I. Cholestasis of pregnancy
- J. Total parenteral nutrition
- K. Non-hepatobiliary sepsis
- L. Benign postoperative cholestasis
- M. Paraneoplastic syndrome
- N. Veno-occlusive disease
- O. Graft-versus-host disease
- P. Infiltrative disease
  1. Tuberculosis
  2. Lymphoma
  3. Amyloidosis
- Q. Infections
  1. Malaria
  2. Leptospirosis

Ans. A

7. Removal of how much terminal ileum causes malabsorption?

A. >50 cm B. >75 cm

C. >100 cm D. >120 cm

Explanation:

- **Removal of ≥1.2 m of terminal ileum causes malabsorption of cobalamin.**
- In some patients after ileal resection, particularly if the ileocecal valve is incompetent, colonic bacteria may contribute further to the onset of cobalamin deficiency.

Ans. D

8. Most common cause of Intermittent impaction of food is:

A. Zenkers diverticulum B. Steakhouse syndrome

C. Achalasia D. Water brash

Explanation:

- Patients typically present older than 40 years, consistent with an acquired rather than congenital origin.
- Schatzki ring is one of the most common causes of intermittent food impaction, also known as "steakhouse syndrome" because meat is a typical instigator.

Ans. B

9. Mayoclinic HISORT Criteria is used for:

A. Acute pancreatitis B. Chronic pancreatitis

C. Hereditary pancreatitis D. Autoimmune pancreatitis

Explanation:

- **Mayo Clinic HISORt criteria indicate that AIP can be diagnosed by the presence of at least one or more of the following:** (1) Histology; (2) Imaging; (3) Serology (elevated serum IgG4 levels); (4) Other organ involvement; and (5) Response to glucocorticoid Therapy, with improvement in pancreatic and extrapancreatic manifestations.

Ans. D

10. A 42-year-old male presents with memory loss over the last several months. He notes antecedent arthralgia, low-grade fevers, skin hyperpigmentation, & frequent diarrhea. On examination he has mild rigidity in his upper extremities, and concurrent slow pendular movements of the eyes and contraction of the masseter. Which of the following is the most likely diagnosis?

A. Wilson disease
B. Neurosyphilis
C. Whipple disease
D. Early-onset Alzheimer disease

Explanation:

- Whipple disease is caused by an infection with Tropheryma whippelii, leading to low-grade fevers, arthralgia, diarrhea, muscle wasting, and hyperpigmentation.
- Neurological symptoms include extrapyramidal symptoms, limitations of vertical gaze, and characteristic oculomasticatory myorhythmia (pendular oscillations of the eyes with rhythmic contractions of the masticatory muscles).
- Wilson disease is an autosomal-recessive disorder resulting in accumulation of copper resulting in liver disease, movement disorders, and dementia.
- Fever and oculomasticatory myorhythmia are not present in Wilson disease.
- Neurosyphilis causes psychosis agitation, aggression, dementia, multiple cranial neuropathies, and multifocal vasculitic infarcts.
- Early-onset Alzheimer disease presents with dementia but without systemic symptoms or movement disorders. Human immunodeficiency virus dementia could present with many of the systemic symptoms described; however, oculomasticatory myorhythmia would not be present.

Ans. C

11. Disease that has patchy specific small intestinal biopsy is:

A. Celiac disease
B. Crohn's disease
C. Bacterial overgrowth
D. Radiation enteritis

Table: Diseases that can be diagnosed by small-intestinal mucosal biopsies

Lesions	Pathologic Findings
Diffuse, Specific	
Whipple's disease	Lamina propria includes macrophages containing material positive on periodic acid-schiff staining
Agammaglobulinemia	No plasma cells; either normal or absent villi ("flat mucosa")
Abetalipoproteinemia	Normal villi; epithelial cells vacuolated with fat postprandially
Patchy, Specific	
Intestinal lymphoma	Malignant cells in lamina propria and submucosa
Intestinal lymphangiectasia	Dilated lymphatics; clubbed villi
Eosinophilic gastroenteritis	Eosinophil infiltration of lamina propria and mucosa
Amyloidosis	Amyloid deposits
Crohn's disease	Noncaseating granulomas
Infection by one or more microorganisms (see text)	Specific organisms
Mastocytosis	Mast cell infiltration of lamina propria
Diffuse, Nonspecific	
Celiac disease	Short or absent villi; mononuclear infiltrate; epithelial cell damage; hypertrophy of crypts

Contd.

Contd.

Tropical sprue	Similar to celiac disease
Bacterial overgrowth	Patchy damage to villi; lymphocyte infiltration
Folate deficiency	Short villi; decreased mitosis in crypts; megalocytosis
Vitamin B_{12} deficiency	Similar to folate deficiency
Radiation enteritis	Similar to folate deficiency
Zollinger-Ellison syndrome	Mucosal ulceration and erosion from acid
Protein-calorie malnutrition	Villous atrophy; secondary bacterial overgrowth
Drug-induced enteritis	Variable histology

Ans. B

12. Identify the endoscopic image:

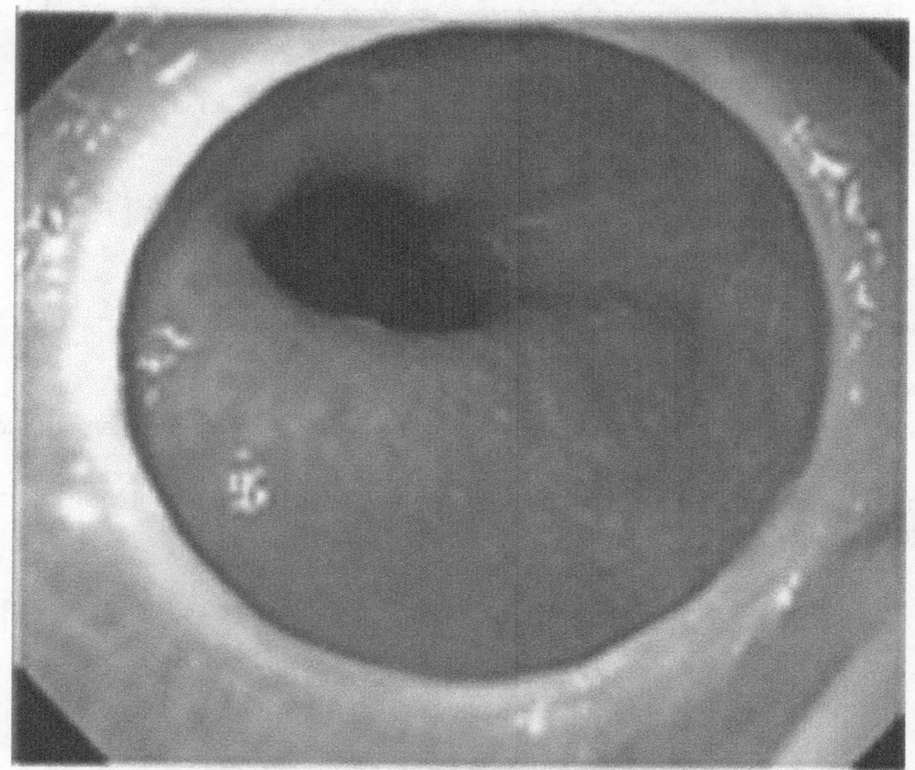

A. Esinophilic esophagitis
B. Cytomegalovirus esophagitis
C. Candida esophagitis
D. Schatzki's ring

Explanation:

- In the image schatzki ring is seen at gastroesophageal junction which can cause episodic dysphagia at beginning meal.
- In cytomegalovirus esophagitis serpigenous ulcers are seen.
- In candida esophagitis white plaque on esophageal mucosa will be seen.
- In eosinophilic esophagitis edema, multiple rings, longitudinally oriented furrows are seen.

Ans. D

13. Identify the image of patient with family history of colon cancer:

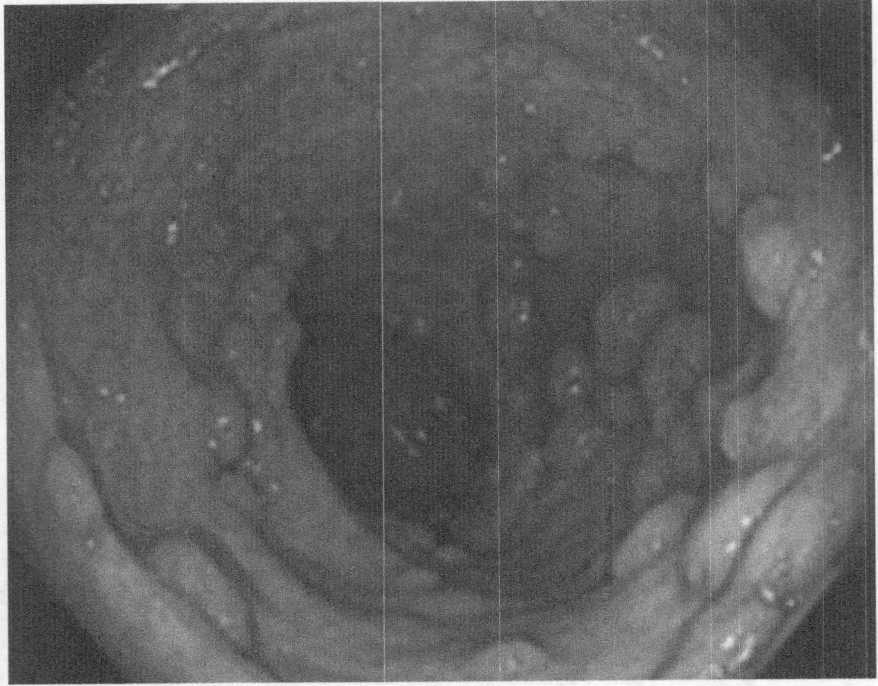

A. Colon polyps

B. Crohn's disease

C. Normal variant

D. Ulcerative colitis

Explanation:

- Colonscopic image of an patient with family history of colon cancer had numerous colon polyps in favour of colon cancer.
- In Crohn's disease there will be most commonly small bowel involvement, transmural involvement and cobblestone appearance.

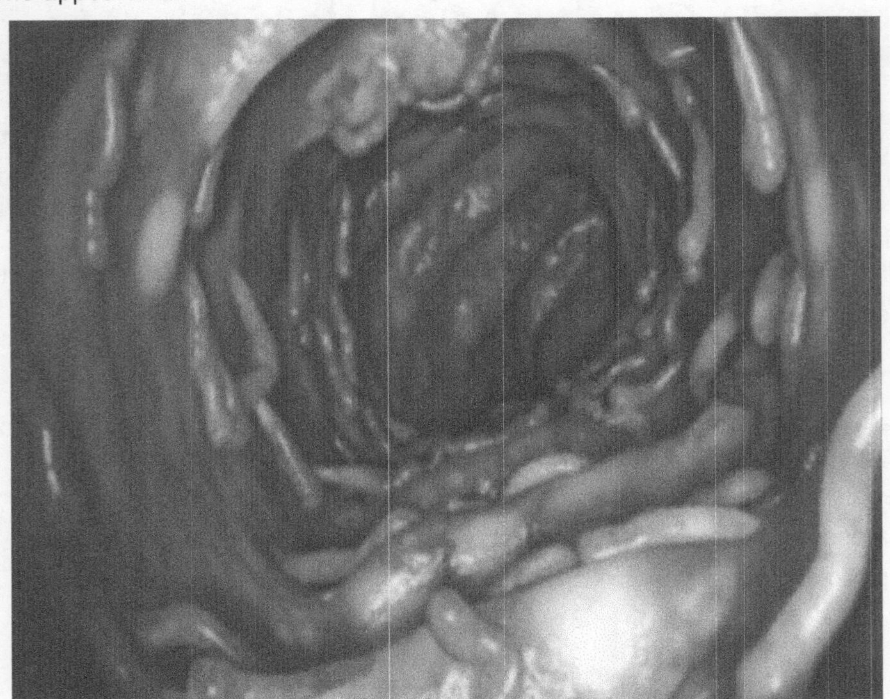

In ulcerative colitis there will be mucosal involvement with ulceration and no cobble stone pattern.

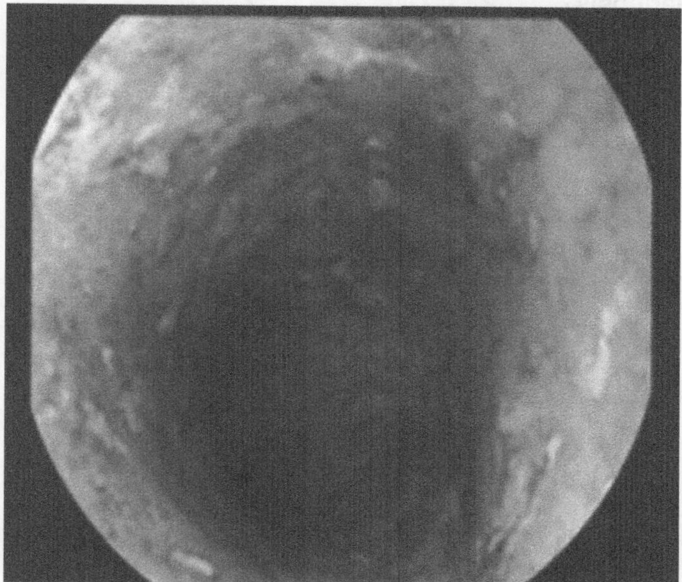

Ans. A

14. Most common cause for Acute hepatitis in Asia:

A. Hepatitis E
B. Hepatitis A
C. Paracetamol induced
D. Autoimmune hepatitis

Explanation:

- HEV is an enterically transmitted virus that causes clinically apparent hepatitis primarily in India, Asia, Africa, and Central America; in those geographic areas, HEV is the most common cause of acute hepatitis; one-third of the global population appears to have been infected.
- This agent, with epidemiologic features resembling those of hepatitis A, is a 27- to 34-nm, non-enveloped, heat-stable, HAV-like virus with a 7200- nucleotide, single-strand, positive sense RNA genome.
- Both IgM anti-HEV during early acute infection and IgG anti-HEV predominating after the first 3 months can be detected.
- Presence of HEV RNA in serum and stool accompanies acute infection; viremia resolves as clinical-biochemical recovery ensues, while HEV RNA in stool may outlast viremia by several weeks.

Ans. A

15. Most common site for gall stone ileus:

A. Third part of duodenum
B. Jejunum
C. Ileum
D. Ileocaecal junction

Explanation:

- Proximal ostomy may be required if unwrapped colon is involved. ***Most common site of intestinal obstruction in patients with gallstone "ileus" is the ileum (60% of patients).***
- Gallstone enters the intestinal tract most often via a cholecystoduodenal fistula.
- It can usually be removed by operative enterolithotomy.
- Addressing gallbladder disease during urgent or emergent surgery is not recommended.

Ans. C

16. Following radiograph of descending taken from the patient with abdominal pain and Difficulty in passing stools. What is the diagnosis?

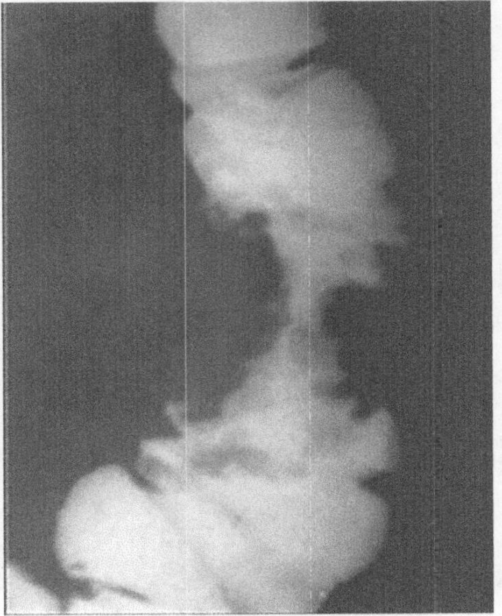

A. Colorectal cancer
B. Diverticulitis
C. Crohn's disease
D. Hirschsprung's disease

Explanation:

- Image shows Annular, constricting adenocarcinoma of descending colon.
- This radiographic appearance is referred to as an "apple-core" lesion and is always highly suggestive of malignancy.
- Because stool becomes more formed as it passes into transverse and descending colon, tumors arising there tend to impede passage of stool, resulting in the development of abdominal cramping, occasional obstruction, and even perforation.
- Radiographs of the abdomen often reveal characteristic annular, constricting lesions ("apple-core" or "napkin-ring").

Ans. A

17. Identify the specimen:

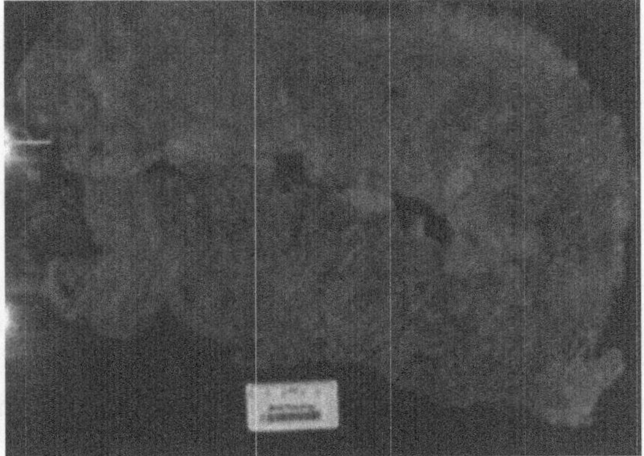

A. Crohn's disease
B. Ulcerative colitis
C. Whipple's disease
D. Normal specimen

Explanation:

- Diffuse (nonsegmental) mucosal disease with broad areas of ulceration. Bowel wall is not thickened and there is no cobble stoning in favour of ulcerative colitis.
- In Crohn's disease thickening of wall, with stenosis, linear serpiginous ulcers and cobblestoning of mucosa.
- Whipple's disease is an bacterial infection most commonly involving small bowel leading to malabsorption.

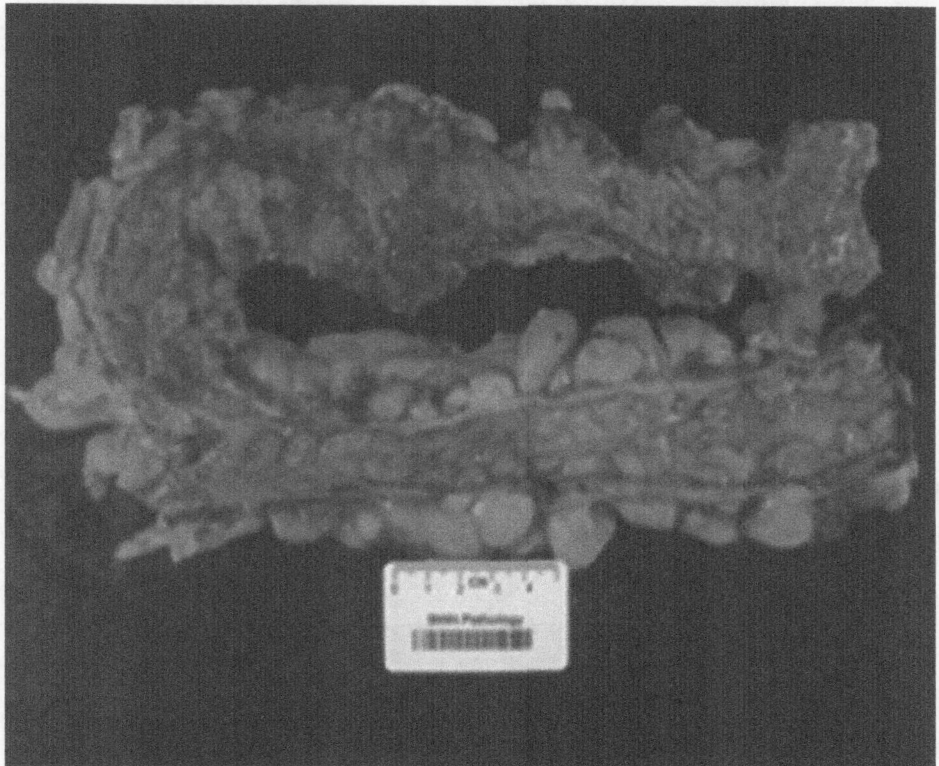

Figure: Crohn's disease of the colon showing thickening of the wall, with stenosis, linear serpiginous ulcer and cobblestoning of the mucosa,

Ans. B

18. Which of the following drug helps in enhancing the response to NSAIDs in case of acute pericarditis and also reduces the risk of recurrent pericarditis?

A. Steroids
B. Azathioprine
C. Colchicine
D. Aspirin

Explanation:

- Colchicine used in the treatment of acute pericarditis enhancers the response to NSAIDs and reduces the chances of recurrent pericarditis. It is given in the dose of 0.5mg OD (< 70 kg) and 0.5 mg BD (> 70 Kg) for 3 months. This acts by concentrating in neutrophils and thereby interferes with migration of neutrophils. Steroids are used when there is no response or failed response to NSAIDs and colchicine. However they increase risk of recurrences, full dose steroids are given only for2-4 days and tapered to low dose. Azathioprine is used in cases of multiple, frequent, and disabling recurrences that continue for more than 2 years and that do not respond to NSAIDs, colchicine or glucocorticoids. Aspirin is used in treatment of acute pericarditis due to its anti-inflammatory activity which helps in reducing pain also.

Ans. C

19. Identify the radiological study:

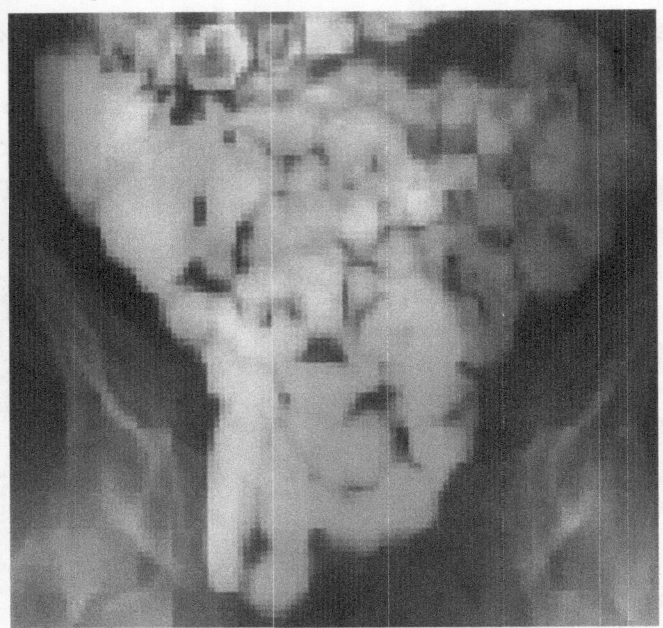

A. Normal study B. Celiac disease

C. Jejunal diverticulosis D. Crohn's disease

Explanation:

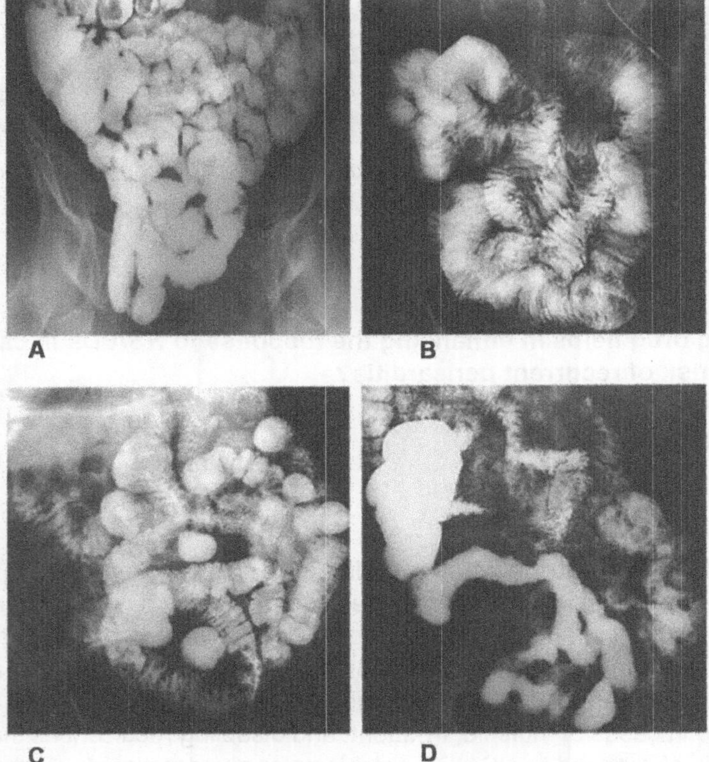

Figure: Barium contrast small-intestinal radiologic examinations. **A.** Normal individual **B.** Celiac disease **C.** Jejunal diverticulosis **D.** Crohn's disease

- In Crohn's disease there will be strictures and fistulas.
- In jejunal diverticulosis there will be filling defects.

Ans. A

20. Identify the image:

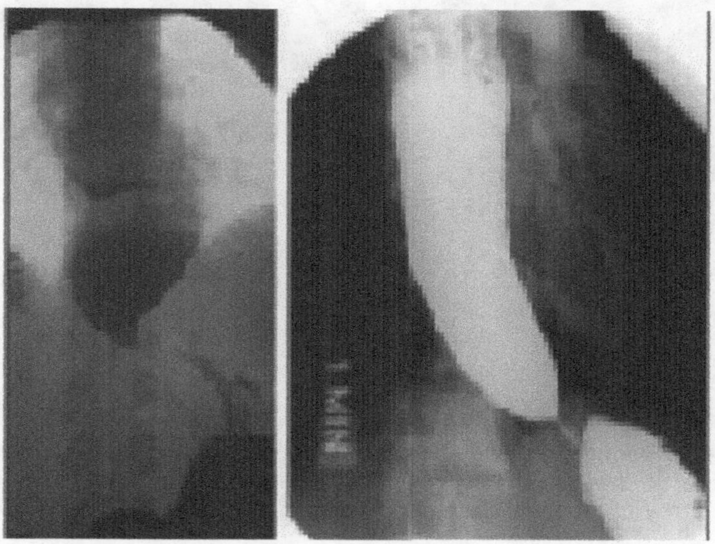

A. Schatzki's ring
B. Achalasia
C. Oesophageal web
D. Diffuse esophageal spasm

Explanation:

- Image shows dilation of esophagus and tappering of gastroesophageal junction and air fluid level within oesophagus.
- Schatzki ring is an indentation shown in lower end of esophagus.

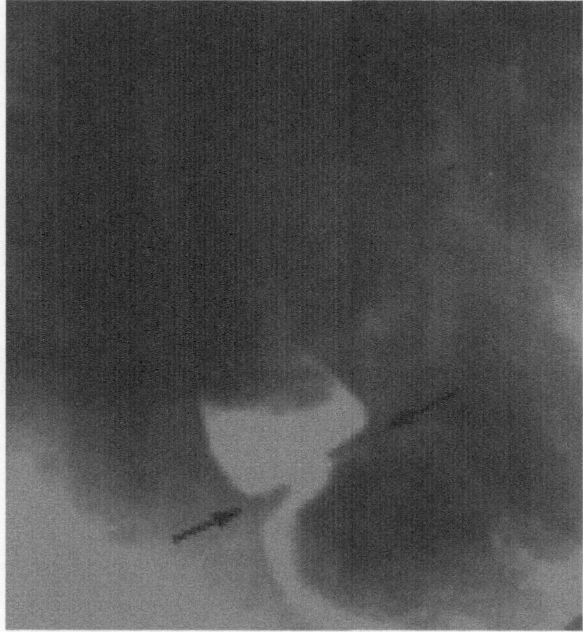

- In diffuse esophageal spasm cork screw appearence of esophagus is seen due to spastic contraction of circular muscle.

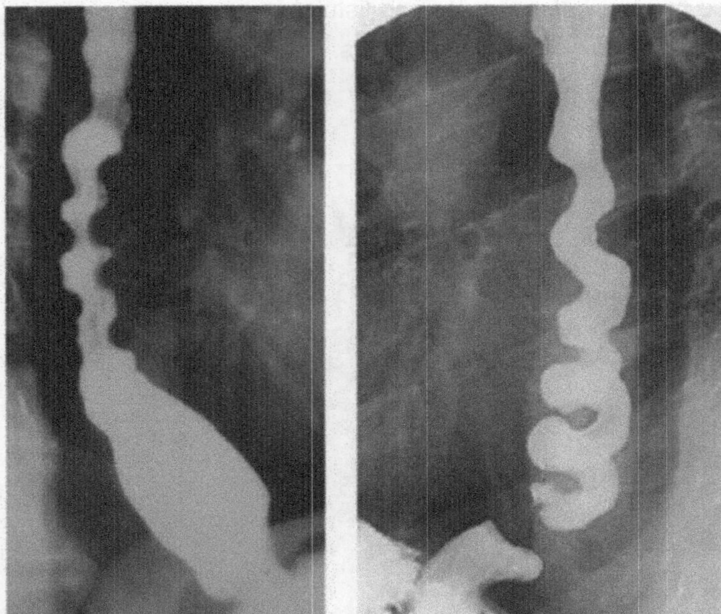

Figure: Diffuse esophageal spasm. The characteristic "corkscrew" esophagus results from spastic contraction of the circular muscle in the esophageal wall; more precisely, this is actually a helical array of muscle. These findings are also seen with spastic achalasia.

Oesophageal web:

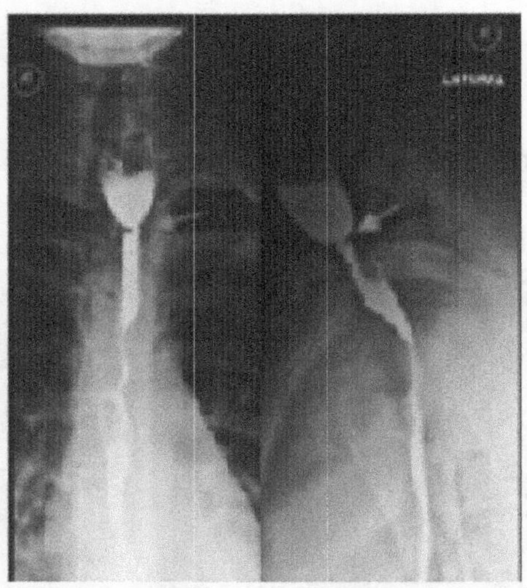

Ans. B

21. About smoking & chronic pancreatitis association, all are true except:

A. Smoking decreased susceptibility to pancreatic autodigestion

B. Predisposes to dysregulation of duct cell CFTR function

C. Smoking is an independent risk factor

D. Dose dependent risk factor for chronic pancreatitis & recurrent acute pancreatitis

Explanation:

- Although alcohol has been believed to be the primary cause of chronic pancreatitis, other factors contribute to the disease because not all heavy consumers of alcohol develop pancreatic disease.

- There is also a strong association between smoking and chronic pancreatitis.
- Cigarette smoke leads to an increased susceptibility to pancreatic autodigestion and predisposes to dysregulation of duct cell CFTR function.
- Smoking is an independent, dose-dependent risk factor for chronic pancreatitis and recurrent acute pancreatitis.
- Both continued alcohol and smoking exposure are associated with pancreatic fibrosis, calcifications, and progression of disease

Ans. A

22. Which gene mutation can most likely cause Inflammatory bowel disease?

A. IL 10 B. IL 13

C. IL 4 D. IL 7

Explanation:

- Multiple mechanisms are involved in induction of oral tolerance and include deletion or anergy of antigen-reactive T cells or induction of CD4+ T cells that suppress gut inflammation (e.g.T-regulatory cells expressing FoxP3 transcription factor) that secrete anti-inflammatory cytokines such as IL-10, IL-35, and transforming growth factor β (TGF-β).
- Oral tolerance may be responsible for the lack of immune responsiveness to dietary antigens and the commensal microbiota in the intestinal lumen.
- In IBD this suppression of inflammation is altered, leading to uncontrolled inflammation.
- Mechanisms of this regulated immune suppression are incompletely known.
- Gene knockout or transgenic (Tg) mouse models of IBD, which include those that are directed at genes demonstrated to be associated with risk for the human disease, have revealed that deleting specific cytokines (e.g.IL-2, IL-10, TGF-β) or their receptors, deleting molecules associated with T-cell antigen recognition (e.g., T-cell antigen receptors), or interfering with IEC barrier function and the regulation of responses to commensal bacteria (e.g., XBP1, mucus glycoproteins, or nuclear factor-κB [NF-κB]) leads to spontaneous colitis or enteritis.

Ans. A

23. All are true about PPI *except:*

A. Duration of inhibition lasts for 72-96 hrs

B. Rebound gastric acid hypersecretion has been described in H.Pylori negative individuals after discontinuation

C. IF Production is also inhibited, so vitamin B12 deficiency anemia is common

D. Long term use of PPI has also been implicated in development of iron, vitamin B12 and magnesium deficiency

Explanation:

- PPI agents are lipophilic compounds; upon entering the parietal cell, they are protonated and trapped within the acid environment of the tubulovesicular and canalicular system.
- These agents potently inhibit all phases of gastric acid secretion.
- Onset of action is rapid, with a maximum acid inhibitory effect between 2 and 6 h after administration and duration of inhibition lasting up to 72–96 h.
- With repeated daily dosing, progressive acid inhibitory effects are observed, with basal and secretagogue-stimulated acid production being inhibited by >95% after 1 week of therapy.
- Half-life of PPIs is ~18 h; thus, it can take between 2 and 5 days for gastric acid secretion to return to normal levels once these drugs have been discontinued.

- Because the pumps need to be activated for these agents to be effective, their efficacy is maximized if they are administered before a meal (except for the immediate-release formulation of omeprazole) (e.g., in morning before breakfast).
- Mild to moderate hypergastrinemia has been observed in patients taking these drugs.
- Carcinoid tumors developed in some animals given the drugs preclinically; however, extensive experience has failed to demonstrate gastric carcinoid tumor development in humans.
- Serum gastrin levels return to normal levels within 1–2 weeks after drug cessation.
- Rebound gastric acid hypersecretion has been described in *H. pylori*–negative individuals after discontinuation of PPIs. It occurs even after relatively short-term usage (2 months) and may last for up to 2 months after the PPI has been discontinued. The mechanism involves gastrin-induced hyperplasia and hypertrophy of histamine-secreting ECL cells.
- Clinical relevance of this observation is that individuals may have worsening symptoms of GERD or dyspepsia upon stopping the PPI.
- Gradual tapering of the PPI and switching to an H2 receptor antagonist may prevent this from occurring.
- *H. pylori*– induced inflammation and concomitant decrease in acid production may explain why this does not occur in *H. pylori*–positive patients.
- If production is also inhibited, but vitamin B12-deficiency anemia is uncommon, probably because of the large stores of vitamin.
- As with any agent that leads to significant hypochlorhydria, PPIs may interfere with absorption of drugs such as ketoconazole, ampicillin, iron, and digoxin. Hepatic cytochrome P450 can be inhibited by earlier PPIs (omeprazole, lansoprazole).
- Rabeprazole, pantoprazole, and esomeprazole do not appear to interact significantly with drugs metabolized by the cytochrome P450 system.
- Overall clinical significance of this observation is not definitely established.
- Caution should be taken when using theophylline, warfarin, diazepam, atazanavir, and phenytoin concomitantly with PPIs.

Ans. C

24. Diseases associated with pernicious anemia include all *except*:

A. Thyroid diseases
B. Vitiligo
C. Hyperparathyroidism
D. Addison disease

Explanation:

- PA may be defined as a severe lack of IF due to gastric atrophy. It is a common disease in northern Europeans but occurs in all countries and ethnic groups. It is more frequent in people of African than Asian ancestry.
- Overall incidence is about 120 per 100,000 population in the United Kingdom (UK).
- Ratio of incidence in men and women among whites is ~1:1.6, and the median age of onset is 70–80 years, with only 10% of patients being <40 years of age.
- However, in some ethnic groups, notably black individuals and Latin Americans, the age at onset of PA is generally lower.
- Disease occurs more commonly than by chance in close relatives and in persons with other organ-specific autoimmune diseases, for example, thyroid diseases, vitiligo, hypoparathyroidism, Type 1 diabetes, and Addison's disease.
- Also associated with hypogammaglobulinemia, with premature graying or blue eyes & persons of blood group A.

- An association with human leukocyte antigen (HLA) 3 has been reported in some but not all series and, in those with endocrine disease, with HLA-B8, -B12, and -BW15.

Ans. C

25. All are true about H. pylori except:

A. Main risk factor for peptic ulceration

B. Risk factor for gastric adenocarcinoma and gastric MALT lymphoma

C. Treatment of H. pylori is the first line therapy for gastric adenocarcinoma

D. Treatment of H. pylori is the first line therapy for Gastric MALT lymphoma

Explanation:

- Treatment of *H. pylori* is of no benefit in the treatment of gastric adenocarcinoma, but prevention of *H. pylori* colonization or eradicative treatment could potentially prevent gastric malignancy and peptic ulceration. In contrast, increasing evidence indicates that lifelong *H. pylori* colonization may offer some protection against complications of gastroesophageal reflux disease (GERD), including esophageal adenocarcinoma. Recent research has focused on whether *H. pylori* colonization is also a risk factor for some extragastric diseases and whether it is protective against some recently emergent medical problems, such as childhood-onset asthma and other allergic and metabolic conditions.

Ans. C

26. All are true about liver except:

A. Basolateral side of the hepatocyte lines space of Disse and is richly lined with microvilli

B. The apical pole of the hepatocyte forms the canalicular membranes through which bile components are secreted

C. Kupffer cells lie within the sinusoidal vascular space and represent largest group of fixed macrophages in body

D. Stellate cells are located in space of Disse and produce collagen and matrix continuously

Explanation:

- Sinusoids are lined by unique endothelial cells that have prominent fenestrae of variable sizes, allowing the free flow of plasma but not of cellular elements. The plasma is thus in direct contact with hepatocytes in the subendothelial space of Disse. Hepatocytes have distinct polarity. The basolateral side of the hepatocyte lines the space of Disse and is richly lined with microvilli; it exhibits endocytotic and pinocytotic activity, with passive and active uptake of nutrients, proteins, and other molecules. The apical pole of the hepatocyte forms the canalicular membranes through which bile components are secreted. The canaliculi of hepatocytes form a fine network, which fuses into the bile ductular elements near the portal areas. Kupffer cells usually lie within the sinusoidal vascular space and represent the largest group of fixed macrophages in the body. The stellate cells are located in the space of Disse but are not usually prominent unless activated, when they produce collagen and matrix. Red blood cells stay in the sinusoidal space as blood flows through the lobules, but white blood cells can migrate through or around endothelial cells into the space of Disse and from there to portal areas, where they can return to the circulation through lymphatics.

Ans. D

27. All are true about HAV except:

A. HAV is a nonenveloped 27-nm, heat-, acid-, and ether-resistant RNA virus in the Hepatovirus genus of the picornavirus family

B. Hepatitis A has an incubation period of ~4 weeks

C. There is longer persistence of virus in the liver, fecal shedding, viremia, and infectivity begins once jaundice becomes apparent

D. The diagnosis of hepatitis A is made during acute illness by demonstrating anti-HAV of the IgM class

Explanation:

- HAV is a nonenveloped 27-nm, heat-, acid-, and ether-resistant RNA virus in the *Hepatovirus* genus of the picornavirus family. Its virion contains four capsid polypeptides, designated VP1–VP4, which are cleaved post-translationally from polyprotein product of a 7500-nucleotide genome. Inactivation of viral activity can be achieved by boiling for 1 min, by contact with formaldehyde and chlorine, or by ultraviolet irradiation. Despite nucleotide sequence variation of up to 20% among isolates of HAV, and despite the recognition of four genotypes affecting humans, all strains of this virus are immunologically indistinguishable and belong to one serotype.
- Human HAV can infect and cause hepatitis in chimpanzees, tamarins (marmosets), and several monkey species. Recently, a hepatotropic *Hepatovirus* related to, and likely to have shared common evolutionary ancestry with, human HAV has been identified in several species of harbor seals, albeit without histologic evidence for liver injury or inflammation. Hepatitis A has an incubation period of ~4 weeks. Its replication is limited to liver, but the virus is present in the liver, bile, stools, and blood during late incubation period and acute preicteric/presymptomatic phase of illness. Despite slightly longer persistence of virus in the liver, fecal shedding, viremia, and infectivity diminish rapidly once jaundice becomes apparent. HAV can be cultivated reproducibly in vitro.
- Antibodies to HAV (anti-HAV) can be detected during acute illness when serum aminotransferase activity is elevated and fecal HAV shedding is still occurring. This early antibody response is predominantly of the IgM class and persists for several (~3) months, rarely for 6–12 months. During convalescence, however, anti-HAV of the IgG class becomes the predominant antibody.
- Therefore, diagnosis of hepatitis A is made during acute illness by demonstrating anti-HAV of the IgM class. After acute illness, anti-HAV of the IgG class remains detectable indefinitely, and patients with serum anti-HAV are immune to reinfection. Neutralizing antibody activity parallels appearance of anti-HAV, and the IgG anti-HAV present in immune globulin accounts for the protection it affords against HAV infection.

Ans. C

28. All below are some NOTES procedures except:

A. Percutaneous endoscopic gastrostomy (PEG) for pancreatic necrosis

B. EUS for staging and biopsy of tumor

C. Peroral endoscopic myotomy (POEM) for achalasia

D. Endoscopic full-thickness resection (EFTR) of gastrointestinal mural lesions

Explanation:

- NOTES is an evolving collection of endoscopic methods that entail passage of an endoscope or its accessories into or through the wall of the gastrointestinal tract to perform diagnostic or therapeutic interventions.
- Some NOTES procedures, such as percutaneous endoscopic gastrostomy (PEG) or endoscopic necrosectom, pancreatic necrosis, are well-established clinical procedures, others such as peroral endoscopic myotomy (POEM) for achalasia, peroral endoscopic tumorectomy (POET) and endoscopic full-thickness resection (EFTR) of gastrointestinal mural lesions are emerging as minimally invasive therapeutic options.
- NOTES is an area of continuing innovation and endoscopic research

Ans. B

29. Least common peptic ulcer related complication is:

A. Gastric outlet obstruction
B. Perforation
C. GI bleeding
D. Gastric atrophy

Explanation:

- Gastric outlet obstruction is the least common ulcer-related complication, occurring in 1–2% of patients.
- A patient may have relative obstruction secondary to ulcer-related inflammation and edema in the peripyloric region.
- This process often resolves with ulcer healing. A fixed, mechanical obstruction secondary to scar formation in the peripyloric areas is also possible.
- Latter requires endoscopic (balloon dilation) or surgical intervention. Signs and symptoms relative to mechanical obstruction may develop insidiously.
- New onset of early satiety, nausea, vomiting, increase of postprandial abdominal pain, and weight loss should make gastric outlet obstruction a possible diagnosis.

Ans. A

30. All are true about diagnosis of GI disease except:

A. Measurement of breath hydrogen while fasting and after oral mono- or oligosaccharide challenge can assesses for persistent Helicobacter pylori infection
B. Deep rectal biopsies facilitate diagnosis of Hirschsprung's disease or amyloid
C. Esophageal manometry is useful for suspected achalasia
D. Gastric emptying breath test is an alternative to scintigraphy for gastroparesis diagnosis

Explanation:

- Tests of gut function provide important data when structural testing is nondiagnostic.
- Functional testing of motor activity is provided by newer high resolution manometric techniques.
- Esophageal manometry is useful for suspected achalasia, whereas small-intestinal manometry tests for pseudo-obstruction and colon manometry evaluates for colonic inertia.
- A wireless motility capsule measures transit and contractile activity in the stomach, small intestine, and colon in a single test. Anorectal manometry with balloon expulsion testing is used for unexplained incontinence or constipation from outlet dysfunction.
- Biliary manometry tests for sphincter of Oddi dysfunction with unexplained biliary pain. A novel endoluminal functional lumen imaging probe is available to measure heightened distensibility in the lower esophageal sphincter in achalasia and pylorus in gastroparesis.
- Measurement of breath hydrogen while fasting and after oral mono- or oligosaccharide challenge can screen for carbohydrate intolerance and small-intestinal bacterial overgrowth. Urea breath testing assesses for persistent *Helicobacter pylori* infection, while a recently approved gastric emptying breath test is an alternative to scintigraphy for gastroparesis diagnosis.

Ans. A

31. Diffuse specific lesions on small intestinal mucosal biopsy seen in all except:

A. Celiac disease
B. Whipple's disease
C. Agammaglobulinemia
D. Abetalipoproteinemia

Explanation:

Table: Diseases that can be diagnosed by small-intestinal mucosal biopsies	
Lesions	**Pathologic Findings**
Diffuse, Specific	
Whipple's disease	Lamina propria includes macrophages containing material positive on periodic acid-schiff staining
Agammaglobulinemia	No plasma cells; either normal or absent villi ("flat mucosa")
Abetalipoproteinemia	Normal villi; epithelial cells vacuolated with fat postprandially
Patchy, Specific	
Intestinal lymphoma	Malignant cells in lamina propria and submucosa
Intestinal lymphangiectasia	Dilated lymphatics; clubbed villi
Eosinophillic gastroenteritis	Eosinophill infiltration of lamina propria and mucosa
Amyloidosis	Amyloid deposits
Crohn's disease	Noncaseating granulomas
Infection by one or more microorganisms (see text)	Specific organisms
Mastocytosis	Mast cell infiltration of lamina propria
Diffuse, Nonspecific	
Celiac disease	Short or absent villi; mononuclear infiltrate; epithelial cell damage; hypertrophy of crypts
Tropical sprue	Similar to celiac disease
Bacterial overgrowth	Patchy damage to villi; lymphocyte infiltration
Folate deficiency	Short villi; decreased mitosis in crypts; megalocytosis
Vitamin B_{12} deficiency	Similar to folate deficiency
Radiation enteritis	Similar to folate deficiency
Zollinger-Ellison syndrome	Mucosal ulceration and erosion from acid
Protein-calorie malnutrition	Villous atrophy; secondary bacterial overgrowth
Drug-induced enteritis	Variable histology

Ans. A

32. **All are true about peritoneal inflammation except:**
   A. Patient with peritonitis characteristically lies quietly in bed
   B. Characteristic feature of peritoneal irritation is tonic reflex spasm of the abdominal musculature
   C. Spasm over a perforated retrocecal appendix is always severe
   D. A slowly developing process also often greatly attenuates the degree of muscle spasm

Explanation:

- *Pain of peritoneal inflammation is invariably accentuated by pressure or changes in tension of the peritoneum,* whether produced by palpation or by movement such as with coughing or sneezing.
- Patient with peritonitis characteristically lies quietly in bed, preferring to avoid motion, in contrast to the patient with colic, who may be thrashing in discomfort.
- Another characteristic feature of peritoneal irritation is tonic reflex spasm of the abdominal musculature, localized to the involved body segment.
- Its intensity depends on the integrity of nervous system, location of inflammatory process, & rate at which it develops.
- Spasm over a perforated retrocecal appendix or perforation into the lesser peritoneal sac may be minimal or absent because of the protective effect of overlying viscera.

- Catastrophic abdominal emergencies may be associated with minimal or no detectable pain or muscle spasm in obtunded, seriously ill, debilitated, immunosuppressed, or psychotic patients.
- Slowly developing process also often greatly attenuates degree of muscle spasm.

Ans. C

33. All are features of severe ulcerative colitis except:

A. Endoscopy showing spontaneous bleeding/ulcerations

B. ESR of more than 20

C. Bowel movements more than 6/day

D. Less than 75% of hemoglobin

Explanation:

- Active disease can be associated with a rise in acute-phase reactants (C-reactive protein [CRP]), platelet count, and erythrocyte sedimentation rate (ESR), and a decrease in hemoglobin.
- Fecal lactoferrin, a glycoprotein present in activated neutrophils, is a highly sensitive and specific marker for detecting intestinal inflammation.
- Fecal calprotectin is present in neutrophils and monocytes and levels correlate well with histologic inflammation, predict relapses, and detect pouchitis.
- Both fecal lactoferrin and calprotectin are becoming an integral part of IBD management and are used frequently to rule out active inflammation versus symptoms of irritable bowel or bacterial overgrowth.
- In severely ill patients, the serum albumin level will fall rather quickly.
- Leukocytosis may be present but is not a specific indicator of disease activity.
- Proctitis or proctosigmoiditis rarely causes a rise in CRP.
- Diagnosis relies on the patient's history; clinical symptoms; negative stool examination for bacteria, *C. difficile* toxin, and ova and parasites; sigmoidoscopic appearance and histology of rectal or colonic biopsy specimens.
- Sigmoidoscopy is used to assess disease activity and is usually performed before treatment.
- If the patient is not having an acute flare, colonoscopy is used to assess disease extent and activity.
- Endoscopically mild disease is characterized by erythema, decreased vascular pattern, and mild friability. Moderate disease is characterized by marked erythema, absent vascular pattern, friability and erosions, and severe disease by spontaneous bleeding and ulcerations.
- Histologic features change more slowly than clinical features but can also be used to grade disease activity.

Ans. B

34. Most common source of liver abscess is:

A. Ruptured appendicitis

B. Pylephlebitis

C. Disease of the biliary tract

D. Pancreatitis

Explanation:

- Liver is the organ most subject to the development of abscesses.
- In one study of 540 intra abdominal abscesses, 26% were visceral. Liver abscesses made up 13% of the total number, or 48% of all visceral abscesses.
- Liver abscesses may be solitary or multiple; they may arise from hematogenous spread of bacteria or from local spread from contiguous sites of infection within the peritoneal cavity.
- In past, appendicitis with rupture and subsequent spread of infection was the most common source for a liver abscess.

- **Currently, associated disease of the biliary tract is most common.**

Ans. C

35. All are true about esophagitis except:

A. Odynophagia is very common with reflux esophagitis

B. The characteristic endoscopic findings in herpes simplex esophagitis are vesicles and small, punched-out ulcerations

C. CMV lesions appear as serpiginous ulcers in an otherwise normal mucosa, particularly in the distal esophagus

D. Biopsies from the ulcer bases have the greatest diagnostic yield for finding the pathognomonic large nuclear or cytoplasmic inclusion bodies in CMV esophagitis

Explanation:

- Regardless of the infectious agent, odynophagia is a characteristic symptom of infectious esophagitis; dysphagia, chest pain, and hemorrhage are also common. Odynophagia is uncommon with reflux esophagitis, so its presence should always raise suspicion of an alternative etiology.

Ans. A

36. Possible Drugs for a Dominant Symptom in IBS include all except:

A. IBS D can be treated by Alosetran

B. IBS C can be treated by linaclotide alone

C. IBS with predominant gas and bloating can be treated with high FODMAP diet

D. Abdominal pain can be treated with SSRI

Explanation:

- Linaclotide is a minimally absorbed 14-amino-acid peptide guanylate cyclase-C (GC-C) agonist that binds to and activates GC-C on the luminal surface of intestinal epithelium.
- Activation of GC-C results in generation of cyclic guanosine monophosphate (cGMP), which triggers secretion of fluid, sodium, and bicarbonate.
- In animal models, linaclotide accelerates GI transit and reduces visceral nociception.
- Analgesic action of linaclotide appears to be mediated by cGMP acting on afferent pain fibers innervating the GI tract.
- Treatment usually involves education, reassurance, and dietary/ lifestyle changes.
- Smaller portion have moderate symptoms that are usually intermittent and correlate with altered gut physiology, e.g., worsened with eating or stress and relieved by defecation.
- For IBS-D patients, treatments include gut-acting pharmacologic agents such as antispasmodics, antidiarrheals, bile acid binders, and the newer gut serotonin modulators
- **In IBS-C patients, increased fiber intake and the use of osmotic agents such as polyethylene glycol may achieve satisfactory results.**
- For patients with more severe constipation, a chloride channel opener (lubiprostone) or GC-C agonist (linaclotide) may be considered.
- For IBS patients with predominant gas and bloating, a low-FODMAP diet may provide significant relief. Some patients may benefit from probiotics and rifaximin treatment.
- A small proportion of IBS patients have severe and refractory symptoms, are usually seen in referral centers, and frequently have constant pain and psychosocial difficulties.
- This group of patients is best managed with antidepressants and other psychological treatments.

Ans. B

37. Overexpression of all these proteins cause IBD except:

A. IL-7
B. IL-10
C. STAT-3
D. STAT-4

Explanation:

Table: Immune system molecule defects in animals or human that cause autoimmune or malignant syndromes

Protein	Defect	Disease or Syndrome	Observation in Animal Models or Humans
Cytokines and Signaling Proteins			
Tumor necrosis factor (TNF) α	Overexpression	Inflammatory bowel disease (IBD), arthritis, vasculitis	Mice
TNF-α	Underexpression	Systemic lupus erythematosus (SLE)	Mice
Interleukin (IL)-1-receptor antagonist	Underexpression	Arthritis	Mice
IL-2	Overexpression	IBD	Mice
IL-7	Overexpression	IBD	Mice
IL-10	Overexpression	IBD	Mice
IL-2 receptor	Overexpression	IBD	Mice
IL-10 receptor	Overexpression	IBD	Mice
IL-3	Overexpression	Demyelinating syndrome	Mice
Interferon-δ	Overexpression in skin	SLE	Mice
STAT-3	Underexpression	IBD	Mice
STAT-4	Overexpression	IBD	Mice
Transforming growth factor (TGF)β	Underexpression	Systemic wasting syndrome and IBD	Mice
TGF-β receptor in T cells	Underexpression	SLE	Mice
Programmed death (CD279, PD-1)	Underexpression	SLE-like syndrome	Mice
Cytotoxic T lymphocyte, antigen-4 (CTLA-4)	Underexpression	Systemic lymphoproliferative disease	Mice
IL-10	Underexpression	IBD (mouse), type 1 diabetes, thyroid disease, primary (human)	Mice and humans
Major Histocompatibility Locus Molecules[a]			
HLA-B27	Allele expression or overexpression	Inflammatory bowel disease	Rats and humans
Complement deficiency of C1, 2, 3 or 4	Underexpression		Humans
LIGHT (TNF superfamily 14)	Overexpression	Systemic lymphoproliferative (mouse) and autoimmunity	Mice

Contd.

Contd.

HLA class II DQB10301, DQB10302	Allele expression	Juvenile-onset diabetes	Humans
HLA class II DQB10401, DQB10402	Allele expression	Rheumatoid arthritis	Human
HLA class I B27	Allele expression	Ankylosing spondylitis, IBD	Rats and humans
Apoptosis Proteins			
TNF receptor 1 (TNF-R1)	Underexpression	Familial periodic fever syndrome	Humans
Fas (CD95; Apo-1)	Underexpression	Autoimmune lymphoproliferative syndrome type 1 (ALPS 1); malignant lymphoma; bladder cancer	Humans
Fas ligand	Underexpression	SLE (only one case identified)	Humans
Perforin	Underexpression	Familial hemophagocytic lymphohistiocytosis (FHL)	Humans
Caspase 10	Underexpression	Autoimmune lymphoproliferative syndrome type II (ALPS II)	Humans
Bcl-10	Underexpression	Non-Hodgkin's lymphoma	Humans
P53	Underexpression	Various malignant neoplasms	Humans
Bax	Underexpression	Colon cancer; hematopoietic malignancies	Humans
Bcl-2	Underexpression	Non-Hodgkin's lymphoma	Humans
c-IAP2	Underexpression	Low-grade MALT lymphoma	Humans
NAIP 1	Underexpression	Spinal muscular atrophy	Humans

Ans. C

38. Symptoms and findings suggesting small bowel disease include all except:

A. Large-volume watery stools
B. Substantial weight loss
C. Malabsorption of iron, calcium, or fat
D. Leukocytes in stool

Explanation:

- Patients with symptoms and findings suggesting small bowel disease, such as large-volume watery stools, substantial weight loss, and malabsorption of iron, calcium, or fat, may undergo upper endoscopy with duodenal aspirates for assessment of bacterial overgrowth and biopsies for assessment of mucosal diseases, such as celiac sprue.

Ans. D

39. Regarding Ulcerative colitis all are true except:

A. Age of onset is second to fourth decade
B. More common in Jewish
C. Smoking and appendectomy increases risk
D. No increased risk with oral contraceptives

Explanation:

- In Caucasian populations, smoking is an important risk factor in IBD with opposite effects on UC (odds ratio [OR] 0.58) and CD (OR 1.76), whereas in other ethnic groups with different genetic susceptibility, smoking may play a lesser role.
- There is a protective effect of previous appendectomy with confirmed appendicitis (risk reduction of 13–26%), particularly at a young age, on the development of UC across different geographical regions and populations. There is a modest association with the development of CD but this may be due to diagnostic bias.
- Oral contraceptive use is associated with the risk of CD with a reported hazard ratio as high as 2.82 among current users and 1.39 among past users.
- Association between oral contraceptive use and UC is limited to women with a history of smoking. There is an association between antibiotic use and the development of childhood IBD with children who received one or more dispensations of antibiotics during first year of life having a 2.9-fold increase in the risk of developing IBD during childhood.
- Breastfeeding may also protect against the development of IBD. Infectious gastroenteritis with pathogens (e.g., *Salmonella*, *Shigella*, *Campylobacter* spp., *Clostridium difficile*) increases IBD risk by two- to threefold. Diets high in animal protein, sugars, sweets, oils, fish and shellfish, and dietary fat, especially ω-6 fatty acids, and low in ω-3 fatty acids have been implicated in increasing the risk of IBD.
- Protective effect of vitamin D on the risk of CD has been reported.

Ans. C

40. Rectal sparing of pseudomembranous of PMC is seen in:

A. 10%
B. 20%
C. 30%
D. 40%

Explanation:

- Pseudomembranous of PMC are confined to the colonic mucosa and initially appear as 1- to 2-mm whitish-yellow plaques.
- Intervening mucosa appears unremarkable, but, as disease progresses, pseudomembranous coalesce to form larger plaques and become confluent over entire colon wall
- **Whole colon is usually involved, but 10% of patients have rectal sparing.**
- Viewed microscopically, the pseudomembranes have a mucosal attachment point and contain necrotic leukocytes, fibrin, mucus, and cellular debris.
- Epithelium is eroded and necrotic in focal areas, with neutrophil infiltration of the mucosa.

Ans. A

41. All are correct about ulcerations of esophagus as seen by endoscopy except:

A. Peptic esophagitis are usually solitary and distal
B. Malignant ulcerations are punctate and diffuse
C. EoE characteristically exhibits multiple esophageal rings, linear furrows, white punctate exudate, and strictures
D. Esophageal ulcerations from pill esophagitis are usually singular and deep at points of luminal narrowing, especially near the carina, with sparing of the distal esophagus

Explanation:

- In terms of endoscopic appearance, the ulcerations seen in peptic esophagitis are usually solitary and distal, whereas infectious ulcerations are punctate and diffuse.
- EoE characteristically exhibits multiple esophageal rings, linear furrows, white punctate exudate, and strictures.

- Esophageal ulcerations from pill esophagitis are usually singular and deep at points of luminal narrowing, especially near the carina, with sparing of the distal esophagus.

Ans. B

42. All are true about extra intestinal manifestations of IBD except:

A. Uveitis is associated with both UC and Crohn's colitis, may be found during periods of remission, and may develop in patients following bowel resection

B. ~5% of patients with UC have PSC, but 50–75% of patients with PSC have IBD

C. PSC occurs less often in patients with CD

D. Patients with IBD have an increased risk of both venous and arterial thrombosis only if the disease is active

Explanation:

- Patients with IBD have an increased risk of both venous and arterial thrombosis even if the disease is not active.
- Factors responsible for the hypercoagulable state have included abnormalities of platelet-endothelial interaction, hyperhomocysteinemia, alterations in coagulation cascade, impaired fibrinolysis, involvement of tissue factor-bearing microvesicles, disruption of the normal coagulation system by autoantibodies, and a genetic predisposition.
- A spectrum of vasculitides involving small, medium, and large vessels has also been observed.

Ans. D

43. All are true about HCV except:

A. HCV is the only member of the genus Hepacivirus in the family Flaviviridae

B. The replication rate of HCV is very high, 1012 virions per day; its half-life is 2.7 h

C. Genotypes differ from one another in sequence homology by ≥10%, and subtypes differ by ~20%

D. Most sensitive indicator of HCV infection is presence of HCV RNA

Explanation:

- Hepatitis C virus, which, before its identification was labeled "non-A, non-B hepatitis," is a linear, single-strand, positive-sense, 9600-nucleotide RNA virus, the genome of which is similar in organization to that of flaviviruses and pestiviruses;
- HCV is the only member of the genus Hepacivirus in the family Flaviviridae.
- HCV genome contains a single, large open reading frame (ORF) (gene) that codes for a virus polyprotein of ~3000 amino acids, which is cleaved after translation to yield 10 viral proteins.
- 5′ end of genome consists of an untranslated region (containing an internal ribosomal entry site [IRES]) adjacent to the genes for three structural proteins, the nucleocapsid core protein, C, and two envelope glycoproteins, E1 and E2.
- 5′ untranslated region and core gene are highly conserved among genotypes, but the envelope proteins are coded for by the hypervariable region, which varies from isolate to isolate and may allow the virus to evade host immunologic containment directed at accessible virus-envelope proteins.
- *3′ end of genome also includes an untranslated region and contains the genes for seven nonstructural (NS) proteins:* p7, NS2, NS3, NS4A, NS4B, NS5A, and NS5B. p7 is a membrane ion channel protein necessary for efficient assembly and release of HCV.
- NS2 cysteine protease cleaves NS3 from NS2, and the NS3-4A serine protease cleaves all downstream proteins from the polyprotein.

- Important NS proteins involved in virus replication include NS3 helicase; NS3-4A serine protease; multifunctional membrane-associated phosphoprotein NS5A, an essential component of the viral replication membranous web (along with NS4B); and the NS5B RNA-dependent RNA polymerase.

Ans. C

44. Complications of Eosinophilic esophagitis include all except:

A. Esophageal stricture

B. Narrow caliber esophagus

C. Esophageal perforation

D. Esophageal adenocarcinoma

Explanation:

- Complications of EoE include esophageal stricture, narrow-caliber esophagus, food impaction, and esophageal perforation.

Ans. D

45. All the statements are true except:

A. Turner's syndrome associated with eosinophilic colitis

B. Hermansky pudlak syndrome associated with Granulomatous colitis

C. Wiskott Aldrich syndrome associated with thrombocytopenia

D. Glycogen storage disease associated with neutropenia

Explanation:

Table: Primary genetic disorders associated with ibd

Name	Genetic Association	Phenotype
Turner's syndrome	Loss of part of all of X chromosome	Associated with UC and colonic CD
Hermansky-Pudlak	Autosomal recessive chromosome 10q23	Granulomatous colitis, oculocutaneous albinism, platelet dysfunction, pulmonary fibrosis
Wiskott-Aldrich syndrome (WAS)	X-linked recessive disorder, loss of WAS protein function	Colitis, immunodeficiency, severely dysfunctional platelets, and thrombocytopenia
Glycogen storage disease	Deficiency of the glucose-6-phosphate transport protein type B1	Granulomatous colitis, presents in infancy with hypoglycemia, growth failure, hepatomegaly and neutropenia
Immune dysregulation polyendocrinopathy, enteropathy X-linked (IPEX)	Loss of FoxP3 transcription factor and T regulatory cell function	UC-like autoimmune enteropathy, with endocrinopathy (neonatal type 1 diabetes or thyroiditis), dermatitis
Early-onset IBD	Deficient IL-10 and IL-10 receptor function	Severe, refractory IBD in early life

Ans. A

46. Fibrosing cholestatic hepatitis is due to choking of the cell with overwhelming quantities of:

A. HBsAg B. HBeAg

C. HDV D. HBcAg

Explanation:

- Precore genetic mutants of HBV have been associated with the more severe outcomes of HBV infection (severe chronic and fulminant hepatitis), suggesting that, under certain circumstances, relative pathogenicity is a property of the virus, not the host.
- Facts that concomitant HDV and HBV infections are associated with more severe liver injury than HBV infection alone and that cells transfected in vitro with the gene for HDV antigen express HDV antigen and then become necrotic in the absence of any immunologic influences are also consistent with a viral effect on pathogenicity.
- Similarly, in patients who undergo liver transplantation for end-stage chronic hepatitis B, occasionally, rapidly progressive liver injury appears in the new liver.
- This clinical pattern is associated with an unusual histologic pattern in the new liver, *fibrosing cholestatic hepatitis*, which, ultrastructurally, appears to represent a choking of the cell with overwhelming quantities of HBsAg.

Ans. A

47. Causes of cirrhosis include all except:

A. Hepatitis B B. Hepatitis C

C. Hepatitis D D. Alcohol

Explanation:

Table: Causes of cirrhosis	
Alcoholism Chronic viral hepatitis • Hepatitis B • Hepatitis C Autoimmune hepatitis Nonalcoholic steatohepatitis Biliary cirrhosis • Primary biliary cholangitis • Primary sclerosing cholangitis • Autoimmune cholangiopathy	Cardiac cirrhosis Inherited metabolic liver disease • Hemochromatosis • Wilson's disease • α_1 Antitrypsin deficiency • Cystic fibrosis Cryptogenic cirrhosis

Ans. C

48. Regarding Pernicious anemia all are true except:

A. Lack of IF/HCl/Pepsin B. M W – 1:1.6

C. Serum gastrin level is low D. CD4 directed against gastric H/K –ATPase

Explanation:

- PA may be defined as a severe lack of IF due to gastric atrophy. It is a common disease in northern Europeans but occurs in all countries and ethnic groups.
- It is more frequent in people of African than Asian ancestry

- Overall incidence is about 120 per 100,000 population in the United Kingdom.
- Ratio of incidence in men and women among whites is ~1:1.6, and median age of onset is 70–80 years, with only 10% of patients being <40 years of age.
- However, in some ethnic groups, notably black individuals and Latin Americans, the age at onset of PA is generally lower.
- Disease occurs more commonly than by chance in close relatives and in persons with other organ-specific autoimmune diseases, for example, thyroid diseases, vitiligo, hypoparathyroidism, Type 1 diabetes, and Addison's disease.
- It is also associated with hypogammaglobinemia, with premature graying or blue eyes, and persons of blood group A.
- An association with human leukocyte antigen (HLA) 3 has been reported in some but not all series and, in those with endocrine disease, with HLA-B8, -B12 and -BW15.

Ans. C

49. Fulminant hepatitis is common in all except:

A. HBV B. HCV

C. HDV D. HEV

Explanation:

- Most feared complication of viral hepatitis is fulminant hepatitis (massive hepatic necrosis); fortunately, this is a rare event.
- Fulminant hepatitis is seen primarily in hepatitis B, D, and E, but rare fulminant cases of hepatitis A occur primarily in older adults and in persons with underlying chronic liver disease, including, according to some reports, chronic hepatitis B and C.
- Hepatitis B accounts for >50% of fulminant cases of viral hepatitis, a sizable proportion of which are associated with HDV infection and another proportion with underlying chronic hepatitis C.
- Fulminant hepatitis is hardly ever seen in hepatitis C, but hepatitis E, as noted above, can be complicated by fatal fulminant hepatitis in 1–2% of all cases and in up to 20% of cases in pregnant women.

Ans. B

50. Hepatic steatosis and insulin resistance appear to be associated with:

A. HBV B. HCV

C. HDV D. HEV

Explanation:

- Attention has been drawn as well to associations between hepatitis C and such cutaneous disorders as porphyria cutanea tarda and lichen planus. A mechanism for these associations is unknown.
- Finally, related to the reliance of HCV on lipoprotein secretion and assembly pathways and on interactions of HCV with glucose metabolism, HCV infection may be complicated by hepatic steatosis, hypercholesterolemia, insulin resistance (and other manifestations of the metabolic syndrome), and type 2 diabetes mellitus; both hepatic steatosis and insulin resistance appear to accelerate hepatic fibrosis and blunt responsiveness to interferon-based antiviral therapy.

Ans. B

51. Confocal laser endomicroscopy and optical coherence tomography is used for:

A. Colon metaplasia and cancer surveillance

B. Barrett's esophagus and gastric cancer surveillance

C. Evaluation of colitis and IBD

D. Evaluation of small intestinal pathology like celiac disease

Explanation:

- Methods employed include narrow band imaging and chromoendoscopy in colitis and confocal laser endomicroscopy and optical coherence tomography in Barrett's esophagus and gastric cancer surveillance.

Ans. B

52. All support Rotor syndrome except:

A. Accumulation in the lysosomes of centrilobular hepatocytes of dark, coarsely granular pigment

B. The gallbladder is visualized on oral cholecystography

C. Total urinary coproporphyrin excretion is increased

D. No reflux of conjugated BSP back into the circulation

Explanation:

Rotor Syndrome

- This benign, autosomal recessive disorder is clinically similar to DJS, although it is seen even less frequently.
- A major phenotypic difference is that the liver in patients with Rotor syndrome has no increased pigmentation and appears totally normal.
- Only abnormality in routine laboratory tests is an elevation of total serum bilirubin, due to a predominant rise in conjugated bilirubin. This is accompanied by bilirubinuria.
- Several additional features differentiate Rotor syndrome from DJS. In Rotor syndrome, gallbladder is usually visualized on oral cholecystography, in contrast to the nonvisualization that is typical of DJS.
- Pattern of urinary coproporphyrin excretion also differs.
- Pattern in Rotor syndrome resembles that of many acquired disorders of hepatobiliary function, in which coproporphyrin I, the major coproporphyrin isomer in bile, refluxes from the hepatocyte back into the circulation and is excreted in urine.
- Thus, total urinary coproporphyrin excretion is substantially increased in Rotor syndrome, in contrast to the normal levels seen in DJS.
- Although the fraction of coproporphyrin I in urine is elevated, it is usually <70% of the total, compared with ≥80% in DJS.
- Disorders also can be distinguished by their patterns of BSP excretion.
- Although clearance of BSP from plasma is delayed in Rotor syndrome, there is no reflux of conjugated BSP back into the circulation as seen in DJS.
- Kinetic analysis of plasma BSP infusion studies suggests the presence of a defect in intrahepatocellular storage of this compound.

- This has never been demonstrated directly. Recent studies indicate that the molecular basis of Rotor syndrome results from simultaneous deficiency of hepatocyte plasma membrane transporters OATP1B1 and OATP1B3.
- This results in reduced reuptake by these transporters of conjugated bilirubin that has been pumped out of the hepatocyte into the portal circulation by MRP3.

Ans. A

53. Medications associated with hepatic steatosis are all except:

A. Azithromycin B. Doxycycline

C. Bleomycin D. Tamoxifen

Explanation:

Table: Medications associated with hepatic steatosis
• Cytotoxic and cytostatic drugs – L-Asparaginase – Azacitidine – Azaserine – Bleomycin – Methotrexate – Puromycin – Tetracycline – Doxycycline • Metals – Antimony – Barium salts – Chromates – Phosphorus – Rare earths of low atomic number – Thallium compounds – Uranium compounds • Other drugs and toxins – Amiodarone – 4,4'-Diethylaminoethoxyhexesterol – Ethionine – Ethyl bromide – Estrogens – Glucocorticoids – Highly active antiretroviral therapy – Hydralazine – Hypoglycin – Orotate – Perhexiline maleate – Safrole – Tamoxifen

Ans. A

54. Cause of Presinusoidal portal hypertension is:

A. Schistosomiasis B. Alcoholic hepatitis

C. Budd-Chiari syndrome D. Inferior vena caval webs

Explanation:

Table: Classification of portal hypertension
Prehepatic
• Portal vein thrombosis
• Splenic vein thrombosis
• Massive splenomegaly (Banti's syndrome)
Hepatic
• Presinusoidal
– Schistosomiasis
– Congenital hepatic fibrosis
• Sinusoidal
– Cirrhosis–many causes
– Alcoholic hepatitis
• Postsinusoidal
– Hepatic sinusoidal obstruction (venoocclusive syndrome)
Posthepatic
• Budd-Chiari syndrome
• Inferior vena caval webs
• Cardiac causes
– Restrictive cardiomyopathy
– Constrictive pericarditis
– Severe congestive heart failure

Ans. A

55. Mild, transient, non-progressive serum aminotransferase elevations that resolve with continued drug use can be seen with all below drugs except:

A. Isoniazid
B. Valproate
C. Ciprofloxacin
D. Statins

Explanation:

- Drug-induced cholestasis ranges from mild to increasingly severe: (1) bland cholestasis with limited hepatocellular injury (e.g., estrogens, 17,α-substituted androgens); (2) inflammatory cholestasis (e.g., amoxicillin-clavulanic acid [the most frequently implicated antibiotic among cases of DILI], oxacillin, erythromycin estolate); (3) sclerosing cholangitis (e.g., after intrahepatic infusion of the chemotherapeutic agent floxuridine for hepatic metastases from a primary colonic carcinoma); and (4) disappearance of bile ducts, "ductopenic" cholestasis, similar to that observed in chronic rejection following liver transplantation (e.g., carbamazepine, levofloxacin).

Ans. C

56. All are true statements except:

A. Anti LKM 1 in autoimmune hepatitis
B. Anti LKM 4 in chronic hepatitis C
C. Anti LKM 2 in drug induced hepatitis
D. Anti LKM3 in Chronic hepatitis D

Explanation:

- **Type I autoimmune hepatitis** is the classic syndrome prevalent in North America and northern Europe occurring in young women, associated with marked hyperglobulinemia, lupoid features, circulating ANAs, and HLA-DR3 or HLA-DR4 (especially B8-DRB1*03).

- Also associated with type I autoimmune hepatitis are autoantibodies against actin and atypical perinuclear antineutrophilic cytoplasmic antibodies (pANCA). Included in the spectrum of type-I autoimmune hepatitis is a subset of patients who lack ANA and anti-LKM1, but who have circulating antibodies to soluble liver antigen. Most of these patients are women and have clinical features similar to, perhaps more severe than, those of other patients with type I autoimmune hepatitis.
- Type II autoimmune hepatitis, often seen in children, more common in Mediterranean populations, and linked to HLA- DRB1 and HLA-DQB1 haplotypes, is associated not with ANA but with anti-LKM. Actually, anti-LKM represent a heterogeneous group of antibodies. In type II autoimmune hepatitis, the antibody is anti-LKM1, directed against cytochrome P450 2D6. This is the same anti-LKM seen in some patients with chronic hepatitis C. Anti-LKM2 is seen in drug-induced hepatitis, and anti-LKM3 (directed against uridine diphosphate glucuronyl transferases) is seen in patients with chronic hepatitis D. Another autoantibody observed in type II autoimmune hepatitis is directed against liver cytosol formimino transferase cyclodeaminase (anti-liver cytosol 1).

Ans. B

57. All are true statements except:

A. Hereditary hemorrhagic telangiectasia and Osler-Weber-Rendu

B. Dieulafoy lesion and aberrant vessel bleeds

C. Watermelon stomach and vascular ectasia

D. Prolapse gastropathy and prolapse of distal stomach into esophagus

Explanation:

- Less common causes of Upper GI Bleeding include neoplasms, vascular ectasias (including hereditary hemorrhagic telangiectasias [Osler-Weber-Rendu] and gastric antral vascular ectasia ["watermelon stomach"]), Dieulafoy's lesion (in which an aberrant vessel in the mucosa bleeds from a pinpoint mucosal defect), **prolapse gastropathy (prolapse of proximal stomach into esophagus with retching, especially in alcoholics),** aortoenteric fistulas, and hemobilia or hemosuccus pancreaticus (bleeding from the bile duct or pancreatic duct).

Ans. D

58. Factors that weigh against the diagnosis of autoimmune hepatitis include all except:

A. Response to treatment

B. Histologic evidence of bile duct injury

C. Mitochondrial antibodies

D. History of hepatotoxic drugs or excessive alcohol

Explanation:

- Factors that weigh in favor of the diagnosis include female gender; predominant aminotransferase elevation; presence and level of globulin elevation; presence of nuclear, smooth muscle, LKM1, and other autoantibodies; concurrent other autoimmune diseases; characteristic histologic features (interface hepatitis, plasma cells, rosettes); HLA-DR3 or DR4 markers; and response to treatment
- A more simplified, more specific scoring system relies on four variables: autoantibodies, serum IgG level, typical or compatible histologic features, and absence of viral hepatitis markers.
- Weighing against the diagnosis are predominant alkaline phosphatase elevation, mitochondrial antibodies, markers of viral hepatitis, history of hepatotoxic drugs or excessive alcohol, histologic evidence of bile duct injury, or such atypical histologic features as fatty infiltration, iron overload and viral inclusions.

Ans. A

59. Highly infectious among below:

A. HBsAg positive serum containing HBeAg
B. HBsAg positive serum containing HBeAg negative
C. HBsAg positive serum containing anti-HBe-positive serum
D. Anti HBsAg positive and anti-HBe-positive serum

Explanation:

- HBsAg-positive serum containing HBeAg is more likely to be highly infectious and to be associated with the presence of hepatitis B virions (and detectable HBV DNA, see below) than HBeAg-negative or antiHBe-positive serum.
- For example, HBsAg-positive mothers who are HBeAg-positive almost invariably (>90%) transmit hepatitis B infection to their offspring, whereas HBsAg-positive mothers with anti-HBe rarely (10–15%) infect their offspring.

Ans. A

60. Hepatotoxicity of aspirin, methotrexate can be more common patient has chronic hepatitis with:

A. HBV
B. HCV
C. HDV
D. HEV

Explanation:

- Generally, drug hepatotoxicity is not more frequent in persons with underlying chronic liver disease, although the severity of the outcome may be amplified.
- Reported exceptions include hepatotoxicity of aspirin, methotrexate, INH (only in certain experiences), antiretroviral therapy for HIV infection, and certain drugs such as conditioning regimens for bone marrow transplantation in the presence of hepatitis C.

Ans. B

61. Patients who are at risk for variceal hemorrhage include:

A. Wedge to free gradient more than 5 mmHg
B. Wedge to free gradient more than 8 mmHg
C. Wedge to free gradient more than 12 mmHg
D. Wedge to free gradient more than 18 mmHg

Explanation:

- Average normal wedged-to-free gradient is 5 mmHg, and patients with a gradient >12 mmHg are at risk for variceal hemorrhage.

Ans. C

62. Sodium intake recommended to cirrhotic patients is:

A. <5gm/d
B. <2g/d
C. <3g/d
D. <4g/d

Explanation:

- Patients with small amounts of ascites can usually be managed with dietary sodium restriction alone.
- Most average diets in the United States contain 6–8 g of sodium per day, and if patients eat at restaurants or fast-food outlets, the amount of sodium in their diet can exceed this amount.

- Thus, it is often extremely difficult to get patients to change their dietary habits to ingest <2 g of sodium per day, which is the recommended amount.

Ans. B

63. All are true about ERCP procedure related complications except:

A. Pancreatitis occurs in ~5% of patients undergoing the procedure

B. 30% of patients develop sphincter of Oddi dysfunction

C. Old patients with diseased ducts are at increased risk

D. Post-ERCP pancreatitis is usually mild and self-limited, but it may result in prolonged hospitalization, surgery, diabetes, or death when severe

Explanation:

- ERCP carries additional risks. Pancreatitis occurs in ~5% of patients undergoing the procedure and in up to 30% of patients with sphincter of Oddi dysfunction. Young anicteric patients with normal ducts are at increased risk.
- Post-ERCP pancreatitis is usually mild and self-limited, but it may result in prolonged hospitalization, surgery, diabetes, or death when severe.
- Significant bleeding occurs after endoscopic sphincterotomy in ~1% of cases. Ascending cholangitis, pseudocyst infection, duodenal perforation, and abscess formation may occur as a result of ERCP.

Ans. C

64. Peptic ulcer character with highest risk of bleeding is:

A. A clean-based ulcer

B. Flat pigmented spots

C. Adherent clots

D. Sentinel clot

Explanation:

- The endoscopic appearance of peptic ulcers provides useful prognostic information and guides the need for endoscopic therapy in patients with acute hemorrhage
- A clean-based ulcer is associated with a low risk (3–5%) of rebleeding; patients with melena and a clean-based ulcer are often discharged home from emergency room or endoscopy suite if they are young, reliable, and otherwise healthy.
- Flat pigmented spots and adherent clots covering the ulcer base have a 10% and 20% risk of rebleeding, respectively. Endoscopic therapy may be considered for an ulcer with an adherent clot.
- When a fibrin plug is seen protruding from a vessel wall in base of an ulcer (so-called sentinel clot or visible vessel), the risk of rebleeding from the ulcer is 40%. This finding generally leads to endoscopic therapy to decrease the rebleeding rate. When active spurting from an ulcer is seen, there is a 90% risk of ongoing bleeding without therapy.

Ans. D

65. All the below statements are true except:

A. Autoimmune hepatitis associated with SMA

B. Wilson disease associated with decreased serum ceruloplasmin

C. Primary biliary cholangitis associated with elevated IgG levels

D. Hemochromatosis associated with elevated iron saturation

Explanation:

Table: Important diagnostic tests in common liver diseases	
Disease	**Diagnostic Test**
Hepatitis A	Anti-HAV IgM
Hepatitis B • Acute • Chronic	 HBsAg and anti-HBc IgM HBsAg and HBeAg and/or HBV DNA
Hepatitis C	Anti-HCV and HCV RNA
Hepatitis D (delta)	HBsAg and anti-HDV
Hepatitis E	Anti-HEV IgM and HEV RNA
Autoimmune hepatitis	ANA or SMA, elevated IgG levels and compatible histology
Primary biliary cholangitis	Mitochondrial antibody, elevated IgM levels, and compatible histology
Primary sclerosing cholangitis	P-ANCA, cholangiography
Drug-induced liver disease	History of drug ingestion
Alcoholic liver disease	History of excessive alcohol intake and compatible histology
Nonalcoholic steatohepatitis	Ultrasound or CT evidence of fatty liver and compatible histology
α_1 antitrypsin disease	Reduced α_1 antitrypsin levels, phenotype PiZZ or PiSZ
Wilson disease	Decreased serum ceruloplasmin and increased urinary copper; increased hepatic copper level
Hemochromatosis	Elevated iron saturation and serum ferrition; genetic testing for *HFE* gene mutations
Hepatocellular cancer	Elevated α-fetoprotein level (to >500 ng/ml); ultrasound or CT image of mass

Ans. C

66. **Unconjugated hyperbilirubinemia:**

A. <10% direct bilirubin
B. <15% direct bilirubin
C. <20% direct bilirubin
D. <5% direct bilirubin

Explanation:

- Bilirubin, a breakdown product of the porphyrin ring of heme-containing proteins, is found in the blood in two fractions—conjugated and unconjugated.
- Unconjugated fraction, also termed the *indirect fraction*, is insoluble in water and is bound to albumin in the blood. The conjugated (direct) bilirubin fraction is water-soluble and can therefore be excreted by the kidney.
- Normal values of total serum bilirubin are reported between 1 and 1.5 mg/dL with 95% of a normal population falling between 0.2 and 0.9 mg/dL.
- If the direct-acting fraction is <15% of the total, the bilirubin can be considered to all be indirect. The most frequently reported upper limit of normal for conjugated bilirubin is 0.3 mg/dL.

Ans. B

67. **Fibrosing cholestatic hepatitis is due to choking of the cell with overwhelming quantities of:**

A. HBsAg
B. HBeAg
C. HDV
D. HBcAg

Explanation:

- Facts that concomitant HDV and HBV infections are associated with more severe liver injury than HBV infection alone and that cells transfected in vitro with the gene for HDV antigen express HDV antigen and then become necrotic in the absence of any immunologic influences are also consistent with a viral effect on pathogenicity.

- Similarly, in patients who undergo liver transplantation for end-stage chronic hepatitis B, occasionally, rapidly progressive liver injury appears in the new liver.
- This clinical pattern is associated with an unusual histologic pattern in the new liver, *fibrosing cholestatic hepatitis*, which, ultrastructurally, appears to represent a choking of the cell with overwhelming quantities of HBsAg.
- This observation suggests that, under the influence of the potent immunosuppressive agents required to prevent allograft rejection, HBV may have a direct cytopathic effect on liver cells, independent of the immune system.

Ans. A

68. There is cross-reactivity between viral antigens HCV NS3 and NS5A with:

A. CYP 2D6
B. CYP 3D8
C. CYP C16
D. CYP 2D9

Explanation:

- Finally, cross-reactivity between viral antigens (HCV NS3 and NS5A) and host autoantigens (cytochrome P450 2D6) has been invoked to explain the association between hepatitis C and a subset of patients with autoimmune hepatitis and antibodies to liver-kidney microsomal (LKM) antigen (anti-LKM).

Ans. A

69. Celiac disease is associated with all except:

A. IgA deficiency
B. Diabetes Mellitus type II
C. Down's syndrome
D. Turner's syndrome

Explanation:

- Celiac disease is also associated with diabetes mellitus type 1, IgA deficiency, Down's syndrome, and Turner's syndrome. The clinical importance of the association with diabetes is that, although severe watery diarrhea without evidence of malabsorption is most often diagnosed as "diabetic diarrhea", assay of antiendomysial antibodies and/or a small-intestinal biopsy must be considered to exclude celiac disease.

Ans. B

70. Therapies that improve symptoms but do not reverse organic abnormalities include all except:

A. Gluten-free diet for celiac disease
B. Lactose restriction for lactase deficiency
C. Carbohydrate restrictions with dumping syndrome
D. Low-FODMAP (fermentable oligo-di-monosaccharides and polyols) diets in IBS

Explanation:

- Dietary modifications for GI disease include treatments that only reduce symptoms, therapies correct pathologic defects, or replace normal food intake with enteral or parenteral formulations.
- Changes that improve symptoms but do not reverse organic abnormalities include lactose restriction for

lactase deficiency, liquid meals in gastroparesis, carbohydrate restrictions with dumping syndrome and low-FODMAP (fermentable oligo-di-monosaccharides and polyols) diets in IBS.

- Gluten-free diet for celiac disease exemplifies a primary therapy to reduce mucosal inflammation.

Ans. A

71. Peptic ulcer character with highest risk of bleeding is:

A. A clean-based ulcer
B. Flat pigmented spots
C. Adherent clots
D. Sentinel clot

Explanation:

- Endoscopic therapy may be considered for an ulcer with an adherent clot.
- When a fibrin plug is seen protruding from a vessel wall in the base of an ulcer (so-called sentinel clot or visible vessel), the risk of rebleeding from the ulcer is 40%.
- This finding generally leads to endoscopic therapy to decrease the rebleeding rate.
- When active spurting from an ulcer is seen, there is a 90% risk of ongoing bleeding without therapy.

Ans. D

72. A 54 year old patient describes vague right sided abdominal discomfort. He is also having intermittent spells of flushing, diarrhoea, palpitations and wheezing. What investigation is likely to give the diagnosis?

A. Urinary 5 hydroxyindoleacetic acid levels
B. Urinary catecholamines
C. Serum cortisol
D. CT abdomen

Explanation:

- The patient has carcinoid syndrome. These tumours excrete 5 hydroxytryptamine which is metabolised to 5 hydroxyindoleacetic acid which is excreted in the urine and these levels should be measured. The underlying diagnosis may be a colorectal cancer and a CT abdomen may be useful in the staging.

Ans. A

73. While testing for ZES, PPI should be stopped atleast _____.

A. 7 days before testing
B. 5 days before testing
C. 10 days before testing
D. 3 days before testing

Explanation:

- Effect of the PPI on gastrin levels and acid secretion will linger several days after stopping the PPI; therefore, it should be stopped for a minimum of 7 days before testing.
- During this period, the patient should be placed on a histamine H2 antagonist, such as famotidine, twice to three times per day.
- Although this type of agent has a short-term effect on gastrin and acid secretion, it needs to be stopped 24 h before repeating fasting gastrin levels.
- Patient may take antacids for the final day, stopping them ~12 h before testing is performed.
- Heightened awareness of complications related to gastric acid hypersecretion during the period of PPI cessation is critical

Ans. A

74. Most important complication of celiac disease is:

A. Development of cancer
B. Intestinal ulceration
C. Refractory sprue
D. Collagenous sprue

Explanation:

- Most important complication of celiac disease is the development of cancer.
- Incidences of both gastrointestinal and non gastrointestinal neoplasms as well as intestinal lymphoma are elevated among patients with celiac disease. For unexplained reasons, the frequency of lymphoma in patients with celiac disease is higher in Ireland and the United Kingdom than in the United States.
- Possibility of lymphoma must be considered whenever a patient with celiac disease who has previously done well on a gluten-free diet is no longer responsive to gluten restriction or a patient who presents with clinical and histologic features consistent with celiac disease does not respond to a gluten-free diet.
- Other complications of celiac disease include the development of intestinal ulceration independent of lymphoma and so-called refractory sprue and collagenous sprue.
- In *collagenous sprue*, a layer of collagen-like material is present beneath the basement membrane; patients with collagenous sprue generally do not respond to a gluten-free diet and often have a poor prognosis.

Ans. A

75. All are true about treatment of IBD except:

A. Glucocorticoids play no role in maintenance therapy in either UC or CD
B. Antibiotics have no role in the treatment of active or quiescent UC
C. Adalimumab is approved for treatment of moderate to severe CD and UC
D. Golimumab is fully human IgG1 antibody against TNF-α and is given orally

Explanation:

- Golimumab is another fully human IgG1 antibody against TNF-α and is currently approved for the treatment of moderately to severely active UC. Like adalimumab and certolizumab, golimumab is injected SC.

Ans. D

76. All are true about HAV except:

A. HAV is a non-enveloped 27-nm, heat-, acid-, and ether-resistant RNA virus in the Hepatovirus genus of the picornavirus family
B. Hepatitis A has an incubation period of ~4 weeks
C. There is longer persistence of virus in the liver, fecal shedding, viremia, and infectivity begins once jaundice becomes apparent
D. The diagnosis of hepatitis A is made during acute illness by demonstrating anti-HAV of the IgM class

Explanation:

- HAV is a non-enveloped 27-nm, heat-, acid-, and ether-resistant RNA virus in the *Hepatovirus* genus of the picornavirus family.
- Its virion contains four capsid polypeptides, designated VP1–VP4, which are cleaved post-translationally from polyprotein product of a 7500-nucleotide genome.
- Inactivation of viral activity can be achieved by boiling for 1 min, by contact with formaldehyde and chlorine, or by ultraviolet irradiation.
- Despite nucleotide sequence variation of up to 20% among isolates of HAV, and despite recognition of four genotypes affecting humans, all strains of this virus are immunologically indistinguishable and belong to one serotype.

- Human HAV can infect and cause hepatitis in chimpanzees, tamarins (marmosets), and several monkey species. Recently, a hepatotropic *Hepatovirus* related to, and likely to have shared common evolutionary ancestry with, human HAV has been identified in several species of harbor seals, albeit without histologic evidence for liver injury or inflammation.
- Hepatitis A has an incubation period of ~4 weeks. Its replication is limited to the liver, but the virus is present in the liver, bile, stools, and blood during the late incubation period and acute preicteric/presymptomatic phase of illness.
- Despite slightly longer persistence of virus in the liver, fecal shedding, viremia, and infectivity diminish rapidly once jaundice becomes apparent. HAV can be cultivated reproducibly in vitro.

Ans. C

77. In HCV–clinical progression and hepatic steatosis are more common in:

A. Genotype 1
B. Genotype 2
C. Genotype 3
D. Genotype 4

Explanation:

- At least six distinct major genotypes (and a minor genotype 7), as well as >50 subtypes within genotypes, of HCV have been identified by nucleotide sequencing.
- Genotypes differ from one another in sequence homology by ≥30%, and subtypes differ by ~20%.
- Because divergence of HCV isolates within a genotype or subtype and within the same host may vary insufficiently to define a distinct genotype, these intragenotypic differences are referred to as *quasispecies* and differ in sequence homology by only a few percent.
- Genotypic and quasispecies diversity of HCV, resulting from its high mutation rate, interferes with effective humoral immunity.
- Neutralizing antibodies to HCV have been demonstrated, but they tend to be short-lived, and HCV infection does not induce lasting immunity against reinfection with different virus isolates or even the same virus isolate.
- Thus, neither *heterologous* nor *homologous* immunity appears to develop commonly after acute HCV infection.
- Some HCV genotypes are distributed worldwide, whereas others are more geographically confined.
- In addition, differences exist among genotypes in responsiveness to antiviral therapy but not in pathogenicity or clinical progression (except for genotype 3, in which hepatic steatosis and clinical progression are more likely).

Ans. C

78. All are true about hepatorenal syndrome except:

A. Particularly poor prognosis is seen in the case of type 2 hepatorenal syndrome
B. Type 1 hepatorenal syndrome defined as >twofold increase in SCr to >2.5 mg/dL, within 2 weeks without an alternate cause
C. Type 2 hepatorenal syndrome is characterized by refractory ascites
D. The hepatorenal syndrome is difficult to distinguish from prerenal azotemia

Explanation:

- Many individuals with advanced liver disease exhibit a hemodynamic profile that resembles prerenal azotemia in the setting of total-body volume overload.
- Systemic vascular resistance is markedly reduced due to primary arterial vasodilation in the splanchnic circulation, resulting ultimately in activation of vasoconstrictor responses similar to those seen in hypovolemia.

- AKI is a common complication in this setting, and it can be triggered by volume depletion and spontaneous bacterial peritonitis.
- Particularly poor prognosis is seen in case of type 1 hepatorenal syndrome, in which AKI, defined as >twofold increase in SCr to >2.5 mg/dL, within 2 weeks without an alternate cause (e.g., shock and nephrotoxic drugs), persists despite volume administration and withholding of diuretics.

Ans. A

79. Antibiotic prophylaxis in patients with cirrhosis and acute GI bleeding include:

A. Only those who are undergoing upper GI endoscopy for diagnostic purpose
B. For those who are undergoing upper GI endoscopy for diagnostic and therapeutic purpose
C. For all patients who have self limiting upper GI bleeding which doesn't require admission
D. For all patients with upper GI bleeding at the time of admission irrespective of procedure being done or not

Explanation:

Table: Antibiotic prophylaxis for endoscopic procedures

Patient Condition	Procedure Contemplated	Goal of Prophylaxis	Periprocedural Antibiotic Prophylaxis
All cardiac conditions	Any endoscopic procedure	Prevention of infective endocarditis	Not indicated
Bile duct obstruction in the absence of cholangitis	ERCP with complete drainage	Prevention of cholangitis	Not recommended
Bile duct obstruction in absence of cholangitis	ERCP with anticipated incomplete drainage (e.g., sclerosing cholangitis, hilar strictures)	Prevention of cholangitis	Recommended; continue antibiotics after the procedure
Sterile pancreatic fluid collection (e.g., pseudocyst, necrosis), which communicates with pancreatic duct	ERCP	Prevention of cyst infection	Recommended; continue antibiotics after the procedure
Sterile pancreatic fluid collection	Transmural drainage	Prevention of cyst infection	Recommended
Solid lesion along upper GI tract	EUS-FNA	Prevention of local infection	Not recommended[a]
Solid lesion along lower GI tract	EUS-FNA	Prevention of local infection	Not recommended[a]
Cystic lesions along GI tract (including mediastinum and pancreas)	EUS-FNA	Prevention of cyst infection	Recommended
All patients	Percutaneous endoscopic feeding tube placement	Prevention of peristomal infection	Recommended[b]
Cirrhosis with acute GI bleeding	Required for all such patients, regardless of endoscopic procedures	Prevention of infectious complications and reduction of mortality	Recommended, upon admission[c]
Continuous peritoneal dialysis	Lower GI tract endoscopy	Prevention of bacterial peritonitis	Recommended
Synthetic vascular graft and other nonvalvular cardiovascular devices	Any endoscopic procedure	Prevention of graft and device infection	Not recommended[d]
Prosthetic joints	Any endoscopic procedure	Prevention of septic arthritis	Not recommended[e]

Ans. D

80. Bridging therapy before endoscopic procedure should be considered in all below conditions except:

A. Atrial fibrillation with a CHA2DS2-VASc score ≥2

B. Mechanical mitral valve

C. Mechanical aortic valve without other thromboembolic risk factors

D. Venous thromboembolism within the past 3 months

Explanation:

Table: Management of antithrombotic drugs prior to endoscopic procedures

Drug	Bleeding Risk of Procedure	Management	Interval between Last Dose and Procedure	Comments
Warfarin	Low[a]	Continue	N/A	Ensure that INR is not supratherapeutic
	High[b]	Discontinue	3-7 days (usually 5), INR should be ≤1.5 for procedure	Consider bridging therapy with heparin;[c] usually safe to resume warfarin on the same or next day
Dabigatran, rivaroxaban, apixaban, edoxaban	Low[a]	Continue or hold morning dose on day of procedure	N/A	
Dabigatran	High[b]	Discontinue	2-3 days if GFR is ≥ 50 ml/min, 3-4 days if GFR is 30-49 ml/min	Bridging therapy not recommended; resume drug when bleeding risk is low
Rivaroxaban, apixaban, edoxaban	High[a]	Discontinue	2 days if GFR is ≥ 60 ml/min, 3 days if GFR is 30-59 ml/min 4 days if GFR is < 30 ml/min	Bridging therapy not recommended; resume drug when bleeding risk is low
Heparin	Low[a]	Continue	N/A	
	High[b]	Discontinue	4–6 hours for unfractionated heparin	Skip one dose if using low-molecular-weight heparin
Aspirin	Any	Continue	N/A	Low-dose aspirin does not substantially increase the risk of endoscopic procedures
Aspirin with dipyridamole	Low[a]	Continue	N/A	
	High[b]	Discontinue	2-7 days	Consider continuing aspirin monotherapy
P2Y12 receptor antagonists (clopidogrel, prasugrel, ticlopidine, ticagrelor, cangrelor)	Low[a]	Continue	N/A	
	High[b]	Coronary stent in place: discuss with cardiologist	5 days (clopidogrel or ticagrelor), 7 days (prasugrel), 10-4 days (ticlopidine)	Risk of stent thrombosis for 12 months after insertion of drug-eluting coronary stent or 1 month after insertion of bare metal coronary stent
		No coronary stent: Discontinue, consider substituting to aspirin		

Ans. C

81. Grading activity in chronic liver disease include all except:

A. METAVIR
B. Histology activity index
C. Ishak fibrosis scale
D. FODPED scoring system

Explanation:

- Several well-verified numerical scales for grading activity in chronic liver disease, most commonly used are the METAVIR, histology activity index and Ishak fibrosis scale.
- Amount of fibrosis is generally staged on a scale of 0 to 4+ (METAVIR scale) or 0 to 6+ (Ishak scale).

Ans. D

82. Vitamin B12 deficiency can cause all except:

A. Hallucinations
B. Paresthesia
C. Memory disturbances
D. Hyporeflexia

Explanation:

Perioral examination	Perioral findings are indicative of certain nutrient deficiencies Angular stomatitis and cheilosis: B complex, iron and protein Glossitis: Niacin, folate and vitamin B_{12} Magenta tongue: Riboflavin Bleeding gums, gingivitis, tooth loss: Vitamin C Angular stomatitis, cheilosis and glossitis are associated with vitamin and mineral deficiencies. Note poor dentition, caries and tooth loss. Difficulty swallowing and impairment of gag should also be recognized
Extremity examination	Extremity findings indicate certain nutrient deficiencies Arthralgia: Vitamin C Calf pain: thiamine Extremities may also exhibit loss of muscle mass and/or peripheral edema. Neurological findings in the extremities may also result from deficiencies described below.
Mental status/nervous system examination	Mental and nervous system findings indicate certain nutrient deficiencies Ophthalmoplegia and foot drop: Thiamine Paresthesia: Thiamine, vitamin B_{12} and biotin Depressed vibratory and position senses: Vitamin B_{12} Anxiety, depression and hallucinations: Niacin Memory disturbance: Vitamin B_{12} Hyporeflexia, loss of lower extremity deep tendon reflexes: Thiamine and vitamin B_{12} Conduct formal cognitive and depressed assessments as appropriate. Dementia and depression are common cause of malnutrition among older persons. Wernicke-Korsakoff syndrome may be observed with severe thiamine deficiency
Functional assessment	Observe and test physical performance as indicated; gait, chair stands, stair steps and balance. These provide complex measures of integrated neurological status, coordination and strength

Ans. A

83. All below chronic disorders have been shown to have a strong association with PUD except:

A. α1-antitrypsin deficiency
B. Polycythemia vera
C. Systemic mastocytosis
D. Cirrhosis

Explanation:

- Specific chronic disorders have been shown to have a strong association with PUD: (1) advanced age, (2) chronic pulmonary disease, (3) chronic renal failure, (4) cirrhosis, (5) nephrolithiasis, (6) α1-antitrypsin deficiency, and (7) systemic mastocytosis.
- Disorders with a possible association are (1) hyperparathyroidism, (2) coronary artery disease, (3) polycythemia vera, (4) chronic pancreatitis, (5) former alcohol use, (6) obesity, (7) African American race, and (8) three or more doctor visits in a year.

Ans. B

84. 22 year old female presented with secondary amenorrhea and pigmentation which she is noticed to be progressive. On examination she was found to have hepatomegaly. She was recently diagnosed with diabetes. With all the above feature diagnosis of hemochromatosis was made. Genetic mutation was +ve for C282 Y homozygosity. Diagnosed with HFE related hemochromatosis. All are reversible with phlebotomy in hemochromatosis except:

A. Hypogonadism
B. Small joint arthropathy
C. All of the above
D. None of the above

Explanation:

Mentation of skin decreases, and cardiac failure may be reversed. Diabetes improves in ~40% of patients, **but removal of excess iron has little effect on hypogonadism or arthropathy. Hepatic fibrosis may decrease, but established cirrhosis is irreversible. Hepatocellular carcinoma occurs as a late sequela in patients who are cirrhotic at presentation.**

Ans. C

85. All are true about PPI use except:

A. Because the pumps need to be activated for these agents to be effective, their efficacy is maximized if they are administered before a meal except for immediate release formulation of omeprazole
B. Mild to moderate hypergastrinemia has been observed in patients taking these drugs
C. Serum gastrin levels return to normal levels within 1–2 weeks after drug cessation
D. Rebound gastric acid hypersecretion has been described in H. pylori–positive individuals after discontinuation of PPIs

Explanation:

- Carcinoid tumors developed in some animals given the drugs preclinically; however, extensive experience has failed to demonstrate gastric carcinoid tumor development in humans.
- Serum gastrin levels return to normal levels within 1–2 weeks after drug cessation.
- Rebound gastric acid hypersecretion has been described in *H. pylori*–negative individuals after discontinuation of PPIs. It occurs even after relatively short-term usage (2 months) and may last for up to 2 months after the PPI has been discontinued.

Ans. D

86. All are true about diverticular disease except:

A. Pseudo diverticulum involves only a protrusion of the mucosa and submucosa through the muscularis propria of the colon

B. The type of diverticulum most commonly affecting the colon is the true diverticulum

C. In Asian populations, 70% of diverticula are seen in the right colon and cecum as well

D. Higher-amplitude contractions combined with constipated, high-fat-content stool within the sigmoid lumen in an area of weakness in the colonic wall results in the creation of these diverticula

Explanation:

- Two types of diverticula occur in the intestine: true and false (or pseudo diverticula).
- True diverticulum is a saclike herniation of the entire bowel wall, whereas pseudodiverticulum involves only a protrusion of mucosa & submucosa through muscularis propria of colon.
- Type of diverticulum most commonly affecting the colon is the pseudo diverticulum. Diverticula commonly affect the left and sigmoid colon; the rectum is always spared. However, in Asian populations, 70% of diverticula are seen in the right colon and cecum as well. Yamanda et al. found right-side colonic diverticulosis in 22% of Japanese patients undergoing colonoscopy.
- *Diverticulitis* is inflammation of a diverticulum.

Ans. B

87. A 39-year-old male presented to the obesity clinic with h/o excessive weight gain from last 4 years. On evaluation his BMI was found to be 29 kg/m^2. On investigation he was diagnosed to have diabetes mellitus. The treating physician decides to start anti obesity drug. True about orlistat are a/e:

A. Reduced fat absorption by 30%

B. Its effects are irreversible.

C. Adverse effects include fatty/oily stools

D. Side affects are counter acted by psyllium mucilloid

Explanation:

Orlistat acts in the lumen of the stomach and small intestine by forming a covalent bond with the active site of these lipases. Taken at a therapeutic dose of 120 mg tid, orlistat blocks the digestion and absorption of ~30% of dietary fat. After discontinuation of the drug, fecal fat content usually returns to normal within 48-72 hours.

Ans. B

88. True regarding CT finding of diverticulitis include all except:

A. Sigmoid diverticula

B. Thickened colonic wall >2 mm

C. Inflammation within the periodic fat with collection of contrast material or fluid

D. Inflammation within the periodic fat without collection of contrast material or fluid

Explanation:

- Diagnosis of diverticulitis is best made on CT with the following findings: Sigmoid diverticula, thickened colonic wall >4 mm, and inflammation within the periodic fat ± the collection of contrast material or fluid. In up to 20% of patients, an abdominal abscess may be present.
- Symptoms of irritable bowel syndrome may mimic those of diverticulitis.
- Therefore, suspected diverticulitis that does not meet CT criteria or is not associated with a leukocytosis or fever is not diverticular disease.
- Other conditions that can mimic diverticular disease include an ovarian cyst, endometriosis, acute appendicitis, and pelvic inflammatory disease.

Ans. B

89. Factors that weigh against the diagnosis of autoimmune hepatitis include all except:

A. Response to treatment
B. Histologic evidence of bile duct injury
C. Mitochondrial antibodies
D. History of hepatotoxic drugs or excessive alcohol

Explanation:

- An international group has suggested a set of criteria for establishing a diagnosis of autoimmune hepatitis.
- Exclusion of liver disease caused by genetic disorders, viral hepatitis, drug hepatotoxicity, and alcohol are linked with such inclusive diagnostic criteria as hyperglobulinemia, autoantibodies, and characteristic histologic features.
- This international group has also suggested a comprehensive diagnostic scoring system that, rarely required for typical cases, may be helpful when typical features are not present.
- Factors that weigh in favor of the diagnosis include female gender; predominant aminotransferase elevation; presence and level of globulin elevation; presence of nuclear, smooth muscle, LKM1, and other autoantibodies; concurrent other autoimmune diseases; characteristic histologic features (interface hepatitis, plasma cells, rosettes); HLA-DR3 or DR4 markers; and response to treatment.
- A more simplified, more specific scoring system relies on four variables: autoantibodies, serum IgG level, typical or compatible histologic features, and absence of viral hepatitis markers.
- Weighing against the diagnosis are predominant alkaline phosphatase elevation, mitochondrial antibodies, markers of viral hepatitis, history of hepatotoxic drugs or excessive alcohol, histologic evidence of bile duct injury, or such atypical histologic features as fatty infiltration, iron overload and viral inclusions.

Ans. A

90. A more simplified, more specific scoring system for diagnosis of autoimmune hepatitis relies on four variables including all except:

A. Autoantibodies
B. Serum IgM level
C. Typical or compatible histologic features
D. Absence of viral hepatitis markers

Explanation:

- Polyclonal hypergammaglobulinemia (>2.5 g/dL) is common in autoimmune hepatitis, as is the presence of rheumatoid factor.
- Circulating autoantibodies are also prevalent, most characteristically ANAs in a homogeneous staining pattern.
- Smooth-muscle antibodies are less specific, seen just as frequently in chronic viral hepatitis.
- Because of the high levels of globulins achieved in the circulation of some patients with autoimmune hepatitis, occasionally the globulins may bind nonspecifically in solid-phase binding immunoassays for viral antibodies.
- This has been recognized most commonly in tests for antibodies to hepatitis C virus, as noted above. In fact, studies of autoantibodies in autoimmune hepatitis have led to the recognition of new categories of autoimmune hepatitis.
- *Type I autoimmune hepatitis* is the classic syndrome prevalent in North America and northern Europe occurring in young women, associated with marked hyperglobulinemia, lupoid features, circulating ANAs, and HLA-DR3 or HLA-DR4 (especially *B8-DRB1*03*).
- Also associated with type I autoimmune hepatitis are autoantibodies against actin and atypical perinuclear antineutrophilic cytoplasmic antibodies (pANCA).
- Included in the spectrum of type-I autoimmune hepatitis is a subset of patients who lack ANA and anti-LKM1, but who have circulating antibodies to soluble liver antigen.

- Most of these patients are women and have clinical features similar to, perhaps more severe than, those of other patients with type I autoimmune hepatitis.
- *Type II autoimmune hepatitis*, often seen in children, more common in Mediterranean populations, and linked to HLA- DRB1 and HLA-DQB1 haplotypes, is associated not with ANA but with anti-LKM.
- Actually, anti-LKM represent a heterogeneous group of antibodies.
- In type II autoimmune hepatitis, the antibody is anti-LKM1, directed against cytochrome P450 2D6. This is the same anti-LKM seen in some patients with chronic hepatitis C. Anti-LKM2 is seen in drug-induced hepatitis, and anti-LKM3 (directed against uridine diphosphate glucuronyltransferases) is seen in patients with chronic hepatitis D.
- Another autoantibody observed in type II autoimmune hepatitis is directed against liver cytosol formiminotransferase cyclodeaminase (anti-liver cytosol 1).

Ans. B

91. Parietal cells located in oxyntic gland secrete all except:

A. HCl
B. IL11
C. Intrinsic factor
D. TNF

Explanation:

- Acid-secreting parietal cell is located in the oxyntic gland, adjacent to other cellular elements (ECL cell, D cell) important in gastric secretory process.
- This unique cell also secretes intrinsic factor (IF) and IL-11.

Ans. D

92. All are true about peptic ulcers except:

A. GUs tend to occur later in life than duodenal lesions, with a peak incidence reported in the sixth decade
B. More than one-half of GUs occur in females and are less common than DUs
C. DUs occur most often in first portion of duodenum (>95%), with ~90% located within 3 cm of pylorus
D. In contrast to DUs, GUs can represent a malignancy and should be biopsied upon discovery

Explanation:

- GUs tend to occur later in life than duodenal lesions, with a peak incidence reported in the sixth decade.
- More than one-half of GUs occur in males and are less common than DUs, perhaps due to the higher likelihood of GUs being silent and presenting only after a complication develops.
- Autopsy studies suggest a similar incidence of DUs and GUs.

Ans. B

93. False-positive test for IgM anti-HBc may be encountered in patients with high-titer of:

A. Anti CCP
B. Rheumatoid factor
C. ANA
D. SMA

Explanation:

- In patients with hepatitis B surface antigenemia of unknown duration (e.g., blood donors found to be HBsAg-positive) testing for IgM anti-HBc may be useful to distinguish between acute or recent infection (IgM anti-HBc-positive) and chronic HBV infection (IgM anti-HBcnegative, IgG anti-HBc-positive).
- A false-positive test for IgM anti-HBc may be encountered in patients with high-titer rheumatoid factor.
- Also, IgM anti-HBc may be re-expressed during acute reactivation of chronic hepatitis B.

Ans. B

94. All are true about peritoneal inflammation except:

A. Patient with peritonitis characteristically lies quietly in bed

B. Characteristic feature of peritoneal irritation is tonic reflex spasm of the abdominal musculature

C. Spasm over a perforated retrocecal appendix is always severe

D. A slowly developing process also often greatly attenuates degree of muscle spasm

Explanation:

- Another characteristic feature of peritoneal irritation is tonic reflex spasm of the abdominal musculature, localized to the involved body segment.
- Its intensity depends on the integrity of the nervous system, location of the inflammatory process, and the rate at which it develops.
- Spasm over a perforated retrocecal appendix or perforation into the lesser peritoneal sac may be minimal or absent because of the protective effect of overlying viscera.
- Catastrophic abdominal emergencies may be associated with minimal or no detectable pain or muscle spasm in obtunded, seriously ill, debilitated, immunosuppressed, or psychotic patients.
- A slowly developing process also often greatly attenuates degree of muscle spasm.

Ans. C

95. All are true about abdominal examination in abdominal pain patients except:

A. Careful pelvic and rectal examinations are mandatory in every patient with abdominal pain

B. Much attention has been paid to the presence or absence of peristaltic sounds, their quality, and their frequency

C. Auscultation of the abdomen is one of the most revealing aspects of the physical examination of a patient with abdominal pain

D. Abdominal signs may be virtually or totally absent in cases of pelvic peritonitis

Explanation:

- Auscultation of the abdomen is one of the least revealing aspects of the physical examination of a patient with abdominal pain.
- Catastrophes such as a strangulating small intestinal obstruction or perforated appendicitis may occur in presence of normal peristaltic sounds.
- Conversely, when the proximal part of the intestine above obstruction becomes markedly distended and edematous, peristaltic sounds may lose characteristics of borborygmi and become weak or absent, even when peritonitis is not present.
- It is usually the severe chemical peritonitis of sudden onset that is associated with the truly silent abdomen.

Ans. C

96. Identify the endoscopic lesion:

A. Barrett's esophagus

B. Duodenal ulcer

C. Gastric antral vascular disease

D. Polyp

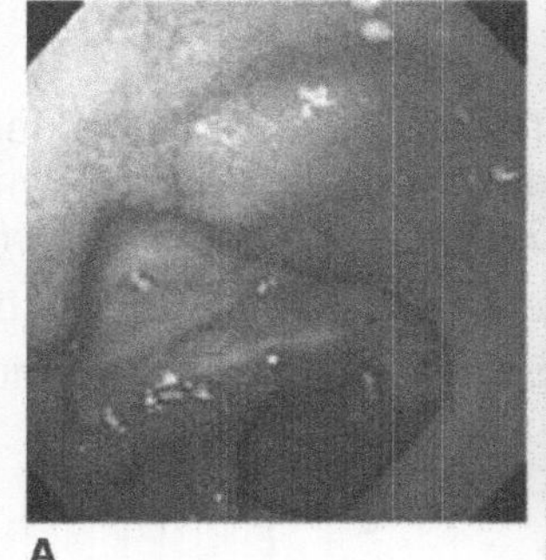

A

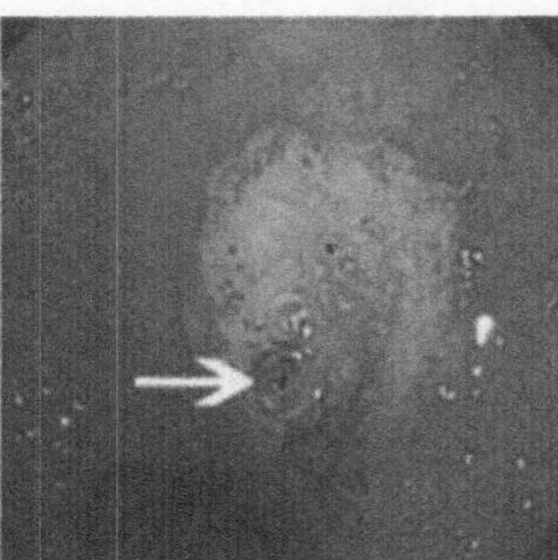

B

Explanation:

- Image A shows ulcer with clean base.

- Image B shows visible vessel from lesion.
- In Barrett's esophagus Barrett's mucosa will be seen from gastroesophageal junction.
- In gastric antral vascular disease the mucosa will have flat or raised vascular ectasia resulting in water melon stomach appearance.

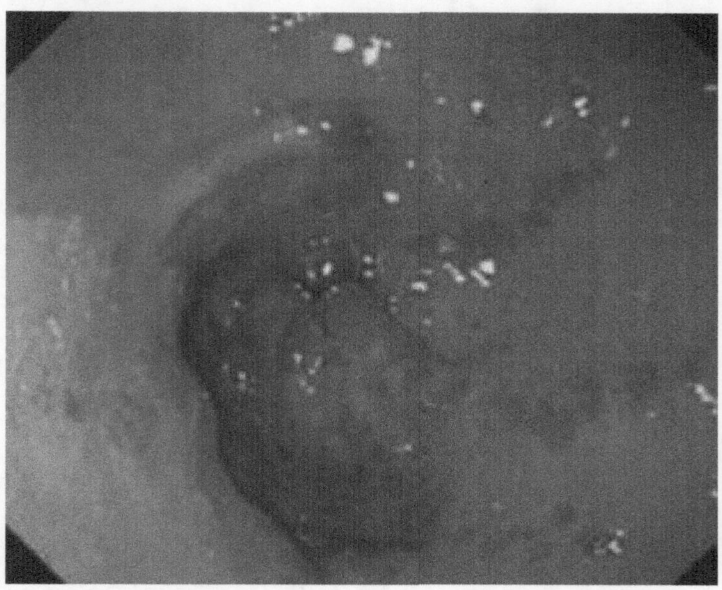

Ans. B

97. Most common position for the anatomic variations of appendix is:

A. Retrocecal B. Preileal

C. Post ileal D. Pelvic

Explanation:

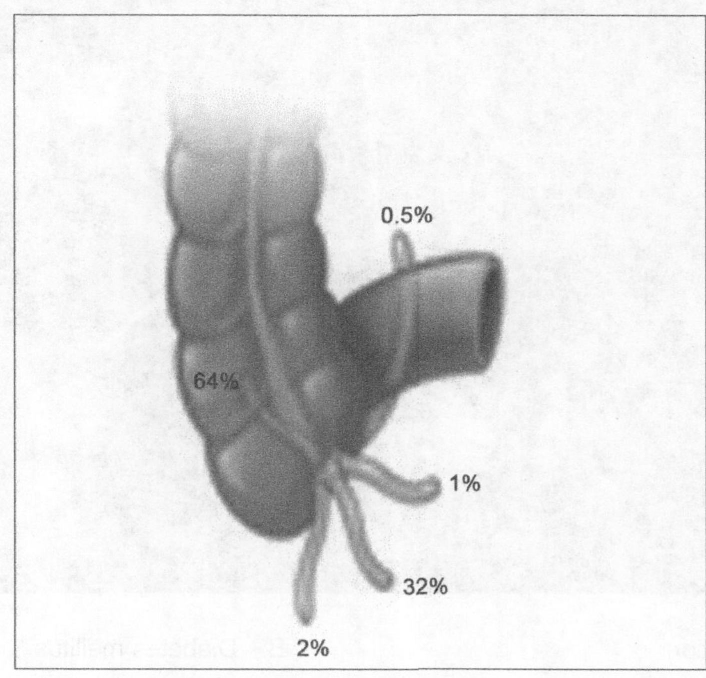

- Retrocecal is the most common position for the appendix situation as shown in image in 64% cases.

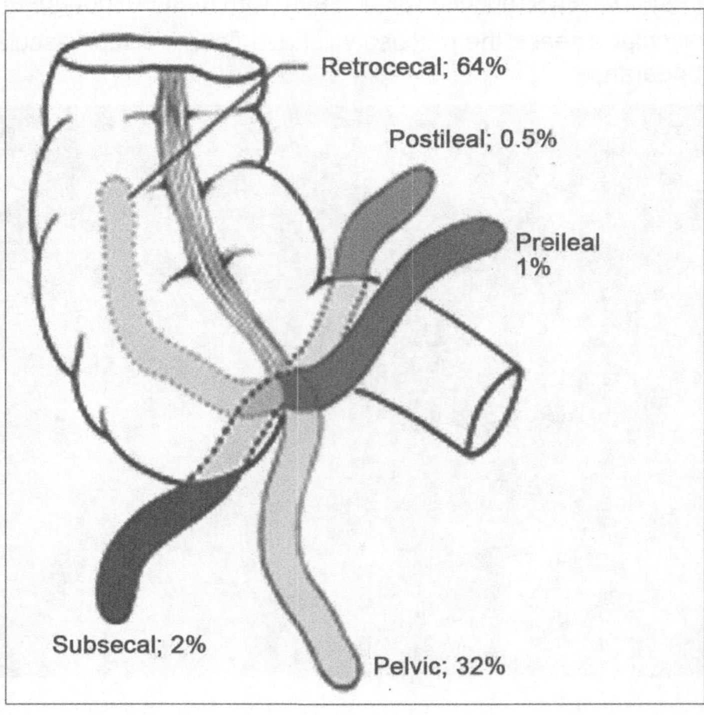

Ans. A

98. A 47 year old chronic alcoholic male presented with complaints of recurrent abdominal pain. lab reports reveals serum amylase-248 IU/L.CT contrast abdomen done, Following image shown MRCP of patient. Which of the following is not complication of the following condition?

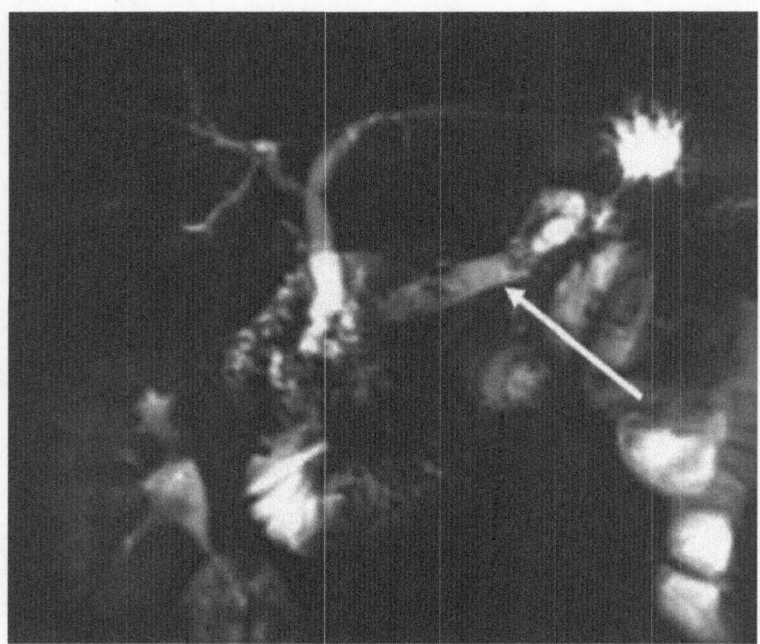

A. Intestinal obstruction
B. Diabetes mellitus
C. Pseudocyst
D. Biliary cirrhosis

Explanation:

- Based on above case and MRCP shows dilated duct and filling defects in favor of chronic pancreatitis. Intestinal obstruction is not usual complication of chronic pancreatitis.

Table: Complications of chronic pancreatitis	
Chronic abdominal pain	Jaundice
Narcotic addiction	Biliary stricture and/or biliary cirrhosis
Diabetes mellitus/impaired glucose tolerance	Pseudocyst
Gastroparesis	Metabolic bone disease
Malabsorption/maldigestion	Pancreatic cancer

Ans. A

99. Most common cause for following condition is:

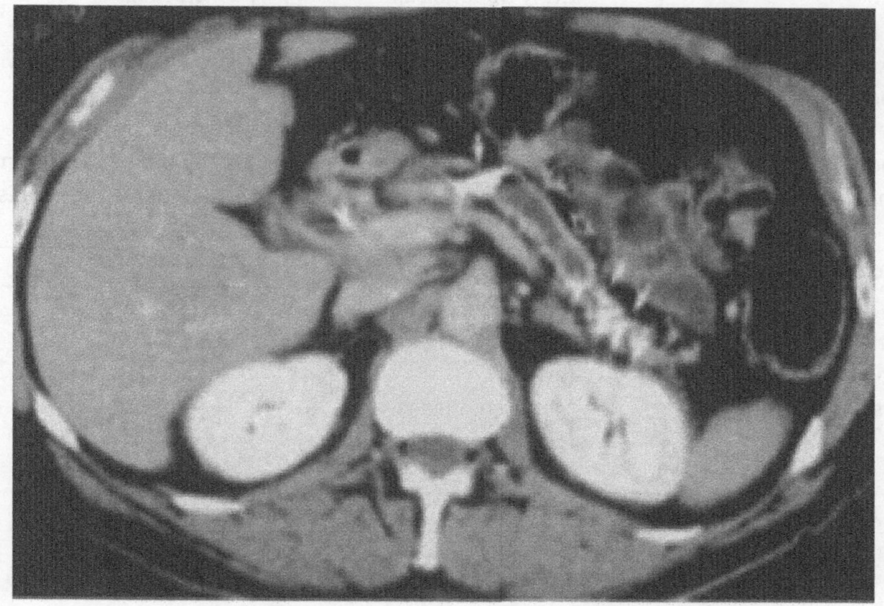

A. Gall stones
B. Alcohol
C. Autoimmune related
D. Genetic mutations

Explanation:

- Contrast CT shows atrophic pancreas, multiple calcifications, dilated pancreatic duct through head and tail in favor of chronic pancreatitis.
- Alcohol is leading and most common cause of chronic pancreatitis world wide.

Ans. B

100. In case of ruptured aortic aneurysm which of the following part of the abdomen perceives the pain?

A. Right upper quadrant
B. Left upper quadrant
C. Peri umbilical region
D. Right lower quadrant

Explanation:

Table: Differential diagnoses of abdominal pain by location		
Right Upper Quadrant	**Epigastric**	**Left Upper Quadrant**
Cholecystitis Cholangitis Pancreatitis Pneumonia/empyema Pleurisy/pleurodynia Subdiaphragmatic abscess Hepatitis Budd-Chiari syndrome	Peptic ulcer disease Gastritis GERD Pancreatitis Myocardial infarction Pericarditis Ruptured aortic aneurysm Esophagitis	Splenic infarct Splenic rupture Splenic abscess Gastritis Gastric ulcer Pancreatitis Subdiaphragmatic abscess
Right Lower Quadrant	**Periumbilical**	**Left Lower Quadrant**
Appendicits Salpingitis Inguinal hernia Ectopic pregnancy Nephrolithiasis Inflammatory bowel disease Mesenteric lymphadenitis Typhlitis	Early appendicitis Gastroenteritis Bowel obstruction Ruptured aortic aneurysm	Diverticulitis Salpingitis Inguinal hernia Ectopic pregnancy Nephrolithiasis Irritable bowel syndrome Inflammatory bowel disease
Diffuse Nonlocalized Pain		
Gastroenteritis Mesenteric ischemia Bowel obstruction Irritable bowel syndrome Peritonitis Diabetes	Malaria Familial Mediterranean fever Metabolic diseases Psychiatric diseases	
Abbreviation: GERD, gastroesophageal reflux disease.		

Ans. C

101. All are true about IBD and cancer except:

A. Risk of neoplasia in chronic UC increases with duration and extent of disease

B. Patients with CD may have an increased risk of NHL, leukemia and myelodysplastic syndromes

C. CD patients may be associated with an increased risk of cancer in the lower rectum and anal canal (adenocarcinoma)

D. Although absolute risk of small-bowel adenocarcinoma in CD is low patients with long-standing, extensive small-bowel disease should consider screening

Explanation:

- IBD patients are also at greater risk for other malignancies.
- Patients with CD may have an increased risk of NHL, leukemia, and myelodysplastic syndromes.
- Severe, chronic, complicated perianal disease in CD patients may be associated with an increased risk of cancer in the lower rectum and anal canal (squamous cell cancers).
- Although the absolute risk of small-bowel adenocarcinoma in CD is low (2.2% at 25 years in one study), patients with long-standing, extensive, small-bowel disease should consider screening.

Ans. C

102. All are true about mesenteric ischemia except:

A. Intestinal angina is generally more acute in onset and often seen in valvular heart disease patients

B. Nonocclusive mesenteric ischemia is also seen in patients receiving high-dose vasopressor infusions

C. Incidence of ischemic colitis following elective aortic repair is 5–9%, and incidence triples in patients following emergent repair

D. Mesenteric venous thrombosis is less common & is associated with presence of hypercoagulable state

Explanation:

- Risk factors for arterioocclusive mesenteric ischemia are generally acute in onset that include atrial fibrillation, recent myocardial infarction, valvular heart disease, and recent cardiac or vascular catheterization, all of which result in embolic clots reaching the mesenteric circulation.
- Nonocclusive mesenteric ischemia, also known as "intestinal angina," is generally more insidious and often seen in the aging population affected by atherosclerotic disease.
- Patients with chronic atherosclerotic disease could also suffer an acute insult from emboli leading to complete occlusion.
- Nonocclusive mesenteric ischemia is also seen in patients receiving high-dose vasopressor infusions, patients presenting with cardiogenic or septic shock, and cocaine overdose. It is the most prevalent gastrointestinal disease complicating cardiovascular surgery.
- Incidence of ischemic colitis following elective aortic repair is 5–9%, and the incidence triples in patients following emergent repair.
- Mesenteric venous thrombosis is less common and is associated with presence of a hypercoagulable state including protein C or S deficiency, antithrombin III deficiency, polycythemia vera, and carcinoma.

Ans. A

103. All may resolve an esophageal food impaction except:

A. Sips of fatty beverage

B. Sublingual nifedipine

C. Sublingual nitrates

D. Intravenous glucagon

Explanation:

- Esophageal obstruction by impacted food or an ingested foreign body is a potentially life-threatening event and represents an endoscopic emergency.
- Left untreated, the patient may develop esophageal ulceration, ischemia, and perforation.
- Patients with persistent esophageal obstruction often have hypersalivation and are usually unable to swallow water.
- Sips of a carbonated beverage, sublingual nifedipine or nitrates, or intravenous glucagon may resolve an esophageal food impaction, but in most patients an underlying web, ring, or stricture is present and endoscopic removal of the obstructing food bolus is necessary.

Ans. A

104. All are true statements except:

A. Patients vomit partially digested food within hour after eating in gastric outlet obstruction

B. Diagnosis of gastric outlet obstruction can be confirmed with a saline load test

C. If the suspicion for a bile duct stone is high and urgent treatment is required ERCP is the procedure of choice

D. Reynolds's pentad is Charcot's triad with the additional presence of shock and confusion

Explanation:

- While transabdominal ultrasound diagnoses only a minority of bile duct stones, MRCP and EUS are >90% accurate and have an important role in diagnosis. If the suspicion for a bile duct stone is high and urgent treatment is required (as in a patient with obstructive jaundice and biliary sepsis), ERCP is procedure of choice since it remains the gold standard for diagnosis and allows for immediate treatment. If a persistent bile duct stone is relatively unlikely (as in a patient with gallstone pancreatitis), ERCP may be supplanted by less invasive imaging techniques, such as EUS, MRCP, or intraoperative cholangiography performed during cholecystectomy, sparing some patients risk and discomfort of ERCP.
- Charcot's triad of jaundice, abdominal pain, and fever is present in ~70% of patients with ascending cholangitis and biliary sepsis. These patients are managed initially with fluid resuscitation and intravenous antibiotics. Abdominal ultrasound is often performed to assess for gallbladder stones and bile duct dilation. However, the bile duct may not be dilated early in the course of acute biliary obstruction. Medical management usually improves patient's clinical status, providing a window of ~24 h during which biliary drainage should be established, typically by ERCP. Undue delay can result in recrudescence of overt sepsis and increased morbidity and mortality rates. In addition to Charcot's triad, the additional presence of shock and confusion (Reynolds's pentad) is associated with a high mortality rate and should prompt urgent intervention to restore biliary drainage.
- Obstruction of the gastric outlet is commonly caused by gastric, duodenal, or pancreatic malignancy, or chronic peptic ulceration with stenosis of the pylorus. Patients vomit partially digested food many hours after eating. Gastric decompression with a nasogastric tube and subsequent lavage for removal of retained material is the first step in treatment. Diagnosis can then be confirmed with a saline load test, if desired. Endoscopy is useful for diagnosis and treatment. Patients with benign pyloric stenosis may be treated with endoscopic balloon dilation of the pylorus, and a course of endoscopic dilation results in long-term relief of symptoms in ~50% of patients. Removable, fully covered lumenapposing metal stents (LAMS) may also be used to treat benign pyloric stenosis. Malignant gastric outlet obstruction can be relieved with endoscopically placed expandable stents in patients with inoperable malignancy.

Ans. C

105. Investigation used for joint vascularity in RA is:

A. Plain X-ray
B. USG
C. CT Joint
D. MRI

Explanation:

- Ultrasound, including power color Doppler, has the ability to detect more erosions than plain radiography, especially in easily accessible joints. It can also reliably detect synovitis, including increased joint vascularity indicative of inflammation.
- Usefulness of ultrasound is dependent on the experience of the sonographer; however, it does offer the advantages of portability, lack of radiation, and low expense relative to MRI, factors that make it attractive as a clinical tool.

Ans. B

106. A 20 year old presented with dystonia, tremors. Examination showed KF ring. Past history of jaundice present. Genetic testing revealed ATP7B mutations. Which is true regarding his disease?

A. Autosomal dominant
B. KF ring is more common in patients with hepatic presentation than neurological symptoms
C. Type of hepatolenticular degeneration
D. Disorder of Iron metabolism

Explanation:

Wilson's Disease

- AR, copper metabolism defective
- ATP7B gene, chro 13
- Parkinsonism with bradykinesia, dystonia, dysarthria, and dysphagia, psychiatric disturbances, wing beating tremor
- Kayser-Fleischer (KF) rings, in Descemets membrane of cornea, seen in 80% of patients with hepatic form of Wilsons and almost all patients with neurological manifestations

Ans. C

107. Genes involved in acute pancreatitis are all except:

A. PRSS1 B. SPINK
C. GATA D. CASR

Explanation:

- All of the major genetic susceptibility factors center on the control of trypsin activity within the pancreatic acinar cell, in part because they were identified as candidate genes linked to intrapancreatic trypsin control. Five genetic variants have been identified as being associated with susceptibility to pancreatitis.
- Genes that have been identified include (1) cationic trypsinogen gene (*PRSS1*), (2) pancreatic secretory trypsin inhibitor (*SPINK1*), (3) the cystic fibrosis transmembrane conductance regulator gene (*CFTR*), (4) the chymotrypsin C gene (*CTRC*), and (5) the calcium-sensing receptor (*CASR*). Investigations of other genetic variants are currently under way, and new genes will be added to this list in the future. Multiple medical, ethical, and psychological issues arise when these genes are discovered, and referral to genetic counselors is recommended.

Ans. C

108. Invasive, direct tests of pancreatic secretory function are most sensitive & specific tests to detect early chronic pancreatic disease when imaging is equivocal or normal is:

A. Secretin tests B. Fecal elastase
C. Quantitative stool fat determination D. Pancreatic biopsy with USG or CT guidance

Explanation:

- Noninvasive, indirect tests of pancreatic exocrine function (fecal elastase) are much more likely to give abnormal results in patients with obvious advanced pancreatic disease (i.e., pancreatic calcification, steatorrhea, or diabetes mellitus) than in patients with occult disease.
- Invasive, direct tests of pancreatic secretory function (secretin tests) are the most sensitive and specific tests to detect early chronic pancreatic disease when imaging is equivocal or normal.

Ans. A

109. In chronic pancreatitis, ERCP abnormalities in main pancreatic duct & side branches have been outlined by:

A. Cambridge classification B. Revised Atlanta criteria
C. Mayoclinic HISORT criteria D. Balthazar grade

Explanation:

- In chronic pancreatitis, ERCP abnormalities in the main pancreatic duct and side branches have been outlined by the Cambridge classification.

- Presence of ductal stenosis and irregularity can make it difficult to distinguish chronic pancreatitis from carcinoma.
- It is important to be aware that ERCP changes interpreted as indicating chronic pancreatitis actually may be due to the effects of aging on the pancreatic duct or sequelae of a recent attack of acute pancreatitis.

Ans. A

110. Not a component of BISAP Score is:

A. Blood sugar >125 mg/dl
B. Impaired mental status
C. SIRS: >/=2 of 4 present
D. Age >60 yrs

Explanation:

Table: Severe acute pancreatitis
Risk Factors for Severity
• Age > 60 years • Obesity, BMI >30 • Comorbid disease (Charlson Comorbidity Index)
Markers of Severity at Admission or with 24 hours
• SIRS–defined by presence of 2 or more criteria: • Core temperature < 36° or > 38°C • Heart rate > 90 beats/min • Respirations > 20/min or PCO_2 < 32 mm Hg • White blood cell count > 12,000/µl, < 4000/µl, or 10% bands • APACE II • Hemoconcentration (hematocrit > 44%) • Admission BUN (>22 mg/dl) • BISAP Score – (B) BUN > 25 mg/dl – (I) Impaired mental status – (S) SIRS: $\geq$ 2 of 4 present – (A) Age > 60 years – (P) Pleural effusion • Organ failure (Modified Marshall Score) • Cardiovascular: Systolic BP < 90 mm Hg, heart >130 beats/min • Pulmonary: PaO_2 < 60 mm Hg • Renal: Serum creatinine >2.0 mg %
Markers of Severity During Hospitalization
• Persistent organ failure • Pancreatic necrosis

Ans. A

111. A patient has undergone gastric bypass surgery has presented with vitamin B12 deficiency. Which of the following symptoms cannot be attributed to vitamin B12 deficiency?

A. Small fibre neuropathy
B. Optic atrophy
C. Behavioural problems
D. Myelopathy

Explanation:

- B12 deficiency causes large-fiber sensory loss affecting proprioception and vibration

- Optic atrophy
- Behavioral changes ranging from mild irritability and forgetfulness to severe dementia and frank psychosis
- Clinical picture of subacute combined degeneration may occur

Ans. A

112. Identify the most probable diagnosis:

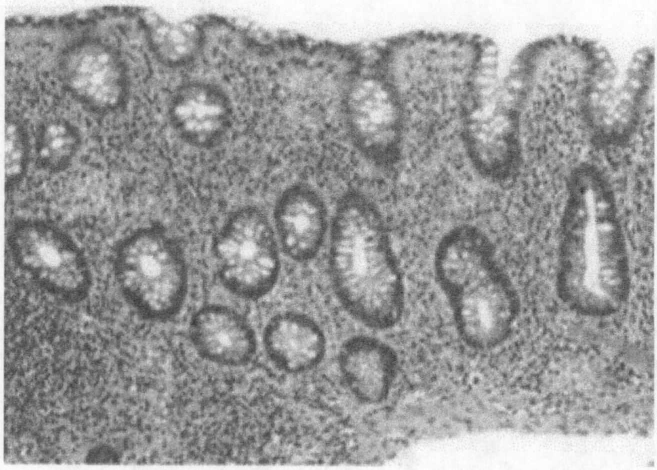

A. Crohn's colitis
B. Eosinophilic esophagitis
C. Ulcerative colitis
D. Whipple's disease

Explanation:

- Image shows mixed acute chronic inflammation, crypt atrophy, multiple small epitheloid granulomas.
- In Eosinophilic esophagitis there infiltration of esophageal mucosa with more than 15 esinophils per high power field.

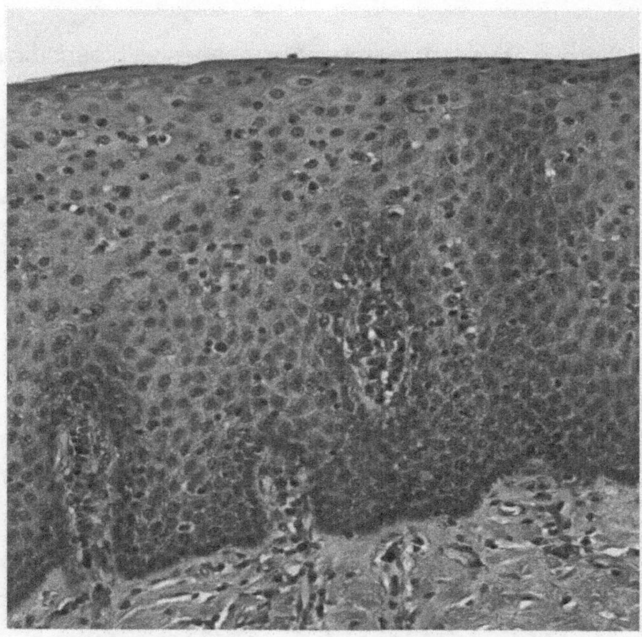

- In ulcerative colitis diffuse mixed inflammation, basal lymphoplamacytosis, crypt atrophy and irregularity and superficial erosion.

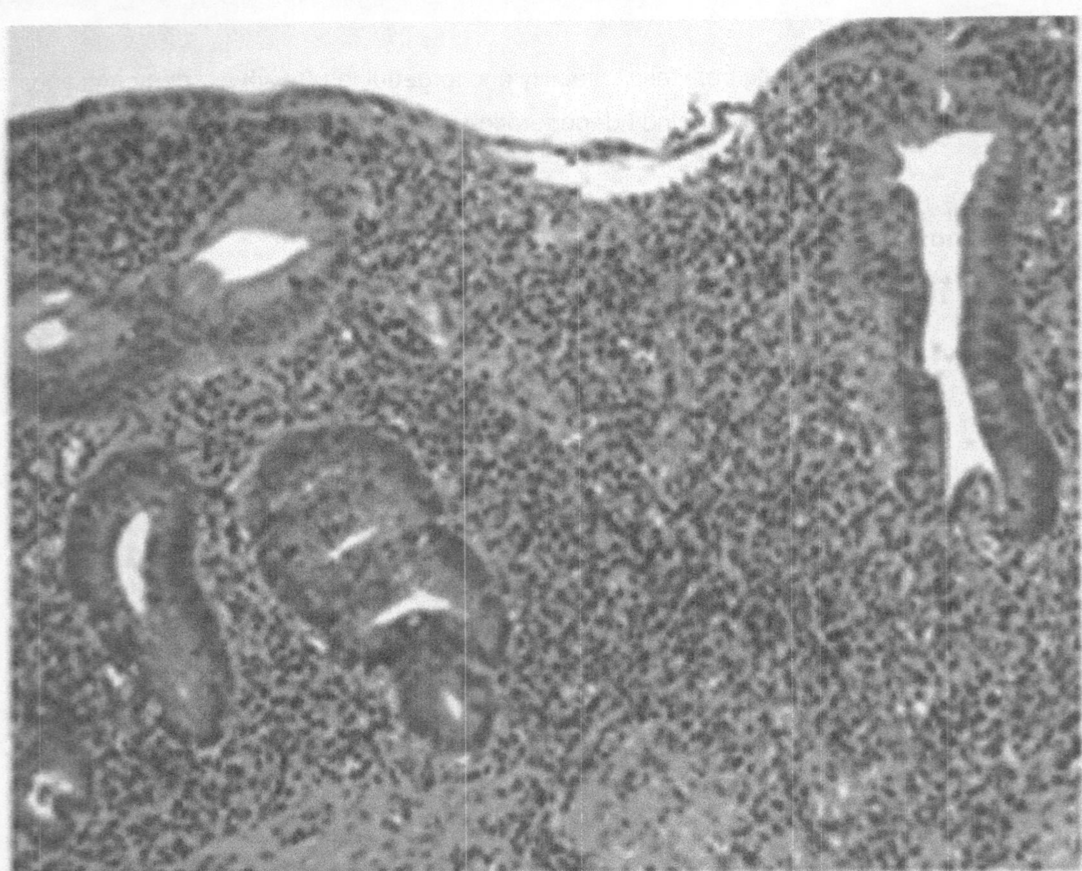

Figure: Medium-power view of colonic mucosa in ulcerative colitis showing diffuse mixed inflammation, basal lymphoplasmacytosis, crypt atrophy and irregularity and superficial erosion. These features are typical of chronic active ulcerative colitis *(Courtesy of Dr. R. Odze, Division of Gastrointestinal Pathology, Department of Pathology, Brigham and Women's Hospital, Boston, Massachusetts; with permission)*

- In Whipple's disease there is abundant foamy macrophages with periodic acid schiff stain (PAS) positive organisms.

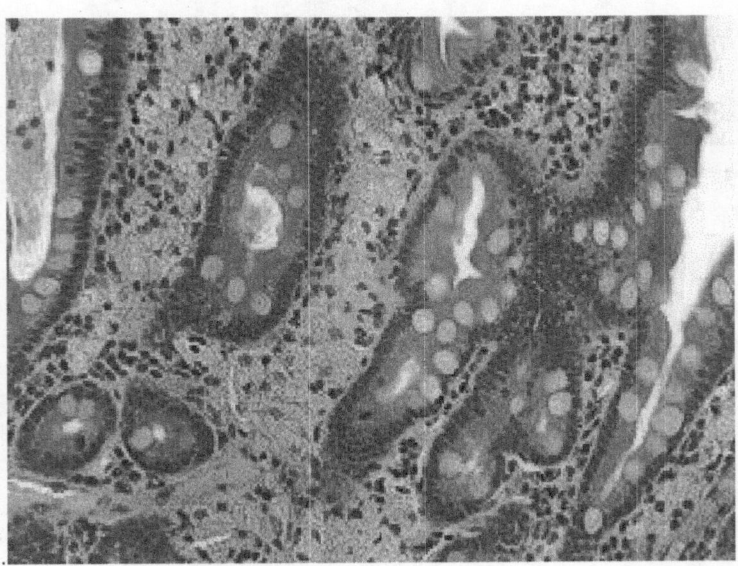

Ans. A

113. Identify the slide shown below & diagnose this condition:

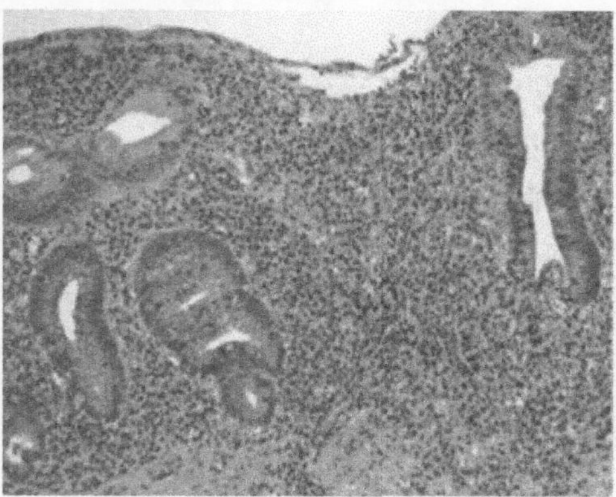

A. Whipple's disease
B. Crohn's colitis
C. Ulcerative colitis
D. Eosinophilic esophagitis

Explanation:

- In the slide, Diffuse mixed inflammation, basal lymphoplasmacytosis, crypt atrophy and irregularity and superficial erosin typical of ulcerative colitis.
- In Whipple's disease foamy macrophages with periodic acid positive in it.

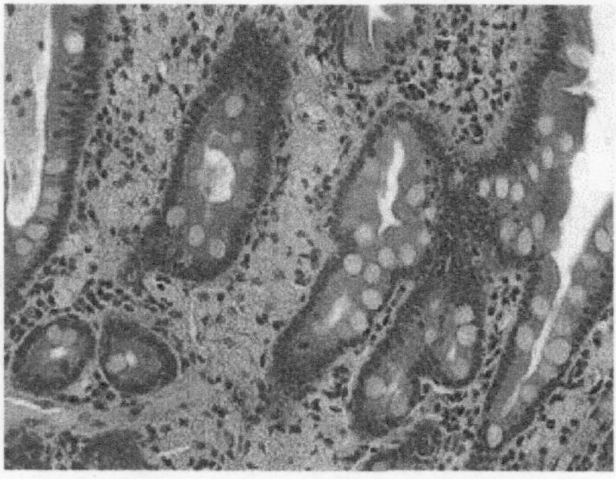

- In Eosinophilic esophagitis there is diffuse infiltration of esophageal mucosa with more than 15 esinophils per high power field.

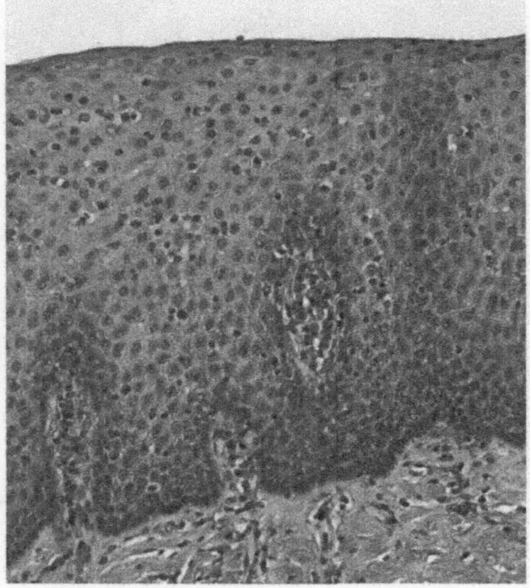

Ans. C

114. Risk factors for Post ERCP Pancreatitis include all except:

A. Age >60 yrs
B. Minor papilla sphincterotomy
C. >2 Contrast injections into pancreatic duct
D. Endoscopic trainee involvement

Explanation:

- Acute pancreatitis occurs in 5–10% of patients following endoscopic retrograde cholangiopancreatography (ERCP). Use of a prophylactic pancreatic duct stent and rectal nonsteroidal anti-inflammatory drugs (NSAIDs, indomethicin) has been shown to reduce pancreatitis after ERCP.
- Risk factors for post ERCP pancreatitis include minor papilla sphincterotomy, sphincter of Oddi dysfunction, prior history of post-ERCP pancreatitis, age <60 years, >2 contrast injections into the pancreatic duct, and endoscopic trainee involvement.

Ans. A

115. Most common Chronic liver disease overall is:

A. Non alcoholic fatty liver disease
B. Alcoholic liver disease
C. Hepatitis C
D. Wilson's disease

Explanation:

- Nonalcoholic fatty liver disease (NAFLD) is the most common chronic liver disease in many parts of the world, including the United States.
- NAFLD encompasses a spectrum of liver pathology with different clinical prognoses.
- Simple accumulation of triglyceride within hepatocytes (hepatic steatosis) is on the most clinically benign extreme of the spectrum.
- On the opposite, most clinically ominous extreme, are cirrhosis and primary liver cancer.
- NAFLD is strongly associated with overweight/obesity and insulin resistance.
- However, it can also occur in lean individuals and is particularly common in those with a paucity of adipose depots (i.e., lipodystrophy).

Ans. A

116. Identify the procedure:

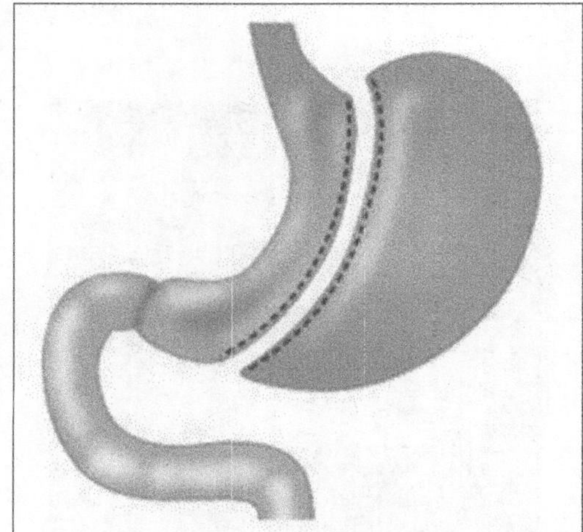

A. Sleeve gastrectomy
B. Roux-en-Y gastric bypass
C. Biliary pancreatic diversion with duodenal switch
D. Biliopancreatic diversion

Explanation:

Bariatric procedures

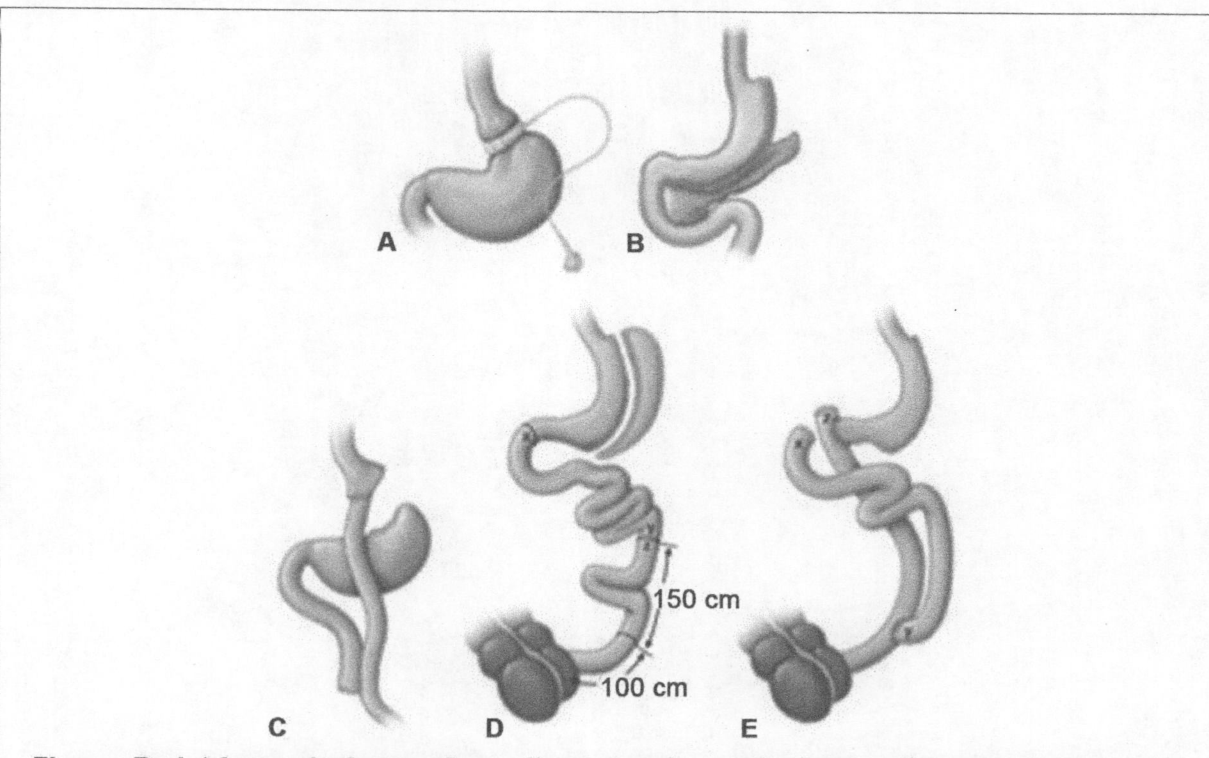

Figure: Bariatric surgical procedures. Examples of operative interventions used for surgical manipulation of the gastrointestinal tract. **A.** Laparoscopic adjustable gastric banding. **B.** Laparoscopic sleeve gastrectomy. **C.** The Roux-en-Y gastric bypass. **D.** Biliopancreatic diversion with duodenal switch. **E.** Biliopancreatic diversion

Ans. A

117. How much fat absorption is inhibited by Orlistat?

A. 20%
B. 5%
C. 30%
D. 15%

Explanation:

Orlistat

- Synthetic lipase inhibitor
- Reversible inhibitor of pancreatic, gastric, and carboxyl ester lipases.
- Taken at a therapeutic dose, orlistat blocks the digestion and absorption of ~30% of dietary fat.
- After discontinuation of the drug, fecal fat content usually returns to normal within 48–72 h.
- Adverse GI effects, including flatus with discharge, fecal urgency, fatty/oily stool, and increased defecation.
- When taken concomitantly, psyllium mucilloid is helpful in controlling orlistat-induced GI side effects.

Ans. C